PHARMACOLOGY FOR RESPIRATORY CARE PRACTITIONERS

PHARMACOLOGY FOR RESPIRATORY CARE PRACTITIONERS

Gregory P. Cottrell, BSc
Professor of Science
Respiratory Therapy Program
School of Health Sciences
Health Technology Division
Fanshawe College
London, Ontario

and

Howard B. Surkin, MA, RRT
Director, Respiratory Care Services
Doylestown Hospital
Doylestown, Pennsylvania

 F. A. DAVIS COMPANY•PHILADELPHIA

F. A. Davis Company
1915 Arch Street
Philadelphia, PA 19103

Printed in the United States of America

Last digit indicates print number: 10 9 8 7 6 5 4 3 2

Publisher: Jean-François Vilain
Editors: Lynn Borders Caldwell
Production Editors: Arofan Gregory and Marianne Fithian
Cover Designer: Steven R. Morrone

As new scientific information becomes available through basic and clinical research, recommended treatments and drug therapies undergo changes. The authors and publisher have done everything possible to make this book accurate, up to date, and in accord with accepted standards at the time of publication. The authors, editors, and publisher are not responsible for errors or omissions or for consequences from application of the book, and make no warranty, expressed or implied, in regard to the contents of the book. Any practice described in this book should be applied by the reader in accordance with professional standards of care used in regard to the unique circumstances that may apply in each situation. The reader is advised always to check product information (package inserts) for changes and new information regarding dose and contraindications before administering any drug. Caution is especially urged when using new or infrequently ordered drugs.

Library of Congress Cataloging-in-Publication Data
Cottrell, Gregory P.
    Pharmacology for respiratory care practitioners / Gregory P.
Cottrell and Howard B. Surkin.
        p.   cm.
    Includes bibliographical references and index.
    ISBN 0-8036-1989-8 (alk. paper)
    1. Pulmonary pharmacology.   2. Respiratory agents.   3. Respiratory
therapy.   I. Surkin, Howard B.   II. Title.
    [DNLM: 1. Pharmacology.   2. Drug Therapy.   QV 4 C851p 1995]
RM388.C68   1995
615'.7—dc20
DNLM/DLC
for Library of Congress   94-41358
                                                                     CIP

This book is dedicated to my wife, Judy, whose supreme patience, unwavering support, and continued enthusiasm made it all possible. You make it all worthwhile.

GPC

This book is dedicated to the following people for their caring, support, and understanding through the good times and the bad.
The Doylestown Hospital Respiratory Care Associates
My parents—Daniel and Mildred Surkin
My sister and brothers and their families—Paula, Marc, and Kenny
My wonderful wife—Ann Marie Surkin
My children—Sara, Jenifer, and the z-man (Zachary)
Especially to Lynn who got me involved with the project.

HBS

The whole art of teaching is only the art of awakening the natural curiosity of young minds.

Anatole France

Foreword

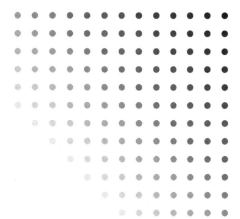

Information concerning the drug classes used in the management of airway patency has always formed the backbone of respiratory pharmacology textbooks as well as the knowledge base for students training to care for pulmonary patients. Respiratory care practitioners of the next century, however, will need more.

Pharmacology for Respiratory Care Practitioners anticipates the needs of future practitioners and meets the challenge head-on. It provides both the fundamentals and the pedagogic aids and reinforcement needed by the beginning reader struggling with a dynamic and complex subject. It also provides valuable information on emerging drug therapies, new concepts of airway mediator and receptor function, and the changing goals of pharmacotherapy in pulmonary medicine. Often, these topics are found only in the more esoteric works on experimental and clinical pharmacology, but in this textbook, the information is presented rather painlessly. And this is precisely the type of information that future respiratory care practitioners will need. Students entering respiratory therapy, cardiopulmonary nursing, or other specialty fields will benefit enormously from the wealth of information and unique organizational style offered by this textbook. In addition, there is enough depth and breadth of coverage to appeal to both the graduate respiratory care practitioner and the respiratory pharmacology educator. It has been my privilege to witness the development of this work. *Pharmacology for Respiratory Care Practitioners* will likely become a standard textbook in pulmonary pharmacology because it has something for everyone. It is truly a learning system whose time has come.

Yvon G. Dupuis, RRT
Coordinator
Respiratory Therapy Program
Fanshawe College
London, Ontario
Associate Editor of *RRT: The Canadian Journal of Respiratory Therapy*,
and author of *Ventilators: Theory and Clinical Applications, ed 2.*

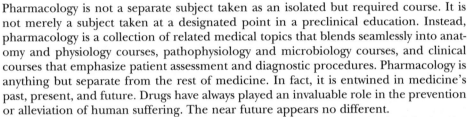

Preface

Pharmacology is not a separate subject taken as an isolated but required course. It is not merely a subject taken at a designated point in a preclinical education. Instead, pharmacology is a collection of related medical topics that blends seamlessly into anatomy and physiology courses, pathophysiology and microbiology courses, and clinical courses that emphasize patient assessment and diagnostic procedures. Pharmacology is anything but separate from the rest of medicine. In fact, it is entwined in medicine's past, present, and future. Drugs have always played an invaluable role in the prevention or alleviation of human suffering. The near future appears no different.

Pharmacology is an *applied* physiology discipline. Knowledge of basic physiologic principles makes pharmacologic topics easier to grasp. Conversely, an understanding of the drug actions that alter body functions serves to reinforce fundamental physiologic concepts. Clinical simulations as well as real life scenarios invariably describe a patient's drug history. For these reasons, an understanding of basic pharmacology is not only a requirement for those who have chosen to become respiratory care practitioners, it is an invaluable asset that helps one understand other aspects of pulmonary medicine.

Pharmacology for Respiratory Care Practitioners is expressly designed for the reader who is introduced to pharmacology concurrently with other preclinical sciences such as anatomy, physiology, and pathophysiology. The text assumes the reader has no prior pharmacology background. It is designed to give that reader a solid academic base in pharmacology and, in so doing, instill the confidence needed to master other medical disciplines. The entire philosophy behind the text as well as the writing, organization, and production of the text has been focused on this single goal. We wish you outstanding success in your chosen field.

ORGANIZATION

The 28 chapters of the text are organized into five units that group chapters related to the same general area of therapeutics.

Unit 1—The Physiologic Basis of Drug Action

This unit assembles three chapters that introduce some of the fundamental principles of pharmacology. Topics such as pharmacokinetics, structure-activity relationships, drug-receptor interactions, and pharmacologic mechanisms such as mimicry and blockade are discussed.

Unit 2—Drugs Affecting the Peripheral Nervous System

Five chapters comprise this unit. Basic concepts of neurochemical transmission are explained prior to an in-depth discussion of the organization and activity of the autonomic nervous system. A discussion of cholinergic drugs plus the nicotinic and muscarinic antagonists completes the unit. Drug actions affecting the respiratory system are emphasized where applicable.

Unit 3—Drugs Affecting the Respiratory System

This unit is the most extensive in the book. Nine chapters covering pulmonary agents are grouped together to provide a comprehensive look at the most common drugs currently in use to treat dysfunctions of the respiratory system. Mediators of the allergic response are introduced first, followed by a chapter covering antiallergic and antihistaminic drugs. Antimuscarinic, β-adrenergic, and xanthine bronchodilators are examined in depth in separate chapters. Glucocorticoids and surface-active agents affecting the respiratory sytem are covered next, followed by two chapters that discuss the antimicrobials used to treat respiratory tract infections.

Unit 4—Drugs Affecting the Cardiovascular System

Unit 4 consists of six chapters that cover the cardiotonics, antianginals, diuretics, antihypertensives, and antiarrhythmics plus the antithrombotics and thrombolytics. Cardiopulmonary effects are emphasized where appropriate.

Unit 5—Drugs Affecting the Central Nervous System

Five chapters covering the drugs that alter central nervous system function are organized into the final unit of the book. These chapters cover many of the drugs that alter ventilation by either depressing or stimulating the central nervous system: psychopharmacologic and hypnotic drugs, analgesics, local anesthetics, general anesthetics, and ventilatory stimulants. Each drug class is discussed in a separate chapter.

PEDAGOGIC AIDS

A variety of instructional aids of proven effectiveness are included in the text. These include chapter outlines, learning objectives, and summaries. Such aids help the reader locate information, associate related facts, and assess mastery of the material. Pedagogic aids are discussed in detail under the heading, *To the Reader.*

READABILITY

Pharmacology for Respiratory Care Practitioners provides a highly-organized, concise description of pharmacologic agents employed in pulmonary medicine. Consistent style, generous use of subheadings, and extensive use of lists and tables within the text narrative add to the readability of the book. The original manuscript was extensively revised after expert reviewers in respiratory pharmacology education pointed out difficult passages and unclear concepts. The result is clearer writing and a better, more focused text. Readability of the text is also enhanced by the use of boldface type for new terms when they are first introduced, a phonetic pronunciation guide for new terms, and a designation for U.S. and Canadian drug names where appropriate. Boxed information describing topics of historical, current, or future pharmacologic importance spark interest in the subject and add immensely to the readability of the text.

SUPPLEMENTARY MATERIAL

Ancillary material for *Pharmacology for Respiratory Care Practitioners* is available as an **Instructor's Guide** and a computerized **Test Bank.** The Instructor's Guide accompanies the text and is designed to help the instructor in adapting the book to the course. Each chapter in the Instructor's Guide contains a **Chapter Synopsis,** which provides a concise summary of textbook contents, and a section called **Relationship to Other Chapters.** The latter feature discusses how the chapter fits into the overall scheme of the book and helps link the chapter with those in related areas. This helps in course design, especially if the course length prevents a "cover-to-cover" approach. Suggestions concerning sections of text that can be minimized and those that are absolutely vital allow an instructor to custom-tailor the text material to individual course requirements.

- Extensive **Review Questions** in a variety of formats such as essay, short-answer, true or false, and matching are included in printed form in the Instructor's Guide. These can be used for student drill, homework, or test exercises.
- **Cybertest™, a computerized test bank** of approximately 600 multiple choice questions, is available to adopters of the text.

TO THE READER

Innovative learning aids have been incorporated into this respiratory pharmacology text. These aids are designed to reinforce the information and concepts presented in the book.

Chapters are grouped into five units. Each unit begins with a concise **Unit Introduction** that previews the general concepts to be introduced. The Unit Introduction briefly describes the common characteristics of the chapters that allow them to be grouped together as a unit. A **Chapter Outline** at the beginning of each chapter details major topics and subheadings to assist the reader in locating areas of interest. **Chapter Introductions** provide a brief overview of chapter contents and relate the chapter to others in the unit.

The most important learning aid to the reader is the list of **Chapter Objectives** presented at the beginning of each chapter. These performance objectives detail the learning expectations of the chapter and are proven devices that promote mastery of the material. Performance objectives allow readers to assess their understanding of the information presented in the text. The reader is encouraged to study small segments of the text and then refer back to the appropriate chapter objectives to determine if the material has been understood. By using the Chapter Objectives as both study guide and feedback, the reader remains focused on a smaller amount of material before moving on to new topics.

Key Terms unique to the topics introduced in the chapter are previewed at the beginning of each chapter and printed in boldface type when they first appear in the text. Where applicable, a phonetic **pronunciation guide** is included with the list of Key Terms. Consult this list as often as necessary. If you cannot pronounce a word, you cannot remember the word. The pronunciation guide uses the following format:

- The most strongly accented syllable is shown in bold, capital letters with secondary accented syllables indicated with a prime (′) symbol as in *pharmacology* (farm′-a-**KOL**-ō-jē)
- Long vowels are indicated by a line over the letter and pronounced with the long sound as in the following common words:

  ā *pain* (pān)
  ē *sleep* (slēp)
  ī *ripe* (rīp)
  ō *sole* (sōl)

- Short vowels are unmarked and are pronounced with a short sound as in the following common words:

  e *bed* (bed)
  i *lid* (lid)
  o *rot* (rot)
  u *tub* (tub)

▪ Other phonetic sounds are shown as:

a	*alone*	(a-lōn)
oo	*cue*	(coo)
yoo	*flute*	(flyoot)
oy	*soil*	(soyl)

Extensive use of **figures** and **tables** helps reinforce important pharmacologic concepts. Readers who are visual learners will appreciate this particular feature of the text. Some tables summarize text contents and are useful for quick reference. Others present additional information to enhance text material. Drug names are grouped into tables and include a pronunciation guide for the generic names. The text also differentiates between **drug names** that are unique to the United States or to Canada. When a drug name is used exclusively in the United States or Canada, it will be designated as such with an appropriate superscript as in *albuterol*[US] or *salbutamol*[CAN]. If no superscript is indicated, the drug name is used and recognized in both countries.

Most chapters include highlighted information in a boxed format. These **perspectives,** although not mandatory reading, discuss interesting and enjoyable topics within the chapter narrative. Some topics are of historical interest, others relate text contents to clinical applications, while some offer a glimpse of future trends in pharmacology. These diversions provide insight into how pharmacology affects our lives. A **Chapter Summary** at the end of each chapter succinctly reviews the major topics discussed in the chapter. Each chapter concludes with a **bibliography.** This collection of pertinent information serves as both a list of suggestions for additional reading as well as a reference for citations in the text narrative.

The **appendices** at the end of the book contain valuable reference information. Appendix A includes tips on performing pharmaceutical calculations and gives tables of measurements and abbreviations for various measurement units. Appendix B discusses prescriptions and the common abbreviations used in prescriptions. The **index** at the end of the book allows you to locate the page reference where specific pharmacologic terms, concepts, and agents can be found. Use it often, especially when studying for exams.

The reader should strive to be interactive with the text. Do not read the material passively. Go back and check off objectives as they are achieved. Study the figures and ask yourself what is being shown. Test yourself before moving on. Understand new terms and their pronunciation. Only by investing such time and effort can your study of pharmacology reap the rewards you deserve.

Acknowledgments
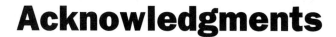

I am deeply grateful to Yvon G. Dupuis, RRT, Professor and Coordinator of the Respiratory Therapy Program at Fanshawe College, for his inspiration and encouragement throughout this project. His outstanding success as an author in the respiratory care field served as a powerful example and motivating force for me. My other colleagues have been supportive and helpful and, although there are too many to acknowledge individually, I would like to thank the faculty of the Respiratory Therapy Program in particular: Professors Richard Rosenthall, MSc; Paul A. Williams, EMCA, RRT; Dennis J. Hunter, EMCA, RRT; and Rob Leathley, RRT.

I would also like to acknowledge Josh G. Cottrell and Ryan P. Cottrell for their excellent line art contributions to the book's illustration program.

Finally, the entire editorial and production staff at F. A. Davis Company is gratefully acknowledged. My appreciation is especially offered to Lynn Borders Caldwell, Allied Health Editor, who enthusiastically took on this project and competently performed all editorial tasks associated with the book. This included the recruitment and coordination of an expert group of reviewers. Her many editorial tasks were made easier by the organizational efforts of Ona Kosmos, Editorial Assistant. My appreciation is also extended to Ralph Zickgraf, Allied Health Senior Developmental Editor, who recognized something of interest in the original textbook proposal and convinced others to take a look at it. A final acknowledgement and thanks are extended to the Art and Production Departments at F. A. Davis Company, in particular, to Arofan Gregory and Herbert J. Powell, Jr.

An outstanding team of respiratory therapy educators was assembled to review the original manuscript for the book. Their critical comments and suggestions for improvement helped shape the final product. I am indebted to them for keeping the book focused and pointing out areas that could be clarified through rewriting. The entire manuscript was thoroughly reviewed for accuracy and respiratory relevance by:

H. Fred Hill, MA, RRT
Assistant Professor
Department of Respiratory Care and Cardiopulmonary Sciences
College of Allied Health Professions
University of South Alabama
Mobile, AL

Jackie Long, MEd, RRT
Director
Respiratory Therapy
Massachusetts Bay Community College
Wellesley, MA

Kenneth D. McCarty, MS, RRT, RCP
Assistant Professor
Director of Clinical Education
Department of Respiratory Therapy
Loma Linda University
Loma Linda, CA

Stanley M. Pearson, MSEd, RRT, C-CPT
Program Coordinator
Respiratory Therapy Program
Southern Illinois University
College of Technical Careers
Carbondale, IL

Portions of the manuscript were reviewed by:

Jan Bohlmann, BS, RRT
Director
Respiratory Care Program
Mt. Hood Community College
Eagle Creek, OR

John Lawrence Coldiron, BA, RRT, CRTT, RCP
Director
Respiratory Care Clinical Education
American River College
Sacramento, CA

Lawrence A. Dahl, RRT, EdD
Instructor and Program Director
Respiratory Technology Program
Hawkeye Community College
Waterloo, IA

—Gregory P. Cottrell

Contents

Unit 1. The Physiologic Basis of Drug Action 1

Chapter 1. Pharmaceutical Phase 3

Chapter 2. Pharmacokinetic Phase 29

Chapter 3. Pharmacodynamic Phase 44

Unit 2. Drugs Affecting the Peripheral Nervous System 55

Chapter 4. Neurochemical Transmission 57

Chapter 5. Autonomic Pharmacology 72

Chapter 6. Cholinergic Agonists 95

Chapter 7. Nicotinic Antagonists 105

Chapter 8. Muscarinic Antagonists 114

Unit 3. Drugs Affecting the Respiratory System 121

Chapter 9. Allergic Mediators 123

Chapter 10. Antiallergics and Antihistamines 138

Chapter 11. Antimuscarinic Bronchodilators   148

Chapter 12. Adrenergic Agonists   158

Chapter 13. Xanthine Bronchodilators   175

Chapter 14. Glucocorticoids   184

Chapter 15. Mucokinetic, Surface-Active, and Antitussive Agents 201

Chapter 16. Antibacterials 220

Chapter 17. Antivirals, Antifungals, and Antiprotozoals 238

Unit 4. Drugs Affecting the Cardiovascular System

Chapter 18. Cardiotonics

Chapter 19. Antianginals

Chapter 20. Diuretics

Chapter 21. Antihypertensives

Chapter 22. Antiarrhythmics 298

Chapter 23. Antithrombotics and Thrombolytics 307

Unit 5. Drugs Affecting the Central Nervous System 319

Chapter 24. Psychopharmacologic and Hypnotic Drugs 321

Chapter 25. Analgesics 334

Chapter 26. Local Anesthetics 349

Chapter 27. General Anesthetics 355

Chapter 28. Ventilatory Stimulants 370

Appendix A: Pharmaceutical Calculations 377

Appendix B: Prescriptions 386

Index 391

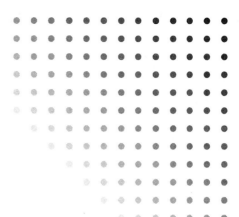

Drug Name Tables

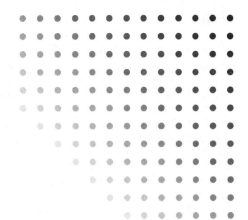

List of Perspectives

Pharmacologic information of historical or clinical relevance as well as topics dealing with future trends in pharmacology are set apart from the text in highlighted boxes.

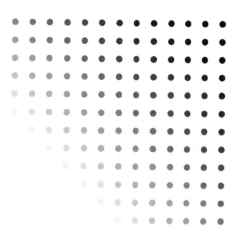

Symbols and Abbreviations Used in the Text

The following list includes symbols and abbreviations other than those directly related to units of measurement or those used as prescription abbreviations.

SYMBOLS

α	alpha
β	beta
γ	gamma
δ	delta
ε	epsilon
η	eta (viscosity)
κ	kappa
λ	lambda (blood-gas partition coefficient)
μ	mu
π	pi (mathematical constant)
σ	sigma

F	bioavailability
$\dot{Q}$	cardiac output
$t_{1/2}$	half-life
$\dot{V}_A$	alveolar ventilation
V_d	volume of distribution

ABBREVIATIONS

AARC	American Association for Respiratory Care
ACE	angiotensin-converting enzyme
ACE-I	angiotensin-converting enzyme inhibitor
ACh	acetylcholine
ACTH	adrenocorticotropic hormone
5'-ADP	5'-adenosine diphosphate

Ab	antibody
Ag	antigen
AIDS	acquired immune deficiency syndrome
ANS	autonomic nervous system
ARDS	adult respiratory distress syndrome
ASA	acetylsalicylic acid
AT III	antithrombin III
ATP	adenosine triphosphate
AV node	atrioventricular node
AP	action potential
BZD	benzodiazepine
cAMP	cyclic adenosine 3′,5′-monophosphate
CCHF	chronic congestive heart failure
CD	collecting duct
CVA	cerebral vascular accident
CFC	chlorofluorocarbon; chlorinated fluorocarbon
cGMP	cyclic guanosine 3′,5′-monophosphate
CHF	congestive heart failure
CNS	central nervous system
C.O.	cardiac output
COMT	catechol-*o*-methyltransferase
COPD	chronic obstructive pulmonary disease
CPZ	chlorpromazine
CRF; CRH	corticotropin releasing factor/hormone
CSRT	Canadian Society of Respiratory Therapists
DA	dopamine
DCT	distal convoluted tubule
DEA	Drug Enforcement Agency
DFP	diisopropyl fluorophosphate
DNA	deoxyribonucleic acid
DPI	dry-powder inhaler
D-R	dose-response; drug-receptor
ECF-A	eosinophil chemotactic factor of anaphylaxis
ECG; EKG	electrocardiogram
ECMO	extracorporeal membrane oxygenation
ED50	median effective dose
EDRF	endothelium-derived relaxing factor (nitric oxide; NO)
EDTA	ethylenediaminetetraacetic acid (or tetraacetate)
5′-GMP	5′-guanosine monophosphate
GTP	guanosine triphosphate
HCFC	hydrochlorofluorocarbon
HFA	hydrofluoroalkane

HIV	human immunodeficiency virus
HPA	hypothalamic-pituitary-adrenal
5-HT	5-hydroxytryptophan; serotonin
IRDS	respiratory distress syndrome of infants
LD50	median lethal dose
LMWH	low molecular weight heparin
LRI	lower respiratory infection
LT	leukotriene
MAC	minimum anesthetic concentration; minimum alveolar concentration
MAO	monoamine oxidase
MAO-I	monoamine oxidase inhibitor
MDI	metered-dose inhaler
NBAAD	nonbronchodilator antiallergic drug
NCF-A	neutrophil chemotactic factor of anaphylaxis
NE	norepinephrine; noradrenaline
NMJ	neuromuscular junction
NREM	nonrapid eye movement
NSAID	nonsteroidal anti-inflammatory drug
OSA	obstructive sleep apnea
PAF	platelet activation factor
PCP	*Pneumocystis carinii* pneumonia; phencyclidine
PCT	proximal convoluted tubule
PDE	phosphodiesterase
PETN	pentaerythritol tetranitrate
PG	prostaglandin
pH	potency of hydrogen
PPHN	persistent pulmonary hypertension of the newborn
PVR	pulmonary vascular resistance
PNS	peripheral nervous system
RAS	reticular activating system
RCP	respiratory care practitioner
REM	rapid eye movement
RDS	respiratory distress syndrome
RMP	resting membrane potential
RNA	ribonucleic acid
RSV	respiratory syncytial virus
SA node	sinoatrial node
S-AR	structure-activity relationship

SIDS	sudden infant death syndrome
SPAG	small-particle aerosol generator
SRP	sustained-release preparation
"SRS-A"	"slow-reacting substance of anaphylaxis"
SVN	small-volume nebulizer
SVR	systemic vascular resistance
TCA	tricyclic antidepressant
T.I.	therapeutic index
tPA	tissue plasminogen activator
TX	thromboxane
URI	upper respiratory infection
USAN	United States Adopted Names (Council)
USFDA	United States Food and Drug Administration
USP	United States Pharmacopeia
USP-NF	United States Pharmacopeia-National Formulary
VMA	vanillylmandelic acid; vanilmandelic acid

UNIT ONE

THE PHYSIOLOGIC BASIS OF DRUG ACTION

UNIT INTRODUCTION

Thousands of years ago a primitive hunter learns too late that the seeds just swallowed are not the ones that impart courage and strength, but are instead lethal. Modern medical researchers in the waning years of the 20th century finally unravel the molecular configuration of the poisonous substance in the seeds. A subtle change in the molecule's shape yields a promising new drug to begin the next millennium.

"The desire to take medicine is perhaps the greatest feature which distinguishes man from the animals."
SIR WILLIAM OSLER, SCIENCE AND IMMORTALITY (1904)

The inherent craving so eloquently described by Osler, a Canadian-born professor of medicine at Johns Hopkins University, has fueled pharmacologic curiosity as well as research. Both the primitive and the modern experimenter have been driven by the same unseen force. This unit examines the roots of modern pharmacology and introduces the fundamental principles behind drug administration, distribution, metabolism, elimination, and actions.

CHAPTER 1

Pharmaceutical Phase

CHAPTER OUTLINE

CHAPTER OBJECTIVES

After studying this chapter the reader should be able to:

- Define the following terms:
  - Drug, pharmacology, pharmaceutical chemistry, pharmacy.
- Distinguish between pharmacotherapeutics and toxicology and between therapeutic and chemotherapeutic agents.
- List the basic sources of drugs and give one example of a drug from each classification.
- Differentiate between the empiric and rational methods of drug development.
- Describe the characteristics of the following names applied to a drug:
  - Chemical, experimental, generic, official, trade.
- Outline the role of the USAN Council and the USFDA in naming drugs in the United States.
- Describe an official drug in Canada.
- Name two drug reference sources and describe the kind of information obtained from such sources.
- Describe the use of drug schedules in the regulation of drugs.
- Differentiate between the pharmaceutical, pharmacokinetic, and pharmacodynamic phases of drug action.
- Define dosage form and outline the characteristics of the following formulations:
  - Oral, injectable, aerosol or micronized powder, suppository, sublingual, miscellaneous.
- Define bioavailability and discuss the advantages and disadvantages of the following routes of administration:
  - Enteral, parenteral, topical, inhalational.
- Compare the advantages and disadvantages of the following aerosol generators for the delivery of drugs:
  - Metered-dose inhaler (MDI), dry powder inhaler (DPI), small-volume nebulizer (SVN), small-particle aerosol generator (SPAG).

KEY TERMS

bioavailability
chemotherapeutic agents
dosage form (formulation)
drug
drug delivery
empirical method
nomenclature
  chemical name
  experimental name
  generic name (nonproprietary
    name [NPN])
  official name (USAN)
  official drug^{CAN}
  trade name (brand name,
    proprietary name, trademark)

pharmaceutical chemistry
pharmaceutical design
pharmacodynamics
pharmacokinetics
pharmacology
pharmacotherapeutics
pharmacy
phases of drug action
  pharmaceutical
  pharmacodynamic
  pharmacokinetic
propellant toxicity
rational method
routes of administration
  dry powder inhaler (DPI)

enteral
inhalational
  metered-dose inhaler (MDI)
parenteral
  small-particle aerosol generator
    (SPAG)
  small-volume nebulizer (SVN)
  topical
schedules of drugs
sources of drugs
  bioengineered
  natural
  synthetic
sulfite sensitivity
toxicology

CHAPTER INTRODUCTION

Basic pharmacologic principles governing the introduction of drugs into the body compose the **pharmaceutical phase** of drug action and the subject of this chapter. The history and sources of drugs and the ways in which they are named and regulated are examined first. This section is followed by a discussion of different formulations of drugs and the various methods available for administration. Because of the special needs of the respiratory care practitioner in delivering pulmonary drugs, the inhalational route of administration is emphasized. The events occurring in the body after a drug has been delivered are discussed in subsequent chapters.

BACKGROUND

Drugs are substances capable of changing a living system. For countless years such substances have been smeared on the skin, inhaled as vapors, ingested as various concoctions, and injected directly into the body. The outcome of the experiments has been passed on by word of mouth, cryptic handwritten records, and medical journals. The information became an integral part of **pharmacology,** the study of the interaction between drugs and the body.

When drugs are found to possess beneficial traits, they are said to have therapeutic effects. When detrimental effects are observed, the drug is described as having toxic effects. The study of such poisonous drug effects is called **toxicology.** Knowledge pertaining to the extraction of a drug or to its chemical synthesis eventually led to modern **pharmaceutical chemistry. Pharmacy** deals with the formulation of drugs, their dispensing, and their legal aspects. **Pharmacotherapeutics** is concerned with the use of drugs to

treat pathophysiologic conditions. A distinction is made between *therapeutic agents,* such as aspirin, that provide symptomatic treatment, and *chemotherapeutic agents,* such as penicillin, that treat causes. **Chemotherapeutic agents** include *antimicrobials,* used to treat infections, and *antineoplastics,* used in anticancer therapy. Other specialties exist within the field of pharmacology. For instance, the study of the movement of drugs between different compartments in the body is called **pharmacokinetics** and is the subject of Chapter 2. The study of the biochemical and physiologic mechanisms of drug action is known as **pharmacodynamics** and is examined in Chapter 3. These subdivisions of pharmacology are shown in Figure 1–1.

SOURCES OF DRUGS

Classic drug sources such as plants, animals, and minerals were the only source of drugs until comparatively recent times. In fact, until the 19th century, all available medications were found in **natural sources,** especially plants. Crude extracts from these sources typically contained many compounds. Identification of the natural source, plus cultivation, extraction, and in some cases an attempt at purification of the active ingredient, was a very difficult process. It was also inexact. Potency of the drug obtained from a natural source was impossible to control, and purity of the sample was erratic at best. Not until the beginning of the 1800s were chemists successful in isolating an active drug (morphine) from a natural source (the opium poppy). Standardization of potency, purity, and other pharmacologic characteristics was then possible with some of the naturally derived drugs. A few modern pharmaceuticals are still obtained from nat-

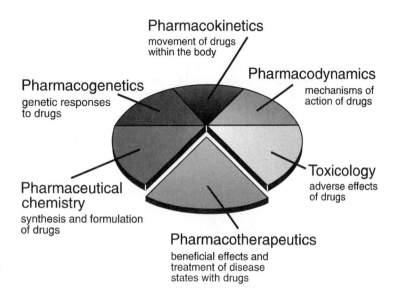

FIGURE 1–1 Subdivisions of pharmacology, the study of the interactions between drugs and the body.

Pharmacokinetics
movement of drugs within the body

Pharmacogenetics
genetic responses to drugs

Pharmacodynamics
mechanisms of action of drugs

Pharmaceutical chemistry
synthesis and formulation of drugs

Toxicology
adverse effects of drugs

Pharmacotherapeutics
beneficial effects and treatment of disease states with drugs

---

TABLE 1–1 SOURCES OF DRUGS: REPRESENTATIVE SAMPLE ONLY

Source	Drug	Medical Use
PLANT		
Purple foxglove (*Digitalis* spp.)	Digitalis parent compound (eg, digoxin)	Increases strength of heart contraction in certain cardiovascular disorders
Deadly nightshade (*Atropa* spp.)	Belladonna alkaloids (eg, atropine)	Decreases gastrointestinal activity; suppresses glandular secretion
Opium poppy	Morphine and other opiates	Relief of severe pain
ANIMAL		
Bovine thyroid gland	Thyroxine	Thyroid hormone deficiencies
Porcine pancreas	Natural-source insulin	Diabetes mellitus
MICRO-ORGANISM		
Molds: *Penicillium* spp.	Penicillins	Various microbial infections
Bacteria: *Streptomyces* spp.	Streptomycins	
MINERAL		
Mineral	Iron	Various anemias
SYNTHETIC		
Artificially produced through chemical synthesis	Albuterol[US] (Salbutamol[CAN])	Bronchodilation (relaxes airway smooth muscle)
BIOENGINEERED		
Cell culture	Urokinase	Thrombolysis (dissolves blood clots)
Recombinant DNA	r-Hirudin	Antithrombosis (prevents coagulation)

ural sources but the number is relatively small. A representative sample of naturally derived drugs is shown in Table 1–1.

Once organic chemistry techniques had progressed to the point where new compounds could be readily produced, **synthetic sources** quickly became the storehouse of potential new drugs. Pharmaceutical chemists could turn out ever-increasing numbers of artificially produced compounds, such as *alkaloids,* which are basic or alkaline substances, sugar-containing compounds called *glycosides,* and nitrogen-containing *amines.* It was up to medical researchers to find a use for them. This requirement is a peculiarity of pharmacology. Often a drug already exists in the natural state or has been synthesized in the laboratory. What remains is further study to find out if the drug has any useful medical applications. In some ways, the saying, "The cure is already on the shelf" applies here, although it is a gross oversimplification.

Basically, new drugs are discovered in two ways: the **empirical method** and the **rational method.** Virtually all drug research occurs today through the *empirical method,* a trial-and-error approach that is costly, time-consuming, and inefficient. It also does not require prior knowledge of the precise way in which a bodily function operates. Physiologists and pharmacologists today understand infinitely more than their predecessors did. However, they rarely understand enough of a mechanism to recommend the specific type of drug required to correct an imbalance of that mechanism. Therefore, the only real alternative is to laboriously investigate and screen sources of drugs, such as folk medicine, plants, animals, minerals, and synthetics, for potential new drugs. Next, the investigator must attempt to determine the mechanism of action. This phase is followed by chemical modification of the drug molecule if required. Extensive animal and human testing follows to establish clinical safety and effectiveness (see Box 3–3). Everything considered, the empiric method of drug development is very complicated and very slow.

By contrast, the rational method of drug development sounds elegantly simple. However, it is deceptively difficult in practice because every intricate detail and nuance of a physiologic mechanism must be known. In other words, with exact knowledge of a body function, it is theoretically possible to decide the goal of therapy beforehand and then determine what type of drug will accomplish that goal. All that remains is synthesis of the necessary drug molecule. The method is quick and economical. The drawback

to the rational method of drug development is our limited knowledge of body function. Although the rational method is difficult to execute, researchers are rapidly gaining expertise in the techniques required. The structure-based drug design method is already supplementing the more traditional empiric method of drug development (Bugg et al, 1993) (Box 1–1).

A final drug source warrants separate attention because it does not conveniently fit the other categories. **Bioengineered sources** of drugs are rapidly growing in importance because they provide a reliable supply of high-purity drugs that are difficult or expensive to produce by conventional means. For example, continuous cell-culturing techniques are being used to produce urokinase, a relatively rare drug used to dissolve blood clots. Another novel bioengineered source for drugs involves recombinant DNA technology, which induces living organisms (bacteria) to create tailor-made drug molecules. The process is a synthesis of sorts because the drug is actually being produced, rather than being derived from a natural source in which it already exists in a preformed state. However, the method involves extraction of a drug from a living source. The confusion in terms stems from the fact that the biologic source, although unquestionably alive, does not exist naturally. It is "artificial" because the bacteria are genetically altered. The biotechnology and pharmaceutical firms that develop such mutants through recombinant DNA techniques hold patent rights on both the organisms and the drugs produced by these unnatural sources. Two of the drugs currently being produced by this technique are insulin, the hormone used in the treatment of diabetes mellitus, and r-hirudin, a promising new drug used to prevent the formation of blood clots (see Box 23–2). Therapeutic agents produced through recombinant DNA techniques exhibit fewer allergic side effects than are seen with some drugs, especially those derived from animals. Sources of drugs are summarized in Table 1–1.

NAMING OF DRUGS

Nomenclature is the process of systematically applying a name to something. Drugs have multiple names (Fig. 1–2). Some names are used primarily by chemists, whereas others are used mainly in pharmaceutical research. Some names are recognized throughout the world; others are familiar to us through media advertising. Nothing can be done about the multiplicity of names. However, the drugs presented in the following

BOX 1–1 VIRTUAL REALITY

Kenneth Wilson, American Nobel physicist, outlined several ambitious goals. Many of his "Grand Challenges," as they came to be known, are well beyond the capabilities of today's supercomputers. The US Office of Science and Technology estimated the computer performance required to meet the Grand Challenges and mapped out a strategy that extends past the turn of the century. The goals include the study of chemical dynamics, aircraft design, long-range weather forecasting, fluid turbulence, ocean circulation, **pharmaceutical design,** the human genome, and other phenomenona. These studies require computational capability being developed in *massively parallel supercomputers.* These machines run mathematical models at speeds that generate nearly exact representations of reality. Performing rapid calculations of the chemical, conformational, electronic, and energetic properties of molecules may enable researchers to design drug molecules with desired characteristics. Such computational needs are measured in teraflops—one trillion floating-point operations per second! It is hoped that by the year 2000, the superfast machines will be able to replace some of the trial-and-error testing and *in vitro* screening of drug samples, thus shifting drug development away from empiric methods toward the rational design of drugs.

Computer-aided design, coupled with sophisticated X-ray crystallography studies of the structure of membrane proteins, is already yielding promising new drugs to enter into clinical trials. These include drugs to treat HIV infections, dissolve blood clots, and control the lung damage caused by emphysema. Most large pharmaceutical firms maintain drug design research teams that are becoming increasingly adept at custom designing a molecular shape to precisely fit a membrane receptor. As researcher CE Bugg explains, "By somewhat simplistic analogy, standard tactics of drug discovery are akin to making and testing many keys in order to find one that happens to fit a lock of unknown shape. In contrast, prior study of the shape and arrangement of tumblers in a lock would lead to rapid design of an effective key" (Bugg et al, 1993). The drugs produced through this rational method are generally more potent, more specific, and less toxic than those developed through the traditional discovery routes of chance observation or screening of large numbers of drug samples.

Bugg CE, Carson WM, and Montgomery JA: Drugs by design. Sci Am 269:92–98, Dec 1993.
Grossman M: Modeling reality. IEEE Spectrum 29:56–58, Sep 1992.

chapters have been organized in a systematic way to aid the reader in becoming familiar with their generic and trade names. This method of presentation also differentiates drug names that are unique to either the United States or Canada.

Chemical Name

The **chemical name** of a drug is a specific means of describing the drug's chemical components and molecular structure. An international standard is used to name all chemical compounds, including drugs. The name is applied consistently and is universally recognized. Therefore, the chemical name of a drug is the same in the United States as it is in Canada. Unfortunately, most chemical names are very complex.

Experimental Name

During early development of a drug, an alphanumeric **experimental name,** or Drug Code Number, is applied. The initials identify the pharmaceutical company developing the drug, as in MSD 999 (Merck, Sharp, and Dohme), AH 3365 (Allen & Hanburys), or Sch 1000 (Schering-Plough). The experimental name is eventually replaced once the generic name of the drug has been approved and assigned.

Generic Name

Another name used universally and therefore applicable in both the United States and Canada is the **generic** or **nonproprietary name** (NPN). In Canada the generic name is occasionally

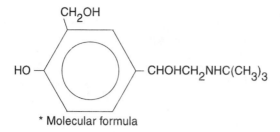

* Molecular formula

Chemical name: α′–[[(1,1–Dimethylethyl)amino]methyl]–4–hydroxy–1,3–
   benzenedimethanol
Experimental name: AH 3365 (drug code number for Allen & Hanburys)
Official name: Albuterol^{US} (USP); other name: Salbutamol^{CAN}
Generic name: albuterol^{US}/salbutamol^{CAN}
Trade name(s): Aerolin, Asmaven, Brochovaleas, Cestin, Cobutolin,
   Ecovent, Proventil, Salbulin, Salbumol, Salbutine,
   Salbuvent, Sultanol, Venetlin, Ventodisk, Ventolin,
   Volmax

*Note: In this text, a benzene ring will be shown as a hexagon with a
   circle inside. This indicates that the electrons are shared by the
   six carbon atoms in the ring.

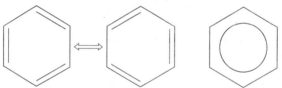

FIGURE 1–2 Drug names and formula of a representative drug (albuterol^{US}/salbutamol^{CAN}).

called the "proper name," but the term is seldom used. The United States Adopted Names (USAN) Council is made up of the American Medical Association and other medical groups. It decides on and "adopts" a specific generic name for a drug. This name is shorter and easier to pronounce than the associated chemical name. Generic names may be used in all countries and by all manufacturers because they are not the property of any person or company. The generic name (USAN) is generally used and accepted in Canada. Occasionally, however, a drug reaches Canada after being developed and named in Europe. In some of these cases, the generic name used in Canada may not be the same as the USAN generic name used in the United States. Fortunately, this does not happen very often. When such dual generic names appear in this text they are designated with an appropriate superscript. For example, albuterol^{US} and salbutamol^{CAN} are generic names for the same drug, a common bronchodilator used in asthma therapy. If no superscript is indicated, the generic name is the same in both countries.

Official Name

The United States Food and Drug Administration (USFDA) is the federal regulatory body responsible for officially naming drugs used in human medicine. The FDA generally accepts the generic (USAN) name as the **official name** of the drug. The official name is used in the USFDA listing of acceptable drugs that meet specified standards of quality, potency, and purity. These manufacturing standards are set forth in a combined reference book called the *United States Pharmacopeia–National Formulary (USP–NF)*.

In Canada, federal legislation called the Food and Drugs Regulations outlines the standards for some drugs. Standards pertaining to drugs not covered specifically by this legislation are defined indirectly through the Food and Drugs Act. The Food and Drugs Act formally recognizes and sanctions several international reference works on drug standards, including the *USP-NF*. **Official drugs** in Canada are those for which a standard exists in these reference works or is specified in the Canadian Food and Drugs Regulations.

In general there is remarkable similarity between drug names used in the United States and Canada, probably more so than between any other two countries in the world. The reason for the similarity can be seen in the link through the *USP–NF* involving official drugs in Canada and official names in the United States. Official drugs in Canada are designated by the Department of National Health and Welfare because an acceptable standard for them exists in an officially recognized United States reference book, the *USP–NF*. The *USP–NF* is also the official standard used by the USFDA to assign official names to drugs. Recall that USFDA-applied official names are almost always the same as the generic names assigned by the USAN Council. The USAN-adopted generic names are almost always the same as the generic names originally submitted by a drug manufacturer. Therefore, generic names in the United States and Canada are nearly always the same.

Trade Name

The **trade name** of a drug is a legally registered drug name. It is also known as the **brand name, proprietary name,** or **trademark.** The name is owned, usually by the company that developed the drug. It is literally the property of the drug company and cannot be used by others. The name is capitalized and often has the registered® symbol associated with it. As with generic names, this text uses superscripts to denote different American and Canadian trade names. For example, Lopressor[US] and Betaloc[CAN] are trade names for a cardiovascular drug known as metoprolol in both countries. If no superscript is specified in the text, the trade name applies in both countries. In this text, a capital letter is used for the trade name of a drug, but the registered symbol, as in Valium®, is not included.

At the end of each chapter, a table lists generic and trade names and offers a phonetic pronunciation guide for the generic names introduced in the chapter. Common adult dosages for selected respiratory drugs administered by inhalation are included where applicable. The objectives at the beginning of each chapter list only

the generic names of drugs to be discussed. Appropriate trade names are included in the text.

Figure 1–2 summarizes the various names that may be applied to a drug. The drug names of clinical relevance are the generic and trade names. Chemical, experimental, and official names are important in certain aspects of pharmacology but are largely omitted from this text.

Some reference works, such as *The Merck Index,* have a pronounced chemistry emphasis, or bias. These references commonly indicate the salt form of the drug, as in atropine sulfate or epinephrine hydrochloride. Medication labels usually indicate drug names in a similar manner. For our purposes, however, this degree of nomenclature detail is unnecessary. In most instances, generic names will be listed in this text without an indication of the salt. The generic name gives the chemical entity responsible for producing the observed pharmacologic effects of a drug. In short, the generic drug is the active ingredient. The salt name merely designates the acid that was used in the synthesis of the drug— hydrochloric acid in the case of epinephrine hydrochloride. Different salts of the same drug are sometimes available. Often, these different versions determine different dosage forms and trade names. For example, epinephrine hydrochloride is an injectable solution called Adrenalin, whereas epinephrine bitartrate is available as an inhaler called Medihaler-Epi (Goth, 1984). Both products contain epinephrine as the active ingredient. Due to characteristic rates of ionization in solution, different salts of the same drug are usually absorbed differently. This variation in absorption results in a product having a slightly different onset or duration of action. Basic pharmacologic effects, however, are unchanged. In an introductory-level pharmacology text, the salts of drugs can be largely ignored.

DRUG PROTOTYPES

To simplify material for teaching purposes, this textbook is organized so that a prototypical drug is introduced in each therapeutic classification and discussed at some length. Often this is one of the original drugs in the therapeutic class. The prototype is usually a drug for which long-term, reliable clinical data are available. General pharmacologic characteristics, indications and contraindications for use, and precautions and adverse reactions pertaining to the prototype are examined. This discussion is followed by more concise overviews of drugs related to the prototype.

DRUG REFERENCE SOURCES

Pharmacology textbooks provide an objective discussion of the pharmacologic characteristics of drugs. Several such texts having a clinical or medical pharmacology emphasis are listed in the bibliographies of various chapters in this book. It is the nature of all textbooks that the information contained in them is somewhat dated by the time of publication (Box 1–2).

Numerous medical journals specialize in clinical pharmacology. These reference sources, like pharmacology textbooks, offer objective comparisons, analyses, and descriptions of drugs in a variety of therapeutic classes. Typically, journals are more focused than textbooks and their information is more timely.

Manufacturers of drugs must submit package inserts or product monographs to the USFDA

BOX 1–2 BEST SELLER

In terms of textbook longevity, a modern book in its 15th edition is a rarity. One that reached its fifteenth century of publication is quite impressive—the equivalent of 75,000 weeks on *The New York Times* Nonfiction Book List! *De Materia Medica,* an illustrated, five-volume encyclopedic work, was written circa AD 77 by the Greek physician and pharmacologist Pedanius Dioscorides. The authoritative reference work contains information concerning the preparation, uses, dosage, and effects of approximately 900 medicinal compounds, only a few of which have survived to the present day. The legacy of Dioscorides, however, lives on. For example, the US Library of Congress uses the general subject heading "Materia Medica" to catalogue a wide range of information relating to drugs. This category includes pharmacopeias, therapeutics, legislation, and sources of drugs. The name itself, Materia Medica, has become an integral part of the language. This gives some hint of the impact the original book has had on medicine. It also indicates a work of significant historical interest.

The original text, *De Materia Medica,* was revised and enlarged through the 1500s. Commentaries were expanded and rewritten by successive editors and translations were completed. A sixth volume was added in 1544 to include new drug information of the day. The text has been republished several times in this century and is available in Greek, Latin, Italian, Spanish, French, English, and Japanese. However, all these translations do not mean that an upgraded, modern edition of Dioscorides' work is available as a timely reference source. These books are facsimile editions—reprinted for their historical importance in the fields of pharmacology, botany, and medicine.

No attempt has been made in recent times to update the information in the original work. In fact, even by 1860 the venerable book was showing its age. This prompted the famous American physician and author Oliver Wendell Holmes to state that except for "opium . . . wine . . . and the vapors which produce the miracle of anesthesia—I firmly believe that if the whole *Materia Medica,* as now used, could be sunk to the bottom of the sea, it would be all the better for mankind—and all the worse for the fishes." This quotation tells us, with eloquent sarcasm, that the practical value of the ancient book had all but disappeared over a century ago. Its historical value, however, has continued to grow.

Dioscorides Pedanius: De Materia Medica (facsimile). In Gunther RT (ed): The Greek Herbal of Dioscorides. Hafner, London, 1968.

Encyclopædia Britannica, ed 15: Micropædia, Vol III. Helen Hemingway Benton, Chicago, 1974.

Lewis R and Jeffrey G: Personal Communication. Oxford County Library System, Ingersoll, ON, Aug 1993.

Library of Congress: Subject Headings, ed 16, Vol III (K–P). Library of Congress, Cataloguing Distribution Service, Washington, DC, 1993.

Modell W, Lansing A, and eds of Time-Life Books: Drugs. Life Science Library. Time, New York, 1969.

Moraca-Sawicki A: History, legislation, and standards. In Kuhn, MM (ed): Pharmacotherapeutics: A Nursing Process Approach, ed 2. FA Davis, Philadelphia, 1990.

for approval. These concise descriptions are prepared according to USFDA guidelines and must outline characteristics such as toxicity, adverse effects, precautions, and other criteria. In a product monograph, manufacturers characteristically include every adverse effect ever reported in the literature, no matter how trivial or rare. This policy effectively shifts most of the burden of responsibility from the pharmaceutical firm to the physician prescribing the drug if an undesirable response is noted in a patient.

Several well-known drug reference sources are basically alphabetical listings of selected package inserts. In the United States, the *Physicians' Desk Reference (PDR)* is available as an annual edition. In Canada, a similar book is the *Compendium of Pharmaceuticals and Specialties (CPS)*. Drug manufacturers submit selected product monographs to be included in these works. Therefore, information on certain pharmaceuticals may not be found. As a result, these reference works possess a degree of subjectivity, or industry bias, not seen in pharmacology textbooks or medical journals. In addition, different drugs are not assessed in a given therapeutic category. This lack of analysis and comparison is probably the greatest distinction between compendia and pharmacology textbooks. However, despite these shortcomings, references such as *PDR* and *CPS* are very popular, drawing on their strengths of timeliness and convenient organization.

Electronic databases offer a convenient means of rapidly locating drug information. Online computer searches by author, subject, or journal title allow retrieval of pertinent data. One of the most extensive computerized information retrieval systems is MEDLARS, the MEDical Literature Analysis and Retrieval System which operates the MEDLINE database. MEDLARS was developed by the United States National Library of Medicine to electronically catalogue references to much of the world's published literature in most medical disciplines. In addition to MEDLINE, specific databases such as TOXLINE and AIDSLINE are available. All are accessible by modem and personal computer. MEDLINE information is also available at many college and university libraries in a CD-ROM format called SilverPlatter.

DRUG REGULATION

Stringent federal laws regulating the manufacture, sale, importation, and dispensing of certain drugs exist in the United States and Canada.

United States

In 1970, the Comprehensive Drug Abuse Prevention and Control Act, popularly known as the Controlled Substances Act, was passed by Congress. This law repealed and superseded older drug laws that had accumulated since the Harrison Narcotic Act of 1914. Interestingly, US federal drug laws controlling *any* substances were almost nonexistent prior to 1914 (see Box 25–3). In the current legislation, various substances are classified into five categories, or **schedules,** ranging from Schedule I C drugs, such as lysergic acid diethylamide (LSD), which have very high abuse potential and no medical use, to less dangerous Schedule V C drugs, such as codeine-containing cough suppressants, which have low potential for abuse and a currently acceptable medical use. Enforcement of the Controlled Substances Act is the responsibility of the Drug Enforcement Administration, a branch of the Department of Justice.

Canada

Controlled substances in Canada are the jurisdiction of the Health Protection Branch of the Department of National Health and Welfare Canada. Regulations regarding the production, marketing, and availability of drugs with a high abuse potential are established by the Food and Drug Act (1927) and the Food and Drug Regulations (1953, 1954). Prescription drugs other than narcotics are categorized into two schedules. Schedule F drugs, such as *corticosteroids,* are prescribed only by qualified practitioners. Schedule G includes controlled drugs, such as *barbiturates,* which must be accounted for by inventory control (record keeping) and, like the Schedule F drugs, can only be prescribed by qualified practitioners. Medical narcotic use of drugs such as morphine is regulated in Canada through the Narcotic Control Act (1960–1961) and the Narcotic Control Regulations (a 1978 amendment to the Narcotic Control Act).

Several drug examples categorized into Schedules I–V controlled substances (United States) plus Schedules F and G and the narcotics (Canada) are presented in Appendix B (Tables B–2 and B–3).

DOSAGE FORMS OF A DRUG

Drugs are manufactured in a variety of **dosage forms,** or **formulations,** for introduction into the body. The **pharmaceutical phase** of the interaction between drugs and the body concerns the administration of different dosage forms through various routes of administration. Once in the body, drugs enter the **pharmacokinetic phase** and move between different compartments. Production of effects at target cells and tissues characterizes the **pharmacodynamic phase** (Fig. 1–3). Not every drug can be made in all forms. For example, a drug formed into a tablet that may be perfectly suitable for oral administration may be too irritating to be offered in a rectal suppository form. Drugs such as aspirin, however, are extremely versatile and can be given orally, rectally, or topically as a related substance, salicylic acid.

Oral Form

The oral form is the most common of the different dosage formulations. *Tablets* are compressed into a soft pill that can be scored for easy division of dose or covered with an enzyme-re-sistant hard shell called an enteric coating. *Capsules* usually consist of a gelatin coating around the active ingredient. Tablets and capsules are often colored to aid in drug and dose identification. Various *liquids* (syrups, suspensions, elixirs) are available for many drugs. Drug forms may be designed to break down slowly or rapidly in the gastric environment to modify the length of time over which they can be absorbed. In general, oral formulations result in a relatively slow onset of drug action. The rate of drug entry into the bloodstream is erratic and difficult to control. However, by altering the type of coating on an oral preparation, pharmaceutical chemists can make a drug more resistant to acidic conditions to allow the drug to reach the small intestine and be absorbed. Sustained-release preparations (SRPs) provide active drug over a period of time and are produced by adding various coatings to drug particles or by varying their sizes and placing them in a soluble gelatin capsule.

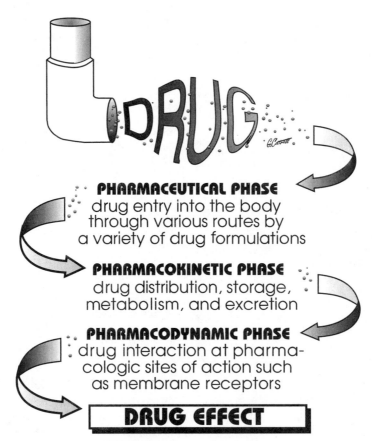

FIGURE 1–3 Phases of drug action.

TABLE 1–2 PHARMACEUTICAL ADDITIVES AND INHALATIONAL DRUGS

PRESERVATIVES

Used as antioxidants and chelating agents to deactivate and control metallic ions and stabilize product
Common in multidose nebulizer solutions
Unit-dose products of common inhalation drugs are usually preservative free
    Benzalkonium chloride
    Disodium ethylenediamine tetra-acetic acid (EDTA-disodium; edetate disodium)
    Example: Ipratropium—Atrovent Inhalation Solution 0.025%; contains benzalkonium chloride and EDTA-disodium
    Sulfites*
        Sodium bisulfite
        Potassium bisulfite
        Sodium metabisulfite
        Potassium metabisulfite
        Sodium sulfite
        Sulfur dioxide
        Example: Isoproterenol—Isuprel Inhalation Solution 0.5%; contains sulfites

PROPELLANTS

CFCs used as delivery gases to power most MDIs
    CFC 11 (trichlorofluoromethane)
    CFC 12 (dichlorodifluoromethane)
    CFC 114 (dichlorotetrafluoroethane)
    (A mixture of these CFCs is known as Freon)
    Example: Albuterol[US] (Salbutamol[CAN])—Ventolin Aerosol; oral MDI contains mixture of CFCs

SURFACTANTS

Used to facilitate the spread of medication in the airways
Found in some MDIs
    Sorbitan trioleate
    Oleic acid
    Lecithin
    Example: Nedocromil—Tilade[CAN]—oral MDI contains sorbitan trioleate

CARRIERS

Used to produce uniform micronized powders in DPIs and reduce drug aggregates
Aid in dispersing the medication during inhalation
    Lactose
    Glucose
    Example: Cromolyn—Intal Spinhaler turbo-inhaler; oral DPI contains lactose particles

*Sulfites may be converted to sulfurous acid and sulfur dioxide in saliva. Sulfur dioxide may cause bronchoconstriction in susceptible asthmatics (Rau, 1989).
CFC—chlorofluorocarbon; DPI—dry powder inhaler; MDI—metered-dose inhaler.

Injectable Form

Various injectable *solutions* and *suspensions* are formulated. If used for intravenous injection, the substance must be water soluble. Some injectable solutions are formulated so that they are separate from a diluent and then reconstituted, or mixed, immediately prior to injection. Water-insoluble or oil-based liquids are suitable for other routes, such as intramuscular injection. Many injectable medications are available in a unit-dose formulation. This method provides a premeasured amount of drug for injection. The unit-dose form is generally more expensive than injectable solutions drawn from a bulk source. However, no unused drug is left after the injection, and the technique is more accurate than calculating doses and drawing a drug sample for injection.

Aerosol and Micronized Powder Form

Several classes of inhalational drugs, such as *bronchodilators,* are formulated as liquids suspended with a delivery gas that is under pressure. The resulting form is called an *aerosol.* Aerosol mists may be delivered by the self-administered **metered-dose inhaler (MDI)** or by nebulizer. Most currently available metered-dose inhalers are pressurized by chlorofluorocarbon (CFC) propellants (Table 1–2). The amount of these CFCs, also called fluorocarbons, in a typical pharmaceutical aerosol canister is quite low. However, abuse of MDI propellants can be hazardous, not to mention the risk due to overdosing with the actual drug being delivered by the aerosol. Deliberate inhalation of high concentrations of propellants under hypoxic conditions may produce adverse reactions. These responses may include toxic cardiovascular effects, central nervous system disturbances, or death. Rational use of an MDI presents relatively few **propellant toxicity** risks compared to the intentional inhalation of large volumes of CFCs. However, bronchoconstriction due to fluorocarbons may occur in hypersensitive individuals using metered-dose inhalers in the proper manner at the prescribed dosage.

The Montreal Protocol is an international agreement that calls for a total worldwide ban, by 1996, on manufacturing processes and products that use chlorofluorocarbons. Clorine molecules from CFCs destroy ozone molecules in the upper atmosphere. The Earth's ozone layer provides protection from damaging ultraviolet radiation; therefore, the integrity of this protective layer is of prime environmental concern. For this reason, alternative propellants having limited impact on the ozone layer are being developed for use with metered-dose inhalers (see Box 12–1).

Drugs often contain preservatives to stabilize the product, prevent chemical or physical decomposition, and maintain shelf life. Some of the preservatives used in drugs include benzalkonium chloride and the sulfites (see Table 1–2). Sulfite additives serving as antioxidants in drugs are typically found in small concentrations. In spite of the small amounts, however, some individuals exhibit unusual **sulfite sensitivity.** This is especially true of some asthmatics. Inhaled sulfites in these patients may be life threatening. Hypersensitivity reactions to sulfites include nausea, diarrhea, wheezing, and dyspnea.

In some patients, the magnitude of the hypersensitivity response to pharmaceutical additives is far in excess of the actual amount of offending substance contained in a therapeutic dose of aerosolized drug. For this reason, respiratory care practitioners and patients should be aware of the potential risk posed by additives such as fluorocarbons and sulfites. Information on additives contained in a specific drug can be obtained from product monographs or directly from the drug manufacturer. Patients who find they have an unusual sensitivity to a drug additive should inform any medical staff of their drug history.

In addition to the development of CFC-free metered-dose inhalers, concerns over patient and environmental safety are shifting attention to the nonaerosol delivery of very finely powdered forms of drugs to the airways (see Box 12–1). *Micronized powders,* such as cromolyn, are delivered by a **dry powder inhaler (DPI).** A current advantage of the dry powder form over the aerosol form is lack of fluorocarbon propellant toxicity. One of the challenges of developing dry powder forms of drugs is that the powder must be produced in a uniform way to ensure reliable deposition of the particles in the airways. Variations in humidity may also cause clumping of drug and adversely affect deposition of particles (AARC, Aerosol Consensus Statement, 1991).

Suppository Form

Several drugs are offered in a *rectal suppository* form ideal for patients who are nauseated, unconscious, or unable to swallow oral medication for some other reason. The disadvantage of this dose form is that many drugs are too irritating to the rectal mucosa to be delivered in this fashion.

Sublingual Form

Sublingual tablets, such as nitroglycerin, are formulated to enter the bloodstream via the rich plexus of blood vessels beneath the tongue. Extensive use of this dose form, however, is restricted by irritation of mucosal linings due to the alkaline nature of many drugs.

Miscellaneous Forms

A variety of *powders,* and *sprays* such as topical anesthetics, are available for application to the skin. *Drops* are used to deliver drugs to the eyes, ears, or nose (Box 1–3).

ROUTES OF ADMINISTRATION

A variety of methods exist to introduce drugs into the body. Some **routes of administration** involving injections produce rapid onset of effect, but the technique itself requires skill. Other administration routes, such as the oral route, require no skill, but the onset of action is much slower and is difficult to control. The concept of **bioavailability** (F) refers to the amount of drug made available in the bloodstream following administration. Routes such as intravenous injection provide essentially 100% of the admin-

BOX 1–3 DRUGS WITH A HOMING INSTINCT

In the 1960s, research into the structure of cell membranes led to the creation of synthetic spheres called *liposomes*. Phospholipid molecules used in the synthesis automatically align themselves when placed in water so that alternating water-soluble and fat-soluble compartments are formed. For several decades, the **drug delivery** potential of liposomes has intrigued researchers. This is because water-soluble and fat-soluble drugs can theoretically be incorporated into the separate compartments. Drugs that have been successfully encapsulated include polyene antifungals such as amphotericin B, aminoglycoside antibacterials like gentamicin, and prostaglandins, such as prostaglandin E_1.

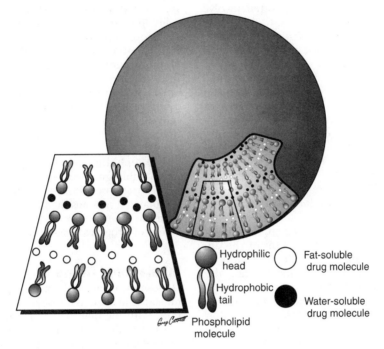

Hydrophilic head

Hydrophobic tail

Phospholipid molecule

Fat-soluble drug molecule

Water-soluble drug molecule

Schematic of internal
structure of liposome
showing alternating layers
and drug compartments

Following administration of liposomes through enteral or parenteral routes, the drug-laden spheres are ingested as foreign material by phagocytic cells such as macrophages. These cells tend to accumulate in organs such as the liver, spleen, lungs, lymph nodes, and bone marrow, thus carrying the drug to these tissues.

Clinical trials are yielding promising results with liposomal drug delivery of anticancer, antibacterial, antifungal, and anti-inflammatory agents. The transfer of drug at high concentration to specifically targeted tissue by these pharmacologic "guided missiles" reduces the unwanted systemic side effects caused by some of the more toxic agents. Other applications of liposomes in medicine include their potential use as oxygen-carrying surrogate red blood cells and as friction-reducing linings for eroded synovial joints.

Bangham AD: Liposomes: Realizing their promise. Hosp Prac (Off Ed) 27:51–62, Dec 1992.

istered dose (F = 1), whereas all other routes provide less than 100% (F < 1). Some advantages and disadvantages of common routes of administration are presented below.

Enteral Route

The **enteral route** refers to the oral route with an ingested drug introduced into the digestive system. The enteral route method is simple and convenient, and allows patient self-medication. However, with a high degree of ease and convenience comes a potential risk. Accidental or intentional drug overdoses most often involve the oral route. Following administration, drug entry into the bloodstream is difficult to control. Advances in drug delivery technology have given us slow-release preparations that stabilize blood levels of orally administered drugs over time. The pH of the stomach can affect oral drug metabolism and absorption, as can the presence of food in the gastrointestinal (GI) tract. Some oral preparations are irritating; therefore, the presence of food in the stomach helps lessen the irritation. Food in the stomach, however, may impede the action of other drugs. For example, tetracycline antibiotics are inactivated by calcium-containing dairy products when they are present in the stomach.

Orally administered drugs reach the bloodstream as a relatively small fraction of the administered dose. This result is due to factors already mentioned, such as metabolism, the presence of food in the GI tract, and the rate of absorption into the bloodstream. An advantage of the oral route in overdose cases is that a portion of the drug can be retrieved by emptying the stomach.

Parenteral Route

Technically speaking, drugs introduced beyond, or outside, the intestine are administered through the **parenteral route** (Gr. *para* [beyond]). As commonly used, the term "parenteral" is a clinical classification referring to all injection routes. Figure 1–4 shows some of the more common parenteral routes such as intravenous (IV), intramuscular (IM), and subcutaneous (SC). In general, these techniques require far more skill than the oral route. The process of accurately drawing a drug dose, locating a suitable injection site, and injecting the drug requires considerably more training than swallowing a pill.

In 1853 the hypodermic syringe and needle was invented and forever changed the way in which drugs could be introduced. Benefits as well as liabilities increased dramatically. Table 1–3 summarizes some advantages and disadvantages of the parenteral routes of administration.

Topical Route

Application of a drug directly to a mucous membrane and dermal application directly to the skin surface are both **topical routes** of administration. Both avoid gastric enzymes and extensive hepatic enzyme activity. Not many drugs can be formulated for topical delivery because of solubility limitations and irritation of tissues. However, topical steroid cremes and lotions and topical anesthetics are available. Transdermal administration is available for nitroglycerin, a drug used in angina therapy. Certain *antihistaminics* used to combat motion sickness are also available in a transdermal form. In these techniques, the drug is slowly absorbed through the intact skin from drug-impregnated dermal patches.

The application of drugs topically through the nasal, sublingual, or rectal route depends on rapid drug absorption through the thin, highly vascularized mucous membranes of the cavities. Like the other nonenteral routes, topical application of drugs avoids gastric enzymes.

Inhalational Route

Deposition of aerosols or fine powders via the **inhalational route** is a type of topical administration. With the delivery of high drug concentrations directly to the respiratory mucosa, local therapeutic effects are optimized and systemic side effects are minimized. The onset of drug action and absorption is rapid because of the large surface area of the lung. In addition, the action of gastric, intestinal, and hepatic enzymes is largely avoided. Drugs formulated and delivered through the inhalational route include several classes of *bronchodilators* plus *corticosteroids* and *antiallergics*. The inhalational route is also used for the delivery of some aerosol *antimicrobials* and *mucokinetics,* and for the delivery of *general anesthetic* gases. A unique feature of the inhalational route is that it is the only route of administration that also serves as a route of elimination. A portion of a given dose is essentially unchanged and may be exhaled.

The inhalational route allows the administration of high doses of drugs and the administration of drugs that are too toxic to be administered systemically. Also, aerosol delivery using

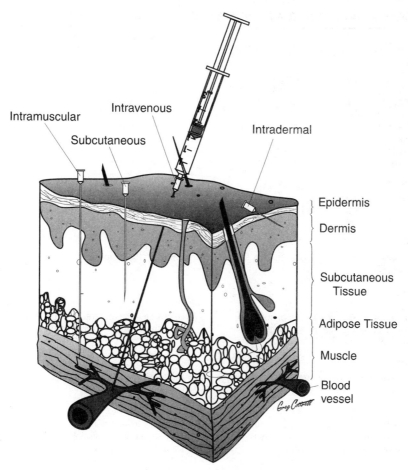

Intramuscular

Intravenous

Subcutaneous

Intradermal

Epidermis

Dermis

Subcutaneous Tissue

Adipose Tissue

Muscle

Blood vessel

FIGURE 1–4 Parenteral routes of administration.

devices such as the small-volume nebulizer (SVN), discussed below, allows prolonged duration of drug therapy. Aerosol delivery, however, can be wasteful because not all of a given drug may reach the site of activity. Small particles allow deeper penetration of the lung, whereas larger ones fail to reach the distal airways, impacting instead in the oropharynx. Systemic absorption, drug inactivation, or both may follow. Table 1–4 outlines some of the advantages and disadvantages of the inhalational route of administration.

Types of Aerosol Generators

Characteristics of various aerosol generators determine the particle size produced. Proper administration technique maximizes therapeutic effect while minimizing waste.

The MDI (Fig. 1–5A) is available for the administration of common respiratory agents

such as albuterol[US] (salbutamol[CAN]), a *bronchodilator*, and beclomethasone, an inhaled *glucocorticoid*. The MDI was developed by Riker Laboratories (now 3M Pharmaceuticals) in 1956. For nearly four decades, the device has proved to be a convenient, reliable, and safe delivery system for administration of pulmonary drugs to the respiratory tract. About 70 million MDIs are currently produced worldwide (3M Pharmaceuticals, 1994). The MDI offers the advantage of precise dosage administration and portability but requires proper technique for maximal effectiveness. Multiple studies have shown that improper MDI technique may result in wasted drug and suboptimal therapy (Epstein et al, 1979; Crompton and Duncan, 1989; Bailey et al, 1990). In addition, most of the MDIs currently available are powered by a mixture of several CFC propellants (see Table 1–2). The mixture is used to control a given vapor pressure in the MDI can-

TABLE 1–3 ADVANTAGES AND DISADVANTAGES OF PARENTERAL ROUTES

Advantages	Disadvantages
INTRAVENOUS ROUTE	
Blood levels reached almost instantaneously	High skill level required for injection
IV bolus of drug delivered to venous system with nearly 100% of dose intact (F = 1)	Irreversibility of drug effect once drug enters circulation
Rapid distribution to all tissues	Not all drugs are compatible with plasma (must be water soluble or in a water-soluble carrier)
Precise control of drug entry to match patient's metabolism and excretion	
Large volumes of water-soluble drug can be administered	
INTRAMUSCULAR ROUTE	
Ideal for injecting water-insoluble drugs	Drug must enter lymphatic system from tissue spaces
Relatively little skill required for injection	Slow absorption and distribution due to sluggish action of lymphatic system
SUBCUTANEOUS ROUTE	
Rapid introduction of drug into subcutaneous tissue below the dermis	Same as for IM route
SPECIALIZED ROUTES	
EPIDURAL	
Access to epidural space around spinal cord produces localized, regional anesthesia with local anesthetics	High skill level required
	Only select drugs administered through this route
INTRAPERITONEAL	
Allows introduction of large volume of dialyzing fluid into peritoneal cavity for peritoneal dialysis	High skill level required
	Only select drugs administered through this route
INTRA-ARTERIAL	
Creates sites for arterial blood gas sampling	High skill level required
Allows administration of a drug that directly targets a tissue through a specific artery	Only select drugs administered through this route
	Deep location of arteries and high pressure within them makes route difficult

F—bioavailability; I-A—intra-arterial; IM—intramuscular; IP—intraperitoneal; IV—intravenous; SC—subcutaneous.

ister (Witek and Schachter, 1994). Evaporation of liquefied propellant provides the energy to discharge medication out of the MDI canister. As was mentioned previously, these propellants are linked to possible toxicity in some patients and to ozone layer destruction (See Box 12–1).

Improvement in delivery of drug from a conventional MDI occurs when extension devices are connected to the inhaler. The addition of certain types of auxiliary or extension devices such as spacers and holding chambers adds to the bulkiness of the MDI (Fig. 1–5B). Spacers, however, enhance the generation of small-diameter, slow-velocity aerosols. This increases the efficacy of drug delivery and decreases the amount of patient coordination required for proper administration of drug.

Proper administration technique using a conventional MDI without a spacer requires that in-halation be synchronized with actuation of the MDI valve (hand-lung coordination). The problem of technique-dependent delivery of medication from a conventional press-and-breathe MDI is significantly reduced with the Autohaler delivery system developed by 3M Pharmaceuticals (Larsen et al, 1993; Newman, 1991). This innovative breath-actuated MDI delivers the *bronchodilator* pirbuterol. The inhaler employs a special valve that holds a metered dose in a chamber until the patient inhales. The patient primes the device by actuating a lever that depresses the pressurized MDI canister and releases medication into a holding chamber. Inspiratory flow triggers a release spring to open a vane that synchronizes delivery of drug with inspiration (Fig. 1–5C). The Autohaler MDI contains 400 metered doses compared to the typical 200 metered doses contained in a conventional MDI.

TABLE 1–4 ADVANTAGES AND DISADVANTAGES OF THE INHALATIONAL ROUTE

Advantages	Disadvantages
Ease of administration and portability of some devices (MDI without spacer, DPI)	Applicability—not all drugs can be formulated as aerosols or micronized powders
Delivery of high drug concentration to the site of action	May be wasteful even with proper technique; MDI delivers 10%–15% of dose, whereas nebulizer only delivers 2%–10%*
Certain aerosol delivery devices (SVN, SPAG) ideal for delivering drug to infants or debilitated patients	Deposition of aerosols in the airways depends on *aerosol physics* (particle diameter, velocity), *patient administration technique* (MDI, DPI), and the *aerosol generator* (most DPIs require large inspiratory flow rates; MDI with spacer device provides more uniform particle diameter)
Localized and topical (at the respiratory mucosa) administration of drug minimizes undesirable systemic effects; absorption into the bloodstream is reduced	
Avoidance of gastric enzymes and extensive hepatic metabolism and renal clearance (pharmacokinetics are not complex compared with other routes)	Some drugs, and delivery gases used to administer them, irritate the airways and may cause drying, coughing, bronchospasm, or nausea
Delivery of drugs that may be toxic if delivered by other routes	CFC propellant toxicity with most MDIs; preservative toxicity (sulfites) with some nebulizer solutions.
Administration of expensive drugs (eg, ribavirin—$400/d)	Open systems release medication aerosol into immediate environment of patient and practitioner; health risk due to passive exposure to aerosolized drug†
Continuous drug delivery with sustained plasma levels with SVN and SPAG	Nosocomial infection risk from inhalation routes (SVN, SPAG) that bypass normal host defenses†
Respiratory care practitioner can instruct the patient regarding proper administration technique and provide care for airways while patient is in the hospital	

*AARC, 1991.
†See Chapter 17.
CFC—chlorofluorocarbon; DPI—dry powder inhaler; MDI—metered-dose inhaler; SPAG—small-particle aerosol generator; SVN—small-volume nebulizer.

A total worldwide ban on CFC usage will be in place by January 1, 1996, to comply with the international standards set down by the Montreal Protocol (see Box 12–1). Countries of the European Union have voluntarily moved this date forward to January 1, 1995. Replacement of CFCs with alternative propellants in pharmaceutical aerosols is equivalent to the introduction of a new drug into the body. For this reason, safety and toxicity studies and full clinical testing must be carried out on new CFC-free inhalers. MDIs have been granted a temporary exemption from the current CFC requirements of the Montreal Protocol to allow sufficient time for the extensive testing that must be done on their replacements. Ultimately, all MDIs in use will have to be CFC-free. The first metered-dose inhaler employing non-CFC propellants is the Airomir system announced in Europe in mid-1994 by 3M Pharmaceuticals. Application for European regulatory approval of albuterol[US] (salbutamol[CAN]), delivered by Airomir, will occur by the end of 1994. This totally redesigned MDI uses hydrofluoroalkanes (HFAs) such as HFA-134a as a replacement propellant and employs special dual seals in the device in conjuction with new valves, a metering chamber, and mouthpiece design (see Fig. 1–6D). HFAs, also known as hydrofluorocarbons (HFCs), have relatively low environmental impact on the ozone layer because they do not liberate chlorine as they break down in the atmosphere. Once USFDA application is made and approval is granted, this novel CFC-free delivery system could be available in the US between mid-1996 and mid-1997 (3M Pharmaceuticals, 1994).

Pressurized propellants and drug preservatives are not used in the DPI. Consequently, toxic effects are lessened. A major limitation to DPIs, however, is that not all medications are available in a dry powder formulation. DPIs do not require coordination between inspiration and depression of a valve because the devices are breath-actuated. A drawback to some DPIs is that relatively large inspiratory flow rates (IFRs) are necessary to deliver the powdered medication to the lung. Some DPIs require IFRs in the range of 60–120 Lpm for maximal efficacy (Witek and Schachter, 1994). Certain patients with respiratory dysfunctions may have difficulty developing IFRs of this magnitude. Single-dose DPIs such as Spinhaler (Fisons) are available for administration of such drugs as the *antiallergic* cromolyn (Fig. 1–6A). This inhaler depends on high inspiratory flow to revolve an impeller. The rotating vanes disperse the powdered medica-

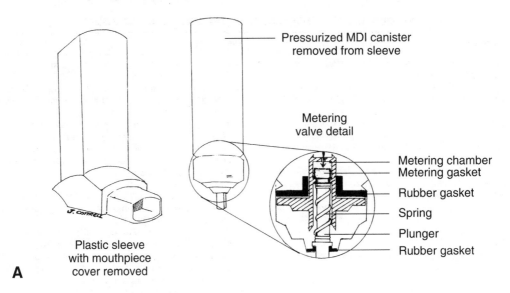

Pressurized MDI canister
removed from sleeve

Metering
valve detail

Metering chamber
Metering gasket

Rubber gasket

Spring

Plunger

Rubber gasket

Plastic sleeve
with mouthpiece
cover removed

A

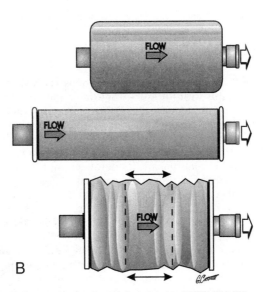

FLOW

FLOW

FLOW

B

FIGURE 1–5 (*A*) Conventional metered-dose inhaler (MDI). (*B*) MDI auxiliary devices.

tion in the airstream after a drug capsule has been pierced by needles.

Another single-dose DPI that depends on the release of powder from a capsule is Glaxo's Rotahaler, used for delivery of albuterol[US] (salbutamol[CAN]) and for beclomethasone. Rotating the device breaks open a hard gelatin capsule against a partition. Dispersal of the contents oc-

curs as the inspiratory airflow passes through a fine screen (Fig. 1–6*B*).

Diskhaler is a multidose DPI marketed by Glaxo and used for administration of the *bronchodilators* albuterol[US] (salbutamol[CAN]) and salmeterol and the inhaled *glucocorticoid* beclomethasone. This DPI employs a flat dosing disk with evenly spaced medication blisters contain-

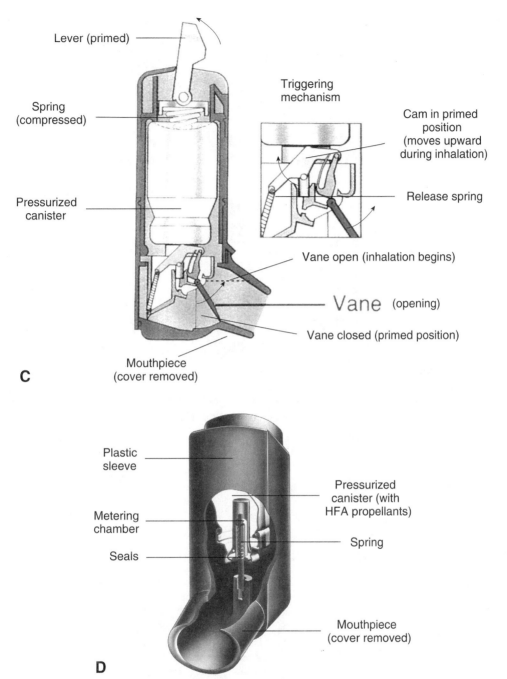

FIGURE 1–5 (*C*) Autohaler breath activated MDI and (*D*) Airomir CFC–free MDI; Courtesy of 3M Pharmaceuticals, used with permission.

ing powdered drug in a measured dose (Fig. 1–6*C*). Raising the lid on the DPI causes a plastic needle to pierce a foil blister so that a precise amount of medication is released and entrained in the inspiratory airflow. The disk contains 8

doses (4 doses of salmeterol) and may be advanced to the next medication blister if additional drug is required.

A convenient multidose DPI first released in Europe, currently available in Canada, and

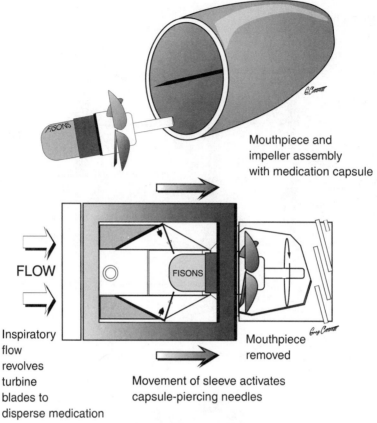

Mouthpiece and
impeller assembly
with medication capsule

FLOW

Mouthpiece
removed

Inspiratory
flow
revolves
turbine
blades to
disperse medication

Movement of sleeve activates
capsule-piercing needles

A

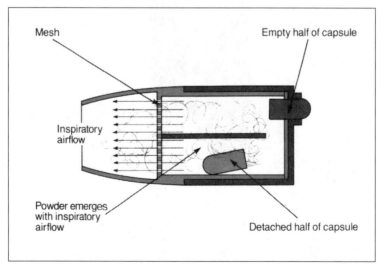

Mesh

Empty half of capsule

Inspiratory
airflow

Powder emerges
with inspiratory
airflow

Detached half of capsule

B

FIGURE 1–6   (*A*) Spinhaler single-dose DPI. (*B*) Rotahaler single-dose DPI. Rotahaler schematic is protected by copyright in favor of Glaxo Group Companies; permission granted by Glaxo Canada Inc.

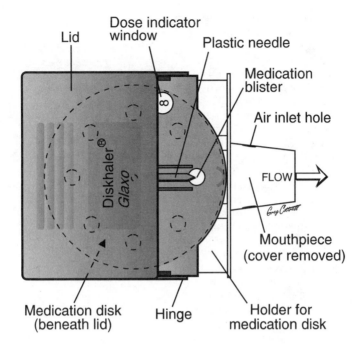

C

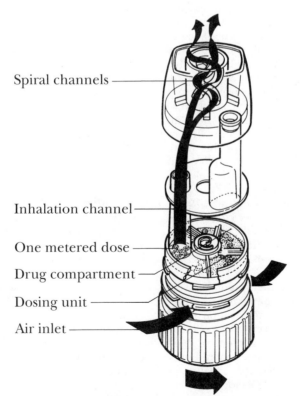

D

FIGURE 1–6 (*C*) Diskhaler multidose DPI. (*D*) Turbuhaler multidose DPI; courtesy of Astra Pharma Inc., used with permission.

awaiting USFDA approval for distribution in the United States, is Turbuhaler. This novel device from Astra Pharmaceuticals is used for administration of terbutaline, a common *bronchodilator,* and for budesonide, an inhaled *glucocorticoid.* The DPI is available for either pulmonary drug as a 200-dose unit in a variety of dosages. This second generation DPI combines compact size and ease of use with production of small particles in the respirable range (5 μm), multiple dosing capability, and a relatively low inspiratory flow rate (Engle et al, 1990). Twisting the grip back and forth primes the device so that powdered drug is released from a medication blister. The drug is broken up and dispersed in the inspiratory airflow as it passes through spiral channels in the mouthpiece (Fig. 1–6D).

Another innovative turn in DPI technology is seen with the development of Dryhaler by Dura Pharmaceuticals. This delivery system is poised to begin clinical studies in 1994 and 1995 with the filing of an Investigational New Drug (IND) application with the USFDA (see Box 3–3). Preliminary trials will use albuterol[US] (salbutamol[CAN]). USFDA application for Dryhaler delivery of the *bronchodilators* bitolterol and ipratropium, will follow. Additional drugs may include the *glucocorticoids,* beclomethasone, triamcinolone, budesonide, and flunisolide, and the *antiallergic* cromolyn. Nonrespiratory drugs such as proteins and peptides, including insulin, may eventually be approved by the USFDA for inhalational delivery by Dryhaler. This versatile third-generation DPI offers multidose convenience via a drug storage cassette and features a high-RPM impeller and special air channeling to break up drug aggregates. The design results in efficient generation of uniformly-sized respirable particles over a large dosage range. In addition, it provides consistent and precise delivery of powdered medication over a wide range of inspiratory flow rates (Dura Pharmaceuticals, 1994). Data from initial clinical testing of Dryhaler will be used in filing a New Drug Application (NDA) with the USFDA by the end of 1995 (see Box 3–3). Potential USFDA approval is projected for 1996 or 1997.

Continuous and precise medication delivery of drugs such as aerosolized pentamidine is possible with a small-volume jet medication nebulizer, or **small-volume nebulizer (SVN)** (Fig. 1–7). This antiprotozoal drug is used to treat *Pneumocystis carinii* pneumonia (PCP). Generation of a consistent-sized aerosol particle is a feature of the SVN, but the device is less portable than other aerosol generators. Other concerns with

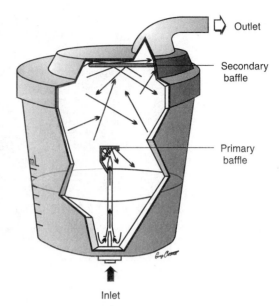

FIGURE 1–7 Small-volume nebulizer (SVN).

the SVN and delivery of aerosols in PCP infections are discussed fully in Chapter 17.

The generation of uniform, very small diameter (1.3 μm) aerosols is a unique feature of the evaporative **small-particle aerosol generator (SPAG)** (Fig. 1–8). The SPAG-2 unit (ICN Pharmaceuticals, Costa Mesa, CA) is used to deliver aerosolized ribavirin. This antiviral agent is used in infants and children with serious lower respiratory infections caused by the *respiratory syncytial virus.* This virus infection and the SPAG are discussed further in Chapter 17.

A comparison of the MDI, DPI, and SVN is given in Table 1–5.

Information Sources for Techniques of Aerosol Delivery

This respiratory pharmacology textbook is not a *respiratory care* text offering guidelines on current aerosol administration protocols. Nor is it a *respiratory equipment* text providing technical details and comparisons of different types and brands of aerosol generators. Treatment protocols covering the techniques of aerosol delivery undergo constant refinement and clinical evaluation. As a result, they frequently change. Instructions covering the "proper" use of an MDI, for example, can become quickly outdated (and no longer "proper") as more effective procedures are developed. For this reason, treatment pro-

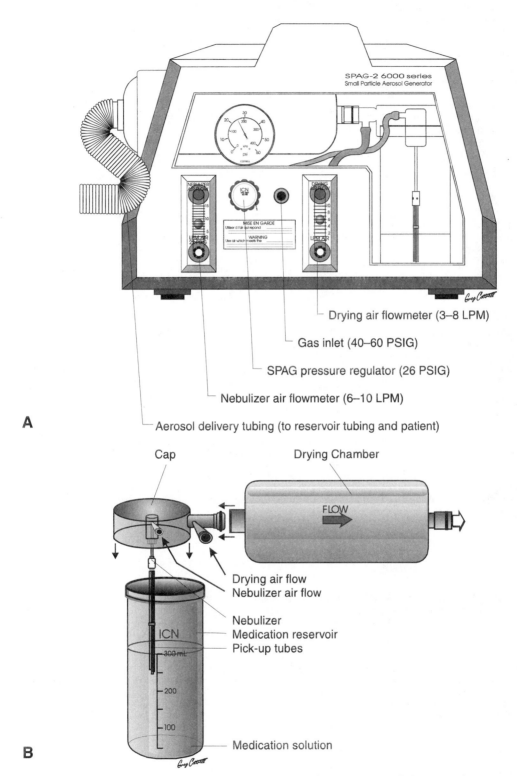

A

Drying air flowmeter (3–8 LPM)

Gas inlet (40–60 PSIG)

SPAG pressure regulator (26 PSIG)

Nebulizer air flowmeter (6–10 LPM)

Aerosol delivery tubing (to reservoir tubing and patient)

Cap

Drying Chamber

FLOW

Drying air flow
Nebulizer air flow

Nebulizer
Medication reservoir
Pick-up tubes

ICN

300 mL

200

100

Medication solution

B

FIGURE 1–8 Small-particle aerosol generator (SPAG). (*A*) Front panel view. (*B*) Rear view of components.

TABLE 1–5 COMPARISON OF DIFFERENT AEROSOL GENERATORS:
Small-Volume Nebulizer, Metered-Dose Inhaler, and Dry Powder Inhaler

Advantages	Disadvantages
SMALL-VOLUME NEBULIZER	
Less patient coordination required	Expensive
Allows medication delivery to infants and young children	Wasteful
High doses possible	Contamination possible if not properly cleaned; potential medium for microbial growth
Modification of drug concentration possible	Not all medications available
Potential to aerosolize nearly any drug	Pressurized gas source required for most units
Continuous drug delivery possible	More treatment time required
No CFC propellants used	
METERED-DOSE INHALER	
Convenient	Patient coordination required with conventional MDIs
Portable	Patient activation required
Inexpensive	Oropharyngeal deposition possible
Short preparation and administration time	Potential for abuse
Some MDIs are breath activated and require less patient coordination	Difficult delivery of high doses
Some MDIs are CFC-free	Not all medications available
	Fixed drug concentrations
	Most MDIs release CFC propellants into environment (potential ozone layer depletion)
	Possible foreign body aspiration from mouthpiece
CONVENTIONAL METERED-DOSE INHALER WITH AUXILIARY DEVICE	
Less patient coordination required	More expensive than MDI
Reduced oropharyngeal deposition	Less portable than MDI; some types are large and cumbersome
Reduced incidence of oropharyngeal candidiasis with inhaled steroids	Poor patient compliance with use of conspicuous device in public
DRY POWDER INHALER	
Less patient coordination required	High inspiratory flow rate required for some DPIs
Breath holding not required	Some units are single dose and require loading
No CFC propellants used	Pharyngeal deposition possible
Breath activated	Cannot be used with intubated patients
Some units are multidose	Not all medications available
Easy count of drug doses	Difficult delivery of high doses
Efficient drug delivery	Possible airway irritation from dry powder
Short preparation and administration time	Possible reaction to lactose or glucose carrier

Source: Adapted from Kacmarek and Hess, 1991; Newman, 1991; Rau, 1991.
CFC—chlorofluorocarbon; DPI—dry powder inhaler; MDI—metered-dose inhaler.

TABLE 1–6 RESPIRATORY CARE TEXTS CONTAINING TECHNICAL ASPECTS OF AEROSOL MEDICATION DELIVERY

Respiratory Care Textbook	AEROSOL PHYSICS		AEROSOL GENERATOR SCHEMATICS				
	Mass Median Aerodynamic Diameter	Deposition of Particles	Metered-Dose Inhaler	Metered-Dose Inhaler with Spacer	Dry Powder Inhaler	Small-Volume Nebulizer	Small-Particle Aerosol Generator
Scanlon et al, 1990	X	X	X			X	X
Eubanks and Bone, 1990		X	X		X	X	
Burton et al, 1991	X	X	X	X	X	X	X
Barnes, 1988	X	X					

tocols are better suited for respiratory technique or therapy courses with reinforcement in the clinical setting. Such information is mandatory for the education of the respiratory care practitioner. Without a doubt, such instruction is an important practical component of respiratory care. It is of doubtful value, however, as a topic in an introductory textbook that focuses on the pharmacologic activity of drugs rather than on the technical aspects of how to administer them.

Information Sources for Technical Aspects of Aerosol Generators

The reader desiring additional information regarding the technical aspects of aerosol drug delivery should consult sources that provide in-depth discussions of aerosol-generating devices. Several respiratory equipment texts and general respiratory care texts are listed in the expanded bibliography at the end of this chapter. These informative sources discuss topics such as the effects of temperature, humidity, and mass median aerodynamic diameter (MMAD) of particles on the deposition of aerosols in the respiratory tract. Many provide schematics of different aerosol devices and compare the efficacy of different brands of aerosol generators. Table 1–6 compares aerosol generator technical information contained in several well-known respiratory care references.

An excellent source of technical information concerning aerosol generators and aerosol drug delivery techniques can be found in the September 1991 issue of *Respiratory Care,* the science journal of the American Association for Respiratory Care (AARC). This special issue covers the AARC Consensus Conference on Aerosol Delivery and includes several valuable research articles. These cover medication delivery systems, protocols for aerosol administration by different generators, aerosol physics, and evaluation of different brands of aerosol generators. Many of the articles have extensive bibliographies and references.

CHAPTER SUMMARY

This chapter presents a brief historic overview of the origins of pharmacology and examines the major sources of drugs. It also outlines the similarities and differences in the naming and regulation of drugs in the United States and Canada. In addition, it introduces the fundamental principles regulating the entry of drugs into the body by exploring different drug formulations and routes of administration. The inhalational route is examined in some detail because of its importance to the respiratory care practitioner in the delivery of pulmonary agents.

BIBLIOGRAPHY

Ariens EJ and Simonis AM: Drug action: Target tissue, dose-response relationships and receptors. In Teorell T, Dedrick RL, and Condliffe PG (eds): Pharmacology and Pharmacokinetics. Plenum Press, New York, 1974.

Balmes JR: Propellant gases in metered dose inhalers: Their impact on the global environment. Respiratory Care 36:1037–1044, 1991.

Benet LZ and Sheiner LB: Pharmacokinetics: The dynamics of drug absorption, distribution, and elimination. In Goodman AG et al (eds): Goodman and Gilman's The Pharmacologic Basis of Therapeutics, ed 7. Macmillan, New York, 1985.

Blaschke TF, Nies AS, and Mamelok RD: Principles of therapeutics. In Goodman AG et al (eds): Goodman and Gilman's The Pharmacologic Basis of Therapeutics, ed 7. Macmillan, New York, 1985.

Budavari S (ed): The Merck Index: An Encyclopedia of Chemicals, Drugs, and Biologicals, ed 11. Merck and Company, Rahway, NJ, 1989.

Bugg CE, Carson WM, and Montgomery JA: Drugs by design. Sci Am 269:92–98, Dec 1993.

Clark WG, Brater DC, and Johnson AR: Goth's Medical Pharmacology, ed 12. CV Mosby, St Louis, 1988.

Clayton BD and Stock YN: Basic Pharmacology for Nurses, ed 9. CV Mosby, St Louis, 1989.

Executive Committee of the American Academy of Allergy and Immunology. Position statement: Inhaled β₂-agonists in asthma. J Allergy Clin Immunol 91:1234–1237, 1993.

Goth A: Medical Pharmacology: Principles and Concepts, ed 11. CV Mosby, St Louis, 1984.

Katzung BG: Introduction. In Katzung BD (ed): Basic and Clinical Pharmacology. Lange Medical Publications, Los Altos, 1982.

Krogh CM (ed): Compendium of Pharmaceuticals and Specialties, ed 28. Canadian Pharmaceutical Association, Ottawa, 1993.

Liska K: Drugs and the Human Body: With Implications for Society. Macmillan, New York, 1981.

MEDLARS MEDLINE Database. US Department of Health and Human Services, Public Health Service, National Institutes of Health, US National Library of Medicine. Bethesda, MD, 1994.

Modell W, Lansing A, and eds of Time-Life Books: Drugs. Life Science Library. Time, New York, 1969.

Moraca-Sawicki A: History, legislation, and standards. In Kuhn, MM (ed): Pharmacotherapeutics: A Nursing Process Approach, ed 2. FA Davis, Philadelphia, 1990.

Musto, DF: Opium, cocaine and marijuana in American history. Sci Am 265:40–47, Jul 1991.

Physicians' Desk Reference: PDR, ed 48. Medical Economics Co. Oradell, NJ, 1994.

Rau JL: Respiratory Care Pharmacology, ed 3. Yearbook Medical Publishers, Chicago, 1989.

The United States Pharmacopeia-The National Formulary (USP-NF). USP 22nd revision. NF 17th ed. The United States Pharmacopeial Convention. Rockville, MD, 1990.

Williamson HE: General principles of drug action and pharmacokinetics. In Conn PM and Gebhart GF (eds):-

Essentials of Pharmacology. FA Davis, Philadelphia, 1989.

EXPANDED BIBLIOGRAPHY: INHALATIONAL ROUTE

PERIODICALS

Aerosol Guidelines Committee, American Association for Respiratory Care: AARC Clinical practice guideline: Selection of aerosol delivery device. Respiratory Care 37:891–897, 1992. (69 references; 26 bibliography entries)

Bailey WC et al: A randomized trial to improve self-management practices of adults with asthma. Arch Intern Med 150:1664–1668, 1990.

Crompton G and Duncan J: Clinical assessment of a new breath actuated inhaler. Practitioner 223:268–269, 1989.

Engle T et al: Peak inspiratory flowrate and inspiratory vital capacity of patients with asthma measured with and without a new dry powder inhaler device (Turbuhaler). Eur Respir J 3:1037–1041, 1990.

Epstein, SW et al: Survey of the clinical use of pressurized aerosol inhalers. Can Med Assoc J 120:813–816, 1979.

Faculty and Writing Committee, American Association for Respiratory Care: Aerosol Consensus Statement—1991. Respiratory Care 36:916–921, 1991.

Kacmarek RM and Hess D: The interface between patient and aerosol generator. Respiratory Care 36:952–976, 1991. (163 references)

Larsen JS et al: Administration errors with a conventional metered dose inhaler versus a novel breath actuated device. Ann Allergy 71:103–106, 1993.

Newman SP: Aerosol generators and delivery systems. Respiratory Care. 36:939–951, 1991. (115 references)

Newman SP et al: Improvement of drug delivery with a breath-actuated pressurized aerosol for patients with poor inhaler technique. Thorax 46:712–716, 1991.

Rau JL: Delivery of aerosolized drugs to neonatal and pediatric patients. Respiratory Care 36:514–542, 1991. (221 references)

PRODUCT INFORMATION

Astra Pharma Inc (Turbuhaler). Mississauga, ON.
Dura Pharmaceuticals (Dryhaler). San Diego, CA.
Fisons Corporation Ltd (Spinhaler). Pickering, ON.
Glaxo Canada Inc (Diskhaler; Rotahaler). Mississauga, ON.
3M Pharmaceuticals (Airomir; Autohaler). St Paul, MN.

TEXTBOOKS

Eubanks DH and Bone RC: Comprehensive Respiratory Care: A Learning System, ed 2. CV Mosby, St Louis, 1990.

Newman SP: Delivery of drugs to the respiratory tract. In Chung KF and Barnes PJ (eds): Pharmacology of the Respiratory Tract: Experimental and Clinical Research. Marcel Dekker, New York, 1993.

Rau JL: Humidity and aerosol therapy. In Barnes TA (ed): Respiratory Care Practice. Year Book Medical Publishers, Chicago, 1988.

Scanlon CL: Humidity and aerosol therapy. In Scanlon CL, Spearman CB, and Sheldon RL (eds): Egan's Fundamentals of Respiratory Care, ed 5. CV Mosby, St Louis, 1990.

Ward JJ and Helmholz HF: Applied humidity and aerosol therapy. In Burton GG, Hodgkin JE, and Ward JJ (eds): Respiratory Care: A Guide to Clinical Practice, ed 3. JB Lippincott, Philadelphia, 1991.

Witek TJ and Schachter EN: Pharmacology and Therapeutics in Respiratory Care. WB Saunders, Philadelphia, 1994.

CHAPTER 2

Pharmacokinetic Phase

CHAPTER OUTLINE

CHAPTER OBJECTIVES

After studying this chapter the reader should be able to:

- Explain how the pH of body fluids can influence absorption of a drug.
- Describe the following mechanisms of absorption:
  - Simple diffusion, filtration, active transport, facilitated diffusion, bulk transport.
- Explain how blood, lymph, and cerebrospinal fluid differ in their ability to distribute drugs.
- Explain why drugs that are free in the plasma can leave the vascular compartment but protein-bound drugs tend to remain.
- Explain the pharmacokinetic concepts of plasma half-life ($t_{1/2}$) and clearance.
- Explain why there is uneven distribution of drugs in the body by describing the role of the blood-brain barrier.
- Describe the outcome of tissue storage on the pharmacokinetics of a drug.
- Differentiate between detoxication and biotransformation.
- Describe biotransformation in the liver by explaining the role of the mixed-function oxidase enzymes.
- Define the following terms:
  - First-pass effect, tolerance, tachyphylaxis, enterohepatic cycling.
- Describe the role of the lung in biotransformation.
- Describe drug elimination through the kidney.
- Describe the role of the following physiologic factors in the modification of drug responses:
  - Age, weight, pathophysiologic state, drug interactions, pharmacogenetics.
- Define the following terms:
  - Additive effect, synergism, potentiation.
- Differentiate between the following types of antagonism:
  - Chemical, physiologic, pharmacologic, pharmacokinetic.
- Define the following terms:
  - Drug allergy, hapten, atopic, immediate hypersensitivity, delayed hypersensitivity, drug idiosyncrasy.

KEY TERMS

absorption
  active transport
  bulk transport
  facilitated diffusion
  filtration
  simple diffusion
antagonism
  chemical
  pharmacokinetic
  pharmacologic
  physiologic
atopic

biotransformation
blood-brain barrier
clearance
distribution
  blood
  cerebrospinal fluid (CSF)
  lymph; lymphatic fluid
drug allergy
drug idiosyncrasy
enterohepatic cycling
first-pass effect
half-life ($t_{1/2}$)

hapten
hypersensitivity
  delayed
  immediate
interactions
  additive or summation effects
  potentiation
  synergism
pharmacogenetics
pharmacokinetic phase
tachyphylaxis
tolerance

CHAPTER INTRODUCTION

As was outlined in the preceding chapter, drugs go through several phases, starting with the pharmaceutical phase, which introduces a drug to the body. Once within the body, drugs often move from one compartment to another, where they are subject to storage, metabolic changes, and elimination. These various movements collectively make up the **pharmacokinetic phase** of drug action and the subject of this chapter.

BASICS OF PHARMACOKINETICS

Absorption

Effect of pH on Absorption of Drugs

Unless directly injected, most drug molecules must undergo **absorption,** or passage through cell membranes, to reach the bloodstream. For example, an orally administered drug must enter luminal cells of the gastrointestinal tract and then pass through endothelial cells of nearby capillaries (Fig. 2–1). Drugs must again pass through cell membranes to leave the bloodstream so that they can be metabolized or eliminated or produce their effect.

Drugs that are weak acids or bases are dramatically affected by the pH of the environment in which they are placed. The pH is the negative logarithm (base 10) of the hydrogen ion concentration of a solution. Therefore, a low pH value, such as pH = 2, represents a relatively large number (1×10^{-2}) that corresponds to the hydrogen ion concentration. Similarly, a larger value, such as pH = 12, represents a much smaller number (1×10^{-12}) corresponding to the hydrogen ion concentration. On the pH scale, values smaller than 7 represent relatively acidic fluids, whereas values higher than 7 represent basic solutions. The pH of several body fluids is given in Table 2–1. Because the pH scale is relative, the pH of one fluid can be compared with that of another. Note that the normal pH

of urine ranges from 5 to 8. Because the pH scale is logarithmic, each whole number increment represents a 10-fold change in hydrogen ion concentration. Therefore, urine with a pH of 5 is 1000 times more acidic than urine with a pH of 8 ($10^3 = 10 \times 10 \times 10 = 1000$). The pH of urine, digestive juice, blood, and cerebrospinal fluid (CSF) can influence the pharmacokinetics of a drug by modifying its absorption.

Weak acids are those that do not ionize readily in aqueous solution. Therefore, they do not yield many hydrogen ions when in equilibrium (nonionized $\rightleftharpoons$ ionized).

Example 1: Ionization of a weak acid in aqueous solution:

$$\underset{\text{acetic acid}}{H_3C\text{-COOH}} \underset{\text{solution}}{\overset{\text{aqueous}}{\rightleftharpoons}} \underset{\substack{\text{hydrogen} \\ \text{ion}}}{H^{1+}} + \underset{\substack{\text{acetate} \\ \text{ion}}}{H_3C\text{-COO}^{1-}}$$

This ionization can be shown generally as:

$$\underset{\text{weak acid}}{HA} \underset{\text{solution}}{\overset{\text{aqueous}}{\rightleftharpoons}} \underset{\text{hydrogen ion}}{H^{1+}} + \underset{\text{anion}}{A^{1-}}$$

When placed in an acidic medium such as gastric juice (pH $\approx$ 2.0) following oral administration, a weak acid drug becomes even *less* ionized. The presence of large numbers of H^{1+} in gastric juice shifts the equilibrium equation to the left. This results in the formation of more nonionized compound:

$$\text{nonionized} \leftarrow \text{ionized}.$$

Example 2: Ionization of weak acid in an acidic medium:

$$\underset{\substack{\text{MORE} \\ \text{ABSORPTION} \\ \text{(nonionized)}}}{HA} \overset{\substack{\text{gastric juice} \\ \text{(pH = 1.6–2.4)}}}{\leftarrow} \underset{\substack{\text{LESS} \\ \leftarrow \text{ABSORPTION} \\ \text{(ionized)}}}{H^{1+} + A^{1-}}$$

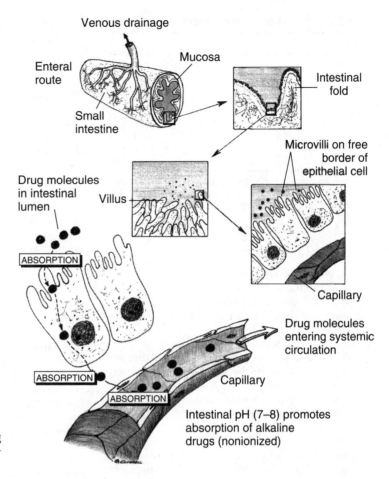

FIGURE 2-1 Schematic—drug entry into the vascular compartment.

Because nonionized drugs are more readily absorbed across lipid-rich cell membranes, the resulting nonionized form of the drug crosses the gastric mucosa and is absorbed into the bloodstream.

Weak bases are those that liberate relatively few hydroxide ions when in equilibrium in aqueous solution.

Example 3: Ionization of a weak base in aqueous solution:

$$\underset{\substack{\text{ammonium}\\\text{hydroxide}}}{NH_4OH} \quad \underset{\substack{\text{aqueous}\\\text{solution}}}{\rightleftharpoons} \quad \underset{\substack{\text{ammonium}\\\text{ion}}}{NH_4^+} \quad + \quad \underset{\substack{\text{hydroxide}\\\text{ion}}}{OH^-}$$

Weak bases become more ionized in an acidic fluid such as gastric juice. The highly reactive hydrogen ions in a fluid with a low pH neutralize the hydroxide ions from the weak base and form molecular water (H_2O or HOH).

This reaction removes product and shifts the equilibrium to the right.

Example 4: Ionization of a weak base in an acidic medium:

$$\underset{}{NH_4OH} \quad \underset{\substack{\text{gastric juice}\\(pH = 1.6\text{–}2.4)}}{\rightarrow} \quad NH_4^{1+} + OH^{1-}$$

$$\underset{\substack{\text{(numerous hydrogen}\\\text{ions from acidic fluid)}}}{H^+ \quad + \quad OH^-} \rightarrow HOH$$

$$\underset{\text{(nonionized)}}{\text{MORE ABSORPTION}} \rightarrow \underset{\text{(ionized)}}{\text{LESS ABSORPTION}}$$

The corresponding shift in equilibrium to the right forces the generation of more ionized product:

$$\text{nonionized} \rightarrow \text{ionized.}$$

A weak base, therefore, becomes more ionized and leaves the stomach without being absorbed.

TABLE 2–1 pH OF BODY FLUIDS

Body Fluid	pH
Gastric juice	1.2–3.0
Vaginal fluid	3.5–4.5
Urine	4.6–8.0
Saliva	6.35–6.85
Blood	7.35–7.45
Semen	7.20–7.60
Cerebrospinal fluid	7.4
Pancreatic juice	7.1–8.2
Bile	7.6–8.6

Source: Adapted from Tortora GJ and Grabowski SR: Principles of Anatomy and Physiology, ed 7. HarperCollins, New York, 1993. Used with permission.

A weak base then enters the small intestine, where the fluid environment is alkaline (pH = 7–8). The higher pH of intestinal fluid generates nonionized drug, shifting the equilibrium to the left:

$$\text{nonionized} \leftarrow \text{ionized.}$$

This reaction occurs because fewer hydrogen ions are available in the intestinal fluid to neutralize the hydroxide ions. The result is that an alkaline drug in an alkaline fluid becomes more nonionized. Therefore, a basic drug is absorbed across the intestinal mucosa to enter the bloodstream.

In general, *cell membranes are more permeable to nonionized substances.* Weak acids become more nonionized and are primarily absorbed in acidic environments. Weak bases, however, become more nonionized and are mainly absorbed in alkaline environments. We will see several examples in which the pH of body fluids such as urine, intestinal juice, CSF, or plasma affects pharmacokinetic rates. For example, elimination of toxic levels of drugs such as *barbiturates* (Chapter 24) or *salicylates* (Chapter 25) can be accelerated by changing the pH of urine. Barbiturates such as phenobarbital are weak acids. Alkalinizing the urine in cases of barbiturate overdose neutralizes excess H^{1+}, causes formation of more ionized product, and shifts the equilibrium to the right:

$$\text{nonionized} \rightarrow \text{ionized.}$$

Recall that absorption across cell membranes is most rapid for the *nonionized* form of a drug. Therefore, alkaline urine slows absorption and recovery of the barbiturate in the kidney and enhances the renal clearance of the excess drug from the body.

For additional information regarding equilibrium reactions, ionization constants of acids

(K_a), and ionization constants of bases (K_b), consult a general chemistry text, such as those listed in the expanded bibliography at the end of this chapter.

Mechanisms of Absorption

Several absorption, or transfer, mechanisms enable drug molecules to cross cell membranes and move between body compartments. Small-diameter lipid-soluble and lipid-insoluble molecules may be passively transferred by **simple diffusion**—movement in response to a concentration gradient. **Filtration** is the passive transfer of substances dissolved in a solvent through a porous membrane. Elimination of many drugs through the kidney involves this process (Chapter 20). **Active transport** is the specialized movement of substances against a concentration gradient and with the aid of carrier molecules. The tubular secretion of penicillin *antibiotics* into the urine is an example of this type of transfer. Active transport is of two types. Primary active transport depends on the sodium-potassium pump mechanism and is described in Chapter 4 in the section on neuronal transmission. Secondary active transport relies on cotransport and countertransport mechanisms and is discussed fully in Chapter 20 with the mechanisms of action of diuretics. Glucose enters cells by means of **facilitated diffusion,** a type of specialized transport that relies on a carrier system to enhance the transfer with a concentration gradient. Finally, some drugs, such as streptomycin antibiotics, are moved through cell membranes in the kidney by **bulk transport** mechanisms such as endocytosis and exocytosis. These mechanisms move relatively large volumes of substances through the membrane. Pinocytosis ("cell drinking") is a type of endocytosis in which a flexible cell membrane folds outward and envelops a drug molecule. The membrane then pinches off and the drug molecule is encased in a vesicle within the cytoplasm of the cell (Fig. 2–2).

Distribution

Vehicles

With the exception of drugs applied topically to produce a localized response, most drugs are introduced into the bloodstream (Fig. 2–3). In Chapter 1, which explains the pharmaceutical phase of drug action, it is seen that dosage forms and routes of administration contribute to bioavailability and determine how readily a drug enters the **blood,** the primary vehicle of **distribution** of drugs.

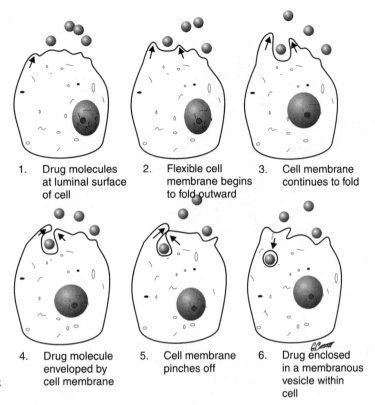

1. Drug molecules at luminal surface of cell

2. Flexible cell membrane begins to fold outward

3. Cell membrane continues to fold

4. Drug molecule enveloped by cell membrane

5. Cell membrane pinches off

6. Drug enclosed in a membranous vesicle within cell

FIGURE 2–2 Pinocytosis—bulk transport of drugs.

Parenteral injections, which use subcutaneous, intradermal, and intramuscular routes, introduce drug into extravascular spaces. These spaces serve as a fluid storage area, or "sump," that is slowly cleared by the lymphatic capillaries. Figure 2–4 shows how these thin-walled vessels operate to pick up excess interstitial fluid and proteins that have been exuded under pressure from blood capillaries. These extravasated substances, and any drug molecules introduced into the interstitial spaces by parenteral administration, are slowly cleared by the lymphatic system. The fluid is returned to general circulation at a point just prior to entry of blood into the right side of the heart. The plasma-derived fluid within lymphatic vessels is called **lymph** or **lymphatic fluid** and represents a secondary vehicle for the distribution of drugs in the body.

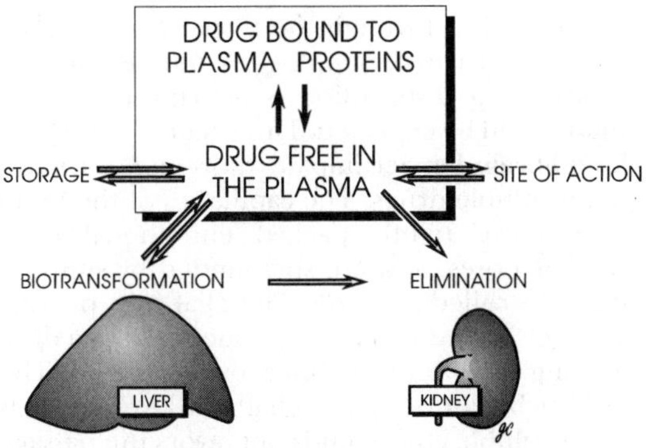

Another plasma derivative, **cerebrospinal fluid (CSF),** plays a minor role as a vehicle for the distribution of drugs into the central nervous system (CNS). This fluid bathes and protects the brain and spinal cord and provides a way to present high concentrations of drug directly to the organs of the CNS.

The Vascular Compartment

Regardless of the route into the bloodstream—direct or indirect—a drug entering general circulation has the potential to reach every cell of the body. (Recall that rapid distribution is both an advantage and disadvantage of the intravenous route.) To leave general circulation, however, a drug molecule must be free in the plasma

DRUG BOUND TO PLASMA PROTEINS

DRUG FREE IN THE PLASMA

STORAGE

SITE OF ACTION

BIOTRANSFORMATION

ELIMINATION

LIVER

KIDNEY

FIGURE 2–3 Pharmacokinetics.

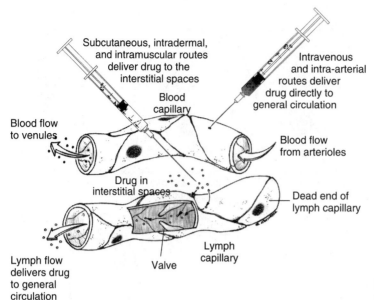

FIGURE 2–4 Lymphatic capillaries and drug in interstitial spaces.

(Fig. 2–3). Drugs bound to plasma proteins, such as albumin, are effectively stored for a time. The rate at which drugs form complexes with and dissociate from plasma protein binding sites is different for every drug. These kinetics determine, in part, how sustained a drug action will be. For example, if 80% of the dose reaching general circulation becomes protein-bound, only the remaining 20% of the dose will be initially available to produce the therapeutic effect. Plasma proteins, therefore, serve as a depot site in the bloodstream. Bound drug slowly becomes unbound and is subsequently metabolized or excreted. This movement induces more drug to leave the protein molecules to maintain the equilibrium with the plasma. If the percentage distribution (80% vs 20%) between bound and unbound forms of the drug persists, the drug is released slowly from plasma storage sites. Everything else being equal, the drug action produced by such a mechanism is prolonged.

The time necessary to reduce an initial dose by half is the **half-life** ($t_{1/2}$) of the drug. Characteristics such as plasma protein binding, metabolism, and elimination all contribute to the half-life because these processes remove drug from the bloodstream. Collectively this removal is referred to as **clearance.** Typically, the clinical effect of a drug disappears before the actual plasma half-life is reached. Another feature to be learned from the schematic of pharmacokinetics

(Fig. 2–3) is that a drug must be free in the plasma to leave the vascular compartment at any appreciable rate. (Protein-bound drugs leak out of capillaries with protein, but do so at a very slow rate.) Plasma protein molecules are simply too large to easily enter the tissue spaces and, as is discussed below in the section on elimination, are not excreted by the kidneys. Therefore, plasma protein–bound drugs tend to have a long half-life and persist in the body, whereas those free in the plasma are more rapidly cleared. An additional variable to consider is that lipid-soluble drugs pass through the cell membrane of the capillary endothelial cells, but lipid-insoluble (water-soluble) drugs must pass through membrane pores. These pores represent a comparatively small fraction of the total capillary surface (Fig. 2–5).

Distribution in most tissues is mainly the result of blood flow through the tissue. In the brain, although it is well supplied by the cerebral arteries, drug distribution is actually much less than would be expected. This occurs because the **blood-brain barrier** impairs movement of many water-soluble drugs. The capillaries of the brain have more tightly packed endothelial cells, smaller pores, and are surrounded by supporting cells called *glial cells.* The glial cells provide another layer that has to be penetrated by a drug gaining entry into the brain (see Fig. 2–5). The lipid-rich nature of the glial cell layer restricts water-soluble compounds but favors the passage

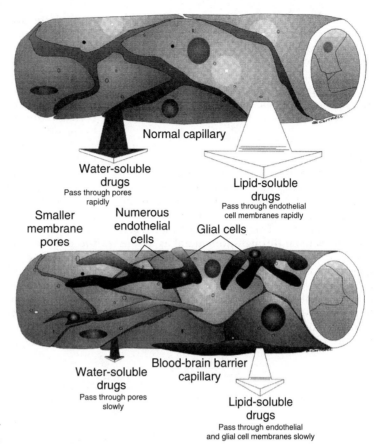

Normal capillary

Water-soluble
drugs
Pass through pores
rapidly

Lipid-soluble
drugs
Pass through endothelial
cell membranes rapidly

Smaller
membrane
pores

Numerous
endothelial
cells

Glial cells

Blood-brain barrier
capillary

Water-soluble
drugs
Pass through pores
slowly

Lipid-soluble
drugs
Pass through endothelial
and glial cell membranes slowly

FIGURE 2–5 Schematic—transfer of drug out of vascular compartment.

of lipid-soluble substances such as certain *general anesthetics* (Chapter 27).

Drug Storage

Various storage sites exist for the deposition of drugs. If a drug is stored, it is not available to produce a drug action. Storage by plasma proteins has already been discussed in relation to distribution of drugs. Some drugs have an affinity for different cellular or tissue components and can go into storage at those sites. Toxic substances (for example, chlorinated hydrocarbon pesticides such as DDT) have a high affinity for adipose tissue and can go into long-term storage. Ultrashort-acting intravenous *anesthetics,* such as the thiobarbiturates thiopental and thiamylal, also have affinity for adipose tissue. They are temporarily stored in the tissue and leave it rapidly during recovery from anesthesia (Chapter 27).

Biotransformation

Most metabolic changes of drug molecules do not directly bring about detoxication, or a decrease in toxicity, but often render a drug or a drug metabolite more water soluble. Once made water soluble, the substance can be rapidly cleared by the kidneys. Some drugs are actually made more toxic during metabolism as a necessary step in the process. For example, aspirin, or acetylsalicylic acid (ASA), is initially converted to salicylic acid, a more toxic metabolite than the parent compound. In general, drug metabolism usually produces less-active compounds from those that are more active. However, some metabolic pathways result in the formation of more active intermediate compounds. **Biotransformation** refers to these varied metabolic events that include changes in toxicity, solubility, or activity of a substance. Biotransformation, therefore, is a general term simply referring to a change in the chemistry of a compound. These chemical changes can alter drug activity. For example, a portion of an oral dose may not even reach the bloodstream because of extensive metabolism in the gastrointestinal (GI) tract or liver. This process is called the **first-pass effect** and is responsible for some of the reduction in drug activity seen with the enteral route.

Liver

Drugs that are free in the plasma may be transported by the hepatic artery to the liver. Drugs administered by mouth are absorbed from the digestive organs and reach the liver by the hepatic portal vein. Therefore, drugs that reach the bloodstream through nonenteral as well as enteral routes are subject to hepatic enzyme systems that bring about biotransformation (Fig. 2–6). The liver's strategic location and versatile activities make it the primary organ of biotransformation. The rate of hepatic biotransformation depends on the percentage of drug free in the plasma, the perfusion of blood through the liver, and the availability and adaptability of hepatic enzymes.

The liver is not only in a strategic location to intercept substances, but is also endowed with a variety of enzymes. Some hepatic enzymes are adaptable and can alter their activity to biotransform different drugs. Several chemical reactions, such as reduction and hydrolysis, are carried out by hepatic enzymes. However, the most versatile and predominant group of enzymes are the cytochrome P-450 enzymes found in hepatic microsomes. These enzymes form the mixed-function oxidase system of the liver and are responsible for converting many lipid-soluble drugs into more water-soluble metabolites. If elimination of drugs through the kidneys were the only means of reducing plasma levels of a drug, lipid-soluble and plasma-bound drugs could circulate almost indefinitely. For this reason, the mixed-function oxidases are important in pharmacokinetics. These enzymes convert drugs into a form that is rapidly cleared by the kidneys. Drugs that are biotransformed by the mixed-function oxidases include phenobarbital

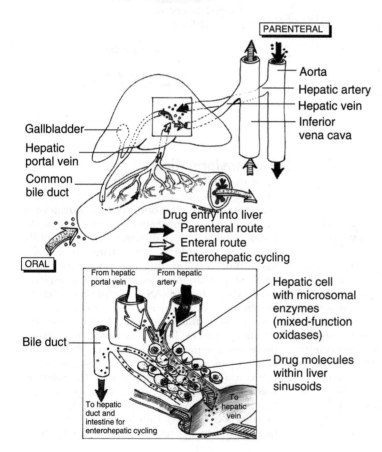

FIGURE 2–6 Hepatic blood flow and enterohepatic cycling.

and pentobarbital *(barbiturates)*, chlorpromazine (an *antipsychotic tranquilizer*), and phenacetin (a pain reliever converted into acetaminophen). Persons with preexisting liver disease often have a deficiency of microsomal enzymes and impaired ability to metabolize drugs. Premature infants also have reduced levels of mixed-function oxidase enzymes. In addition, some drugs, such as the histamine antagonists cimetidine and terfenadine, may inhibit hepatic drug-metabolizing enzymes. **Tolerance** is the phenomenon whereby additional drug is required to produce the same desired effect. Some cases of tolerance can be explained on the basis of induction of microsomal enzymes. Chronic exposure to some drugs may induce or initiate production of additional drug-metabolizing enzyme. This increased enzyme capacity inactivates a particular dose of drug and necessitates administration of a larger dose to produce the same effect. **Tachyphylaxis** is described as rapidly developing tolerance and is often seen with nasal *decongestants* and the *antihistaminics*. Tolerance is also described in terms of receptor regulation (see Chapter 3).

Lungs

Several vasoactive and bronchoactive substances undergo biotransformation in the lung as they pass through pulmonary circulation. For example, pulmonary capillary endothelial cells secrete angiotensin-converting enzyme (ACE). This enzyme activates angiotensin I in the bloodstream, converting it to a powerful vasoconstrictor called angiotensin II. (The renin-angiotensin-aldosterone mechanism of blood pressure control is discussed fully with the *antihypertensive* drugs in Chapter 21.) Substances such as norepinephrine, and potent bronchoconstrictors such as bradykinin and certain prostaglandins, are activated by the lung. The enzyme phospholipase A_2 can be found in the lung, where it acts on cell membrane–bound phospholipids to convert them to arachidonic acid. This substance undergoes further enzymatic action to yield metabolites that are potent inflammatory mediators. Allergic mediators and the arachidonic acid metabolites are discussed in Chapter 9.

Digestive Organs

The digestive organs, especially the small intestines, are well equipped with a variety of enzymes. These enzymes chemically transform orally administered drugs prior to absorption across the intestinal mucosa or elimination with feces.

Elimination

Regardless of the potential therapeutic benefit of a drug, the body treats *all* such compounds as foreign substances to be eliminated (Fig. 2–3). The rate of clearance from the body is different for each compound and depends on such pharmacokinetic characteristics as distribution and metabolism unique to that compound. The lungs and intestines perform a minor role in drug elimination, followed by the skin and salivary glands. Most drug elimination occurs through the kidneys.

Lungs

Recall from the Chapter 1 that some drugs, such as *general anesthetics* delivered through the inhalational route, can also be eliminated through the lungs.

Intestinal-Biliary Route

Orally administered drugs and their metabolites may be eliminated through the intestines. Some drugs may be biotransformed by gastric and intestinal enzymes before entering the hepatic portal system. On reaching the liver they are altered further by hepatic enzymes, especially the mixed-function oxidases. Occasionally, drug metabolites may *re-enter* the digestive system from the liver to undergo further processing before elimination. Such a route involves concentration of metabolites in the gallbladder and biliary excretion into the duodenum of the small intestine. Drug metabolites arriving in the intestine (with the bile rather than with the material leaving the stomach) may be further biotransformed by intestinal enzymes and eliminated with feces. Drugs exposed in this fashion to repeated intestinal and hepatic enzymes have undergone **enterohepatic cycling** (Fig. 2–6).

Exocrine Glands

Elimination of drug metabolites through the sudoriferous glands (sweat glands) of the skin, the salivary glands of the oral cavity, and the breast milk of mammary glands occurs to a minor extent. Most drugs are released in very small amounts through these elimination routes.

Kidneys

During the pharmacokinetic phase of drug action, the kidney is the primary organ of drug elimination (Fig. 2–3). This primary role is the result of several factors. First, the kidneys are highly perfused organs that receive approximately 20% of the cardiac output. Under resting

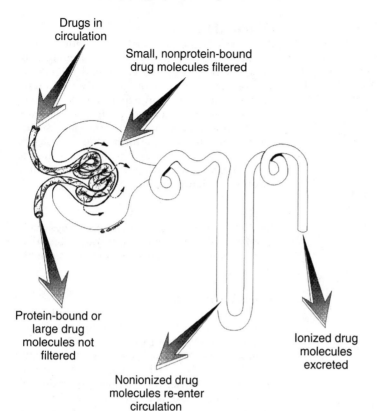

Drugs in circulation

Small, nonprotein-bound drug molecules filtered

Protein-bound or large drug molecules not filtered

Nonionized drug molecules re-enter circulation

Ionized drug molecules excreted

FIGURE 2–7 Elimination of drugs—kidney (schematic of nephron).

conditions, this translates into a renal blood flow of around 1–1.5 L/min. This high flow rate in turn ensures that any substance in the plasma will reach the kidney relatively quickly. Second, the glomerular capillaries of the kidneys operate under roughly twice the pressure of other capillaries in the body. Glomerular filtrate is derived from plasma and is the precursor of urine. Pressure is necessary to form this filtrate. Finally, substances in the plasma that are small enough to be filtered through the membrane pores of the functional units of the kidney tend to leave the bloodstream quickly (Fig. 2–7). High perfusion, high pressure, and selective pore sizes ensure that small, water-soluble drug metabolites are cleared from the body rapidly. Recall that protein-bound drugs tend to not enter the filtrate because plasma proteins are too large to pass through the pores. In addition, ionized metabolites tend to remain in the filtrate and be excreted, whereas nonionized metabolites are reabsorbed, thus re-entering circulation. Drugs that undergo such reabsorption generally have a long half-life.

MODIFICATION OF DRUG RESPONSES

The fate of drugs following their administration includes all the pharmacokinetic factors discussed so far. Differences in distribution, storage, biotransformation, and elimination all contribute to the overall response because only the portion of a dose that remains intact can produce the desired effect. This amount of drug, however, may produce different effects in different people. It may even produce different effects in the same person on different days.

Physiologic factors introduce additional variables that are independent of pharmacokinetic factors. Differences in age, weight, genetics, and other factors are the reasons physicians must individualize dosages and adjust drug treatments for the requirements of a given patient.

Age

Neonatal (<9 months) and geriatric (>60 years) patients, representing the extremes of the age spectrum, exhibit the greatest variation in

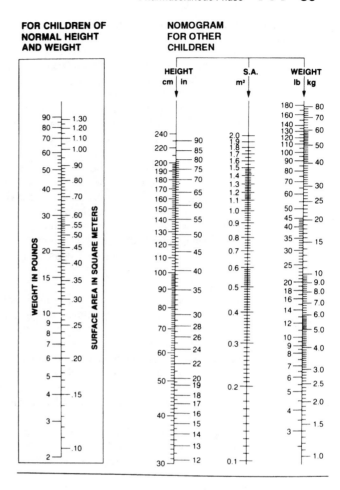

FOR CHILDREN OF NORMAL HEIGHT AND WEIGHT

NOMOGRAM FOR OTHER CHILDREN

FIGURE 2–8 West's nomogram. Plot child's height and weight; draw a line between the two points. The point where this line intersects the surface area line is the child's surface area. (From Nelson Textbook of Pediatrics, ed. 13. W.B. Saunders Co., Philadelphia, with permission.)

drug response. The physiologic factors responsible for the variation are complex and usually interlocking. In a newborn, for example, the ratio of body fluid compartments to total body mass is different from that in an adult. The total amount of albumin-binding sites in a neonate is also different. These variables profoundly affect drug distribution and storage. Neonates also have incomplete hepatic enzyme systems, and their renal mechanisms are not fully developed. For these reasons, the ability of a newborn to metabolize and eliminate drugs is different from that of a mature individual. For a physician, pediatric dosage determination is complex because the patients are not merely "small adults." Various formulas based on age, weight, or surface area have been developed for calculation of safe dosages in children. The most reliable of these systems is based on determination of infant body surface area (BSA) from a nomogram (Figure 2–8). Pediatric dosage is then calculated as a fraction of the adult dosage. The fraction needed is the infant BSA (in m^2) divided by the adult BSA, which is 1.7 m^2 (Box 2–1).

Geriatric patients also present special challenges to the physician because older patients often have both a greater incidence of coexisting pathologic conditions and reduced effectiveness of absorption, distribution, metabolism, and elimination mechanisms. These variables, especially with multiple drug regimens, warrant special consideration. Physicians often begin therapy with minimal doses and then cautiously increase the dose to produce the desired effect.

BOX 2–1 THERAPEUTIC ORPHANS

Ethical considerations prevent the general testing of new drugs in infants and children. However, without the data derived from such a test population, it is difficult or impossible for pharmaceutical companies to provide drug dosage recommendations. Consequently, most drugs carry a statement such as, "Proof of safety and efficacy in children under 12 years of age has not been established." A handful of drugs, such as ribavirin, have been specifically developed for treatment of infants (Chapter 17). These neonatal drugs are special exceptions to the general rule concerning the testing of new drugs in infants and children.

Other than the ethical concerns over drug testing, why are neonatal and pediatric patients "therapeutic orphans" when it comes to drug dosages? More important, how do pediatricians arrive at a safe and effective dosage for their young patients?

The obvious difference between pediatric and adult patients is body weight. However, weight alone does not provide the entire answer to the dosing problem because children of different ages exhibit differences in absorption, distribution, metabolism, and excretion. In addition, pharmacokinetics changes dramatically during the first 6 months of life.

Absorption

Oral absorption of drugs in neonatal and pediatric patients can vary because of variations in gut motility and pH. Blood flow, tissue perfusion, and muscle mass are not fully developed in neonates; therefore, absorption is reduced following intramuscular administration of drugs. The inhalational route is suitable for administration of some drugs to neonatal and pediatric patients, but absorption may be reduced by ineffective technique. For example, proper use of a metered-dose inhaler may be difficult or impossible for the very young patient. In addition, these patients cannot generate the high inspiratory flow rates (>60 L/min) required for delivery of drug from a dry powder inhaler. Absorption of drug from these devices is severely limited. Nebulizers provide reliable delivery and absorption of many drugs for the neonatal or pediatric patient. Ease of convenience, however, is lacking with these aerosol generators. (Table 1–5 compares advantages and disadvantages of different aerosol generators.)

Distribution

Most drugs are distributed in the extracellular fluid. Therefore, pharmacokinetics can be affected by the different proportions of body water. For example, total body fluid and extracellular fluid in relation to body mass are both higher in a neonate than in an adult. As a result, water-soluble drugs in a neonate require higher doses per kilogram of body mass to produce a desired effect.

Biotransformation

Liver function is immature in neonates. Less-effective hepatic enzymes means that a drug's half-life is longer and therapeutic effects persist longer. For example, the half-life of the bronchodilator theophylline is 3–10 hours in a newborn but around 5–6 hours in an adult (Kirsch, 1990).

Excretion

Kidney function is not fully developed in neonates. Glomerular filtration rate, renal blood flow, and tubular secretion are less than in the adult kidney. Therefore, the neonate has reduced ability to concentrate and excrete drugs.

Calculations

The variables discussed above indicate why neonatal and pediatric patients are usually not included in drug dosing recommendations from drug manufacturers. Several calculation methods based on fractions of the average adult dose are available:

Fried's Rule (for patients < 1 year of age):

$$\text{Pediatric Dose} = \frac{\text{Age in months}}{150} \times \text{Adult Dose}$$

Clark's Rule (for patients > 2 years of age):

$$\text{Pediatric Dose} = \frac{\text{Weight in pounds}}{150} \times \text{Adult Dose}$$

Young's Rule (for patients > 2 years of age):

$$\text{Pediatric Dose} = \frac{\text{Age in years}}{\text{Age in years} + 12} \times \text{Adult Dose}$$

Body Surface Area (BSA) Formula:

$$\text{Pediatric Dose} = \frac{\text{Surface area of child (in m}^2)}{1.7} \times \text{Adult Dose}$$

Body surface area calculations for drug dose correlate with the physiologic characteristics of the child better than do formulas based on age or weight. In the BSA method, a child's height and weight are plotted on a nomogram (Fig. 2–8). A line is drawn between the two points and the intersection with the surface area line gives the child's body surface area in square meters. This BSA value is then used in the calculation above to arrive at the pediatric dose.

Deglin JH and Vallerand AH: Davis's Drug Guide for Nurses, ed 3. FA Davis, Philadelphia, 1993.

Kirsch CS: Pharmacotherapeutics for the neonate and the pediatric patient. In Kuhn MM (ed): Pharmacotherapeutics: A Nursing Process Approach, ed 2. FA Davis, Philadelphia, 1990.

Rau JL: Delivery of aerosolized drugs to neonatal and pediatric patients. Respiratory Care. 36:514–542, 1991.

Rau JL: Respiratory Care Pharmacology, ed 3. Year Book Medical Publishers, Chicago, 1989.

Weight

Pharmacologic characteristics of drugs are generally based on actions produced in an ideal 70-kilogram individual. These observations are founded on evidence from experiments in which drugs are administered in the form of milligrams per kilogram of body mass. The distribution of a drug is approximately proportional to body mass. The special case of drug dosages in infants and children is mentioned above.

Pathophysiologic States

Coexisting disease processes that alter absorption, distribution, metabolism, or elimination obviously can affect drug actions on an individual basis. Patients with hepatic or renal disease are sensitive to even normal drug dosages.

Tolerance and Tachyphylaxis

The phenomena of tolerance and tachyphylaxis were discussed previously with biotransforma-tion. The actual mechanisms involved are not completely understood (see Receptor Regulation in Chapter 3).

Drug Interactions

Various drug responses, or **interactions,** may occur in an individual when more than one drug is introduced at the same time. Many drugs produce their effects independently of each other, but in some drug combinations the effect produced by two drugs may be greater or less than that produced by one drug given on its own (monotherapy).

Additive Effects

Additive, or **summation, effects** of two drugs occur if half the dose of drug A and half the dose of drug B produce the same effect as the full dose of either drug administered singly. Additive effects are used in balanced anesthesia, whereby several CNS depressants are given in succession. The additive effects of the drugs produce the desired depth of nervous system depression.

Synergism and Potentiation

Drug **synergism,** unfortunately, is an ambiguous term that can be defined in several ways. First of all, synergism can be viewed simply as an additive effect in which one drug helps or assists another through summation. A more accurate description of drug synergism is that the effect produced by two drugs is greater than an additive effect. Finally, synergism can be defined as a drug interaction whereby one drug increases the potency of another by interfering with its metabolism in some way. The term **potentiation** is also used to describe the latter case: one drug increases the activity of another.

Antagonism

Occasionally two drugs administered together result in decreased activity if the drugs exhibit **antagonism** of some kind. **Chemical antagonism** occurs when one drug chemically combines with another and inactivates it. Antidotes such as dimercaprol (British Anti-Lewisite; BAL) chemically antagonize metals including mercury, lead, or arsenic in cases of poisoning.

Two drugs that produce opposite effects on a physiologic mechanism exhibit **physiologic antagonism.** For example, a CNS depressant and a CNS stimulant functionally oppose each other and may cancel each other's effects.

Pharmacologic antagonism occurs when two drugs compete for the same reactive site. An example of such antagonism is the competition between histamine and antihistaminic drugs for the same histamine receptor.

One drug may interact with another through several mechanisms that affect pharmacokinetics. Such **pharmacokinetic antagonism** may involve modification of absorption, metabolism, or elimination. Either potentiation or antagonism may result from the interaction. For example, calcium-containing dairy products in the digestive system interfere with tetracycline antibiotics by combining with them and decreasing absorption, thus reducing their activity.

Pharmacogenetics

Certain adverse drug reactions, prolonged drug actions, and shortened drug actions can occasionally be attributed to genetic differences. The study of interindividual genetic variation has developed into the pharmacologic discipline of **pharmacogenetics.**

Drug Allergy

A **drug allergy** is an unusual and often severe response to an otherwise safe dose of drug. This same dose fails to produce the unusual reaction or to stimulate the immune mechanism in most people. The specific operation of an antigen-antibody reaction is covered in Chapter 9. It is sufficient at this point to state that some individuals with a hereditary predisposition to allergy may become sensitized following initial exposure to a drug or to a drug bound to a protein molecule. A **hapten** is a drug that binds with a plasma protein. Such a drug–protein complex may act as an antigenic substance to trigger an allergic response (see Fig. 9–1). Persons with a genetic predisposition to allergy are **atopic** and members of the same family often exhibit symptoms of hay fever, asthma, food allergies, or dermatitis. Following initial exposure, subsequent exposure to a small amount of the same drug elicits the unusual and unexpected response of drug allergy. Drug allergies can be identified through the positive reaction to a skin test using the offending substance. Either an immediate or a delayed allergic reaction is seen. **Immediate hypersensitivity** reactions include anaphylaxis, urticaria (hives), drug fever, and asthma. Serum sickness and contact dermatitis are examples of drug allergies of the **delayed hypersensitivity** type.

Drug Idiosyncrasy

Certain unusual drug reactions may occur in individuals having no history of drug allergy. Such a **drug idiosyncrasy** is often due to an enzyme deficiency caused by a genetic defect in the individual. These deficiencies in turn interfere with drug metabolism. This interference may prolong the action of the drug or cause toxicity at a dose level considered safe for the general population. For example, pharmacogenetic studies have determined that some people having a particular enzyme deficiency are unable to metabolize the muscle relaxant succinylcholine at a normal rate. Such individuals are susceptible to prolonged apnea caused by paralysis of ventilatory muscles. This abnormal drug response may occur even when the drug is given at the usual dosage (see Muscle Relaxants in Chapter 7).

CHAPTER SUMMARY

The pharmacokinetic phase of drug action allows drugs to be transferred between various compartments. The fate of drugs entering the body includes absorption through cell membranes, distribution to different tissues and organs, and storage at various plasma, cellular, and tissue sites. In addition, biotransformation in the liver, lungs, or digestive organs and elimination by the kidney, lungs, or intestines contribute to the pharmacokinetics of a drug. The comparatively small fraction of the original dose that persists after the pharmacokinetic phase is the portion of the drug that produces the desired therapeutic effect.

Various physiologic variables such as age, weight, pathophysiologic state, and genetics modify drug responses. These factors operate in addition to pharmacokinetic factors and account for much of the individual variation seen with drug responses.

BIBLIOGRAPHY

Benet LZ: Pharmacokinetics: I. Absorption, distribution, and excretion. In Katzung BD (ed): Basic and Clinical Pharmacology. Lange Medical Publications, Los Altos, 1982.

Benet LZ and Sheiner LB: Pharmacokinetics: The dynamics of drug absorption, distribution, and elimination. In Goodman, AG et al (eds): Goodman and Gilman's The Pharmacologic Basis of Therapeutics, ed 7. Macmillan, New York, 1985.

Blaschke TF, Nies AS, and Mamelok RD: Principles of therapeutics. In Goodman AG et al (eds): Goodman and Gilman's The Pharmacologic Basis of Therapeutics, ed 7. Macmillan, New York, 1985.

Clark WG, Brater DC, and Johnson AR: Goth's Medical Pharmacology, ed 12. CV Mosby, St Louis, 1988.

Correia MA and Castagnoli N: Pharmacokinetics: II. Drug biotransformation. In Katzung BD (ed): Basic and Clinical Pharmacology. Lange Medical Publications, Los Altos, 1982.

West JB: Respiratory Physiology: The Essentials, ed 4. Williams and Wilkins, Baltimore, 1990.

Williamson HE: General principles of drug action and pharmacokinetics. In Conn PM and Gebhart GF (eds): Essentials of Pharmacology. FA Davis, Philadelphia, 1989.

EXPANDED BIBLIOGRAPHY: GENERAL CHEMISTRY

COLLEGE LEVEL

Mortimer CE: Chemistry, ed 6. Wadsworth, Belmont, CA, 1986.

Timberlake KC: Chemistry: An Introduction to General, Organic, and Biological Chemistry, ed 5. Harper-Collins, New York, 1992.

Zumdahl SS: Chemistry, ed 2. DC Heath, Lexington, MA, 1989.

Zumdahl SS: Introductory Chemistry: A Foundation, ed 2. DC Heath, Lexington, MA, 1993.

CHAPTER 3

Pharmacodynamic Phase

CHAPTER OUTLINE

Chapter Introduction
Basics of Pharmacodynamics
  BACKGROUND
  SPATIAL CONFIGURATION

TYPES OF PHARMACOLOGIC
  RECEPTORS
RECEPTOR REGULATION
Dose-Response Relationships

POTENCY AND EFFICACY
AGONISTS AND ANTAGONISTS
TOXICITY AND SAFETY
Chapter Summary

CHAPTER OBJECTIVES

After studying this chapter the reader should be able to:

- Define pharmacologic receptor and describe two types of studies that have been used to discover the existence of such receptors.
- Describe the formation of a drug-receptor complex and the chain of events set in motion by the complexing.
- Name three cellular sites where pharmacologic receptors can be found.
- Define a structure-activity relationship (S-AR) and explain how changes in the structure of a drug can change the specificity of response.
- Describe how changes in drug sensitivity can occur by explaining the concepts of receptor downregulation and upregulation.
- Explain the general concept of dose-response relationships and describe the median effective dose (ED50) of a drug.
- Differentiate between drug potency and drug efficacy.
- Define the following pharmacologic terms: affinity, agonist, partial agonist, antagonist drug.
- Compare the mechanisms of action of competitive and noncompetitive antagonists.
- Describe the interaction between an agonist and a competitive antagonist and between an agonist and a noncompetitive antagonist.
- Define the following pharmacologic terms:
  - Toxicity, median lethal dose (LD50), safety.
- Explain the concept of therapeutic index (T.I.) and relate this to the safety of a drug.

KEY TERMS

affinity
agonist
antagonist
competitive antagonism
downregulation
dose-response relationship
drug-receptor complex

efficacy
median effective dose (ED50)
median lethal dose (LD50)
noncompetitive antagonism
partial agonist
pharmacodynamic phase
pharmacologic receptor

potency
safety
structure-activity relationship
  (S-AR)
therapeutic index (T.I.)
toxicity
upregulation

CHAPTER INTRODUCTION

The preceding chapter introduced the pharmacokinetic phase of drug action responsible for the movement of drugs between different body compartments. Much of a given dose is stored, metabolized, or eliminated, leaving a relatively small amount of drug to enter the **pharmacodynamic phase** of drug action and produce the desired therapeutic effect. This chapter examines the biochemical and physiologic mechanisms by which a drug alters cellular activity.

BASICS OF PHARMACODYNAMICS

Background

Pharmacodynamics deals with the physiologic and biochemical mechanisms of drug action. Drug action takes place at a specialized region known as the **pharmacologic receptor.** The receptor site is complementary to a drug molecule, that is, it has a configuration that is similar to the shape of a drug. The origins of the receptor concept date to the turn of the 20th century with identical observations made by two independent researchers. M. Lewandowsky, in 1898, and J.N. Langley, in 1901, both found that injections of adrenal gland extracts caused organ effects that were similar to those produced through stimulation of sympathetic nerves (Weiner and Taylor, 1985). In 1905, Langley noted that specific sites of drug interaction, or "receptive substances," as he called them, may exist at the surface of effector cells. He observed that some of these sites are excitatory, whereas others are inhibitory, and that the organ response to epinephrine depended on the type of receptive substance present on the effector cell. This view has undergone continuous refinement so that today the receptor theory of interaction is used to explain the action of most drugs, enzymes, hormones, and neurotransmitters (chemical messengers released by nerve cells). Following Langley's work, researchers around the world continued to study the interaction between drugs and binding sites on effector cells. An interesting history of the studies relating to pharmacologic receptors and neurotransmitters is given by Weiner and Taylor (1985). The discovery of the neurotransmitters acetylcholine and norepinephrine is briefly outlined in Box 4–1.

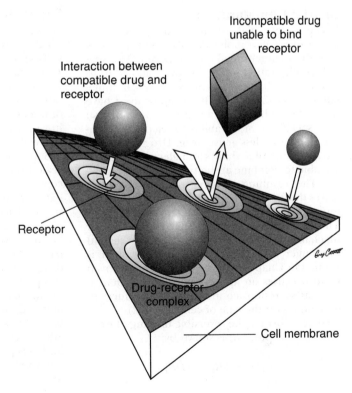

FIGURE 3–1 Schematic—drug-receptor complex.

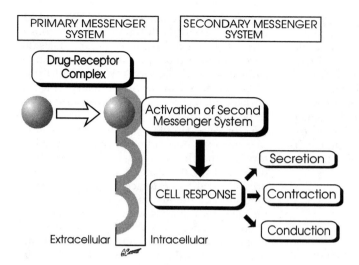

FIGURE 3–2 Initiation of cellular events by drug-receptor complex.

The theory of receptors is based on studies of drug structure and the pharmacologic activity produced, studies of relationships between drugs that produce a response and those that oppose the action, and studies of the selective binding of radioactive-labeled drugs to cell membranes.

Spatial Configuration

Receptors are high-affinity binding sites composed of protein molecules arranged in a specific three-dimensional configuration. The spatial configuration of a receptor allows it to discriminate between various chemical molecules acting as stimuli. The receptor must have the ability to bind with a drug, but it must also have specificity, or the ability to reject the chemical signal of a less active drug. Drug molecules having compatible shapes and electrical charges are able to combine at the receptor site (Fig. 3–1). The resulting **drug-receptor complex** involves the formation of a chemical bond (usually temporary) between the drug and the receptor. The interaction is normally linked to an effector mechanism through an intracellular second messenger system. (This messenger system is studied in Chapter 5.) The effector mechanism in turn causes an appropriate cellular change such as secretion, contraction, or conduction, depending on the type of cell (Fig. 3–2).

At equilibrium, the reversible binding of drug (*D*) and receptor (*R*) is shown by:

$$[D] + [R] \underset{k_2}{\overset{k_1}{\rightleftharpoons}} [DR]$$

where [ ] equals "concentration of" and k_1 and k_2 are the rate constants for the forward and backward reactions, respectively. The ability of a drug to produce an effect is related to its ability to combine at receptors. The extent of the response is proportional to the number of receptors complexed.

Types of Pharmacologic Receptors

Several types of drug receptors exist. Most are on the surface of the cell membrane of target cells and include those that interact with *antihistaminics, narcotics,* and *tranquilizers.* Some receptors, such as those that interact with steroid hormones or drugs, are located in the cytoplasm of target cells. A few substances, such as thyroid hormone, interact at receptors on the nucleus of a cell.

Sophisticated X-ray diffraction studies have revealed the three-dimensional nature of the receptor site. Deeper understanding of the spatial nature of the site may eventually permit the design of drugs with molecular shapes that will *precisely* fit a pharmacologic receptor at a specific location. Discovery of receptor subtypes has paved the way for this future development in drug design. Armed with knowledge of specific receptor characteristics, pharmaceutical chemists will be able to synthesize drugs with the required dimensions to interact at a specific receptor subtype, thus minimizing unwanted side effects. The following description of acetylcholine receptors offers a glimpse of the details known about this class of pharmacologic receptor.

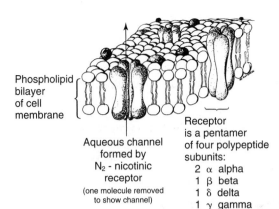

FIGURE 3–3 Schematic—nicotinic acetylcholine receptor.

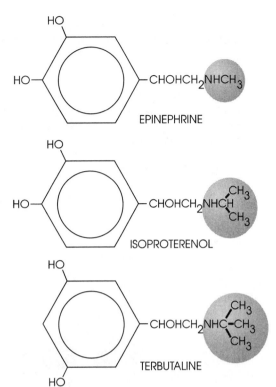

FIGURE 3–4 Structure-activity relationships (S-ARs).

Acetylcholine receptors on skeletal muscle cell membranes are among the most extensively studied receptor populations. (Acetylcholine receptors on skeletal muscle are discussed further in Chapter 7.) Figure 3–3 shows a schematic of the configuration of the acetylcholine receptor at these neuromuscular sites. A procedure called the patch clamp technique electrically isolates a single receptor on a living cell membrane. It has been found that these receptors are composed of five polypeptide subunits that surround a membrane channel. The channel permits the movement of cations through the membrane. When acetylcholine molecules complex with specific subunits of the receptor, the channel opens, thus changing membrane permeability and allowing sodium, potassium, and calcium cations to flow. The three-dimensional nature of the proteins composing this receptor is typical of pharmacologic receptors. Such knowledge concerning receptor structure is essential for researchers attempting to explain the interaction of drugs at receptor sites (Box 3–1).

Relating the three-dimensional characteristics, or *stereochemistry*, of a drug to its receptor interactions are **structure-activity relationships (S-ARs)**. Researchers are becoming increasingly adept at identifying the portion of a drug molecule that is required to allow the drug to complex at a specific receptor. The complexing in turn is responsible for the therapeutic effect. Certain portions of the molecule can be modified without any loss of therapeutic effect to produce a new chemical derivative. This chemical analogue may possess enhanced characteristics, such as fewer or less severe side effects, faster onset of action, or longer duration of action. Figure 3–4 shows the molecular formulas for three drugs having airway-relaxing effects useful in

asthma therapy. (These drugs are discussed in Chapter 12.) All three have similar therapeutic effects in the respiratory system but exhibit decreasing cardiovascular side effects (going from top to bottom in the series). The increase in specificity is due to alteration of drug structure. The desired therapeutic attributes of the original compound are retained, but the derivatives exhibit fewer side effects. Detailed knowledge of S-ARs is an essential part of modern drug design (Box 3–2).

Receptor Regulation

Changes in drug sensitivity may occur following prolonged exposure to a particular drug or hormone. The phenomenon is due to alteration in the *number* of pharmacologic receptors available for drug interaction. Fortunately, this modification of the receptor population and the resulting change in drug response does not occur with every drug. In fact, most drugs can be administered at a uniform dosage on a continuous basis without any change in sensitivity or response.

Continuous drug administration may decrease the number of receptors, a phenomenon called **downregulation.** This change results in

BOX 3–1 PATCH CLAMPS AND RECEPTORS

The 1991 Nobel Prize for Medicine or Physiology was awarded to Erwin Neher and Bert Sakmann for their description of single ion channels in cell membranes using a revolutionary research tool called the *patch clamp technique*. Early studies were done on the electric organ of eels and rays, a tissue with an extremely dense nicotinic acetylcholine receptor population. By touching the cell membrane with a delicate glass microelectrode filled with an acetylcholine (ACh) solution (the patch electrode) and applying gentle suction to form a seal, a *single* nicotinic receptor could be isolated from adjacent areas (see figure). Connecting the electrode to a suitable amplifier revealed the electrical activity

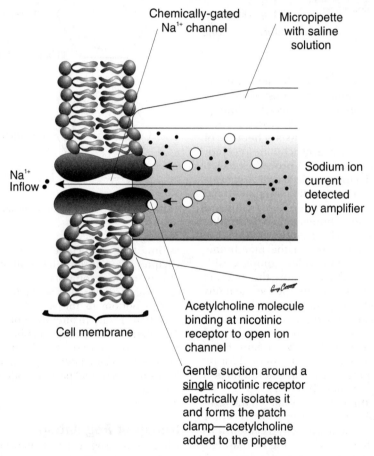

Chemically-gated
Na^{1+} channel

Micropipette
with saline
solution

Na^{1+}
Inflow

Sodium ion
current
detected
by amplifier

Cell membrane

Acetylcholine molecule
binding at nicotinic
receptor to open ion
channel

Gentle suction around a
<u>single</u> nicotinic receptor
electrically isolates it
and forms the patch
clamp—acetylcholine
added to the pipette

evoked by the nicotinic receptor being bombarded by ACh molecules. ACh molecules complexing at two α-subunits of the receptor caused the aqueous channel to open briefly to permit cationic flow. The patch clamp technique permitted the recording of ion fluxes as the channel opened and closed. It also allowed researchers to elucidate the spatial configuration of the nicotinic acetylcholine receptor (Figure 3–3).

Martin AR: Principles of neuromuscular transmission. Physiology in Medicine Series. Hosp Pract (Off Ed) 27:147–158, Aug 15, 1992.

Neher E and Sakmann B: The patch clamp technique. Sci Am 266:44–51, Mar 1992.

Unwin N: The structure of ion channels in excitable cells. Neuron 3:665–676, 1989.

desensitization, or a decrease in drug response. With a reduced receptor population the only way to produce the same number of drug-receptor complexes is with more frequent administration of drug. Tachyphylaxis, as occurs with nasal *decongestants* and *beta-adrenergic stimulants,* is produced through this mechanism. Recall that the mechanism of tolerance and tachyphylaxis is not fully understood. For example, tachyphylaxis with the nitrates does not involve changes in receptor numbers.

Upregulation, or an increase in receptor number, is not as common as downregulation. Upregulation results in heightened drug sensitivity because more receptors are available for interaction at any dosage level. Individuals with a hyperactive thyroid gland oversecrete thyroid hormone, which in turn induces an increase in adrenergic receptors on cell membranes. The upregulation of receptors makes a person with hyperthyroidism very sensitive to the action of drugs and hormones known as *catecholamines.* Therefore, normal doses of these substances produce unwanted side effects. (Catecholamines and adrenergic receptors are studied in Chapter 5.)

DOSE-RESPONSE RELATIONSHIPS

Potency and Efficacy

As the dosage of a drug is increased, the amount of drug entering the pharmacodynamic phase increases. This effect increases the pharmacologic response. A **dose-response relationship,** then, is the proportional change in drug response to a changing drug dosage (Fig. 3–5). At some dosage level, however, *all* of the pharmacologic receptors are complexed by the drug. The receptor population is very large, typically measured in the millions of receptors at a single location. It is, however, a finite number. Once drug molecules have complexed with all available receptors, a maximal pharmacologic response is evoked. Increasing drug dosage beyond this level does not alter the pharmacologic response.

A typical logarithmic dose-response curve is depicted in Figure 3–6, where the drug response is plotted against the logarithm of the drug dose. The **median effective dose (ED50)** is the dose that produces a specified intensity of effect in 50% of individuals. As can be seen, the sigmoid curve has a characteristic plateau corresponding to maximal receptor complexing.

Potency refers to the relative ability of a drug to evoke a particular response at a given dose. If two drugs are capable of causing the same response but Drug A produces the response at a lower dose than Drug B, Drug A is considered more potent than Drug B. Drugs are often described on the basis of potency, but the comparison is meaningless unless *equieffective* doses are considered. Figure 3–7A shows two drugs with the same effectiveness. Drug A, however, is more potent than Drug B because it is producing its maximal effect at a lower dose. In the comparison shown in Figure 3–7B, Drug A is not only more potent than Drug B, but is also more ef-

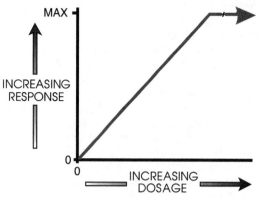

FIGURE 3–5   Generalized dose-response relationship.

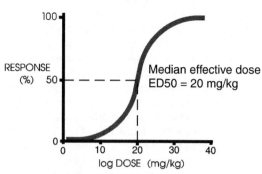

FIGURE 3–6   Log dose-response curve.

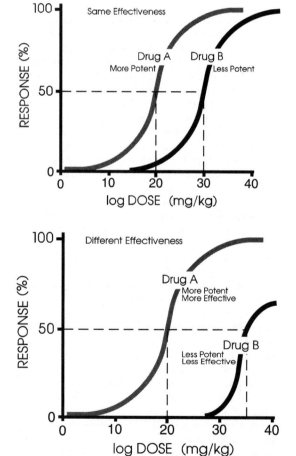

FIGURE 3–7   (A) Comparison of potencies of two drugs with the same effectiveness. (B) Comparison of potencies of two drugs with different effectiveness.

fective because it elicits a maximal response, whereas Drug B fails to do so. Therefore, in clinical applications, the effectiveness of a drug is more important than its potency. A more potent drug can be given in a smaller dose, but if it lacks therapeutic effectiveness, the greater potency is clinically irrelevant.

The ability of a drug to produce a desired therapeutic response is its effectiveness, or intrinsic activity. This characteristic is also known as **efficacy,** or the ability to produce an effect relative to a given number of drug-receptor complexes. Drugs with high efficacy are able to produce a desired therapeutic effect by forming relatively few drug-receptor complexes.

Agonists and Antagonists

An **agonist** is a drug that interacts with receptors to trigger a pharmacologic response. An agonist possesses efficacy and **affinity,** the tendency to combine with certain receptors. The extent of the pharmacologic response is proportional to the number of drug-receptor complexes formed. A drug is called a **partial agonist** if it has affinity for a receptor site but does not elicit the same magnitude of response as a full agonist. A partial agonist cannot produce the same maximal effect as a full agonist because it has less efficacy.

Antagonist drugs interact with a pharmacologic receptor and prevent the action of an agonist. Antagonists possess affinity for the same receptor used by the full agonist but are totally lacking in efficacy.

Competitive antagonism occurs when the antagonist drug binds reversibly at a receptor. Figure 3–8 shows the change produced in the logarithmic dose-response curve when an agonist drug and a competitive antagonist drug contend for the same pharmacologic receptor. There is a parallel displacement to the right of the logarithmic dose-response curve, but no change in the maximal response elicited by the agonist. This effect is caused by the reversibility of the binding between competitive antagonist and receptor. The total receptor population is unchanged, but an increased amount of agonist is required to produce the maximal response. The potency of the agonist, therefore, has been decreased. The chapters to follow discuss many examples of such agonist-antagonist interactions. For instance, acetylcholine is an agonist that exhibits affinity and efficacy and combines at the same receptor as the competitive antagonist atropine. Atropine has affinity but lacks efficacy; therefore, the logarithmic dose-response curve

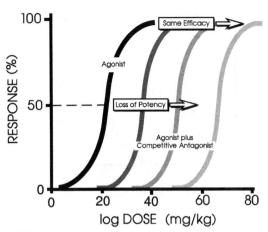

FIGURE 3–8 Log dose-response curve (agonist plus competitive antagonist).

generated by the two drugs in competition would resemble that of Figure 3–8.

Some antagonists combine irreversibly with pharmacologic receptors, producing **noncompetitive antagonism.** These noncompetitive antagonists, like the competitive type, lack efficacy. They also bind permanently to receptors and essentially isolate those receptors from possible interaction with an agonist. The permanently occupied receptors are simply no longer part of the receptor population with which an agonist drug may interact. Therefore, the efficacy of the agonist is reduced—it can no longer elicit a maximal pharmacologic response, no matter what the agonist drug concentration. The typical logarithmic dose-response curve with a noncompetitive antagonist is shifted both to the right

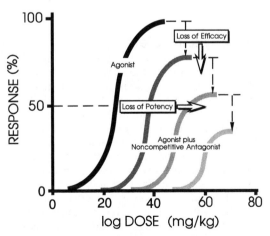

FIGURE 3–9 Log dose-response curve (agonist plus noncompetitive antagonist).

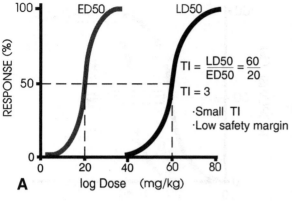

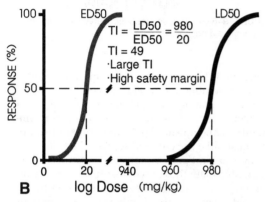

FIGURE 3–10   (*A*) Therapeutic index (TI)—low safety margin. (*B*) Therapeutic index—high safety margin.

and down, indicating not only loss of agonist potency but also loss of agonist efficacy (Fig. 3–9). Examples of this type of antagonism are examined in Chapter 6.

Toxicity and Safety

During development of a new drug an assessment of **toxicity,** or the production of adverse effects, is carried out. The **median lethal dose (LD50)** is the dose that produces lethal effects in half of a test population. For obvious reasons, laboratory animals are used in such tests. Sublethal doses permit an acceptable correlation between some animal and human toxicity effects. (The allergic airway response in guinea pigs, for instance, is very similar to that of humans.) Species differences, however, do exist, and these variables introduce a degree of uncertainty to animal testing of drugs. In addition, many sublethal toxicity effects such as nausea, dizziness,

headache, and fatigue, which are common in humans, are not recognizable in test animals. Nevertheless, animal testing prior to human clinical trials of a new drug provides researchers with invaluable toxicity guidelines (Box 3–3).

It has been said that "all drugs are poisons and all poisons are drugs." A small dose of curare, an arrow poison from tropical rain forests, provides the modern surgeon with precise control over unwanted muscular contractions. The same drug in a larger dose paralyzes respiratory muscles and halts breathing. Stated simply, there exists a lethal amount of virtually any substance. Some drugs are very unforgiving—a certain amount produces the desired therapeutic effect, but slightly more causes toxic effects. Others have a large range between the therapeutic and toxic doses.

Figure 3–10*A* shows ED50 and LD50 curves for the same drug. The distance between the logarithmic doses producing the desired therapeutic effect (ED50) and the lethal effect (LD50) represents the **safety** margin for the drug. This margin is expressed as the therapeutic ratio, or **therapeutic index (T.I.),** where:

$$T.I. = \frac{LD50}{ED50}$$

The ED50 and LD50 doses are usually given in milligrams of drug per kilogram of body mass. Like all indices, the therapeutic index has no units. For example, if the LD50 is 60 mg/kg and the ED50 is 20 mg/kg, as shown in Figure 3–10*A*, the T.I. for the drug is 3 because the dose units cancel:

$$T.I. = \frac{LD50}{ED50} = \frac{\overset{3}{\cancel{60 \text{ mg/kg}}}}{\underset{1}{\cancel{20 \text{ mg/kg}}}} = 3$$

Other features being equal, a drug having a low ED50 and a high LD50 has a large "therapeutic window" (Fig. 3–10*B*). It is this differential that is most important from a clinical standpoint. In fact, for a physician, the actual logarithmic doses involved in laboratory testing of a given drug are relatively unimportant. The clinician is more concerned with knowing by *how much* a therapeutic dosage can be exceeded before toxic effects begin to show in most people. Drugs with low safety margins include *general anesthetics* (T.I. < 2). The dose of anesthetic required to maintain a deep level of central nervous system de-

BOX 3–3 INVESTIGATIONAL NEW DRUGS

The public has always been enthusiastic about the debut of effective new drugs. With contemporary health care concerns such as cancer, AIDS, and the emergence of anti-biotic-resistant strains of micro-organisms, there is an added sense of urgency concerning the development of new drugs. What delays their release?

To start with, limitations are inherent in the empirical method of drug development (see Chapter 1). Screening of drug sources, extraction and identification of active ingredients, synthesis of the actual drug, and preliminary animal studies are very time consuming. Second, a potential new drug must show proven **efficacy** and **safety** in humans. Designing and carrying out tests that prove this is difficult, expensive, and once again time consuming.

To safeguard public health, establish standards for research, and facilitate the development of new drugs, the US Food and Drug Administration (USFDA) administers a set of protocols to cover *Investigational New Drug* (IND) research. The USFDA reviews the preliminary animal study data available for the drug being developed. Such studies give a general pharmacologic profile for the drug, but toxicity findings may not correlate exactly with human data. However, if the efficacy and safety results appear favorable, IND status is granted. Three phases of human clinical trials are then initiated.

Phase 1

Preliminary Pharmacologic Evaluation (Clinical Studies)

This phase involves small studies to determine a pharmacokinetic profile for the drug. In these tests using healthy human volunteers, relatively few investigators are involved and only small doses of the drug are used. With increasing doses, an evaluation is made to see if the effects observed in animals apply to humans.

Phase 2

Basic Controlled Clinical Evaluation (Clinical Studies)

A larger number of clinical investigators perform controlled studies to gain as much pharmacologic information as possible regarding the safety and efficacy of the new drug. During this phase, the potential use of the drug in disease is studied and the proper dosage is determined.

Phase 3

Extended Clinical Evaluation (Clinical Trials)

Comprehensive clinical trials of the new drug are carried out by a much larger group of clinical investigators using a larger number of patients. Double-blind studies are most often employed. In these studies neither the patient nor the investigator knows whether the new drug or a placebo is being given.

Surveillance

If extended clinical evaluation (Phase 3) indicates that the drug has adequate efficacy and safety, a *New Drug Application* (NDA) is approved by the USFDA. The sponsoring drug company then markets the drug and closely monitors its effects in the general population. Occasionally, adverse reactions, such as drug idiosyncrasies or allergies, that were not observed in the clinical testing phases are evident in a large population. If the reactions seen in the post–market surveillance stage are widespread and severe enough, the drug is recalled.

Goth A: Medical Pharmacology: Principles and Concepts. CV Mosby, St Louis, 1984.
Liska K: Drugs and the Human Body: With Implications for Society. Macmillan, New York, 1981.
Moraca-Sawicki A: History, legislation, and standards. In Kuhn MM (ed): Pharmacotherapeutics: A Nursing Process Approach, ed 2. FA Davis, Philadelphia, 1990.

pression is almost as much as the dose that causes lethal depression of vital control centers for cardiac, ventilation, and blood pressure functions. By contrast, *antibiotics* such as penicillin have a generous range between therapeutic and toxic doses (T.I. > 100) and are inherently safe on the basis of therapeutic versus lethal doses. (Other drawbacks, such as penicillin allergy, are dealt with in Chapter 16.)

CHAPTER SUMMARY

This chapter outlines the basics of drug action at pharmacologic receptors: the ability of receptors to discriminate between various chemical signals, the ability of a drug to interact at a receptor, and the importance of structure-activity and dose-response relationships. In addition, the concepts of spatial configuration and affinity, efficacy and potency, and toxicity and safety are presented. Subsequent chapters reinforce these pharmacodynamic principles as various drug classes are discussed.

BIBLIOGRAPHY

Clark WG, Brater DC, and Johnson AR: Goth's Medical Pharmacology, ed 12. CV Mosby, St Louis, 1988.

Horn JP: The heroic age of neurophysiology. Physiology in Medicine Series. Hosp Pract (Off Ed) 27:65–74, Jul 15, 1992.

Martin AR: Principles of neuromuscular transmission. Physiology in Medicine Series. Hosp Pract (Off Ed) 27:147–158, Aug 15, 1992.

Neher E and Sakmann B: The patch clamp technique. Sci Am 266:44–51, Mar 1992.

Roberts JM and Bourne HR: Drug receptors and pharmacodynamics. In Katzung BD (ed): Basic and Clinical Pharmacology. Lange Medical Publications, Los Altos, 1982.

Ross EM and Gilman AG: Pharmacodynamics: Mechanisms of drug action and relationship between drug concentration and effect. In Goodman AG et al (eds): Goodman and Gilman's The Pharmacologic Basis of Therapeutics, ed 7. Macmillan, New York, 1985.

Weiner N and Taylor P: Neurohumoral transmission: The autonomic and somatic motor nervous systems. In Goodman AG et al (eds): The Pharmacologic Basis of Therapeutics, ed. 7. Macmillan, New York, 1985.

Williamson HE: General principles of drug action and pharmacokinetics. In Conn PM and Gebhart GF (eds): Essentials of Pharmacology. FA Davis, Philadelphia, 1989.

UNIT TWO

DRUGS AFFECTING THE PERIPHERAL NERVOUS SYSTEM

UNIT INTRODUCTION

Pharmacologic agents acting on the peripheral nervous system include drugs that stimulate and drugs that inhibit nerve transmission. The pharmacologic action can occur at various locations, including autonomic ganglia, junctions between autonomic nerve fibers and effectors, and junctions between voluntary nerve fibers and skeletal muscles. Chemical mediation of the many junctions, or synapses, controls the *conduction* of nerve impulses, the *contraction* of muscle, and the *secretion* of glands. Therapeutic agents can be employed to dilate the pupils, slow a rapid heart rate, empty the bladder, or block contractions of skeletal muscle. They are an extremely versatile group of drugs that can be best understood within the context of neurochemical transmission and autonomic pharmacology.

CHAPTER 4

Neurochemical Transmission

CHAPTER OUTLINE

CHAPTER OBJECTIVES

After studying this chapter the reader should be able to:

- Briefly describe the function of neuroglial cells.
- Describe the structure and function of the following parts of a typical neuron: cell body, dendrites, axon, myelin, synaptic vesicles.
- Describe the structure of multipolar, bipolar, and pseudounipolar neurons.
- Describe the functions of sensory, motor, and connector neurons.
- Describe the role of the sodium-potassium pump in relation to the resting membrane potential of a nerve cell.
- Explain the role of ion channels in nerve impulse transmission.
- Describe cell membrane electrical changes occurring during the generation of an action potential by explaining polarization, depolarization, and repolarization.
- Explain the differences between the absolute and relative refractory periods.
- Outline the electrical changes produced during propagation of an action potential along an axon.
- Describe the all-or-none principle and explain why most drugs cannot modify axonal transmission.
- Explain how an impulse is transferred across a synaptic gap by describing the role of neurotransmitters and receptors.
- Describe the mechanisms that terminate chemical transmission.
- Compare an excitatory postsynaptic potential (EPSP) and an inhibitory postsynaptic potential (IPSP) as they relate to neurotransmitters.
- Explain the concept of drug-altered function at synapses by describing the pharmacologic actions of mimicry and blockade.

KEY TERMS

action potential (AP)
all-or-none principle
axon
dendrite (**DEN**-drīt)
depolarization
excitatory postsynaptic
    potential (EPSP)
inhibitory postsynaptic potential
    (IPSP)
ion channel
    chemically–gated ion channel
    nongated channels (leakage
        channels)
    voltage-gated ion channel
neurochemical
    (neurotransmitter) (nyoo-rō-
    TRANS-mit-er)

neuroeffector (nyoo-rō-ē-**FEK**-
    tōr); (effector)
neuroglia (nyoo-**ROG**-lē-a);
    (neuroglial cells, glial cells)
neuron (NYOO-ron)
    bipolar neuron
    connector neuron (interneuron)
    motor neuron (efferent neuron)
    multipolar neuron
    pseudounipolar neuron (unipolar
        neuron)
    sensory neuron (afferent neuron)
neuronal transmission (axonal
    transmission)
polarized; polarization
postsynaptic (postjunctional)
presynaptic (prejunctional)

refractory period
    absolute refractory period
    relative refractory period
repolarization
resting membrane potential
    (RMP)
sodium-potassium pump (Na^{1+}/
    K^{1+}/ATPase)
synapse (**SI**-naps)
    axoaxonal synapse
    axodendritic synapse
    axosomatic synapse
synaptic (si-**NAP**-tik) gap
    (synaptic cleft, synaptic
    junction)
synaptic transmission
    (junctional transmission)

CHAPTER INTRODUCTION

The transmission of information within the nervous system is accomplished through two mechanisms, an electrical and a chemical mode. Most drugs modify body functions by altering the chemical means of information transfer in the nervous system. This chapter examines the role played by nervous tissue and the functions carried out by nerve cells. The mechanisms associated with nerve impulse transmission are studied in detail to provide the insight necessary to understand how and where most drugs exert their influence.

NERVOUS TISSUE

A tissue is a group of related cells working together to perform the same function. *Nervous tissue* is one of the four basic tissue types in the body. The other three are *epithelial tissue,* found as coverings of organs and of the body itself and as linings of hollow structures; *muscular tissue,* which performs all contractile functions; and *connective tissue,* consisting of all other tissue types, such as bone, cartilage, fat, and blood.

Subtypes of Cells

Neuroglia perform a variety of key functions in a background, or supportive, role. There are several types of neuroglia, also known as **neuroglial cells** or **glial cells,** functioning in essential roles such as support and protection. Some glial cells form part of the protective blood-brain barrier, others are found as supportive cells wrapped around parts of neurons, and still others function as phagocytic cells and play a scavenger role in nervous tissue.

Neurons exhibit the twin characteristics of *irritability,* the ability to respond to a stimulus, and *conductivity,* the ability to transmit an electrical impulse. These two functions of stimulus response and impulse transmission are developed to a high degree of sophistication in neurons.

A typical neuron, or nerve cell, is a composite cell, possessing all the generalized structural features found in neurons (Fig. 4–1). Nerve cells located in different parts of the nervous system may possess features that deviate from the following generalized description. In the typical neuron the bulk of the cytoplasm is located in the cell body. This component is the expanded portion of the cell that contains the nucleus and the metabolic machinery of the cell. Fiber-like extensions of the cell body are called cell processes and are made up of **dendrites** and an **axon.** Extensively branched dendrites carry impulses toward the cell body and can be found as single or multiple structures. The axon transmits impulses away from the cell body and is always found as a single structure. Typically these cell processes have fine branches at their ends. Most axons branch into several axon terminals, which have synaptic bulbs at their distal ends. Many axons are extremely long and thin. Their structure gives a fibrous appearance to the cell, hence the name "nerve fiber." Myelinated axons are surrounded by a lipid-rich insulating layer called *myelin.* This material is formed by neuroglial cells known as neurolemmocytes, or Schwann cells. These cells wrap around the axon in one location. Successive neurolemmocytes placed

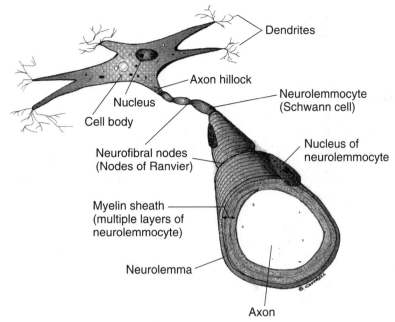

Dendrites

Axon hillock

Neurolemmocyte
(Schwann cell)

Nucleus

Cell body

Nucleus of
neurolemmocyte

Neurofibral nodes
(Nodes of Ranvier)

Myelin sheath
(multiple layers of
neurolemmocyte)

Neurolemma

Axon

FIGURE 4–1 Typical neuron.

end-to-end give the myelinated fiber a characteristic bulged or "sausage link" appearance. The outer layer of the wrapping is called the *neurolemma,* and the gaps between adjacent neurolemmocytes are called *neurofibral nodes* or *nodes of Ranvier.*

CLASSIFICATION OF NEURONS

Structural Classification

Three different morphologic (shape) arrangements are recognized for neurons. The differences are based on the number of dendrites present on the cell body. **Multipolar neurons** possess multiple poles or dendrites; therefore, many information pathways lead into the cell body (Fig. 4–2). Such a structural arrangement contributes to the complex web of interconnections common in multineuronal networks. Diversity of data pathways is advantageous when a large amount of information must be processed. Multipolar neurons are abundant in the brain and spinal cord, where information processing is a prime function. Estimates of the number of multipolar neurons in the brain are staggering, ranging from 10 billion to 15 billion cells. Many of these cells interconnect with thousands of others.

Bipolar neurons have two poles, or extensions. A single dendrite carries information into the

cell body and a single axon conveys information out of the cell body (Fig. 4–2). Such an arrangement provides only one pathway for information transfer in the cell. One of the few locations where bipolar neurons can be found is the retina of the eye. The light-sensitive rods and cones of the retina are specialized bipolar neurons that convert different wavelengths and intensities of light into nervous impulses, which are amplified and then transmitted to visual centers in the brain.

Pseudounipolar, or **unipolar, neurons** *appear* to have one extension that goes a short distance from the cell body before splitting in two. In fact, a single dendrite leads into the cell body and a single axon leads out (Fig. 4–2). The distribution of pseudounipolar neurons in the nervous system is not widespread. Such neurons carry sensations such as pain, touch, and temperature into the spinal cord through a pathway called the dorsal root. Such nerve cells are known as dorsal root ganglion cells and form the sensory limb of spinal reflex arcs.

Functional Classification

A functional classification of neurons is based on the direction in which impulses are transmitted. **Sensory,** or **afferent, neurons** transmit impulses toward the brain and spinal cord (Fig. 4–3).

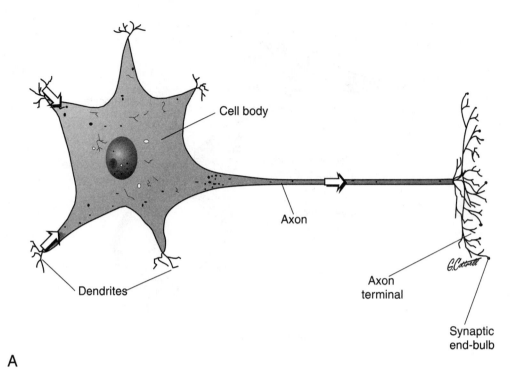

Arrows show the path of information flow
through the neuron

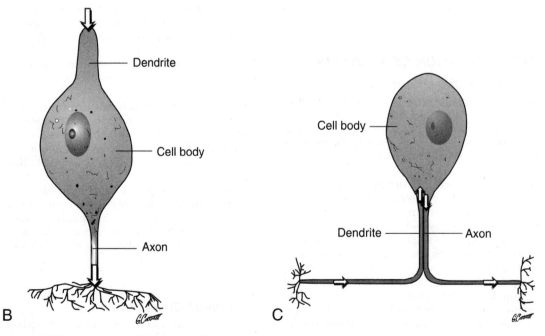

FIGURE 4–2   Structural classification of neurons. (*A*) Multipolar neuron. (*B*) Bipolar neuron. (*C*) Pseudounipolar neuron.

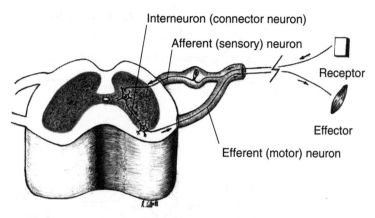

FIGURE 4–3 Functional classification of neurons.

Transverse section of spinal cord showing a three-neuron reflex arc

Some sensory neurons are involved in spinal reflexes, carrying sensations such as pain and touch into the spinal cord.

Motor, or **efferent, neurons** carry impulses away from the brain and spinal cord to **neuroeffectors** throughout the body (Fig. 4–3). Neuroeffectors, also known simply as **effectors,** are target cells or tissues such as muscles, glands, or other nerve cells. Depending on the type of cell, these effectors respond to stimulation by contracting, secreting, or relaying a nerve impulse. In response to a stimulus, some efferent neurons complete the spinal reflex loop by carrying motor impulses from the spinal cord to skeletal muscles.

Connector neurons, or **interneurons,** convey impulses from sensory neurons to motor neurons (Fig. 4–3). This role places them within the central nervous system, where they connect incoming sensory fibers with outgoing motor fibers.

NEURONAL TRANSMISSION

Multineuronal Pathways

In the lumbar region of the spinal cord, thousands of neuronal cell bodies are found. Some of these cells are responsible for sending motor impulses to the muscles of the lower leg, ankle, and foot. Axons of these cells exit from the spinal cord, are bundled together to form a peripheral nerve, and then travel down the leg uninterrupted for more than 1 m. Motor fibers of such nerves are the longest cells in the body. An impulse traveling through such an intact

neuron reaches its destination in the shortest possible time (Fig. 4–4). This fast and efficient method of transmission, however, is atypical because most nerve impulses are transmitted along multineuronal pathways (Fig. 4–4). Impulses still reach their destination, but must now cross fluid-filled gaps between adjacent nerve cells. Thus, nerve impulses consist of **neuronal,** or **axonal, transmission** which occurs within the nerve cell, and **synaptic,** or **junctional, transmission,** which occurs between a nerve cell and a neuroeffector.

Neuronal transmission is a fast-moving mode of transmission that involves a type of *electrical* phenomenon. Synaptic transmission is a relatively slow-moving mode of transmission and depends on a *chemical* type of activity. A nerve impulse crossing several **synaptic gaps** and traveling along a multineuronal pathway, therefore, is made up of a series of neurochemical or electrochemical events. An impulse must be converted from electrical to chemical and back to electrical at each synaptic gap in such a pathway.

Resting Membrane Potential

The cell membrane functions as a bioelectric generator or charge accumulator because it separates two fluids having slightly different electrical characteristics. The **resting membrane potential (RMP)** develops because there is a small buildup of positive charges in the extracellular fluid and a small accumulation of negative charges in the intracellular fluid. The buildup of charge is found only in the fluid immediately adjacent to the cell membrane. Away from the

SINGLE NEURON PATHWAY

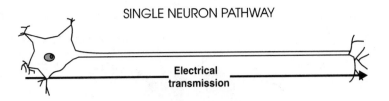

Electrical
transmission

MULTINEURONAL PATHWAY

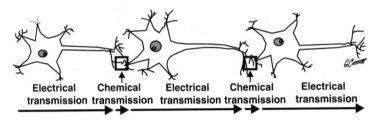

| Electrical | Chemical | Electrical | Chemical | Electrical |
| transmission | transmission | transmission | transmission | transmission |

Neuronal or axonal transmission involves an electrical
(cationic) mechanism whereas synaptic or junctional
transmission depends on a chemical (neurotransmitter)
mechanism

FIGURE 4–4 Neuronal pathways.

cell membrane, no concentration of electrical charges is evident. Separation of positive and negative charges represents an electrical potential that can be measured in millivolts (mV) across the cell membrane ($1\ mV = 1 \times 10^{-3}\ V$). The separation is a type of potential energy. Such resting membrane potentials in neurons range from -40 mV to -90 mV. Because the interior of the cell is electrically negative with respect to the outside, a minus sign is used to express RMP values. A typical RMP for a nerve cell is -70 mV (see Table 22–1). Cell membranes that possess such an electrical potential are **polarized.** Flow of electrical charge is called a *current.* In a nerve cell, moving ions rather than electrons carry the current. The ionic flow occurs through pores or ion channels in the electrically insulated cell membrane.

Development of the resting membrane potential depends on two factors. First, the cation and anion composition of the fluid inside the cell is different from that outside the cell. Extracellular fluid is rich in sodium ions (Na^{1+}) and chloride ions (Cl^{1-}), whereas intracellular fluid has abundant potassium ions (K^{1+}) and anions in the form of amino acids in protein molecules.

Second, the cell membrane is selective, or semipermeable. A completely permeable cell membrane would allow an equilibrium whereby the ionic concentrations would be exactly equal on both sides of the membrane. A semipermeable membrane, by contrast, restricts the movement of some substances while enhancing the movement or allowing free movement of others. The cell membrane is 50 to 100 times more permeable to K^{1+} than it is to Na^{1+}. Consequently, K^{1+} leaves the cell in response to its concentration gradient and the interior becomes increasingly negative. The resulting electrical gradient tends to pull some K^{1+} back into the cell, whereas the Na^{1+} concentration gradient tends to cause some Na^{1+} to leak into the cell. With a freely permeable membrane, these cation movements, plus the exit of anions from the cell's interior (due to an electrical gradient), would eventually create an equilibrium. With the plasma membrane only slightly permeable to sodium, however, Na^{1+} diffuse inward far too slowly to balance the more rapid K^{1+} leakage outward. In addition, most anions of the intracellular fluid are not free to exit because they are part of high molecular weight proteins, which cannot easily pass through the membrane pores. The result of low membrane permeability to both Na^{1+} and anions is that the interior of the cell becomes increasingly negative as K^{1+} exit.

Sodium-Potassium Pumps

Although the cell membrane is only slightly permeable to sodium ions, Na^{1+} continually leak inward in response to a concentration gradient and an electrical gradient. Primary active transport mechanisms called **sodium-potassium pumps** move Na^{1+} that have leaked inward back into the extracellular fluid. The pumps also transport K^{1+} into the cell. However, K^{1+} quickly disperse because of the electrochemical gradients described above. The prime role of the sodium-potassium pumps, therefore, is to transport Na^{1+} out of the cell. Because these small cations continually leak through membrane channels, the pumps must operate continually, expending energy by splitting ATP (adenosine triphosphate) molecules. (The role of ATP is covered in Chapter 5.) Because the pump is a protein that functions like an enzyme, the transport mechanism is sometimes called **$Na^{1+}/K^{1+}/$ ATPase.**

Ion Channels

Several types of **ion channel** allow ions to flow into and out of the cell through the cell membrane. Some ion channels are always open and are called **leakage,** or **nongated, channels.** Such channels account for differences in membrane permeability. **Voltage-gated ion channels,** however, are normally closed, but open in response to a change in voltage at the membrane. Their opening and closing are responsible for generating nerve impulses (see "Action Potential"). Chemical stimuli such as **neurotransmitters,** hormones, and drugs, and ions such as Ca^{2+}, activate **chemically gated ion channels.** Unlike voltage-gated ion channels, chemically gated ion channels allow for a graded response, or potential. This response depends on the number of gated channels opened and the length of time during which they are open. Chemically gated ion channels work in different ways. Some act directly on membrane permeability to open a channel for movement of cations such as Na^{1+}, K^{1+}, and Ca^{2+}. For example, the neurotransmitter acetylcholine acts on certain membrane receptors to cause chemically gated ion channels to open (see Fig. 3–3 and Box 3–1). A few chemically gated ion channels operate indirectly through a second messenger system. (This system is discussed fully in Chapter 5.)

Action Potential

An **action potential** (Fig. 4–5), or nerve impulse, is created by the opening and closing of voltage-

j15

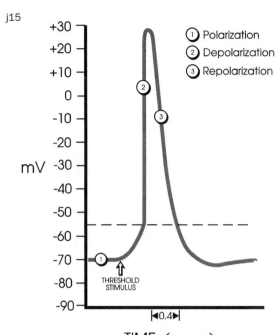

FIGURE 4–5Action potential (typical neuron).-

gated Na^{1+} and K^{1+} channels. **Depolarization** is the loss and reversal of membrane polarization brought about by the rapid opening of voltage-gated Na^{1+} channels. **Repolarization** is the recovery step whereby the resting membrane potential is restored through the opening of voltage-gated K^{1+} channels and the closing of voltage-gated Na^{1+} channels.

Depolarization

At a critical (threshold) level of approximately −55 mV, voltage-gated Na^{1+} channels open (Fig. 4–6A). Sodium ions rapidly flow inward in response to the concentration and electrical gradients established by the Na^{1+}/K^{1+} pumps. The membrane potential becomes less negative with the arrival of each positively charged Na^{1+} in the cell's interior. Inward diffusion continues, finally changing the voltage to +30 mV (Fig. 4–5). An example of drug interference with this mechanism is seen with the *local anesthetic* procaine and the *antiarrhythmic* lidocaine. These drugs block nerve impulses by preventing voltage-gated Na^{1+} channels from opening. As a result the nerve impulse is halted.

Repolarization

Voltage-gated K^{1+} channels begin to open at the same time as voltage-gated Na^{1+} channels, but

Extracellular fluid

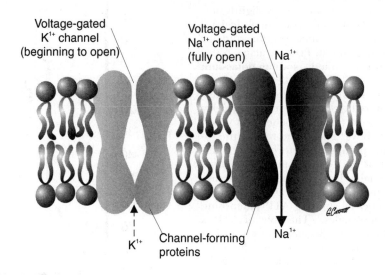

A Intracellular fluid

Extracellular fluid

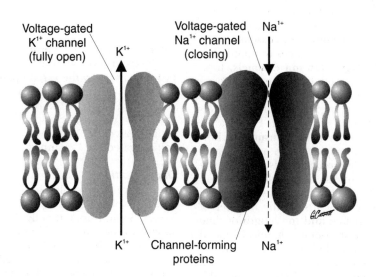

B Intracellular fluid

FIGURE 4–6 Ion channels. (*A*) Depolarization. (*B*) Repolarization.

do so more slowly (Fig. 4–6*A*). As a result the K^{1+} channels open at about the same time that the Na^{1+} channels are closing (Fig. 4–6*B*). Therefore, Na^{1+} inflow is slowed and K^{1+} outflow is increased. These cation movements change the membrane potential from +30 mV to 0 to −70 mV and thus restore the normal resting membrane potential (Fig. 4–5).

Refractory Periods

For a second action potential to be generated, the voltage-gated Na^{1+} channels must be closed and in their resting state. If this has not occurred, even a very strong stimulus cannot trigger another action potential. Such a phase in which the membrane is resistant to further stimuli is called the **absolute refractory period.** It is the rate-limiting step in neuronal transmission. Large-diameter axons have an absolute refractory period of approximately 0.4 milliseconds (ms). This period translates into a frequency of 2500 impulses per second:

$$\frac{1 \text{ impulse}}{0.4 \text{ ms}} \times \frac{1000 \text{ ms}}{1 \text{ s}} = 2500 \text{ impulses/s}$$

This value represents the theoretical upper limit of neuronal performance attained in experimental procedures. In actual operating circuits in the body, however, frequencies of around 600 impulses per second are typical. During the **relative refractory period,** a second action potential can be generated, but a stronger than normal stimulus is required. During this period the Na^{1+} channels have closed but the K^{1+} channels are still open.

Conduction

For an impulse to reach the terminal branches of an axon, it must be conducted along the axon. The localized region of depolarization stimulates an adjacent segment of membrane and opens voltage-gated Na^{1+} channels. The moving wave of depolarization, therefore, is self-propagating as it travels along the axon. The membrane is refractory immediately behind the action potential. Therefore, this moving wave of electrical change sweeps along behind the depolarization wave. Some large-diameter nerve fibers conduct electrical impulses at velocities of around 100 m/second. These impulses, traveling faster than 200 mph, can leave the brain and reach the distal end of the spinal cord in about 0.01 second.

Once a threshold stimulus is applied to a nerve cell membrane, the nerve impulse travels at exactly the same speed in a given nerve fiber every time. This concept, the **all-or-none principle,** is a characteristic of all cell membranes. There is no gradation in response once an action potential has been generated. For example, muscle fibers do not contract with half their strength if a stimulus of half the threshold value is applied. They contract maximally or not at all. Similarly, nerve impulses always travel at the maximum speed for a particular nerve cell once a threshold stimulus has been applied. Structural features such as axon diameter contribute to differing velocities. For example, impulse velocity increases proportionately with axon diameter. For a given nerve cell, however, an impulse will either succeed and travel at top speed within the cell or will fail and will not be transmitted at all. A summary of the steps involved in neuronal transmission is presented in Table 4–1.

As we have seen, neuronal transmission is the high-speed electrical mode of nerve impulse transmission. It is an ideal mechanism for getting information from one end of the nerve cell to the other as quickly as possible. In addition, the resulting impulse is self-propagating and is an all-or-nothing affair. When the wave of electrical change arrives at the terminal end of an axon, however, it is unable to cross the space separating the axon from the next cell in the pathway. Multineuronal pathways with their re-

---

TABLE 4–1 SUMMARY OF NEURONAL TRANSMISSION

1. RMP of approximately -70 mV is generated by the cell membrane, which is polarized.
   K^{1+} permeability is 50–100 times greater than Na^{1+} permeability; therefore, K^{1+} leak outward faster than Na^{1+} diffuse inward.
   Na^{1+}/K^{1+}/ATPase is the active transport mechanism that moves Na^{1+} into the extracellular fluid.
2. A threshold stimulus causes changes in ionic permeability.
   Voltage-gated Na^{1+} channels open rapidly; voltage-gated K^{1+} channels open slowly.
   An action potential (nerve impulse) results.
3. Depolarization occurs as Na^{1+} rapidly diffuse inward and temporarily reverse the electrically negative interior of the cell; Na^{1+} current causes membrane voltage to change from -70 mV to 0 to $+30$ mV.
4. Repolarization occurs as voltage-gated Na^{1+} channels close and voltage-gated K^{1+} channels open fully.
   Outflow of K^{1+} helps restore the negative interior and reestablish normal RMP.
   Absolute refractory period occurs while voltage-gated Na^{1+} channels are still open—no further stimulation possible.
   Relative refractory period follows as voltage-gated Na^{1+} channels close but K^{1+} channels remain open—further stimulation is possible with a strong (suprathreshold) stimulus.
5. Wave of depolarization is self-propagating as it spreads along axonal membrane; a wave of repolarization follows.
   Membrane exhibits all-or-none property in regard to generation of action potentials.

Na^{1+}/K^{1+}/ATPase—sodium-potassium pump; RMP—resting membrane potential.

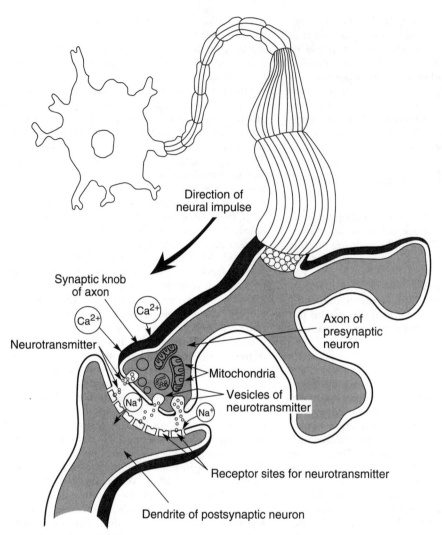

FIGURE 4–7 Impulse transmission at a synapse. (Modified with permission from Scanlon VC and Sanders T: Essentials of Anatomy and Physiology. FA Davis Co, Philadelphia, 1991, p. 166.)

sulting gaps between cells are commonplace in the nervous system. These fluid-filled gaps must be spanned by a totally different mode of impulse transmission. Examination of the chemical nature of impulse transmission at these sites is invaluable because it is through alteration of chemical transmission that many drugs modify the activity of the nervous system.

SYNAPTIC TRANSMISSION

The Synaptic Cleft

The narrow, fluid-filled gap between a nerve cell and another cell is called the **synaptic cleft,** or

synaptic gap (Gr *synapsis*—a connection). The **presynaptic** neuron sends the signal; the **postsynaptic** cell receives the signal. (The terms **prejunctional** and **postjunctional** can be used interchangeably with *presynaptic* and *postsynaptic*.) The distance between cells at a typical synaptic cleft is a mere 20 nm (1 nanometer [nm] = 1 × 10^{-9} m), and yet this incredibly small gap effectively halts the electrical mode of transmission.

Most drugs are unable to modify the mechanisms involved in the electrical events of neuronal transmission. A chemical **synapse,** however, is a functional connection between cells that offers ample opportunities for drugs to alter nerve transmission. In general, the chemical

BOX 4–1 VAGUSSTOFF AND SYMPATHIN: A SHORT HISTORY OF NEUROTRANSMISSION

In 1914, Henry Dale of Great Britain conducted investigations into the pharmacologic properties of acetylcholine. He noticed that the drug seemed to exactly reproduce the responses to stimulation of parasympathetic nerves. Dale introduced the term *parasympathetic* to describe the effects of acetylcholine.

Following Dale's work, a classic study in experimental pharmacology was performed in 1921 by Otto Loewi of Germany. In this elegant experiment, a frog's heart was perfused with a physiologic saline solution and the vagal (parasympathetic) nerves going to the heart were electrically stimulated to slow the contractions. The saline solution was collected and then transferred to a second frog heart, which had been denervated (its nerve connections had been severed). Perfusion of the denervated heart caused an immediate decrease in its contractions. The change paralleled the decreased activity of the electrically stimulated heart. Clearly some substance had been added to the solution collected from the first heart. This substance produced effects in the denervated heart that were identical to those produced by vagal stimulation of the intact heart. A chemical transmitter had been discovered. Loewi named the compound *Vagusstoff;* it was eventually identified as acetylcholine. In 1936, Loewi and Dale received the Nobel Prize for Medicine or Physiology for their study of the chemical transmission of nerve impulses that had led to the discovery of **neurotransmitters.**

The American physiologist Walter B. Cannon and his coworkers continued to investigate the action of compounds recovered from the stimulation of nerves. Their work in the 1930s included study of an adrenaline-like substance that Loewi had recovered after cardiac accelerator nerves were stimulated. Cannon originally named the mediator *sympathin.* Like epinephrine, this substance was capable of raising the heart rate and blood pressure but differed from epinephrine in certain vascular effects. A decade later (1946), the unknown mediator was identified as *norepinephrine* by U.S. von Euler of Sweden. Ulf von Euler was a corecipient of the 1970 Nobel Prize for Medicine or Physiology.

Gerald MC: Pharmacology: An Introduction to Drugs. Prentice-Hall, Englewood Cliffs, NJ, 1981.

Weiner N and Taylor P: Neurohumoral transmission: The autonomic and somatic motor nervous systems. In Goodman, AG et al (eds): Goodman and Gilman's The Pharmacologic Basis of Therapeutics, ed 7. Macmillan, New York, 1985.

---

events of synaptic transmission can be either imitated or inhibited by drugs (see Fig. 4–9 below).

Synaptic transmission between nerve cells illustrates the basics of the chemical mode of transmission. Neuronal synapses are classified on the basis of the cellular connections involved. The **axodendritic synapse** is found between the terminal branches of the axon of a presynaptic neuron and the branches of a dendrite of a postsynaptic neuron. Junctions found between an axon and a neuronal cell body are termed **axosomatic synapses.** Those located between a presynaptic axon and the axon of a postsynaptic nerve cell are called **axoaxonal synapses.** For the purposes of our discussion, the axodendritic synapse is well suited (Fig. 4–7).

Neurotransmitters

Anabolic enzymes are located in the axonal endings of presynaptic neurons. These enzymes are required for the biosynthesis of special molecules known as **neurotransmitters,** or **neurochemicals** (Box 4–1). Different nerve cells synthesize different neurotransmitters and store them in membrane-enclosed saclike structures called *synaptic vesicles* (see Figs. 4–1 and 4–7). When an impulse arrives at the terminal ending of an axon, the depolarization opens both voltage-gated Ca^{2+} channels and voltage-gated Na^{1+} channels. Calcium ions flow from the extracellular fluid into the axon terminals in response to a concentration gradient. The buildup of Ca^{2+} intracellularly causes the membranes of synaptic vesicles to fuse with the cell membrane. They then discharge their neurotransmitter into the synaptic cleft. Neurotransmitter molecules function as chemical messengers and rapidly diffuse across the synaptic gap toward the postsynaptic cell membrane. There is, however, a synaptic delay of approximately 0.5 milliseconds,

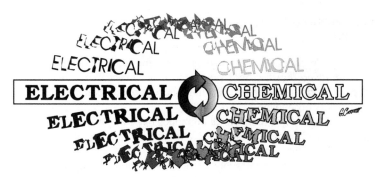

FIGURE 4–8 Conversion of electrical information to chemical information.

making chemical synapses slower acting than electrical synapses, which do not depend on neurotransmitters (Tortora and Grabowski, 1993). The presence of neurotransmitter molecules in the synaptic gap represents the conversion of electrical to chemical transmission and the change from axonal to synaptic mechanisms (Fig. 4–8). The synaptic gap is also the place where most drugs modify the activity of the nervous system. Chemical synapses only allow one-way transmission of information. This occurs because the presynaptic neuron at a given synapse is the source of stored neurotransmitter and the postsynaptic cell is equipped with membrane receptors that bind the neurotransmitter once it has been released by the presynaptic cell.

Receptors

Cell membranes possess specialized surface structures called receptors (Fig. 4–7). At these locations, cell membranes appear slightly thicker because special proteins are inserted into the lipid material of the membrane. These protruding, specialized proteins are the membrane receptors, which bind with neurotransmitters. As was discussed in the previous chapter, membrane receptors have a three-dimensional configuration and a spatial similarity to specific neurotransmitters, hormones, or drugs. As a result of their complementary shape, receptors can discriminate between different molecules and only bind those having a similar configuration.

Because of the random movement of neurotransmitters in the synaptic gap, more and more membrane receptors on the postsynaptic cell are occupied, thus producing a graded response. The temporary chemical bond that forms between the neurotransmitter and the receptor is called a *complex*. It is this neurotransmitter-receptor complex that activates chemical changes in the postsynaptic membrane. As was discussed previously, this activation may be direct, through chemically gated ion channels, or indirect, through a secondary messenger system.

Postsynaptic Potentials

Some neurotransmitters are termed *excitatory*, whereas others are termed *inhibitory*. A few cause inhibition at one location but excitation at another. Obviously, these descriptions do not depend on the neurotransmitter itself, but on the postsynaptic events set in motion by the neurotransmitter complexing with a particular receptor. The neurotransmitter acetylcholine, for example, causes contraction of skeletal muscle but inhibits contraction of cardiac muscle.

If *depolarization* of a postsynaptic membrane occurs, the neurotransmitter is *excitatory*. The neurotransmitter brings the membrane closer to threshold, usually because it has opened a chemically gated ion channel. For example, if neurotransmission causes a chemically gated Na^{1+} channel to open, Na^{1+} inflow is increased and the postsynaptic membrane becomes depolarized (Fig. 4–8). Similarly, opening of a chemically gated Ca^{2+} channel causes Ca^{2+} inflow. This type of change in postsynaptic potential is called an **excitatory postsynaptic potential (EPSP).** Several EPSPs arriving in succession cause a postsynaptic cell membrane to depolarize. This results in nerve conduction, muscle contraction, or glandular secretion, depending on the cell type.

If a postsynaptic membrane is *hyperpolarized* by a neurotransmitter, an **inhibitory postsynaptic potential (IPSP)** has occurred. In this case, the neurotransmitter is termed *inhibitory* because it has made the postsynaptic membrane more difficult to depolarize. This effect can occur if the inside of the membrane is made more negative. A neurotransmitter can generate an IPSP if a

TABLE 4-2 SUMMARY OF SYNAPTIC TRANSMISSION

1. Presynaptic neurons synthesize neurotransmitter from precursors using anabolic enzymes. Neurotransmitter is stored in synaptic vesicles in the terminal endings of neurons.
2. Depolarization of neuron opens voltage-gated Na^{1+} channels and voltage-gated Ca^{2+} channels.
3. Ca^{2+} flows into presynaptic cell, causing synaptic vescicles to fuse with the cell membrane and discharge their stored neurotransmitter into the synaptic junction.
4. Neurotransmitter rapidly diffuses toward postsynaptic cell membrane.
5. Neurotransmitter complexes (binds) with special membrane receptors on postsynaptic cell and either opens chemically gated ion channels or triggers an intracellular secondary messenger system.
6. Postsynaptic cell responds by conducting, contracting, or secreting.
   If EPSPs depolarize the postsynaptic cell, the neurotransmitter is termed *excitatory.*
   If IPSPs hyperpolarize the postsynaptic cell, the neurotransmitter is termed *inhibitory.*
7. Synaptic transmission terminates as neurotransmitter is removed from the synaptic junction by various mechanisms:
   Diffusion out of the synaptic junction
   Inactivation by catabolic enzymes
   Uptake into neuronal or nonneuronal tissues

EPSP—excitatory postsynaptic potential; IPSP—inhibitory postsynaptic potential.

chemically gated K^{1+} channel or Cl^{1-} channel is opened to increase membrane permeability to these ions. Outflow of K^{1+} or inflow of Cl^{1-} along their respective concentration gradients makes the cell's interior more negative. This increases the resting membrane potential and hyperpolarizes the membrane.

Termination of Chemical Transmission
Neurotransmitters must be removed from the synaptic cleft to terminate the chemical transmission phase. If they remain, they continue to influence the postsynaptic cell. Some neurotransmitter simply diffuses out of the synaptic cleft. In addition, catabolic enzymes are present in the synaptic gap to degrade the chemical messengers. In some cases the inactivation takes the form of hydrolysis, whereby the neurotransmitter is split in two by a chemical reaction with water. The resulting breakdown products are inactive and incapable of combining with membrane receptors. (Specific catabolic enzymes are discussed in Chapter 5.) Another means of inactivation involves the transfer, or uptake, of neurotransmitter into presynaptic neurons or into nonneuronal tissues. These two uptake mechanisms are discussed fully in the Chapter 5. A summary of the steps involved in synaptic transmission is presented in Table 4–2.

DRUG-ALTERED FUNCTION AT SYNAPSES
The manipulation of chemical messengers at synapses provides virtually unlimited potential for the modification of nervous system activity. Variables such as synthesis, release, diffusion,

complexing, and inactivation of neurotransmitters present a multitude of ways in which drugs can influence synaptic transmission.

Mimicry
Direct-Acting Drugs
Direct-acting drug molecules possess such a close structural similarity to naturally occurring neurotransmitters that they are able to imitate the action of the neurotransmitter. This action includes the ability to complex at specific receptor sites (Fig. 4–9). The close chemical similarity of the naturally occurring molecule epinephrine and the synthetic molecule isoproterenol is shown by Figure 3–4. Isoproterenol, acting as an agonist, can influence many of the same receptors as epinephrine. This effect triggers an identical response at most synapses. Recall from the previous chapter that pharmacologic agonists possess affinity and exhibit efficacy at receptors. The membrane receptors involved cannot differentiate between the naturally occurring substance and its synthetic equivalent. Many direct-acting drugs have been developed that have highly specific actions, combining with selected receptors in the body. Most exhibit significantly more specificity than their naturally occurring counterparts.

Indirect-Acting Drugs
Indirect-acting drugs produce mimicry because they increase the amount of neurotransmitter available at a synapse. Because naturally occurring neurotransmitter is involved, this effect is not receptor specific. It can be brought about

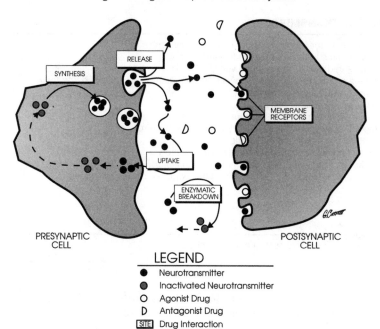

PRESYNAPTIC
CELL

POSTSYNAPTIC
CELL

LEGEND

● Neurotransmitter
◉ Inactivated Neurotransmitter
○ Agonist Drug
D Antagonist Drug
[SITE] Drug Interaction

FIGURE 4–9 Mimicry and blockade—sites of drug interaction.

through several mechanisms, such as enhanced release of neurotransmitter, inhibition of neurotransmitter reuptake, or interference with catabolic enzymes.

Some drugs elevate synaptic levels of neurotransmitter by causing the release of higher than normal amounts of neurotransmitter from storage (see Fig. 4–9). The potent stimulant effect of amphetamines on the brain is due partly to this mechanism.

Another powerful stimulant, cocaine, causes synapses in the brain to be overwhelmed with norepinephrine. This occurs because cocaine blocks the reuptake of norepinephrine into presynaptic axons. *Reuptake* is a misnomer because it implies incorrectly that uptake has already occurred. Some of the norepinephrine molecules released with the arrival of a nerve impulse are taken back into presynaptic axon terminals. Blocking this mechanism elevates the amount of neurotransmitter in the synaptic gap and causes stimulation of the postsynaptic neuron (Fig. 4–9).

Another indirect mechanism to increase neurotransmitter levels in the synapse involves inhibition of enzymes that normally inactivate neurotransmitter molecules (Fig. 4–7). By inhibiting catabolic enzymes, drugs such as physostigmine elevate the amount of acetylcholine neurotransmitter in the synapse.

Blockade

Pharmacologic Antagonism

Impulse transmission at the synapse can be interrupted in several ways, including competition for available pharmacologic receptors. Drugs that can occupy specific receptor sites but cannot activate such sites are known as blocking agents, blockers, or antagonists. Recall from the previous chapter that such antagonists possess affinity but lack efficacy. In other words, they cannot elicit a pharmacologic response. Neurotransmitter molecules released into the synaptic gap must compete with blocking agents for available membrane receptors (Fig. 4–9). Many examples of drugs exhibiting this mechanism of action will be encountered in subsequent chapters. A classic example of pharmacologic antagonism is the interaction between the blocking agent curare and the neurotransmitter acetylcholine released by motor nerve fibers. These two substances have affinity for the same membrane receptors on skeletal muscle cells. Receptor complexes formed with acetylcholine result in depolarization, generate an excitatory postsynaptic potential, and cause muscle contraction. Complexes formed with curare hyperpolarize the membrane, create an inhibitory postsynaptic potential, and cause muscle paralysis.

Inhibition of Neurotransmitter

Interference with the synthesis of neurotransmitter or inhibition of its release from presynaptic nerve endings inhibits synaptic transmission (Fig. 4–9). In such an interaction, there is an insufficient amount of neurotransmitter available to stimulate postsynaptic membrane receptors. The bacterium *Clostridium botulinum* produces botulism toxin and causes botulism food poisoning. This extremely powerful toxin paralyzes muscle activity, including that of respiratory muscles, by blocking the release of acetylcholine from motor nerve endings. With insufficient neurotransmitter at the synapses, muscle contractions become weaker and weaker, finally ending in respiratory collapse and death for the poisoning victim.

CHAPTER SUMMARY

This introductory chapter explores the structure and function of nerve cells and nerve impulse transmission. The underlying mechanisms of axonal and synaptic transmission are examined in some detail. Such information is essential for understanding the effects of many drugs. It is shown that synaptic transmission is the mechanism most often influenced by drug action.

BIBLIOGRAPHY

Carola R, Harley JP, and Noback CR: Human Anatomy and Physiology, ed 2. McGraw-Hill, New York, 1992.

Horn JP: The heroic age of neurophysiology. Physiology in Medicine Series. Hosp Pract (Off Ed) 27:65–74, Jul 15, 1992.

Katz B: Nerve, Muscle, and Synapse. McGraw-Hill, New York, 1966.

Martini F: Fundamentals of Anatomy and Physiology, ed 2. Prentice-Hall, Englewood Cliffs, NJ, 1992.

Stevens CF: The neuron. Sci Am. 241:54–65, Sep 1979.

Thibodeau GA and Patton KT: Anatomy and Physiology, ed 2. Mosby–Year Book, St Louis, 1993.

Tortora GJ and Grabowski SR: Principles of Anatomy and Physiology, ed 7. HarperCollins, New York, 1993.

CHAPTER 5

Autonomic Pharmacology

CHAPTER OUTLINE

CHAPTER OBJECTIVES

After studying this chapter the reader should be able to:

- Outline the parts of the nervous system included in the central nervous system and the peripheral nervous system.
- Describe the flow of information in the afferent and efferent systems and list their parts.
- Compare the two divisions of the autonomic nervous system on the basis of structural and functional differences.
- Explain the role of the fight-or-flight response.
- Explain how sympathetic dominance occurs during the alarm reaction and describe the role of the adrenal medulla.
- Describe the differences between dual and single innervation of organs.
- List the neurotransmitters, receptors, and catabolic enzymes of the autonomic nervous system.
- Describe the mechanisms by which norepinephrine and acetylcholine neurotransmitters are inactivated.
- Compare the pharmacologic response of norepinephrine release at alpha- and beta-adrenergic receptors.
- Compare the pharmacologic response of acetylcholine release at muscarinic and nicotinic cholinergic receptors.
- Outline the pharmacologic mechanisms of action that account for drug classifications based on the ANS divisions.
- Describe the action of G membrane proteins in the secondary messenger system.
- Describe the role of cyclic adenosine-3′,5′-monophosphate (cAMP), cyclic guanosine-3′,5′-monophosphate (cGMP), and calcium as secondary messengers.

72

- Describe the changes in secondary messenger levels when autonomic receptors are stimulated.
- Describe autonomic balance of organs on the basis of cAMP/cGMP levels using bronchiolar smooth muscle as an example.

KEY TERMS

acetylcholine (ACh) (as-SĒ-til-kō-lēn)
acetylcholinesterase (as-SĒ-til-kō-lin-ES-ter-āz)
adenosine (a-DEN-ō-zēn)
adenosine triphosphate (ATP)
adenylate cyclase (a-di-ni-LĀT SĪ-klās)
adrenal medulla (a-DRĒ-nal me-DUL-a)
adrenalin (a-DREN-a-lin) (epinephrine) (epi-NEF-rin)
adrenergic (ad-re-NER-jik) fiber
adrenergic receptor (adrenoceptor) (a-DRĒ-nō-sep-tōr)
afferent system
alpha-adrenergic receptor
  α_1-adrenergic receptor
  α_2-adrenergic receptor
autonomic nervous system (ANS)
beta-adrenergic receptor
  β_1-adrenergic receptor
  β_2-adrenergic receptor
blocker; blocking agent
  alpha blocker (α_1, α_2)
  beta blocker (β_1, β_2)
  muscarinic blocker (M$_1$, M$_2$, M$_3$)
  nicotinic blocker (N$_1$, N$_2$)
calmodulin (kal-MOD-ū-lin)
cascade effect
catecholamine (kat-e-KŌL-a-mēn)
catechol-O-methyltransferase (COMT) (kat-e-kōl-ō-meth-il-TRANS-fer-āz)
central nervous system (CNS)
choline ester (KŌ-lēn ES-ter)
cholinergic (kō-lin-ER-jik) fiber

cholinergic receptor (cholinoceptor) (kō-LIN-ō-sep-tōr)
cholinesterase (kō-lin-ES-ter-āz)
  acetylcholinesterase
  plasma cholinesterase (pseudocholinesterase)
craniosacral (krā-nē-ō-SĀ-kral) outflow
cyclic adenosine-3′,5′-monophosphate (cyclic AMP, cAMP)
cyclic guanosine-3′,5′-monophosphate (cyclic GMP, cGMP)
dopamine receptor (dopaminergic receptor)
  DA$_1$-dopamine receptor
  DA$_2$-dopamine receptor
efferent system
fight-or-flight response (alarm reaction)
fixed-membrane-receptor mechanism (membrane-bound receptor mechanism)
G membrane proteins (G$_s$, G$_i$) (guanine nucleotide–binding regulatory proteins)
ganglion (GANG-lē-on)
guanosine (GWA-nō-zēn)
guanosine triphosphate (GTP)
guanylate cyclase (GWA-ni-lāt SĪ-klās)
innervation
  dual innervation
  single innervation
monoamine oxidase (MAO) (mon-ō-a-MĒN OKS-i-dāz)
muscarine (MUS-ka-rēn)

muscarinic (mus-ka-RIN-ik) receptor
  M$_1$-muscarinic receptor
  M$_2$-muscarinic receptor
  M$_3$-muscarinic receptor
nicotine (NIK-ō-tēn)
nicotinic (NIK-ō-tin-ik) receptor
  N$_1$-nicotinic receptor
  N$_2$-nicotinic receptor
nonadrenergic noncholinergic (NANC) neurotransmission
norepinephrine (nor-ep-i-NEF-rin) (noradrenalin) (nor-a-DREN-a-lin)
nucleoside (NYOO-klē-ō-sīd)
nucleotide (NYOO-klē-ō-tīd)
parasympathetic division
parasympathomimetic (par-a-sim-PATH-ō-mi-me-tik)
peripheral nervous system (PNS)
phosphodiesterase (FAHZ-fō-dī-ess-ter-āz)
plasma cholinesterase (pseudocholinesterase)
postganglionic fiber
preganglionic fiber
protein kinases
rest-and-restorative
secondary messenger
sympathetic division
sympathetic dominance
sympathomimetic (sim-PATH-ō-mi-me-tik)
thoracolumbar (thō-rak-ō-LUM-bar) outflow
uptake mechanisms
  uptake-1 (uptake I, amine I)
  uptake-2 (uptake II, amine II)

CHAPTER INTRODUCTION

The nervous system is concerned with the integration and coordination of body systems. Monitoring physiologic changes, processing information, and controlling organ function helps maintain the stability of the internal environment of the body (homeostasis). Some drugs can restore the stability, whereas others can upset it. The major divisions of the nervous system and the flow of information within those divisions are introduced in this chapter, with emphasis on the role played by the autonomic nervous system (ANS). The structural, functional, and pharmacologic features of the ANS are discussed, including autonomic drug classifications.

A clear understanding of the role played by the divisions of the autonomic nervous system and their neurotransmitters is vital. The concepts that follow are crucial to an understanding of autonomic pharmacology and to a large number of therapeutic drugs discussed in subsequent chapters. The reader must master all of the following material because of the pivotal nature of this information.

NERVOUS SYSTEM

Integrating innumerable bits of information and coordinating diverse activities are essential to maintain the normal functioning of the body. Sensory information from the exterior and the interior of the body is continually received by the brain and is routed to appropriate areas for processing. Some sensory input is compared with information already present in the brain; some is blended with other incoming sensations. Once the data have been integrated or combined, appropriate motor responses are initiated. This elaborate interplay coordinates the various activities of different tissues and organs.

Conceptual Division of the Nervous System

The various parts of the nervous system can be divided into two major categories. The **central nervous system (CNS)** comprises the brain and spinal cord. The **peripheral nervous system (PNS)** comprises all parts of the nervous system outside the brain and spinal cord. Included in this peripheral category are cranial nerves, spinal nerves, and the nerve fibers making up the **autonomic nervous system (ANS).**

An outline of the central and peripheral divisions is presented in Figure 5–1. From the chart, however, it is impossible to determine which nerves carry sensory impulses, which ones carry motor impulses, and which fibers carry a combination of sensory and motor impulses. For example, most cranial nerves are mixed-function nerves composed of sensory and motor fibers. A few, however, are purely sensory, and a few are predominantly motor. Some cranial nerves contain fibers belonging to the autonomic nervous system. All spinal nerves are mixed-function nerves, whereas the autonomic nervous system is made up primarily of motor fibers.

Flow of Information

Because many drugs produce their effects by modifying nervous activity, the reader must have a basic understanding of nervous system function. One of the best ways to understand the workings of the nervous system is to visualize the entire system being composed of two streams of information: an **afferent system** conveying information toward the CNS and an **efferent system** carrying impulses away from it. The flow of information presented in Figure 5–2 reveals that

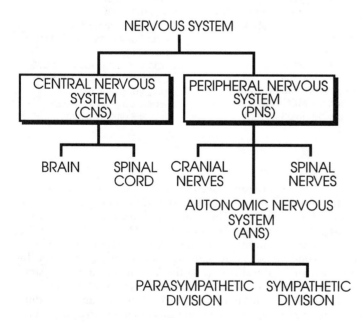

FIGURE 5–1 Conceptual divisions of the nervous system.

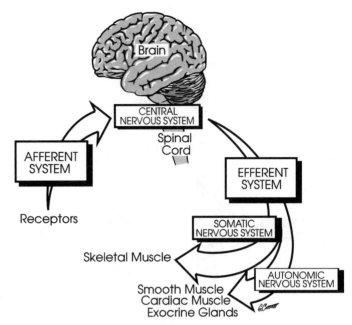

FIGURE 5–2 Flow of information in the nervous system.

the ANS is primarily an efferent system, transmitting motor information to smooth muscle, cardiac muscle, and glands. Because many autonomic control mechanisms can be modified by drugs, we now examine the subdivisions of the ANS by comparing their structural, functional, and pharmacologic features.

STRUCTURAL COMPARISON OF AUTONOMIC NERVOUS SYSTEM DIVISIONS

Origin of Nerve Fibers

The two nerve trunks making up the **sympathetic division** of the ANS originate in the spinal cord between thoracic and lumbar segments T1 and L2. These parallel trunks are found on either side of the spinal cord and form the **thoracolumbar outflow** (Fig. 5–3). The term *outflow* indicates that the nerve impulses carried by these fibers are motor impulses going to the viscera. Thoracic organs, including the airways, are innervated by sympathetic ganglia that originate at T3–6. Fibers of the **parasympathetic division** of the ANS exit from the superior and inferior portions of the CNS. The superior, or cranial, portion of the parasympathetic division is made up of motor fibers that are bundled with several cranial nerves (III—occulomotor, VII—facial, IX—

glossopharyngeal, and X—vagus). The inferior portion is made up of motor fibers that leave the spinal cord in the sacral region. The cranial and sacral portions of the parasympathetic division together form the **craniosacral outflow** (Fig. 5–3).

Location of Autonomic Ganglia and Fiber Length

An autonomic pathway is composed of two neurons. A **preganglionic fiber** carries motor impulses from the spinal cord to an autonomic **ganglion.** A ganglion is a collection of nerve cell bodies located outside the CNS. The nerve cell bodies belong to **postganglionic fibers,** which carry motor impulses from autonomic ganglia to viscera (Fig. 5–3).

Sympathetic ganglia associated with the sympathetic division are found on either side of the spinal cord as parallel chains of interconnected ganglia (Fig. 5–4). Because of the proximity of the sympathetic ganglia to the spinal cord, the preganglionic fibers are relatively short, whereas the postganglionic fibers connecting the ganglia with effectors are relatively long.

Preganglionic fibers of the parasympathetic division are relatively long because parasympathetic ganglia are located distal to the spinal cord, usually near or within the organ innervated. The length of parasympathetic postgan-

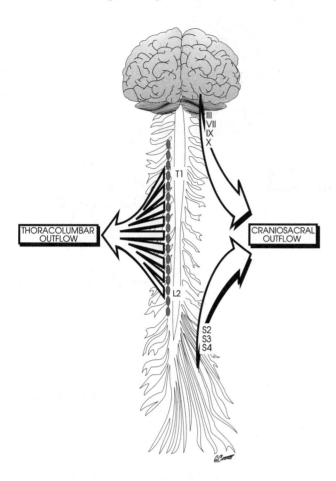

FIGURE 5–3 ANS—origin of autonomic fibers.

glionic fibers is correspondingly short because of the location of the ganglia (Fig. 5–4).

Ratio of Preganglionic to Postganglionic Fibers

An impulse arriving in a preganglionic fiber diverges into several outgoing impulses in the postganglionic fibers that emerge from the ganglion. The ratio of preganglionic fibers to postganglionic fibers determines the extent to which motor information is distributed in the ANS. Within sympathetic ganglia, the ratio of incoming to outgoing fibers is approximately 1:20. This ratio allows for more diverse sympathetic responses. In other words, more organs can respond to sympathetic impulses because of the widespread distribution of postganglionic fibers. In parasympathetic ganglia, the ratio of preganglionic to postganglionic fibers is around 1:4. This arrangement creates a more focused parasympathetic response in organs (Fig. 5–4). These anatomic variations have an important bearing

on many of the functional differences between the two ANS divisions.

FUNCTIONAL COMPARISON OF AUTONOMIC NERVOUS SYSTEM DIVISIONS

The autonomic nervous system controls the activities of diverse effectors such as heart muscle, vascular smooth muscle, bronchiolar smooth muscle, and glandular tissue. Autonomic functions include regulation of heart rate and force of cardiac contraction, peripheral vascular resistance, airway resistance, and glandular secretion.

The two subdivisions of the ANS are physiologic antagonists. In other words, the sympathetic and parasympathetic divisions functionally oppose each other. This mutual antagonism is apparent in organs that receive motor fibers belonging to each division. The antagonism results in a functional autonomic balance of visceral activity in such organs.

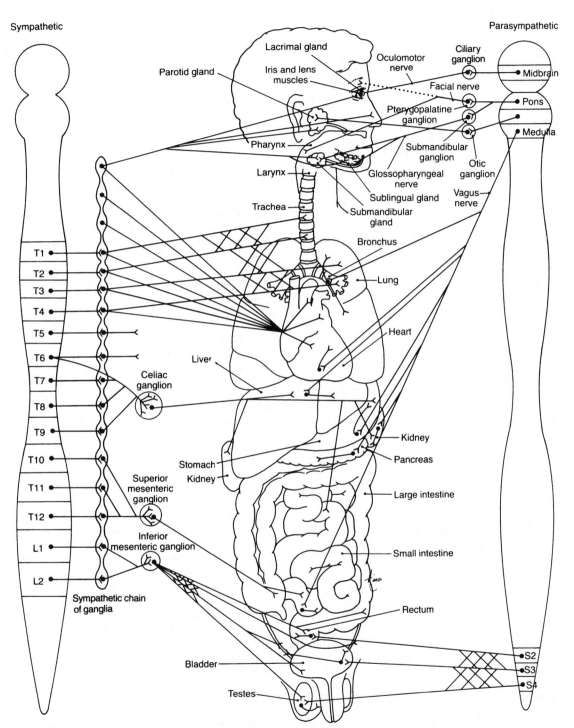

FIGURE 5–4 ANS—autonomic ganglia, fiber length, and organs innervated. (From Scanlon VC and Sanders T: Essentials of Anatomy and Physiology. FA Davis Co, Philadelphia, 1991, p. 186, with permission.)

Sympathetic Division

The sympathetic division of the ANS prepares the body to meet a stressful situation. In response to threatening stimuli, certain physiologic changes in the organs are triggered by efferent impulses delivered by the sympathetic fibers. These changes occur almost instantaneously and represent the classic **fight-or-flight** response to stress (also known as the **alarm reaction**). The response of the sympathetic division is immediate and widespread. The phenomenon is called **sympathetic dominance** and occurs as a result of structural features already discussed, such as interconnected sympathetic ganglia, multiple postganglionic sympathetic fibers, and direct sympathetic stimulation of the **adrenal medulla** gland by preganglionic sympathetic fibers. The functional basis of sympathetic dominance can be explained by several factors, including suppression of nonessential organs, rapid response of vital organs, and secretion by the adrenal medulla.

During the fight-or-flight response, blood is temporarily shunted away from nonvital areas such as the skin and digestive organs. This is done to allocate blood to vital organs that play an important role in the alarm reaction. Contraction of smooth muscle in most portions of the gastrointestinal and urinary tracts is inhibited, and secretion by digestive organs is suppressed. Vital resources such as glucose and blood are reallocated to essential tissues to meet the stress.

Organs such as the heart, lungs, and skeletal muscles must respond rapidly to stress. Essential organs receive a greater flow of blood to meet their increased oxygen and nutrient demands and to remove carbon dioxide and wastes. The ability of these organs to respond quickly to stress is also a result of subtle changes such as an increase in glucose concentration of the blood. This increase is caused by the action of liver cells converting stored glycogen to glucose.

The adrenal medulla is an endocrine gland that develops from a large sympathetic ganglion, complete with a preganglionic sympathetic nerve fiber connecting it with the spinal cord. The gland synthesizes potent hormones called **catecholamines** such as **norepinephrine** and **epinephrine.** (Catecholamines are studied in detail in Chapter 12.) Epinephrine, also known as **adrenalin,** is called the ''alarm reaction hormone'' and is particularly powerful in regard to potentiation of sympathetic effects. Adrenalin sustains and intensifies the fight-or-flight reaction. It is released in larger amounts during stress, when the adrenal medulla is stimulated by sympathetic impulses. Norepinephrine, also known as **noradrenalin,** is a normal constituent of the internal environment. It is secreted by the adrenal medulla at a constant level and helps regulate blood vessel diameter and blood pressure.

Parasympathetic Division

The parasympathetic division of the ANS functionally opposes the sympathetic division. Parasympathetic stimulation of an organ produces an effector response, which is basically the opposite of that caused by sympathetic stimulation. (This relationship is valid only for organs that receive efferent fibers from both ANS divisions.) The parasympathetic division is described in physiologic terms as performing **rest-and-restorative** functions in the body. It is active during periods devoid of stress and restores body processes when not being dominated by the sympathetic division. Some readers may find the acronym *SLUG* useful for remembering dominant parasympathetic responses, which include *salivation, lacrimation, urination,* and *gastric motility.* In general, parasympathetic activity returns organ functions to normal levels. In structural terms, the lack of extensive interconnected parasympathetic ganglia plus the relatively low ratio of preganglionic to postganglionic fibers helps explain the lack of diverse activity in the parasympathetic division.

A summary of organ responses to sympathetic and parasympathetic stimulation is presented in Table 5–1.

Innervation of Viscera

Innervation refers to the nerve connections made with an organ. The majority of organs in the body possess **dual innervation;** that is, they are innervated by fibers from both divisions of the ANS. Impulses arriving through one division cause a characteristic change in visceral function. This change is physiologically antagonized by impulses from the opposing division. In general, the level of activity in such dually innervated organs reflects the *net effect* of the two autonomic divisions (Fig. 5–5). If the nervous activity of one division begins to dominate that of the other, the normal autonomic balance of that organ is changed. During the alarm reaction, sympathetic impulses spread further and cause more profound, longer-lasting changes than those caused by parasympathetic impulses. As a result, sympathetic dominance

TABLE 5–1   AUTONOMIC STIMULATION OF ORGANS

Organ	Sympathetic (Thoracolumbar)	Parasympathetic (Craniosacral)
Eye		
Iris	Dilation	Constriction
Intraocular pressure	Decreased	Decreased
Tear gland secretion		Increased
Glands		
Salivary	Viscous secretion	Watery secretion
Sweat	Secretion, palms	Generalized secretion*
Piloerectors	Contraction	
Bronchioles		
Secretions	Mixed response	Increased
Smooth muscle	Relaxation†	Contraction
Heart		
Rate	Acceleration	Deceleration
Force	Increased	Decreased
Gastrointestinal Tract		
Muscle wall (motility)	Relaxation	Contraction
Sphincters	Contraction	Relaxation
Secretion		Increased secretion
Spleen	Contraction	
Urinary Bladder		
Fundus	Relaxation	Contraction
Trigone and sphincter	Contraction	Relaxation
Blood vessels (arterioles)		
Skeletal Muscle	Dilation	Dilation‡
Coronary	Dilation (β_2)	Dilation
Skin, viscera	Constriction	

Source: Adapted from Long, 1989.

*Many sweat glands have receptors that are stimulated by acetylcholine-like drugs and blocked by atropine-like drugs. The anatomic origin of these nerves is sympathetic and they are often called "cholinergic sympathetic."

†Sympathetic neurons do not innervate smooth muscle found in bronchioles. However, β_2-adrenoceptors are located on airway smooth muscle. When such receptors are stimulated, bronchodilation will result (see Box 5–1).

‡Parasympathetic neurons do not innervate vascular beds found in skeletal muscle, but muscarinic receptors are on the vascular smooth muscle, and when stimulated, dilation will resut.

is responsible for most of the organ changes normally associated with the fight-or-flight response.

A few effectors, such as blood vessels, salivary and sweat glands, and the adrenal medulla, are controlled through **single innervation.** These organs respond to the *total amount* of nervous activity carried by the single autonomic pathway, rather than the net effect of two opposing ANS divisions (Fig. 5–6). The degree of nervous activity determines the baseline organ response. An increase or decrease in this basal amount of neuronal activity results in a characteristic change in organ function. As an example, vascular tone is maintained in the singly innervated smooth muscle of arterioles. An increase in efferent activity causes additional vascular smooth muscle contraction and a state of relative vasoconstriction. Less than the basal amount of nervous activity results in vascular smooth muscle relaxation and vasodilation.

PHARMACOLOGIC COMPARISON OF AUTONOMIC NERVOUS SYSTEM DIVISIONS

Neurotransmitters

Chemical synapses between parasympathetic postganglionic fibers and neuroeffectors depend on the release of **acetylcholine (ACh)** from postganglionic fibers. Fibers that produce and release acetylcholine are called **cholinergic fibers.** Ganglionic synapses of the sympathetic and parasympathetic divisions are mediated by acetylcholine; therefore, the preganglionic fibers of both divisions of the ANS are classified as cholinergic fibers (Fig. 5–7).

The neurotransmitter liberated from the axonal endings of nearly all postganglionic sympathetic fibers is **norepinephrine (NE),** or noradrenalin (Fig. 5–7). Fibers that synthesize and release noradrenaline are referred to as **adrenergic fibers.** Most sympathetic fibers fall into

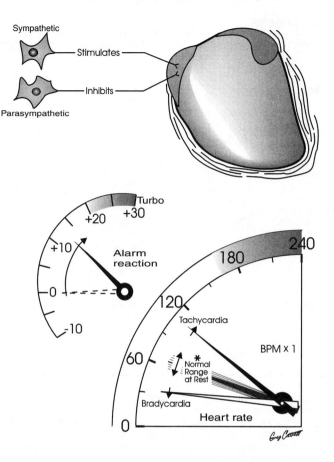

FIGURE 5–5   Dual innervation—the heart.

* Normal range of heart rate at rest represents balance
between sympathetic and parasympathetic effects

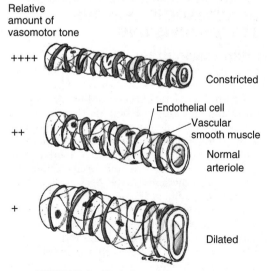

FIGURE 5–6   Single innervation—arteriole.

this classification, but a few release ACh. Such neurons are called *cholinergic sympathetic fibers* and innervate the adrenal medulla.

Certain regulatory substances involved in the control of visceral function are not released by cholinergic *or* adrenergic fibers. The presumed role of these mediators and neuromodulators in airway function is discussed in see Box 5–1.

Autonomic Receptors

Adrenergic Receptors

Receptors that complex with catecholamines, such as norepinephrine, epinephrine, and dopamine, are classified as **adrenergic receptors,** or **adrenoceptors** (Fig. 5–8). Receptors are named according to the neurotransmitter with which they combine, not the type of nerve fiber in the immediate vicinity. For example, adrenergic receptors can be found in both the CNS

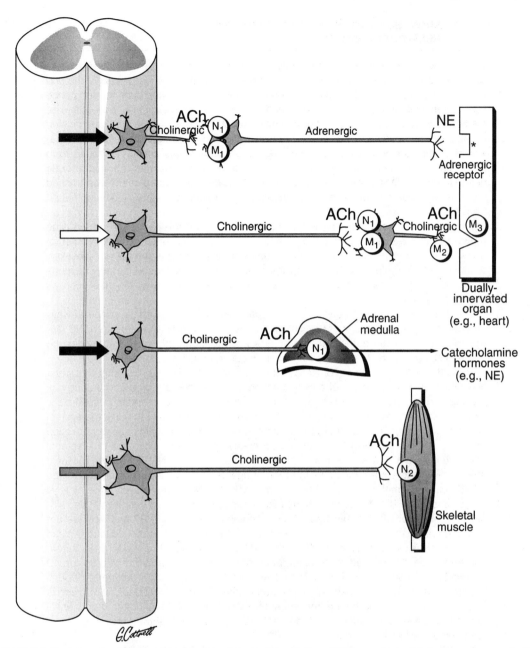

FIGURE 5–7 Neurotransmitters and receptors of the peripheral nervous system. Large black arrow = sympathetic division, ANS; large white arrow = parasympathetic division, ANS; large gray arrow = somatic nervous system. ACh = acetylcholine; NE = norepinephrine. Receptors: N_1 = N_1-nicotinic; N_2 = N_2-nicotinic; M_1 = M_1-muscarinic; M_2 = M_2 muscarinic; M_3 = M_3-muscarinic. (*See Figure 5–8 for functional classification of adrenergic receptors.)

and the ANS. In the ANS, norepinephrine can induce totally different responses at similar effectors. For example, vascular smooth muscle relaxation can occur in one vascular bed while vascular smooth muscle contraction is being triggered simultaneously in a different vascular bed. Vasodilation delivers additional blood to vital regions such as the skeletal muscles; vasoconstriction reduces blood flow to nonessential areas such as the skin (Table 5–2).

Early research into the action of different catecholamines at different sites eventually clarified

BOX 5–1 BRONCHODILATION AND THE ELUSIVE NANC NEUROTRANSMITTER

Various substances play a presumed role in neurotransmission within the nervous system. For instance, NMDA (*N*-methyl-D-aspartic acid) and amino acids such as glycine and GABA (γ-aminobutyric acid) mediate impulses in the CNS. Peptides such as substance P, angiotensin II, and vasoactive intestinal polypeptide (VIP) have also been identified as mediators in various responses. For example, substance P is involved in transmission of the pain response (see Box 25–1); VIP was originally recovered from gastric mucosa, where it inhibits gastric function. These regulatory substances are not released from adrenergic or cholinergic nerves. Some are presumed to be involved in **nonadrenergic noncholinergic (NANC) neurotransmission.** For three decades, researchers have tracked the elusive transmitter or transmitters thought to be involved in NANC inhibitory neural transmission.

Several substances, including VIP, nitric oxide (NO), and the purine ATP (adenosine triphosphate) are being investigated. These substances may function as NANC neurotransmitters in the relaxation response of smooth muscle in the airways and gastrointestinal tract. The role of NANC neurotransmitters in the airway response may have important consequences for the future treatment of reversible airway disease such as bronchial asthma.

Cholinergic innervation through the vagal pathway to smooth muscle of the airways maintains a baseline amount of bronchomotor tone. Inhibitory NANC nerves (i-NANC) are the only bronchodilator pathway in human airways. Therefore, this pathway provides the prime inhibitory innervation to oppose vagally induced bronchoconstriction.

To study the *in vitro* effects of NANC transmission in the airways, investigators must first inhibit known mediators of airway function. For example, atropine and propranolol are used to block postjunctional M_3-muscarinic and β_2-adrenergic receptors, respectively. Indomethacin, an aspirinlike drug, is used to inhibit cyclo-oxygenase to block the synthesis of tissue hormones called prostaglandins. (Certain prostaglandins cause relaxation of airway smooth muscle.) Even with these mediators blocked, chemical or electrical stimulation of the airways results in bronchodilation through i-NANC nerves. The next step involves the systematic administration of agents that specifically block suspected NANC neurotransmitters such as VIP, NO, and ATP. The NANC response on the airways is then observed. The i-NANC bronchodilation response is still intact despite VIP and ATP blockade, but not with NO blockade. These findings suggest that VIP and ATP are not primarily responsible for the inhibitory neural effect that results in bronchodilation. When NO synthesis is blocked, however, the bronchodilator response in the airways is inhibited. The effect can be reversed by administration of L-arginine, a substrate needed for NO synthesis. In addition, removal of NO occurs rapidly in physiologic solutions through spontaneous chemical breakdown of the substance. For these reasons, *nitric oxide* is strongly suspected to be the neurotransmitter in inhibitory NANC-mediated bronchodilation. Other substances, such as VIP and ATP, acting alone or together, may play a neuromodulator, or modifying, role.

Inhaled NO also shows promise as a selective vasodilator in the treatment of pulmonary hypertension (see Box 21–1).

Barnes PJ: Autonomic pharmacology of the airways. In Chung KF and Barnes PJ (eds): Pharmacology of the Respiratory Tract: Experimental and Clinical Research. Marcel Dekker, New York, 1993.

Barnes PJ: Neural mechanisms in asthma. Br Med Bull 48:149–168, 1992.

Belvisi MG et al: Inhibitory NANC nerves in human tracheal smooth muscle: A quest for the neurotransmitter. J Appl Physiol 73: 2502–2510, 1992.

Ellis JL and Undem BJ: Inhibition by L-NG-nitro-L-arginine of nonadrenergic-noncholinergic–mediated relaxations of human isolated central and peripheral airways. Am Rev Respir Dis 146:1543–1547, 1992.

Goth A: Medical Pharmacology: Principles and Concepts, ed 11. CV Mosby, St Louis, 1984.

Lammers JW, Barnes PJ, and Chung KF: Nonadrenergic, noncholinergic airway inhibitory nerves. Eur Respir J 5:239–246, 1992.

Sanders KM and Ward SM: Nitric oxide as a mediator of nonadrenergic noncholinergic neurotransmission. Am J Physiol 262:G379–G392, 1992.

Taylor AE et al: Clinical Respiratory Physiology. WB Saunders, Philadelphia, 1989.

the role of adrenergic receptors. For instance, it was observed that norepinephrine exhibited different potencies at different locations. Also, the action of epinephrine at one location could be blocked by a particular compound, but blockade of its action at another location required a different antagonist. These characteristics ultimately led to the recognition of two distinct groups of adrenergic receptors, each capable of interacting with norepinephrine but each antagonized by a different blocking agent. The receptors are now known as **alpha- (α-)** and **beta- (β-) adrenergic receptors** and are defined by their responses to adrenergic agents such as norepinephrine. In other words, adrenergic receptors are classified *functionally*. Adrenergic recep-

tors are located both pre- and postsynaptically and regulate the actions of native catecholamines, many synthetic catecholamines, and catecholamine derivatives (Table 5–3).

POSTJUNCTIONAL ADRENERGIC RECEPTORS. Adrenergic receptors located on postsynaptic membranes directly mediate effects at organs. Both inhibitory and excitatory subtypes are found.

BETA RECEPTORS. Binding of **β₂-adrenergic receptors** by drugs such as albuterol[US] (salbutamol[CAN]) (a drug used in asthma therapy) results in inhibitory or depressive responses such as relaxation of smooth muscle or inhibition of glandular secretion. Organ responses such as relaxation of bronchiolar or vascular

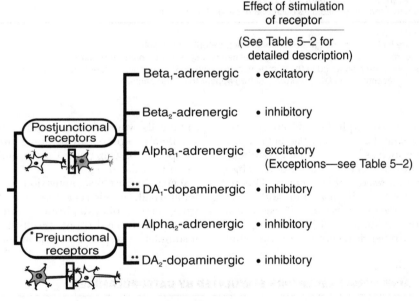

Effect of stimulation
of receptor

(See Table 5–2 for
detailed description)

- Beta₁-adrenergic   • excitatory

- Beta₂-adrenergic   • inhibitory

Postjunctional receptors

- Alpha₁-adrenergic   • excitatory (Exceptions—see Table 5–2)

- ** DA₁-dopaminergic   • inhibitory

*Prejunctional receptors

- Alpha₂-adrenergic   • inhibitory

- ** DA₂-dopaminergic   • inhibitory

* Neuromodulator or autoreceptor role—stimulation of prejunctional receptors suppresses NE release; blockade of receptors enhances NE release

* Classified as "adrenergic" because of structural similarity between norepinephrine and dopamine

FIGURE 5–8 Adrenergic receptors—functional classification.

TABLE 5–2 ADRENERGIC RECEPTORS AND VISCERAL RESPONSES

α_1-Adrenoceptor (excitatory*, postsynaptic)
  Vasoconstriction (cutaneous, renal, etc)
  Myocardial ectopic excitation
  Myometrial contraction
  Iris dilator contraction (mydriasis)
  Intestinal relaxation
  Pilomotor contraction
  Glycogenolysis (liver)
  Splenic contraction
  Ejaculation
α_2-Adrenoceptor (inhibitory, presynaptic†)
  Sympathetic nerve terminal—agonists decrease release of norepinephrine
β_1-Adrenoceptor (excitatory, postsynaptic)
  Increase heart rate (positive chronotropic action)
  Increase heart contractile force (positive inotropic action)
  Increase lipolysis
β_2-Adrenoceptor (inhibitory, postsynaptic)
  Skeletal muscle vasodilation ⎫
  Coronary vasodilation   ⎪
  Myometrium relaxation   ⎬ Smooth muscle relaxation
  Bronchial relaxation   ⎪
  Intestinal relaxation   ⎪
  Ureter relaxation   ⎭
  Lower intraocular pressure
  Increase tremor associated with highly coordinated muscle movements
  Increased glycogenolysis (liver, skeletal muscle)
DA_1-Dopamine adrenoceptor‡ (inhibitory, postsynaptic)
  Vasodilation (renal, mesenteric)
DA_2-Dopamine adrenoceptor‡ (inhibitory, presynaptic)
  Sympathetic nerve terminal—agonists decrease release of norepinephrine

Source: Adapted from Long, 1989.
*α_1 Receptors are inhibitory in the gastrointestinal tract, except for the sphincters.
†Postsynaptic α_2 receptors are present in the central nervous sytem and some other sites.
‡Dopamine receptors are also found in the central nervous system. DA_1 receptors (peripheral) and D_1 receptors (central) are similar; DA_2 receptors and D_2 receptors (central) appear to be the same.

smooth muscle are typical β_2-adrenergic responses. The stimulation of cardiac beta receptors by a drug such as isoproterenol (a synthetic catecholamine) results in a beta response characterized by increased cardiac activity. This response includes a rise in heart rate and an increase in the force of contraction. These special beta receptors are designated **β_1-adrenergic receptors.** (β_1-Adrenergic receptors are also found

on fat cells, where they are involved with lipolysis.) Beta receptors can be antagonized by the nonspecific blocking agent propranolol, an important cardiac drug.

ALPHA RECEPTORS. Activation of postjunctional **α_1-adrenergic receptors** by alpha agonist drugs such as phenylephrine, a mucosal vasoconstrictor in nasal sprays, results in excitatory or stimulatory responses. These include contrac-

TABLE 5–3 ADRENERGIC RECEPTORS STIMULATED BY CATECHOLAMINES

Catecholamine Drug	Adrenoceptors					
Epinephrine	α_1	α_2	β_1	β_2	—	—
Norepinephrine	α_1	α_2	β_1	—	—	—
Dopamine	α_1	—	β_1	—	DA_1	DA_2*
Isoproterenol	α_1†	—	β_1	β_2	—	—

Source: Adapted from Long, 1989.
*Dopamine stimulates DA_2 receptors and inhibits adrenergic transmission only if the amine I transport system is inhibited by agents such as cocaine or tricyclic antidepressants. The reasons for this selectivity are unknown.
†Slight action.

tion of smooth muscle and secretion by glandular tissue. Norepinephrine is released from sympathetic postganglionic nerve fibers that supply gastrointestinal tract smooth muscle and digestive glands. Here it complexes with α_1-adrenergic receptors and inhibits digestive activity. These gastrointestinal tract α_1-adrenergic receptors do not have a specialized name, but are simply α_1-adrenergic receptors that do not respond in the same way as the other postsynaptic α_1-adrenergic receptors in the body. The result of adrenergic stimulation of the gut, therefore, is decreased motility and secretion. α_1-Adrenergic receptors are blocked by phentolamine.

DOPAMINE RECEPTORS. The catecholamines dopamine and norepinephrine have a similar chemical structure. Dopamine functions as a neurotransmitter in the central and peripheral nervous systems, and because of the close structural ties between dopamine and norepinephrine, **dopamine (dopaminergic) receptors** are classified as adrenergic. Peripheral dopamine receptors designated **DA₁–dopamine receptors** are inhibitory. Dopamine activates peripheral DA₁–dopamine receptors and causes vasodilation of renal and mesenteric (intestinal) blood vessels to increase blood flow to these organs.

PREJUNCTIONAL ADRENERGIC RECEPTORS. Presynaptic receptors have an inhibitory effect on the ability of adrenergic nerve fibers to release norepinephrine. Receptors *modulate,* or regulate, the amount of neurotransmitter released into the synapse. Such receptors are termed *autoreceptors.*

ALPHA-ADRENERGIC RECEPTORS. Alpha₂-adrenergic receptors are located on sympathetic presynaptic nerve terminals. When stimulated, such receptors inhibit the release of norepinephrine. This action results in blockade of sympathetic nervous impulses. Some of the norepinephrine released into an adrenergic synapse with the arrival of a nerve impulse normally binds with presynaptic α_2-adrenergic receptors. This negative feedback mechanism autoregulates the neurosecretion of norepinephrine by suppressing the further release of neurotransmitter. α_2-Adrenergic agonists such as clonidine block adrenergic transmission and are useful in the treatment of hypertension. Therapeutic α_2-adrenergic antagonists are not available, but yohimbine is employed as an experimental drug. When α_2-adrenergic blocking agents are developed, they may prove useful in the management of shock because they will facilitate adrenergic transmission by suppressing the autoreceptor role of α_2-adrenergic receptors.

DOPAMINE RECEPTORS. Inhibitory dopamine receptors known as **DA₂-dopamine receptors** are located on sympathetic nerve terminals. Agonists such as bromocriptine can stimulate these DA₂-dopamine receptors, thereby decreasing the release of norepinephrine from adrenergic nerve fibers. Such drugs are useful in the control of hypertension. DA₂-Dopamine receptor antagonists such as haloperidol (an antipsychotic agent) block presynaptic DA₂-dopamine receptors and facilitate adrenergic transmission peripherally. (This drug also acts at dopamine receptors in the CNS.)

Adrenergic receptor subtypes are outlined in a flowchart in Figure 5–8. The response of various organs to the action of adrenergic receptors is summarized in Table 5–2. Major drug receptor agonists and antagonists affecting adrenergic receptors are listed in Table 5–4.

Cholinergic Receptors

Receptors that complex with ACh are known as **cholinergic receptors,** or **cholinoceptors** (Fig. 5–9). ACh activity at such receptors can be antagonized by blocking agents, but a single blocking agent cannot antagonize ACh at all locations (Box 5–2). Like adrenergic receptor responses, this type of activity generally suggests that cholinergic receptors differ in some subtle way and that more than one subtype of cholinergic receptor exists (Fig. 5–9).

POSTJUNCTIONAL CHOLINERGIC RECEPTORS. Cholinergic receptors located on postsynaptic membranes directly mediate effects at organs.

NICOTINIC RECEPTORS. Nicotine, an alkaloid substance found in tobacco, is capable of stimulating specific cholinergic receptors in the body. These receptors are located on the cell membranes of postganglionic neurons within the autonomic ganglia of both divisions, the secretory cells of the adrenal medulla, and skeletal muscle cells found at neuromuscular junctions. Nicotine is a potent toxin that possesses no intrinsic therapeutic value. It is, however, useful for pharmacologic study. Cholinergic receptors stimulated by nicotine are referred to as **nicotinic receptors. N₁-Nicotinic receptors** are postjunctional receptors located within both sympathetic and parasympathetic ganglia. ACh released from preganglionic fibers within autonomic ganglia binds with N₁-receptors to stimulate postganglionic fibers. The receptors are antagonized by ganglionic blocking drugs such as mecamylamine. **N₂-nicotinic receptors** are postjunctional receptors found at neuromuscular junctions. Stimulation of N₂-receptors on skele-

TABLE 5–4 RECEPTOR AGONISTS AND ANTAGONISTS AFFECTING THE PERIPHERAL NERVOUS SYSTEM

Stimulation of Receptor	Inhibition of Receptor
SYMPATHETIC GANGLIA SYNAPSES	
Acetylcholine (N_1)	Curare (N_1) (slight action)
Nicotine (N_1)	Mecamylamine (N_1)
	Pirenzepine (M_1)*
	(experimental)
SYMPATHETIC NEUROEFFECTOR SYNAPSES	
Albuterol[US] (salbutamol[CAN])	Bromocriptine (DA_2)†
($\beta_1 < \beta_2$)	
Dopamine (α_1, β_1, DA_1)	Clonidine (α_2)†
Epinephrine (α_1, β_1, β_2)	Phentolamine (α_1, α_2)†
Haloperidol (DA_2)†	
Isoproterenol (β_1, β_2)	
Norepinephrine (α_1, β_1)	
Phenylephrine (α_1)	
Yohimbine (α_2)†	
(experimental)	
PARASYMPATHETIC GANGLIA SYNAPSES	
Acetylcholine (N_1)	Curare (N_1) (slight action)
Nicotine (N_1)	Mecamylamine (N_1)
	Pirenzepine (M_1)*
	(experimental)
PARASYMPATHETIC NEUROEFFECTOR SYNAPSES	
Acetylcholine (M_3)	Atropine (M_2, M_3)†
Bethanechol (M_3)	Scopolamine (M_2, M_3)†
Pilocarpine (M_2)†	Ipratropium (M_2, M_3)†
	4-DAMP (M_3)‡
	(experimental)
NEUROMUSCULAR JUNCTION SYNAPSES	
Acetylcholine (N_2)	Curare (N_2)
Nicotine (N_2)	Succinylcholine (N_2)

*The role of M_1-muscarinic receptors is not fully understood. They may facilitate N_1-mediated neurotransmission in the ganglia. M_1-receptors are also located in the cerebral cortex.

†Presynaptic receptors—α_2-adrenergic, DA_2-dopaminergic, and M_2-muscarinic—function as autoreceptors to modulate the release of neurotransmitters through a negative feedback mechanism. When such receptors are stimulated, neurotransmission is reduced. When they are blocked, neurotransmission is enhanced.

‡4-Diphenylacetoxy-N-methyl-piperidine methiodide (Barnes, 1993a).

tal muscle cell membranes results in contraction of skeletal muscle. The receptors are blocked by competitive antagonists such as curare. (Curare also exhibits a degree of ganglionic blockade.)

MUSCARINIC RECEPTORS. An alkaloid substance called **muscarine** is derived from certain poisonous mushrooms and can stimulate cholinergic receptors. Muscarine has no therapeutic value but is useful for observing pharmacologic activity at specific cholinergic receptors. Autonomic receptors stimulated by muscarine are referred to as **muscarinic receptors**. **M_1-muscarinic receptors** are postjunctional and are located in both autonomic ganglia and the cerebral cortex. M_1-Muscarinic receptors are selectively antagonized by the experimental drug pirenzepine (see Newer Antimuscarinics in Chapter 11). The physiologic role of M_1-muscarinic receptors is not fully understood. They are believed to act in an excitatory manner by aiding or facilitating neurotransmission mediated by N_1-nicotinic receptors in the ganglia. M_1-muscarinic receptors may be involved in the regulation of cholinergic bronchomotor tone (Barnes, 1993a). For this reason, subtype-selective muscarinic blocking agents may prove to be clinically valuable.

M_3-MUSCARINIC RECEPTORS. Postjunctional muscarinic receptors are sensitive to experimental blocking agents such as 4-DAMP (see Newer Antimuscarinics in Chapter 11) and have been classified as **M_3-muscarinic receptors** (Barnes, 1993a). They are found at synapses between parasympathetic postganglionic fibers and neuroeffectors such as smooth muscle, cardiac muscle, and glands, and at a few sympathetic effector organs, such as sweat glands. Postjunctional muscarinic receptors are stimulated by ACh and ACh derivatives, such as bethanechol chloride. As outlined above, M_3-muscarinic receptors are antagonized by nonselective muscarinic blockers, such as atropine. Muscarinic blocking agents that are selective for M_1- and M_3-muscarinic receptors of airway smooth muscle are under development. Such drugs should prove to be valuable in the treatment of airway disease.

PREJUNCTIONAL CHOLINERGIC RECEPTORS. Presynaptic receptors have an inhibitory effect on the ability of cholinergic nerve fibers to release acetylcholine into the synapse.

M_2-MUSCARINIC RECEPTORS. When prejunctional **M_2-muscarinic receptors** are activated, they inhibit the release of ACh from postganglionic parasympathetic nerves. Through this powerful inhibitory influence on ACh release, the M_2-muscarinic receptors function as autoreceptors in a negative feedback role. Selective stimulation of M_2-muscarinic receptors by pilocarpine inhibits ACh release and limits cholinergic reflex bronchoconstriction (Barnes, 1993a). Nonselective muscarinic antagonist drugs such as atropine and ipratropium block at both prejunctional M_2- and postjunctional M_3-muscarinic receptors. Therefore, blockade of the prejunctional autoreceptors may cause *more* ACh to be released from cholinergic nerve ter-

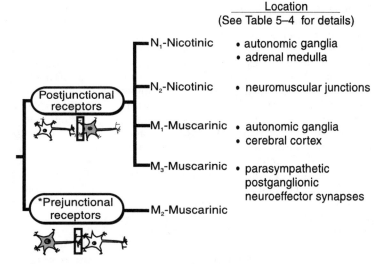

| | Location |
| | (See Table 5–4 for details) |

- N₁-Nicotinic — • autonomic ganglia • adrenal medulla
- N₂-Nicotinic — • neuromuscular junctions
- M₁-Muscarinic — • autonomic ganglia • cerebral cortex
- M₃-Muscarinic — • parasympathetic postganglionic neuroeffector synapses
- M₂-Muscarinic

Postjunctional receptors

*Prejunctional receptors

*Neuromodulator or autoreceptor role—stimulation of prejunctional receptors suppresses ACh release; blockade of receptors enhances ACh release

FIGURE 5–9 Cholinergic receptors—location classification.

minals. This effect may in turn reduce the ACh-blocking action of muscarinic antagonists at postjunctional M₃-muscarinic receptors.

Cholinergic receptor subtypes are outlined in a flowchart in Figure 5–9. Major drug receptor agonists and antagonists affecting cholinergic receptors are listed in Table 5–4 (Box 5–2).

Inactivation of Autonomic Neurotransmitters

The activity of native neurotransmitters is relatively short-lived. This occurs primarily because of the action of catabolic enzymes, but is also brought about by neuronal uptake. As a general rule, drug molecules that are chemically similar to endogenous neurotransmitters are inactivated nearly as quickly as the neurotransmitters. This occurs because the catabolic enzymes recognize and react with key structural features shared by the native molecule and closely related synthetic derivatives.

Catecholamines

The inactivation of catecholamines depends on several uptake and metabolic mechanisms. More than half the norepinephrine released into synapses reenters the presynaptic axon terminals

---

BOX 5–2   ROTATIONAL ABILITY OF ACETYLCHOLINE MOLECULE

Acetylcholine is capable of complexing at muscarinic or nicotinic receptors with equal ease. Cholinergic antagonists, however, exhibit specificity for only one type of receptor. Atropine blocks at muscarinic sites, whereas curare blocks at nicotinic sites. The versatility of the ACh molecule is attributed to its flexibility, which permits it to rotate around some of its chemical bonds. This rotational ability allows ACh to adapt to the slightly different surface configurations of the two types of cholinergic receptors. Atropine and curare apparently lack this rotational feature and their rigidity limits them to one type of receptor. Some synthetic molecules are receptor specific because they have the same type of conformational rigidity. Findings such as these help reinforce the basic principles of structure-activity relationships.

Goth A: Medical Pharmacology: Principles and Concepts, ed 11. CV Mosby, St Louis, 1984.

through the action of an amine pump mechanism. The relative constancy of catecholamine stores in adrenergic nerve fibers is explained by this mechanism. Cocaine can block the **uptake-1 mechanism** and thus enhance the action of norepinephrine. Within the neuron, norepinephrine is enzymatically destroyed by **monoamine oxidase (MAO).** MAO also inactivates any norepinephrine released from storage within the axoplasm of the neuron. The **uptake-2 mechanism** is responsible for transferring circulating catecholamines such as isoproterenol, epinephrine, and norepinephrine into nonneuronal storage sites. These sites include cardiac muscle cells, liver and kidney cells, perisynaptic glial cells, and blood vessels. The uptake-2 mechanism removes exogenous catecholamines from the body. This removal occurs because the substances are enzymatically destroyed within the nonneuronal storage sites by MAO and a second enzyme called **catechol-O-methyltransferase** (COMT). Some corticosteroid drugs can inhibit the uptake-2 mechanism and thus enhance the action of catecholamines.

Choline Esters

The choline ester class of compounds includes the native neurotransmitter ACh as well as synthetic choline esters such as bethanechol. Choline esters are inactivated by the **cholinesterase** group of catabolic enzymes. **Plasma cholinesterase,** or **pseudocholinesterase,** is nonspecific, degrading choline esters that leave the vicinity of the cholinergic synapse. Another enzyme called **acetylcholinesterase** is very specific, inactivating acetylcholine at the synapse.

The fate of norepinephrine and acetylcholine released from adrenergic and cholinergic nerve fibers is summarized in Figure 5–10.

DRUG CLASSIFICATIONS BASED ON AUTONOMIC NERVOUS SYSTEM DIVISIONS

Mechanisms of Action

Mimicry

Drugs that mimic the effects produced by sympathetic or parasympathetic innervation are classified as **sympathomimetics** and **parasympathomimetics,** respectively. Imitation of autonomic activity can be accomplished either directly or indirectly.

Direct-acting drugs possess a close structural similarity to naturally occurring neurotransmitters and simulate the action of the neurotransmitter at specific receptor sites. Agonist drugs, such as isoproterenol, are classified as direct-acting sympathomimetics and are similar in structure to norepinephrine. Direct-acting parasympathomimetics, such as methacholine, are chemically similar to ACh.

Indirect-acting drugs produce mimicry through potentiation to simulate autonomic activity. Potentiation can be brought about through blockade of catabolic enzyme activity as is seen with the cholinesterase-inhibitor physostigmine; or inhibition of neurotransmitter uptake, exhibited by cocaine and the amphetamines (see Fig. 4–7).

Blockade

Adrenergic **blockers** are pharmacologic antagonists that specifically antagonize subtypes of adrenergic receptors. **Alpha blockers,** such as phentolamine, and **beta blockers,** such as propranolol, compete with norepinephrine for respective adrenergic receptors.

Cholinergic blockers produce a pharmacologic blockade at cholinergic receptors. **Nicotinic blockers,** such as mecamylamine, compete with ACh at autonomic ganglia (N_1-nicotinic receptors); pancuronium competes with ACh at neuromuscular junctions (N_2-receptors). **Muscarinic blockers,** such as atropine, competitively block ACh at M_2- and M_3-muscarinic receptors (see Fig. 4–7).

Terms used to describe drugs affecting the peripheral nervous system are summarized in Table 5–5.

ROLE OF SECONDARY MESSENGERS

Fixed-Membrane-Receptor Mechanism

Diverse chemical messengers such as neurotransmitters, hormones, and drugs can produce the same physiologic response in a cell even if some of the messengers bind at completely different receptor sites. For example, norepinephrine neurotransmitters released from adrenergic nerve endings, catecholamine hormones such as epinephrine, and drugs such as β_2-adrenergic sympathomimetics and muscarinic blockers can all produce bronchodilation.

The mechanism by which different extracellular, or primary, messengers produce the same cellular response involves substances known as

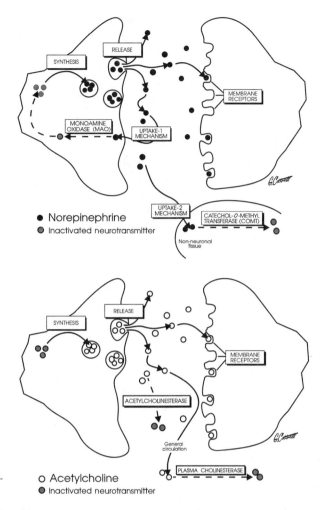

FIGURE 5–10 Fate of norepinephrine and acetyl-choline.

● Norepinephrine
● Inactivated neurotransmitter

○ Acetylcholine
● Inactivated neurotransmitter

TABLE 5–5 TERMS USED TO DESCRIBE DRUG ACTION*

Site of Action	Receptor Agonist	Receptor Antagonist
Autonomic ganglia	Nicotinic	Antinicotinic
	Ganglionic stimulant	Ganglionic depressant
	Preganglionic stimulant	Preganglionic depressant
Postganglionic sympathetic neuroeffector junction	Adrenergic stimulant	Adrenergic blocker
	Sympathetic stimulant	Sympathetic inhibitor
	Sympathomimetic	Sympatholytic
	α_1, β_1, etc, receptor agonist	α_1, β_1, etc., receptor antagonist
Postganglionic parasympathetic neuroeffector junction	Muscarinic agonist	Muscarinic depressant
	Cholinergic	Anticholinergic
	Muscarinic	Antimuscarinic
	Parasympathetic stimulant	Parasympathetic inhibitor
	Parasympathomimetic	Parasympatholytic
	Cholinomimetic	—
Myoneural junction	Myoneural stimulant	Myoneural depressant
	Neuromuscular agonist	Muscle relaxant
	—	Neuromuscular blocking agent

Source: Adapted from Long, 1989.

*The terms *agonist*, *-mimetic*, and *stimulant* are interchangeable. Likewise, the terms *antagonist*, *depressant*, *inhibitor*, and *blocking agent* are often substituted for each other.

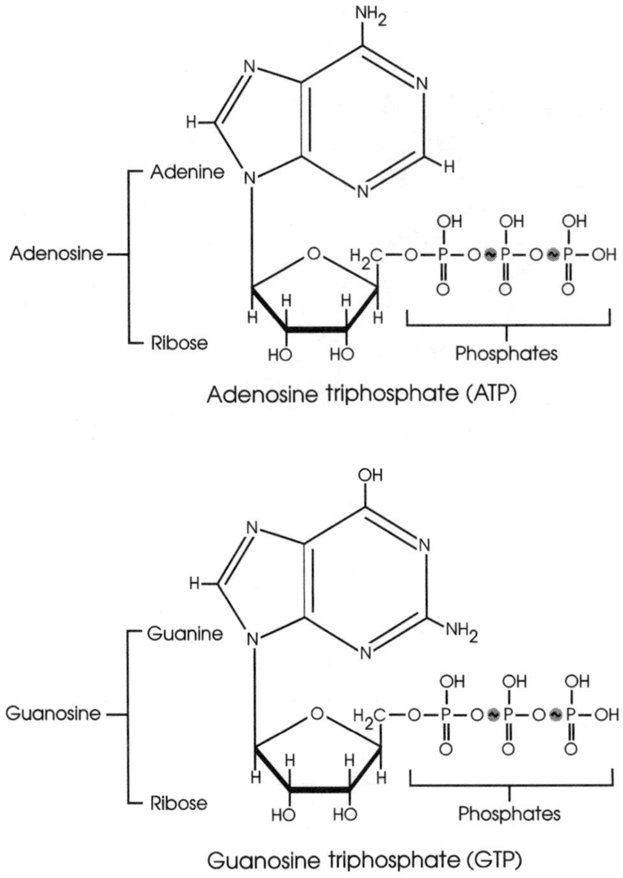

FIGURE 5–11 Nucleotide derivatives (ATP, GTP).

secondary messengers. These messengers are located within effector cells. The hypothesis involving secondary messengers is called the **fixed-membrane-receptor mechanism,** or the **membrane-bound receptor mechanism.** Several different extracellular factors in this mechanism are capable of influencing a common intracellular system. Intracellular, or secondary, messengers are responsible for initiating changes within the effector cells. The changes are characteristic of the action attributed to the primary messenger. In this way, both a β_2-agonist and an M_3-antagonist can be classified as bronchodilator drugs. Both drugs are extracellular substances, but they operate at two different membrane receptors. In fact, one is an agonist and the other is an antagonist. One *promotes* relaxation of airway smooth muscle, whereas the other *prevents* contraction. Both operate through a secondary messenger system that results in an increase in airway diameter.

The Cyclic AMP and Cyclic GMP System

Nucleotides, Nucleosides, and High-Energy Compounds

Nucleotides are compounds that serve as basic building blocks of deoxyribonucleic acid (DNA) and ribonucleic acid (RNA). Nucleotides have three components: a nitrogenous base such as adenine, guanine, cytosine, thymine, or uracil; a five-carbon cyclic sugar molecule known as a *pentose;* and one or more phosphate groups (PO_4^{3-}) referred to as inorganic phosphate (P_i) (Fig. 5–11).

If no phosphate groups are present but a nitrogenous base is bound to a pentose sugar, the resulting compound is called a **nucleoside.** Adenine plus the pentose sugar ribose yields the nucleoside **adenosine.** Guanine plus ribose produces **guanosine.** Adenosine and guanosine are

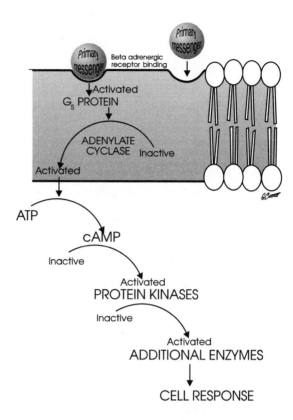

FIGURE 5–12 Secondary messengers and cascade effect.

the building blocks of the secondary messengers known as cyclic nucleotides.

Adenosine triphosphate (ATP) is the main energy-providing chemical in cells. A similar nucleotide derivative is **guanosine triphosphate (GTP).** Both are able to trap, store, and release energy in the chemical bonds that bind their phosphate molecules together in a linear chain (Fig. 5–11). When an energy-rich ATP molecule is hydrolyzed by appropriate enzymes, the phosphate groups on the molecule can be removed one at a time to release stored energy. Initially, ADP (adenosine diphosphate) is formed, followed by the production of AMP (adenosine monophosphate) when a second phosphate group is removed:

$$ATP \rightarrow ADP + P_i + Energy$$
$$\downarrow$$
$$ADP \rightarrow AMP + P_i + Energy$$

Cyclic AMP and Cyclic GMP

The ATP and GTP molecules can be converted in one step to produce nucleotide derivatives that function as secondary messengers. These sec-

ondary messengers are involved in the mechanisms of action of many autonomic drugs.

The binding of a primary messenger at a β-adrenergic receptor initiates the sequence leading to secondary messenger formation. The β-adrenergic receptor interacts with a stimulatory guanine nucleotide–binding regulatory protein (G_s) located in the cell membrane (Fig. 5–12). This **G membrane protein** then binds GTP, and the GTP·G_s complex subsequently interacts with and activates **adenylate cyclase,** an enzyme located on the inner surface of the cell membrane (Weiner and Taylor, 1985). Adenylate cyclase brings about the conversion of ATP directly to **cyclic adenosine 3′,5′-monophosphate (cyclic AMP,** or **cAMP).** The numbers "three prime" and "five prime" indicate specific carbon atoms serving as attachment points for the ring structure of cAMP (Fig. 5–13). Similarly, GTP is enzymatically changed by **guanylate cyclase** to yield **cyclic guanosine 3′, 5′-monophosphate (cyclic GMP** or **cGMP)** (Fig. 5–13). Binding of drug to an inhibitory receptor, such as an α₂-adrenergic receptor, results in decreased cAMP production. The α₂-adrenergic receptor interacts with an in-

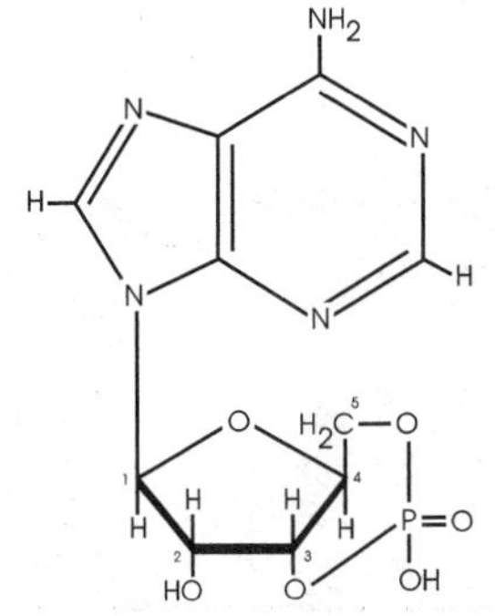

Cyclic adenosine 3′,5′-monophosphate (cAMP)

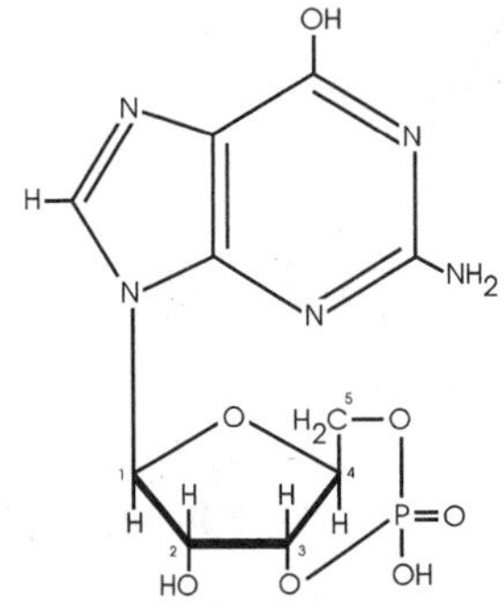

Cyclic guanosine 3′,5′-monophosphate (cGMP)

FIGURE 5–13 Secondary messengers (cAMP, cGMP).

hibitory guanine nucleotide regulatory protein called G_i. G_i then binds GTP, and the $G_i \cdot$GTP complex inactivates adenylate cyclase (Weiner and Taylor, 1985).

In 1971, Earl W. Sutherland of the United States received the Nobel Prize for Medicine or Physiology for the discovery of cAMP. The significance of the discovery has continued to grow during the past two decades as more and more mechanisms are found to involve secondary messengers. For example, cAMP and cGMP represent a final common pathway for several extracellular substances, such as hormones, neurotransmitters, and many drugs. Rapid changes occur within the cell once a primary messenger binds at a surface receptor and activates the second messenger system. The rapid response occurs because the required enzymes do not need to be synthesized. They are already present and can quickly initiate intracellular changes, such as the production of cAMP. Therefore, a single primary messenger molecule can trigger the production of thousands of molecules of secondary messengers through the action of preexisting enzymes. Secondary messen-

gers such as cAMP do not possess any intrinsic activity, but instead activate additional enzymes, which finally produce a characteristic cellular response. For example, cAMP rapidly activates one or more intracellular enzymes collectively called the **protein kinases.** Protein kinases in turn activate additional enzymes to magnify the initial stimulus. This process finally produces a change in the effector cell unique to the primary messenger that activated the sequence. Depending on the receptor type and the cell type, the change might involve decreased tension of smooth muscle, increased contractility of cardiac muscle, increased glandular secretion, or activation of protein synthesis (see Fig. 4–7).

This type of pathway, whereby the product of one reaction catalyzes the next reaction in a sequence, is common in physiologic mechanisms and is termed a **cascade effect.** Cascade effects amplify the initial stimulus because they involve multiple enzymes, each performing its own job and triggering the activation of another (see Fig. 5–12).

Inactivation of the cyclic nucleotides is carried out by **phosphodiesterase (PDE)** enzymes specific for the two secondary messengers. The production and inactivation of cAMP and cGMP are summarized in Figure 5–14.

AUTONOMIC BALANCE OF VISCERAL FUNCTION

Antagonistic Action of Cyclic AMP and Cyclic GMP

The antagonistic nature of the sympathetic and parasympathetic divisions of the ANS can be viewed in terms of the intracellular levels and opposing actions of the cyclic nucleotide secondary messenger system. In summary, sympathetic stimulation causes adrenergic nerve endings to release norepinephrine, which complexes with adrenergic receptors. This receptor binding activates adenylate cyclase. The enzyme then converts ATP to cAMP. Cyclic AMP activates protein kinases, which produce a specific cellular action. In a similar fashion, parasympathetic activity results in the release of acetylcholine from cholinergic fibers. Acetylcholine complexing at cholinergic receptors causes activation of guanylate cyclase and production of cGMP from intracellular stores of GTP. Cyclic GMP then influences protein kinases to produce a characteristic action. In terms of effects in the respiratory system, an increase in the intracellular level of cAMP causes bronchiolar smooth muscle relaxation and bronchodilation and inhibits glandu-

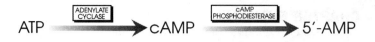

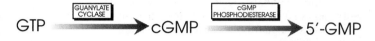

FIGURE 5–14 Production and inactivation of cyclic nucleotides.

lar secretion and histamine release. Elevated levels of cGMP promote shortening of bronchiolar smooth muscle fibers and bronchoconstriction, an increase in glandular activity, and histamine release.

Autonomic Receptors and Secondary Messengers

The binding of primary messengers to various subtypes of autonomic receptors influences secondary messengers. For example, stimulation of β_2-adrenergic receptors produces an increase in cAMP production through activation of G_s regulatory proteins. In smooth muscle activated by such receptors, intracellular Ca^{2+} accumulates in structures such as mitochondria. Without free Ca^{2+} in the cytoplasm of muscle cells, muscle fibers cannot shorten. Therefore, contraction is blocked and relaxation occurs in effectors such as airway smooth muscle. β-Adrenergic stimulation of cardiac (β_1) receptors results in increased cAMP levels and increased strength of contraction.

Activation of M_3-muscarinic cholinergic receptors results in an increase in the production of cGMP and contraction of airway smooth muscle. Conversely, blocking such a muscarinic re-

ceptor inhibits cGMP formation and prevents the shortening of muscle fibers in airway smooth muscle. Thus, a β_2-agonist and an M_3-antagonist can both produce bronchodilation.

Stimulation of presynaptic α_2-adrenergic receptors decreases cAMP production by activating G_i regulatory proteins. This action suppresses the release of norepinephrine from sympathetic nerve endings and inhibits neurotransmission. Stimulation of α_1-adrenergic receptors causes a rapid increase in the concentration of intracellular Ca^{2+}. Calcium functions as an intracellular messenger in some cells. Primary messengers binding at postsynaptic α_1-adrenergic receptors cause chemically gated Ca^{2+} channels in the plasma membrane to open. This allows Ca^{2+} to diffuse into the cell from the extracellular fluid. The Ca^{2+} inflow occurs because of a concentration gradient. The resulting increase in intracellular Ca^{2+} activates a protein enzyme called **calmodulin.** This substance activates various protein kinases. The protein kinases activate or inhibit additional enzymes in a cascade manner to finally bring about a characteristic cellular response such as contraction, conduction, or secretion. The relationship between autonomic receptors and secondary messengers is summarized in Table 5–6.

TABLE 5–6 AUTONOMIC RECEPTORS AND SECONDARY MESSENGERS

Autonomic Receptor Stimulated*	Secondary Messenger Activated	Effect on Muscle
β_1-Adrenergic	↑ cAMP	Increased force of myocardial contraction
β_2-Adrenergic	↑ cAMP	Smooth muscle relaxation
α_1-Adrenergic	↑ Ca^{2+}	Smooth muscle contraction
α_2-Adrenergic	↓ cAMP†	Smooth muscle relaxation
M_2-Muscarinic	Effect unknown	Effect unknown
M_3-Muscarinic	↑ cGMP	Smooth muscle contraction

*Only the autonomic receptors located at postganglionic neuroeffector synapses are included in this comparison.
†Decreased cAMP production in prejunctional fibers suppresses norepinephrine release, which in turn decreases cAMP formation in postjunctional cells to bring about relaxation.
cAMP—cyclic AMP; cGMP—cyclic GMP; ↑—activation; ↓—inhibition.

CHAPTER SUMMARY

This chapter examines the structural, functional, and pharmacologic similarities and differences between the subdivisions of the autonomic nervous system. In addition, concepts such as enzymatic degradation, uptake mechanisms, and secondary messengers are discussed. Subtypes of autonomic receptors are introduced and the basis of autonomic drug classification is outlined. It is stressed that the introductory principles presented in this chapter will prove invaluable in the study of autonomic drugs.

BIBLIOGRAPHY

Barnes PJ: Autonomic pharmacology of the airways. In Chung KF and Barnes PJ (eds): Pharmacology of the Respiratory Tract: Experimental and Clinical Research. Marcel Dekker, New York, 1993a.

Barnes PJ: Molecular biology of receptors in the respiratory tract. In Chung KF and Barnes PJ (eds): Pharmacology of the Respiratory Tract: Experimental and Clinical Research. Marcel Dekker, New York, 1993b.

Berridge MJ: The molecular basis of communication within the cell. Sci Am 253:142–152, Oct 1985.

Carola R, Harley JP, and Noback CR: Human Anatomy and Physiology, ed 2. McGraw-Hill, New York, 1992.

Clark WG, Brater DC, and Johnson AR: Goth's Medical Pharmacology, ed 12. CV Mosby, St Louis, 1988.

Guyton AC: Textbook of Medical Physiology, ed 7. WB Saunders, Philadelphia, 1986.

Johnson GE: PDQ Pharmacology. BC Decker, Toronto, 1988.

Katzung BG: Introduction to autonomic pharmacology. In Katzung BD (ed): Basic and Clinical Pharmacology. Lange Medical Publications, Los Altos, 1982.

Lehnert BE and Schachter EN: The Pharmacology of Respiratory Care. CV Mosby, St Louis, 1980.

Long JP: Drugs Acting on the Peripheral Nervous System. In Conn PM and Gebhart GF (eds): Essentials of Pharmacology. FA Davis, Philadelphia, 1989.

Martini F: Fundamentals of Anatomy and Physiology, ed 2. Prentice-Hall, Englewood Cliffs, NJ, 1992.

Pyne NJ and Rodger IW: Guanine-nucleotide binding regulatory proteins in receptor-mediated actions. In Chung KF and Barnes PJ (eds): Pharmacology of the Respiratory Tract: Experimental and Clinical Research. Marcel Dekker, New York, 1993.

Rau JL: Respiratory Care Pharmacology, ed 3. Yearbook Medical Publishers, Chicago, 1989.

Snyder SH: The molecular basis of communication between cells. Sci Am 253:132–141, Oct 1985.

Thibodeau GA and Patton KT: Anatomy and Physiology, ed 2. Mosby–Year Book, St Louis, 1993.

Tortora GJ and Grabowski SR: Principles of Anatomy and Physiology, ed 7. HarperCollins, New York, 1993.

Weiner N and Taylor P: Neurohumoral transmission: The autonomic and somatic motor nervous systems. In Goodman AG et al (eds): Goodman and Gilman's The Pharmacologic Basis of Therapeutics, ed 7. Macmillan, New York, 1985.

CHAPTER 6

Cholinergic Agonists

CHAPTER OUTLINE

CHAPTER OBJECTIVES

After studying this chapter the reader should be able to:

- Differentiate between a direct- and an indirect-acting cholinergic drug.
- Explain why acetylcholine has no therapeutic value.
- Differentiate between a reversible and an irreversible cholinesterase inhibitor by describing their mechanisms of action.
- Describe the toxicologic effects produced by the organophosphate group of irreversible cholinesterase inhibitors and describe the drugs that are used in the management of such toxicities.
- Describe the pharmacologic activity of the cholinesterase regenerator pralidoxime chloride.
- Describe the effect of cholinergic drugs on secondary messengers.
- Name three indications and three contraindications for use of the cholinergics and explain the rationale behind each of their uses and limitations.
- Differentiate between myasthenic crisis and cholinergic crisis.
- Describe the pharmacologic activity of the following direct-acting cholinergics (choline esters):
  - Bethanechol, carbachol, methacholine.
- Describe the pharmacologic activity of the following indirect-acting cholinergics (anticholinesterases):
  - Physostigmine, neostigmine, pyridostigmine bromide, edrophonium chloride, isoflurophate.

KEY TERMS

anticholinesterase (an-tē-kō-lin-**ES**-ter-āz) (cholinesterase inhibitor) (ChE-I)
  irreversible anticholinesterase
  reversible anticholinesterase
bronchoprovocation testing
  (bronchial challenge testing)

cholinergic (**KŌ**-li-ner-jik) (cholinomimetic) (**KŌ**-li-nō-mi-me-tik)
  direct-acting cholinergic
  indirect-acting cholinergic
cholinergic crisis
glaucoma

ileus (**ILL**-ē-us)
miosis (mī-**Ō**-sis)
myasthenia gravis (mī-a-**STĒ**-nē-a GRA-vis)
myasthenic crisis
organophosphate (O-P)
  compounds

CHAPTER INTRODUCTION

The drugs that mimic acetylcholine neurotransmission belong to a versatile group used to initiate intestinal and bladder contractions, restore skeletal muscle activity, slow the heart, and promote controlled bronchoconstriction. Some members of the group stimulate all cholinergic sites, whereas others exhibit a more selective action at certain cholinergic receptors.

This chapter is the first of many that apply basic physiologic principles to explain the rationale, or reasoning, behind the use of a particular therapeutic agent. The pharmacologic activity of drugs includes the mechanism of action, indications for use, contraindications, precautions, and adverse reactions. These aspects of the autonomic drugs can be easily understood if the reader has a clear perception of the structural, functional, and pharmacologic differences between the two subdivisions of the autonomic nervous system.

CLASSIFICATION OF CHOLINERGIC DRUGS

Terminology

Drugs that imitate the actions of acetylcholine (ACh) are called **cholinergic drugs** or **cholinomimetics.** *Parasympathomimetic* is a more limited term, referring only to those drugs that mimic ACh release at postganglionic *parasympathetic* synapses. Recall from the previous chapter that ACh is also released at other synapses. These additional cholinergic sites include the brain, adrenal medulla, autonomic ganglia, and neuromuscular junctions. Therefore, the more general term *cholinergic* is preferable to *parasympathomimetic.*

Direct-Acting Cholinergics

Direct-acting cholinergic drugs such as the choline esters produce a mimicry of cholinergic activity. This is because their chemical structure is similar to that of ACh and they bind with cholinergic receptors. They exhibit affinity as well as efficacy.

Acetylcholine is the endogenous choline ester and is naturally produced by cholinergic nerve fibers. It directly stimulates all cholinergic receptors because it can conform to the slightly different surface configurations of muscarinic and nicotinic receptors (see Box 5–2). Molecules such as muscarine, nicotine, and some synthetic choline esters lack the conformational flexibility

of ACh and bind at one receptor subtype. Therefore, such agents exhibit either muscarinic or nicotinic specificity. ACh would appear to be the ideal drug to use therapeutically as a direct-acting cholinergic, but it has serious shortcomings. First, ACh *lacks receptor specificity.* The activities of ACh are so varied and widespread that production of a selective therapeutic response is not possible. Second, ACh is *rapidly inactivated* by the cholinesterase enzyme system, including nonspecific plasma cholinesterase (pseudocholinesterase) and specific acetylcholinesterase (Fig. 6–1). Rapid degradation limits its usefulness as a practical therapeutic drug. Last, the *control of dosage* is virtually impossible because ACh administered orally, subcutaneously, or intramuscularly is prone to immediate attack by catabolic enzymes. If it is given intravenously to deliver a larger volume and compensate for the rapid enzymatic activity, ACh may cause fatal bradycardia, acting like massive parasympathetic stimulation of the heart. Recall that some parasympathetic impulses are carried by the vagus nerve, one of the cranial nerves. Therefore, this type of cardiac response is sometimes called *vagal slowing* of the heart. For these reasons, ACh is not useful as a therapeutic agent. However, it is a convenient choline ester to use for comparison purposes.

Synthetic choline esters, such as bethanechol, have been developed that have more specific activity than ACh. In addition, these derivatives resist enzymatic destruction long enough to have a useful duration of action. They have a molecular configuration that slows the enzymatic attack on the molecule while still allowing the drug to interact at certain cholinergic receptors.

Indirect-Acting Cholinergics

Indirect-acting cholinergics (indirect-acting cholinomimetics) elevate ACh levels by inactivating cholinesterase enzymes. Such drugs are known as **anticholinesterases,** or **cholinesterase inhibitors (ChE-I).** The cholinergic drug molecules themselves do not complex with cholinergic receptors, but instead potentiate the level of ACh. ACh then binds at the receptors to cause the stimulation. Because anticholinesterase drugs increase ACh levels at all cholinergic synapses, and because ACh shows no preference for muscarinic or nicotinic receptors, the cholinesterase inhibitor drugs are nonspecific. This is in contrast to some of the choline ester, drugs which show a degree of receptor specificity.

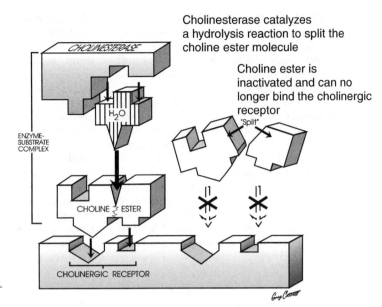

Cholinesterase catalyzes
a hydrolysis reaction to split the
choline ester molecule

Choline ester is
inactivated and can no
longer bind the cholinergic
receptor

FIGURE 6–1 Action of cholinesterase—schematic of mechanism.

Reversible Cholinesterase Inhibitors

Cholinergics such as physostigmine exhibit competitive antagonism of cholinesterase enzymes by temporarily inactivating them (Fig. 6–2). The effect is reversible, relatively short-lived, and controllable. Therefore, this class of cholinergic drug is useful therapeutically. The duration of action ranges from 4 to 8 hours and depends on the rate of dissociation of the drug from the enzyme and the rate of removal of the drug through the normal routes of metabolism and excretion.

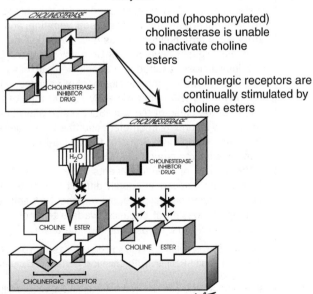

Cholinesterase-inhibitor drug
has affinity for cholinesterase
enzyme

Bound (phosphorylated)
cholinesterase is unable
to inactivate choline
esters

Cholinergic receptors are
continually stimulated by
choline esters

FIGURE 6–2 Action of cholinesterase-inhibitors—schematic of mechanism.

Irreversible Cholinesterase Inhibitors

Some anticholinesterase drugs permanently inhibit cholinesterase enzymes (see Fig. 6–2). This action affects both plasma cholinesterases and acetylcholinesterase. The binding involves noncompetitive antagonism, and the only way cholinesterase enzymes become available again is through synthesis of additional enzyme. Therapeutic uses of irreversible anticholinesterases, such as diisopropyl fluorophosphate (DFP), are rare because of the long-term nature of the effect and the lack of control and reversibility. One of the few medical applications involves the treatment of glaucoma. Nonmedical use of these compounds in agricultural pesticides and chemical warfare agents presents a formidable treatment challenge when severe toxicity symptoms develop (Box 6–1).

Management of Anticholinesterase Toxicities

Potent agricultural pesticides, such as malathion, parathion, and diazinon, have been derived from chemical nerve gases. These neurotoxins, known as **organophosphate compounds,** are lethal to the nervous system of insects. They also present a threat to the human nervous system because their mechanism of action involves the irreversible inhibition of cholinesterase. Individuals at risk from such agents include military personnel, agricultural and chemical workers, and accidental poisoning victims. In fact, the primary interest in the organophosphate compounds is toxicologic because of the widespread use of insecticides in the environment. These agents can be introduced through ingestion, inhalation, or dermal contact. A person exposed

BOX 6–1 NERVE GAS

NBC warfare consists of nuclear, biologic, and chemical weapons. Preparations for offensive strikes and defensive countermeasures have consumed world resources for decades. The specter of global nuclear conflict has become less threatening of late, but total stockpiles of biologic and chemical weapons are enormous. (Estimates of chemical weapons are in the hundreds of thousands of tons!) The weapons are also relatively cheap and often for sale to any country with hard currency.

The most deadly and insidious of the chemical warfare agents are the nerve gases known as organophosphate cholinesterase inhibitors. (Chemically, these organophosphate agents are classified as phosphoric acid–ester compounds.) They elevate ACh levels in the brain to cause central nervous system excitement, confusion, and convulsions. Elevated levels of ACh at muscarinic and nicotinic sites result in peripheral nervous system effects such as decreased heart rate, bronchoconstriction, salivation, and gastrointestinal hypermotility with nausea, vomiting, and diarrhea (Table 6–1). Many of these **irreversible anticholinesterases** have been derived from original stocks of organophosphate nerve gases developed by Germany during the Second World War. Original research with insecticides resulted in a deadly neurotoxin variant called tabun (code letters GA). This was followed by the development of sarin (code letters GB) and soman (code letters GD) (Bryden, 1989). Approximately 12,000 tons of tabun was divided among the Allied Forces at the close of the war. Successive alterations of the original organophosphate nucleus by scientists in different countries have yielded newer and deadlier variations of the parent compound. Some of the derivatives have been employed with lethal results in minor conflicts around the globe.

The amount of chemical agents in storage is difficult to assess. Verification of their removal and disposal is equally difficult to monitor. For these reasons, chemical stockpiles in weapon ordnance depots represent a significant destabilizing factor in the world. Neither possession of chemical warfare technology nor the threat of its use requires superpower status. Anyone can own the terror.

Bryden J: Deadly Allies: Canada's Secret War 1937–1947. McClelland and Stewart, Toronto, 1989.
Meselson M and Robinson JP: Chemical warfare and chemical disarmament. Sci Am 242:38–47, Apr 1980.
Stelzmüler H: NBC defence: NATO needs new devices. Military Technology 2:24–35, Feb 1983.

to such a poison can experience any or all of the physiologic effects caused by massive amounts of ACh in the nervous system. Toxic effects include intense muscarinic and nicotinic cholinergic effects in the peripheral nervous system and cholinergic effects in the brain. These may include excitement, confusion, and convulsions. Respiratory failure may occur through a combination of bronchoconstriction, laryngospasm, increased tracheobronchial secretions, and loss of control of respiratory muscles. Virtually all body systems can be adversely affected to some degree (Table 6–1). Anticholinesterase drugs perma-

nently inactivate the cholinesterase system of enzymes. As a result, synaptic levels of ACh remain above normal for the length of time required by the body to synthesize additional enzyme. This can take approximately 2 weeks for production of plasma cholinesterase and up to 3 months for the replacement of acetylcholinesterase. During this time cholinergic receptors must be "protected" from the effects of excessive ACh (Table 6–2).

Atropine is administered to antagonize ACh at muscarinic receptors. It prevents slowing of the heart, decreases hypermotility of the gut, and reduces tracheobronchial and gastrointestinal tract secretions. Nicotinic stimulation due to elevated ACh levels is not reduced by atropine. Therefore, neuromuscular activity such as skeletal muscle fasciculations (fine tremors of muscle *fascicles,* or bundles) and initial contractions leading to skeletal muscle paralysis are unchanged. With continuous monitoring of the heart, atropine is administered at a dose necessary to restore and maintain a normal heart rate.

Pralidoxime (Protopam) is administered parenterally in the early stages of the toxicity as an antidote to aid in the regeneration of cholinesterase enzymes. Pralidoxime (also called PAM or 2-PAM) is a synthetic drug that is incorporated into cholinesterase after the enzyme has been phosphorylated by an anticholinesterase drug. Phosphorylated cholinesterase is stable, inactive, and incapable of attacking ACh (Fig. 6–2). The addition of pralidoxime reactivates cholinesterase so that the regenerated enzyme can resume its catabolic role and reduce the excess ACh.

TABLE 6–1 SYMPTOMS OF ANTICHOLINESTERASE TOXICITY

Peripheral Nervous System	Central Nervous System
RESPIRATORY SYSTEM	
Bronchoconstriction	Excitement
Laryngospasm	Restlessness
Increased tracheobronchial secretions	Insomnia
Decreased action of ventilatory muscles (see: "skeletal muscles," below)	Confusion
	Convulsions
	Respiratory depression
CARDIOVASCULAR SYSTEM	
Bradycardia (negative chronotropic effect)*	
Decreased force of contraction (negative inotropic effect)	
Hypotension*	
GASTROINTESTINAL TRACT	
Increased glandular secretion	
Increased motility (peristalsis)	
Abdominal cramping	
Nausea, vomiting, diarrhea	
URINARY SYSTEM	
Micturition (emptying of bladder)	
SKELETAL MUSCLE	
Fasciculations (fine tremors)	
Fatigue	
OTHER EFFECTS	
Miosis (pupil constriction)	
Blurred vision	
Lacrimation	
Salivation	
Sweating	

*Bradycardia and hypotension are caused by ACh stimulation of M_2-muscarinic receptors. Excessive ACh at sympathetic ganglia (N_1-nicotinic receptors) may cause tachycardia and increased arteriolar vasoconstriction leading to hypertension.

TABLE 6–2 TREATMENT OF ANTICHOLINESTERASE TOXICITY

SUPPORTIVE THERAPY

Intravenous fluid replacement
Electrolyte replacement
Endotracheal intubation
Assisted ventilation
Suctioning

ANTIMUSCARINIC DRUGS

Parasympatholytic agents such as atropine are administered to block muscarinic receptors.

CHOLINESTERASE REGENERATOR DRUGS

Drugs such as pralidoxime chloride assist in the reactivation of phosphorylated cholinesterase if given early in the management of the toxicity (Clark et al, 1988).

In addition to atropine and pralidoxime therapy, management of anticholinesterase toxicities includes supportive measures such as intravenous fluid and electrolyte replacement, assisted ventilation, endotracheal intubation, and suctioning (Table 6–2).

EFFECT OF CHOLINERGIC DRUG ON SECONDARY MESSENGERS

Regardless of the type of cholinergic drug administered, whether it is a choline ester or an anticholinesterase, the effect on the intracellular system of secondary messengers is the same. Direct- and indirect-acting cholinergics activate guanylate cyclase. Guanylate cyclase then enzymatically converts stored GTP (guanosine triphosphate) to cyclic guanosine-3',5'-monophosphate (cyclic GMP; cGMP). Within the cell, cGMP triggers cholinergic changes such as bronchoconstriction (see Table 5–6). Cholinergics of the choline ester type mimic ACh, bind at cholinergic receptors, and directly induce guanylate cyclase. The cholinesterase inhibitors boost the level of endogenous ACh, which in turn combines in a normal way at cholinergic receptors and activates guanylate cyclase.

THERAPEUTIC AGENTS

Choline Esters

BETHANECHOL (Urecholine). Bethanechol exhibits considerable stability and is not readily hydrolyzed by the cholinesterase enzymes; therefore, it is available for oral use. Muscarinic effects are dominant and a certain degree of selectivity is seen in gastrointestinal and urinary tract effects. This makes bethanechol ideal for treating postoperative abdominal distension and urinary retention. At therapeutic doses, ganglionic and neuromuscular effects (nicotinic) are lacking.

INDICATIONS. Gastrointestinal tract stasis (paralytic **ileus**) is seen postoperatively, especially if a patient received muscarinic antagonist drugs, such as atropine, prior to surgery and if the surgical procedure involved manipulation of abdominal organs. Choline esters with muscarinic activity are usually administered to mimic parasympathetic stimulation and restore normal intestinal motility.

Postoperative retention of urine can be complicated by preoperative administration of muscarinic antagonists. These drugs block parasympathetic impulses normally innervating the smooth muscle of the bladder wall. Direct-acting choline esters with muscarinic activity are usually indicated to initiate emptying of the bladder.

CONTRAINDICATIONS. Because cholinergics mimic parasympathetic effects in the tracheobronchial tree, including bronchoconstriction and increased secretions, preexisting conditions of bronchial asthma can be worsened by the administration of this class of drugs.

If stasis of the gastrointestinal tract is caused by an obstruction of the small intestine, cholinergic drugs are contraindicated. Increased motility could cause trauma to the gut.

Increased urinary system activity caused by a cholinergic drug is useful and desirable only if no obstructions are present in the urinary system. If the decreased motility, however, is a result of obstructions such as renal calculi (kidney stones), the effect of the cholinergic on motility would aggravate the condition.

A condition of bradycardia can be worsened by drugs that mimic the cardioinhibitory effect of parasympathetic stimulation. Therefore, choline esters and anticholinesterases are contraindicated.

CARBACHOL (Carbamylcholine). Muscarinic and nicotinic activity characterize carbachol; therefore, a large amount produces ACh-like effects. Carbachol is not hydrolyzed quickly by the cholinesterases, and its long life in the body permits oral administration.

INDICATIONS. Carbachol produces miosis, or pupil constriction, and is ideal for reducing the intraocular pressure of glaucoma. (See Physostigmine below for additional drug treatments of glaucoma.)

CONTRAINDICATIONS. See Bethanechol.

METHACHOLINE (Mecholyl). Muscarinic activity is exhibited by methacholine. It is chemically similar to ACh (both are acetyl esters) and is therefore hydrolyzed by acetylcholinesterase, but more slowly than native ACh. Methacholine is slowly attacked by the plasma cholinesterases but is not long-acting enough to be administered orally. Few medical uses for methacholine exist. It is used principally in research to assess the efficacy of bronchodilator drug therapy in asthma. The *methacholine challenge test* is a common **bronchoprovocation** or **bronchial challenge test** whereby the drug is administered under strictly monitored and controlled conditions to evoke bronchoconstriction. (The antidote, atropine, is always on hand to reverse the bronchoconstriction if necessary.) Provocation of bronchiolar smooth muscle mimics parasympathetic stimulation and is done in research to simulate bronchoconstriction in asthmatic and nonasthmatic subjects. Studies are made of the differences in

TABLE 6–3 SUMMARY OF CHOLINE ESTER ACTIVITY

Choline Ester	Cholinesterase Susceptibility	Cholinergic Receptor Effects		Duration of Action (min)
		Muscarinic	Nicotinic	
Acetylcholine	Very high	+	+	Very short (5)
Bethanechol	Low	+	*	Long (60–90)
Carbachol	Low	+	+	Long (60–90)
Methacholine	High	+	−	Short (10–15)

Source: Data from Long, 1989.
*At higher doses, ganglionic and neuromuscular effects (nicotinic) may be produced.
+—active; −—inactive.

airway resistance between individuals and of the differences in efficacy of various bronchodilator drugs used to relieve bronchospasm.

CONTRAINDICATIONS. See Bethanechol.

Muscarinic receptor agonists (choline esters) are summarized in Table 6–3 under the headings of Cholinesterase Susceptibility, Cholinergic Receptor Effects, and Duration of Action.

Anticholinesterases

Reversible Cholinesterase Inhibitors

PHYSOSTIGMINE (Eserine). Physostigmine, a **reversible anticholinesterase,** is well absorbed and can be instilled in the eye to treat **glaucoma.** It is also useful for treating **myasthenia gravis** and curare overdoses. Physostigmine is the specific antidote for anticholinergic (antimuscarinic) toxicity. It has an affinity for cholinesterase 10,000 times greater than that of ACh for cholinesterase. Therefore, physostigmine inactivates cholinesterase enzymes easily but in a reversible manner because of the competitive antagonism. The duration of action is around 4 hours.

INDICATIONS. Myasthenia gravis is a neuromuscular disorder characterized by decreased strength of contraction, inability to maintain repeated contractions, and rapid onset of fatigue. It can affect all skeletal muscle, including muscles of ventilation. Myasthenia gravis is an autoimmune disorder with two components:

1. Insufficient ACh in synaptic vesicles
2. Decreased number of nicotinic cholinergic receptors

The condition can be alleviated by increasing the amount of ACh available for neurotransmission. The use of reversible anticholinesterase drugs inhibits the destruction of the relatively small amount of ACh released from somatic motoneurons of patients suffering from myasthenia gravis. The rationale for inhibiting neurotransmitter destruction is to provide enough ACh for normal neuromuscular transmission.

Neuromuscular blocking agents, such as curare and its newer derivatives, are frequently employed as skeletal muscle relaxants prior to surgery. Following surgery, cholinesterase inhibitors are administered to potentiate ACh levels and counter the neuromuscular blockade. Overdoses of the curarelike drugs are also treated by the administration of anticholinesterases.

Muscarinic blockers, such as atropine, are anticholinergic drugs of the antimuscarinic type. These drugs competitively antagonize ACh at muscarinic sites. Drug overdoses or poisoning by the muscarinic blockers can be reversed by cholinergic drugs that elevate ACh levels. Anticholinesterase drugs, such as physostigmine, increase the amount of ACh at synapses. ACh then competes with the muscarinic blocking agent for available muscarinic receptors.

Elevated intraocular pressure can be reduced by promoting increased drainage of aqueous humour from the anterior chamber of the eye. Circular smooth muscle fibers of the iris contract under parasympathetic stimulation to constrict the pupil (**miosis**). As this occurs, the ciliary body (containing ciliary muscle) moves posteriorly to change the tension on the suspensory ligaments that surround the lens, thus changing the thickness of the lens. As the smooth muscle of the ciliary body contracts, the anterior chamber angle increases and the drainage of aqueous humor is enhanced (Fig. 6–3). Because cholinergics cause pupil constriction and increased drainage of aqueous humor, they can be successfully used to reduce the intraocular pressure of glaucoma. Reversible cholinesterase inhibitors, such as physostigmine, are generally employed.

CONTRAINDICATIONS. See Bethanechol (Box 6–2).

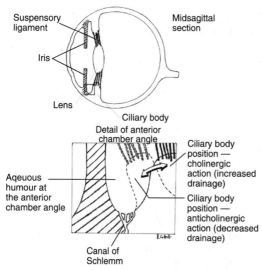

FIGURE 6–3 Cholinergic activity at the eye.

NEOSTIGMINE (Prostigmin). Neostigmine is a synthetic analogue of physostigmine. It produces similar cholinergic effects, such as sweating, salivation, increased gastrointestinal and urinary tract motility, and bradycardia and skeletal muscle fasciculations. Injectable and oral forms exist.

INDICATIONS. Uses include the treatment of glaucoma and myasthenia gravis and the reversal of curare effects.

CONTRAINDICATIONS. See Bethanechol.

EDROPHONIUM. An indirect-acting cholinergic, edrophonium is chemically similar to neostigmine. However, it combines with cholinesterase enzymes for only a few minutes.

INDICATIONS. Edrophonium is useful as an anticurare drug because it has a rapid onset of action. The primary use of such a short-acting (5–10 minutes) cholinergic drug, however, is the edrophonium test. This test is used in diagnosis

of myasthenia gravis and assessment of myasthenic treatment. In the diagnosis of myasthenia gravis, a patient suspected of having the disorder is given edrophonium. After a brief period, the patient with myasthenia gravis exhibits improved muscular strength lasting about 5 minutes. In the myasthenic patient already diagnosed and being treated with an anticholinesterase such as neostigmine or pyridostigmine, muscle weakness can still occur. This paradoxic response is termed **cholinergic crisis** and may be due to the effects of too much cholinergic drug. The muscle weakness is caused by *excess* ACh, which produces a depolarization type of neuromuscular block that can affect muscles of ventilation. Various types of neuromuscular blockade are examined in Chapter 7. Because myasthenia gravis is a disorder involving the N_2-nicotinic receptors of the motor endplate, muscle weakness, including respiratory distress, can also be due to *deficient* ACh. This type of weakness is termed **myasthenic crisis.** Because of respiratory system involvement, differentiation of myasthenic crisis from cholinergic crisis is often necessary to make dosage adjustments. This is done in a hospital with ready access to support systems, such as mechanical ventilation.

The edrophonium test allows a physician to precisely increase or decrease the dosage of the primary myasthenic drug. If the patient briefly exhibits increased strength following edrophonium administration, the improvement is due to the addition of this short-acting cholinesterase inhibitor to the patient's drug regimen. The implication is that the patient has additional ACh for neurotransmission and is presently being undertreated. Such a patient usually benefits from an increase in cholinesterase inhibitor dosage. However, if a cholinergic crisis is responsible for the patient's symptoms, a small amount of edrophonium does not alleviate the distress and

---

BOX 6–2   GUILTY AS CHARGED

Physostigmine is found naturally in the Calabar bean (*Physostigma venenosum*) of West Africa. This tropical vine grows in the Calabar region of Nigeria and has a colorful history as the source of the ordeal bean. Beans containing the active ingredient physostigmine are ingested as a "guilt test" by an individual accused of a crime. A suspect who survives the ordeal is considered innocent. The test is also done to expose witches and witchcraft. (The customary dose for this particular test is eight beans.) Symptoms of the poisoning ordeal include the usual cholinergic effects produced by toxic levels of **cholinesterase inhibitors**—namely, bradycardia, hyperactive bowel, salivation, bronchoconstriction, and others (Table 6–1).

Lewis WH and Elvin-Lewis MPF: Medical Botany. John Wiley and Sons, New York, 1977.

TABLE 6–4   SUMMARY OF CHOLINESTERASE INHIBITOR ACTIVITY

Cholinesterase Inhibitor Drug	Inhibition of Cholinesterase		Increase of Acetylcholine in Brain	Topical Use in Eye	Major Use
	Acetyl	Plasma			
REVERSIBLE CHOLINESTERASE INHIBITORS					
Physostigmine	+ +	+	+ + +	+ + +	Glaucoma, CNS cholinergic, myasthenia gravis, curare antagonist
Neostigmine	+ + +	–	–	–	Cholinergic agonist, myasthenia gravis, curare antagonist
Edrophonium	+ +	–	–	–	Curare antagonist, "edrophonium test" (cholinergic vs myasthenic crisis)
IRREVERSIBLE CHOLINESTERASE INHIBITORS					
Isoflurophate	+	+ + +	+ +	+ +*	None
Malathion	+	+ +	+ +	+*	Insecticide

Source: Adapted from Long, 1989.
*Irreversible inhibitors are no longer used in ocular pharmacology because of damage to the lens and increased frequency of detached retinas.
CNS—central nervous system; +—active; ——inactive.

usually worsens the muscle weakness. Patients in cholinergic crisis also exhibit signs of muscarinic stimulation such as miosis, bronchoconstriction, increased airway secretions, bradycardia, and increased gastrointestinal motility. A reduction in cholinesterase inhibitor dosage is usually indicated in such cases. Recall that anticholinesterases such as neostigmine are nonspecific cholinergic drugs, indirectly stimulating nicotinic as well as muscarinic receptors.

CONTRAINDICATIONS. See Bethanechol.

PYRIDOSTIGMINE (Mestinon). Pyridostigmine is a neostigmine substitute with a duration of action of approximately 4 hours.

INDICATIONS. The primary use of pyridostigmine is in the treatment of myasthenia gravis.

CONTRAINDICATIONS. See Bethanechol.

Irreversible Cholinesterase Inhibitors

Diisopropyl fluorophosphate (DFP). Many potentially poisonous substances, such as neurotoxins and insecticides, are **irreversible anticholinesterases.** Therapeutic agents are rare. DFP, also known as isofluorophosphate or isofluorophate (Floropryl), however, is one of the few notable

exceptions. Isoflurophate is an organophosphate compound that irreversibly inhibits cholinesterase enzymes. The potency, however, is less than that of most other members of the organophosphate group.

TABLE 6–5   DRUG NAMES: CHOLINERGIC AGONISTS

Generic Name	Trade Name
CHOLINE ESTERS	
Bethanechol (be-**THAN**-kol)	Urecholine
Carbachol (**KAR**-ba-kol)	Carbamylcholine
Methacholine (meth-a-**KŌ**lēn)	Mecholyl
REVERSIBLE ANTICHOLINESTERASES	
Physostigmine (fī-zō-**STIG**-mēn)	Eserine
Neostigmine (nē-ō-**STIG**-mēn)	Prostigmin
Edrophonium (ed-rō-**FŌN**-ēum)	Tensilon
Pyridostigmine (pī-rid-ō-**STIG**-mēn)	Mestinon
IRREVERSIBLE ANTICHOLINESTERASES	
Isoflurophate	Floropryl
Diisopropyl fluorophosphate (dī-īsō-**PRO**-pil **FLYOO**-rō-faz-fāt) (DFP or isofluorophosphate)	

INDICATIONS. With careful monitoring, isoflurophate has been administered to reduce intraocular pressure in the treatment of glaucoma; however, this use is controversial (Long, 1989). Because the duration of action of isoflurophate is very long (100 hours), frequent administration of the drug is not required.

CONTRAINDICATIONS. See Bethanechol.

A summary of cholinesterase inhibitor activity and uses of the anticholinesterase drugs is presented in Table 6–4. Generic and trade names of the cholinergic agonists discussed in this chapter are listed in Table 6–5.

CHAPTER SUMMARY

This chapter introduces the drugs that mimic ACh activity. Two classes of cholinergic agent are discussed: the relatively specific group of choline esters and the nonspecific group of cholinesterase inhibitors. Mechanisms of action and the pharmacologic characteristics of cholinergic drugs are examined. Many of the basic pharmacologic principles introduced in the first five chapters of the text are reinforced in this chapter.

BIBLIOGRAPHY

Clark WG, Brater DC, and Johnson AR: Goth's Medical Pharmacology, ed 12. CV Mosby, St Louis, 1988.

Howder CL: Cardiopulmonary Pharmacology: A Handbook for Respiratory Practitioners and Other Allied Health Personnel. Williams and Wilkins, Baltimore, 1992.

Katzung BG: Introduction to autonomic pharmacology. In Katzung BD (ed): Basic and Clinical Pharmacology. Lange Medical Publications, Los Altos, 1982.

Long JP: Drugs acting on the peripheral nervous system. In Conn PM and Gebhart GF (eds): Essentials of Pharmacology. FA Davis, Philadelphia, 1989.

Lopate G and Pestronk A: Autoimmune myasthenia gravis. Hosp Pract (Off Ed) 28:109–131, Jan 15, 1993.

Taylor P: Anticholinesterase agents. In Goodman AG et al (eds): Goodman and Gilman's The Pharmacologic Basis of Therapeutics, ed 7. Macmillan, New York, 1985.

Taylor P: Cholinergic agonists. In Goodman AG et al (eds): Goodman and Gilman's The Pharmacologic Basis of Therapeutics, ed 7. Macmillan, New York, 1985.

Watanabe AM: Cholinergic receptor stimulants. In Katzung BD (ed): Basic and Clinical Pharmacology. Lange Medical Publications, Los Altos, 1982.

CHAPTER 7

Nicotinic Antagonists

CHAPTER OUTLINE

CHAPTER OBJECTIVES

After studying this chapter the reader should be able to:

- Describe the mechanism of action of ganglionic blocking agents.
- State one indication and one contraindication for use of ganglionic blockers and explain the rationale behind the use and limitation.
- Describe the pharmacologic activity of the following ganglionic blocking agent:
  - Mecamylamine.
- Differentiate between central and peripheral skeletal muscle relaxation mechanisms.
- Name the neurotransmitter released from somatic motoneurons and the receptors found at neuromuscular junctions.
- Contrast the mechanisms of action of nondepolarizing and depolarizing blocking agents.
- Explain how a nondepolarizing blockade, a depolarizing blockade, and a desensitizing blockade can be reversed.
- State three indications and three contraindications for use of neuromuscular blockers and explain the rationale behind each of their uses and limitations.
- List two precautions for use of skeletal muscle relaxants.
- Describe the pharmacologic activity of the following skeletal muscle relaxants:
  - D-tubocurarine (curare), metocurine, atracurium, pancuronium, vecuronium, gallamine, succinylcholine.

KEY TERMS

anticholinergic (acetylcholine
  [ACh] antagonist)
antinicotinic (nicotinic
  antagonist)
  N_1-Nicotinic antagonist
    (ganglionic blocker)
  N_2-Nicotinic antagonist
    (neuromuscular blocker)
curare

curariform
depolarizing blocker
desensitization block (dual
  block) (Phases I and II)
motor endplate
muscle action potential (MAP)
neuromuscular junction (NMJ)
  (myoneural junction)

nicotine
nicotinic receptor
  N_1-nicotinic receptor
  N_2-nicotinic receptor
nondepolarizing blocker
sarcolemma
sarcoplasm
sarcoplasmic reticulum

CHAPTER INTRODUCTION

Acetylcholine (ACh) is the neurotransmitter released from nerve fibers at several locations within the peripheral nervous system. Drugs which interfere with acetylcholine neurotransmission are referred to as **acetylcholine antagonists,** or **anticholinergics.** Those that compete with acetylcholine at nicotinic receptors are known as **nicotinic antagonists,** or **antinicotinics.** Two subtypes exist: **ganglionic blockers** affecting ganglionic sites and **neuromuscular blockers** affecting neuromuscular sites.

GANGLIONIC BLOCKERS

Mechanism of Action

Preganglionic neurons are classified as cholinergic fibers because they release acetylcholine (ACh) when a nerve impulse arrives at the ganglion. The cholinergic receptors found postsynaptically within autonomic ganglia of both sympathetic and parasympathetic pathways are designated as N_1-**nicotinic receptors.** A very small number of muscarinic cholinergic and α-adrenergic receptors are also present in ganglia but they play a minor role (Box 7–1).

Drugs that competitively antagonize ACh at the nicotinic receptors of autonomic ganglia are referred to as **ganglionic blockers.** These blocking agents prevent impulse transmission from reaching postganglionic fibers by occupying ganglionic nicotinic receptors and preventing ACh from gaining access to the receptor sites. Ganglionic blockers are limited in therapeutic usefulness mainly because they lack specificity at autonomic ganglia. This is because identical nicotinic receptors are found in the ganglia of both autonomic nervous system divisions (see Fig. 5–7).

Pharmacologic Effects

The amount of pharmacologic activity produced by ganglionic blockade reflects the degree of autonomic innervation at a particular organ. For example, singly innervated organs such as blood vessels tend to respond more predictably than organs receiving sympathetic and parasympathetic impulses. Dually innervated organs such as the heart receive a reduced number of autonomic impulses because both divisions are blocked at the ganglia. This lack of specificity makes control of pharmacologic effects less than satisfactory.

Effects on vasculature are relatively uncomplicated because most blood vessels in the body are innervated through the sympathetic division only. Ganglionic blockade reduces sympathetic tone to these vascular beds, resulting in peripheral vasodilation and a fall in blood pressure, especially in a person who is standing. This posture-related response is caused by reduced venous return. It is called *orthostatic hypotension* and occurs because of venous pooling in the legs. A recumbent patient does not exhibit the same degree of hypotension. Side effects of the ganglionic blocking agents are related to the dominant type of autonomic receptor present on the organ innervated. Dry mouth, pupil dilation, and decreased gastrointestinal and urinary tract motility indicate ganglionic blockade at parasympathetic ganglia. The production of side effects such as constipation and urinary retention points out the difficulties and limitations inherent in this relatively nonselective group of autonomic drugs.

THERAPEUTIC AGENTS

MECAMYLAMINE (Inversine). Mecamylamine is well absorbed from the gastrointestinal

---

BOX 7–1   NEW DRUG FROM THE NEW WORLD

In the mid-20th century, **nicotinic receptors** and their N_1 and N_2 subtypes were elucidated. Four hundred years earlier the tobacco plant of the Americas awaited discovery by European explorers. Jean Nicot (ca. 1560), the French ambassador to Portugal, obtained tobacco seeds that had reached Europe from the newly explored western hemisphere. He sent the seeds to Catherine de Medici, mother of the French king. Through these actions, Europe was introduced to the seductive power of **nicotine,** the alkaloid found in tobacco. The group of plants that includes tobacco was named *Nicotiana* in Jean Nicot's honor.

Ashimov I: Words of Science and the History Behind Them. Riverside Press, Cambridge, MA, 1959.

tract and has a relatively long duration of action (4–12 hours). Therapeutic doses produce ganglionic blocking effects, but higher doses can produce neuromuscular blockade in addition to ganglionic blockade.

INDICATIONS. The primary indication for use of the ganglionic blockers is to lower blood pressure in hypertensive states and produce controlled hypotension during certain procedures, such as vascular surgery. Reduced vascular tone is responsible for the desired drop in blood pressure. Because ganglionic selectivity is essentially lacking with the ganglionic blockers, these are not the drugs of first choice to control hypertension. More effective antihypertensive agents are available and are examined in Chapter 21.

CONTRAINDICATIONS. A preexisting condition of hypotension can obviously be made worse by the administration of drugs that reduce vascular tone.

NEUROMUSCULAR BLOCKERS

Site of Action

Drugs that produce skeletal muscle relaxation can be classified on the basis of their site of action (Fig. 7–1). Some are effective in the brain or spinal cord (central nervous system), others act directly on the skeletal muscle to promote relaxation, and still others produce their effects at the interface between motoneurons and skeletal muscle (peripheral nervous system).

Drugs that produce skeletal muscle relaxation

by interfering with neurotransmission of motor impulses in the brain or spinal cord are designated *centrally acting muscle relaxants*. This group includes tranquilizers such as diazepam (Valium) and is covered in later chapters dealing with the central nervous system.

Peripherally acting skeletal muscle relaxants act either intra- or extracellularly. Only the peripheral agents acting outside the muscle cell are considered in the following discussion. The skeletal muscle relaxants acting at these **neuromuscular,** or **myoneural, junctions** do so through one of two extracellular mechanisms:

1. They competitively antagonize ACh to *prevent* impulse transmission at the neuromuscular junction.
2. They act like an excess of ACh to *promote* impulse transmission, which is then followed by a blocking or relaxation effect. Detailed mechanisms of action are outlined below.

SKELETAL MUSCLE CONTRACTION

The Neuromuscular Junction

The sequence involved in impulse transmission at neuromuscular junctions (NMJ) generally follows that described for synaptic transmission in Chapter 4. The synapses between motoneurons of the somatic nervous system and skeletal muscle have the same general features as synapses

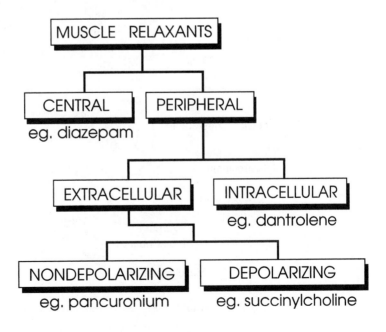

FIGURE 7–1 Muscle relaxants.

found between neurons. For example, NMJs feature presynaptic axons equipped with synaptic vesicles and stored neurotransmitter, postsynaptic receptors, and catabolic enzymes to degrade the neurotransmitter. The basic structural difference is the **motor endplate.** This is a specialized portion of the **sarcolemma,** or skeletal muscle cell membrane, directly adjacent to the terminal branches of the somatic motoneuron (Fig. 7–2). A neuromuscular junction, therefore, consists of axon terminals of the motoneuron and the motor endplate of the muscle fiber.

When a nerve action potential, or impulse, arrives at the axon terminal, ACh is liberated from synaptic vesicles in the manner described in Chapter 4. ACh diffuses across the synaptic cleft toward the motor endplate. The motor endplate contains **N₂-nicotinic receptors,** which bind ACh. Figure 3–3 shows the conformation of this receptor. It is a pentamer of four types of polypeptide subunits: 2 alpha subunits plus one each of beta, delta, and gamma subunits. When ACh molecules bind at both alpha subunits, an aqueous channel (pore) briefly opens through the motor endplate membrane, allowing ionic flux. The N₂-nicotinic receptor is part of a family of channel-forming proteins that alter membrane

permeability. (Later chapters discuss other examples of such channel-forming receptor proteins interacting with drugs, such as benzodiazepine *tranquilizers* and the *barbiturates.*)

Muscle Action Potential

The chemically gated ion channels in the motor endplate allow small cations such as Na^{1+} to pass. As discussed in Chapter 4, sodium inflow changes the resting membrane potential (RMP) of a cell. (RMP values for different cells are given in Table 22–1 in Chapter 22.) This change initiates a **muscle action potential (MAP)** that is quickly transmitted along the sarcolemma and into the interior of the muscle fiber. In the relaxed muscle cell, Ca^{2+} ions are stored in an extensive tubular network called the **sarcoplasmic reticulum (SR).** As the muscle action potential spreads into the sarcoplasmic reticulum, Ca^{2+} ions are released to enter the cytoplasm, or **sarcoplasm,** of the muscle fiber. It is the presence of free Ca^{2+} in the sarcoplasm that triggers the actual shortening of the muscle fiber. Although not classified as a neuromuscular blocker, the skeletal muscle relaxant dantrolene (Dantrium) produces relaxation intracellularly by interfering with this Ca^{2+} release mechanism.

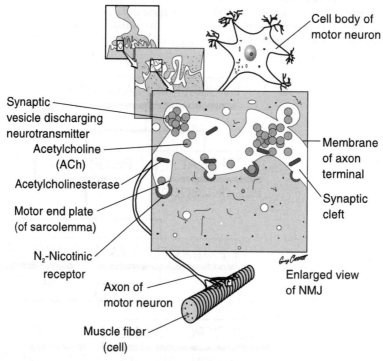

Cell body of motor neuron

Synaptic vesicle discharging neurotransmitter

Acetylcholine (ACh)

Acetylcholinesterase

Motor end plate (of sarcolemma)

N₂-Nicotinic receptor

Axon of motor neuron

Muscle fiber (cell)

Membrane of axon terminal

Synaptic cleft

Enlarged view of NMJ

FIGURE 7–2 Neuromuscular junction (NMJ).

Contraction

The rise in Ca^{2+} concentration in the sarcoplasm added to the availability of ATP (adenosine triphosphate) activates various muscle proteins. Some are regulatory proteins that govern the action of contractile proteins. Others play a support role only. They are organized into thick, thin, and elastic filaments. Because the thick and thin filaments slide past one another to produce shortening of the muscle fiber, the process is called the *sliding filament mechanism*. This mechanism is not essential for understanding the pharmacology of neuromuscular blockers; nevertheless, it is a fascinating topic. The reader wishing more information concerning the physiology of muscle contraction is directed to the general anatomy and physiology texts cited in the chapter bibliography.

Relaxation

Relaxation of a muscle fiber following contraction is caused by two events. If a nerve impulse does not arrive in the motor neuron, additional ACh is not released from synaptic vesicles. Acetylcholinesterase in the synaptic cleft will then rapidly degrade any remaining ACh. Without ACh neurotransmitter, the generation of MAPs ceases and Ca^{2+} ions are no longer released from the sarcoplasmic reticulum. The nondepolarizing neuromuscular blockers discussed below inhibit ACh neurotransmission and halt MAP generation.

Calcium ion active transport pumps in the muscle fiber also contribute to muscle relaxation. The pumps remove free Ca^{2+} from the sarcoplasm and move the ions into the sarcoplasmic reticulum. Here they are stored until the arrival of a new MAP. As Ca^{2+} levels drop in the sarcoplasm, muscle proteins are inactivated. The filaments then slide back to their relaxed positions, thus lengthening the muscle.

MECHANISMS OF ACTION

Nondepolarizing Blockers

Peripherally acting skeletal muscle relaxants that exhibit competitive antagonism with acetylcholine for nicotinic receptors are known as **nondepolarizing blockers.** These drugs have affinity for N_2-nicotinic receptors on motor endplates but do not trigger a contraction in skeletal muscle. In other words, they have affinity but lack efficacy. They prevent the motor endplate from depolarizing, and as can be seen in Figure 7–3, there is a decrease in the ability of skeletal mus-

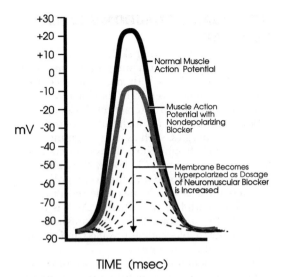

FIGURE 7–3 Muscle action potentials—effect of nondepolarizing blocking agents.

cle to contract. This muscle relaxation state is known as *flaccid paralysis*. The newer agents exhibit a reasonable amount of receptor specificity at neuromuscular (N_2) sites. However, the **curariform,** or curarelike, agents also antagonize ACh at ganglionic (N_1) sites. In addition, the nondepolarizing blockers interact with certain drugs to potentiate skeletal muscle relaxation. Some *antibiotics,* such as streptomycin, and *general anesthetics,* such as halothane, cause prolonged neuromuscular blockade when used in combination with nondepolarizing blockers. These agents are discussed in later chapters.

Depolarizing Blockers

Neuromuscular blocking agents that actually promote depolarization of the motor endplate are known as **depolarizing blockers.** These skeletal muscle relaxants act like an excess of ACh to cause initial stimulation of skeletal muscle, which is then followed by relaxation. Flaccid paralysis is not produced. The initial stimulation is visible as skeletal muscle fasciculations, or fine tremors in muscle bundles. Irreversible cholinesterase inhibitors such as the organophosphates elevate ACh levels to such an extent that a depolarization type of neuromuscular block is produced. These drugs are neither classified nor employed as depolarizing blocking agents. However, they produce fasciculations, tremors, and muscle weakness (see Table 6–1).

REVERSAL OF NEUROMUSCULAR BLOCKADE

Because nondepolarizing skeletal muscle relaxants are competitive ACh antagonists, they form reversible complexes with nicotinic receptors. The effect can be reversed by making more ACh available for receptor interaction. This objective is best accomplished through the use of indirect-acting cholinergics, such as physostigmine, neostigmine, or edrophonium. These anticholinesterase drugs elevate ACh levels, thus allowing more ACh to compete with the nondepolarizing blockers for available N_2-nicotinic receptors on the motor endplate. If sufficient ACh is made available for neuromuscular transmission, the skeletal muscle blockade is reversed and normal muscle contraction returns.

If an anticholinesterase, such as physostigmine, is used in an attempt to reverse neuromuscular blockade caused by a depolarizing blocker, the relaxation becomes even more pronounced. In fact, cholinesterase inhibitor–type drugs are contraindicated in the reversal of a depolarizing block because the blockade is already being caused by an excess of ACh. Additional ACh provided by the drug action of an anticholinesterase would only make matters worse. Instead, reversal is accomplished by protecting the nicotinic receptors from the excess ACh. A nondepolarizing blocking agent provides the competitive antagonism needed to counter the action of the depolarizing blocking agent. As will be seen later, it is not practical to reverse the muscle relaxation normally produced by a *short-acting* depolarizing blocker.

A desensitization, or dual block, is an anomaly defined as an abnormal response to the depolarizing block produced by the drug succinylcholine. Reversal of this unusual succinylcholine blockade will be examined further in this chapter.

THERAPEUTIC AGENTS

Nondepolarizing Blockers

D-TUBOCURARINE. The prototype for nondepolarizing blockers is curare, or D-tubocurarine (Tubarine). Newer derivatives of curare exhibit fewer side effects. The greatest drawback of curare is its lack of receptor specificity. The drug is a potent neuromuscular blocker but also produces ganglionic blockade. Therefore, it may cause reduction of sympathetic vascular tone leading to hypotension. Additional side effects include the release of histamine from storage cells. Histamine release causes vasodilation and a further drop in blood pressure (see Table 9–3).

INDICATIONS. Neuromuscular blockers of the nondepolarizing type are routinely used preoperatively to produce flaccid paralysis of skeletal muscle. This state is desirable because it allows the surgeon to perform incisions and close wounds more easily during the course of surgery. The flaccid state can be achieved with general anesthetics alone but requires a deep level of anesthesia to totally abolish skeletal muscle contraction. Therefore, anesthesia is made safer by the preoperative use of nondepolarizing blockers because lighter anesthesia can then be used.

A patient with thoracic trauma such as flail chest who requires assisted ventilation may exhibit asynchronous breathing ("fighting the ventilator") caused by muscle spasms or neurologic problems. These patients may be given nondepolarizing blockers in an attempt to produce skeletal muscle relaxation to match patient effort with the ventilator.

Nondepolarizing blockers are administered to produce flaccid paralysis to protect skeletal muscle from being damaged during violent contractions. Such contractions may be caused by seizure disorders or electroconvulsant therapy.

In cases of normal depolarizing neuromuscular blockade, the use of nondepolarizing agents to competitively antagonize ACh allows resumption of skeletal muscle contractions. The use of a nondepolarizing blocker as a reversal agent is only beneficial, however, in cases of depolarizing block uncomplicated by a dual, or desensitization, block (see Succinylcholine below).

CONTRAINDICATIONS. Myasthenia gravis is characterized by insufficient amounts of ACh for neuromuscular transmission. The administration of a nondepolarizing blocking agent further reduces the amount of ACh available for neurotransmission and is therefore contraindicated.

A certain variability is seen in the response of individuals to some neuromuscular blocking agents. Cardiovascular and respiratory system differences are most common. Because of the possibility of bronchoconstriction, respiratory muscle paralysis, and prolonged apnea, artificial ventilation facilities, including airway management, ventilatory support, and oxygen, must be available. Lack of airway control and resuscitation facilities are contraindications for the use of neuromuscular blockers. The drugs are potentially hazardous and are generally administered only by anesthesiologists and other clinicians who have had extensive training in their use (Taylor, 1985).

Because nondepolarizing blockade is a feature of Phase II of a desensitizing block, the condition may be worsened by the administration of a nondepolarizing agent (see Succinylcholine below).

PRECAUTIONS. Histamine-liberating neuromuscular blockers, such as curare, may worsen a condition of bronchial asthma because histamine is a potent bronchoconstrictor.

The paralyzing action of skeletal muscle relaxants on respiratory muscles is always a precaution to be considered with this powerful class of drugs. The potential of the drugs to cause ventilatory depression and apnea demands that resuscitation equipment be near at hand.

Skeletal muscle relaxants have absolutely no effect on pain perception or on the level of consciousness in a patient. Other drug classes, such as *analgesics* and *sedatives,* are required

to alter these conditions. This precaution must be considered with the neuromuscular blockers.

If succinylcholine, a depolarizing blocker, has been administered previously, its effects must be allowed to diminish before a nondepolarizing blocker is given (Box 7–2).

METOCURINE (Metubine). Metocurine is similar to curare but possesses approximately two to three times the potency and fewer cardiovascular system side effects. Like curare it may cause the release of histamine, with all attendant side effects such as bronchoconstriction, vasodilation, and hypotension.

INDICATIONS, CONTRAINDICATIONS, AND PRECAUTIONS. See D-tubocurarine.

ATRACURIUM (Tracrium). Atracurium besylate is a nodepolarizing blocker similar to curare. It may cause histamine release.

BOX 7–2 ONE-TREE CURARE

"One-tree curare" is the best naturally produced **curare** in the world. South American Indians, on observing a monkey hit by a muscle-paralyzing, curare-tipped dart or arrow, rate the poison as being of excellent quality if the monkey only makes it from one tree to the next after being struck by the lethal missile.

After the influx of Spanish explorers, samples of curare began reaching Europe, but it was not until the early 19th century that the neuromuscular blocking properties of curare were systematically studied by the French researcher François Magendie and his successor Claude Bernard. These pioneers of the experimental method in pharmacology accurately described the mechanism of action of the drug at the NMJ and were able to demonstrate its paralyzing effect on animals.

Indians in the Amazon Valley and in the tropical rain forests of Guiana prepare darts and arrows with a resinous extract often containing poisonous substances from several plant sources. The method of preparation and the ingredients contained in the end-product are unique for different tribes in the region. The gummy residue rubbed on arrows and darts, to be used on animal and human prey alike, is made from a boiled extract of bark and wood taken from creeping vines, or "bushropes," called *pareira* (*Chondodendron tomentosum*) in Ecuador and Peru, and from *Strychnos lethalis* and other *Strychnos* species in more easterly areas. The residue of crude curare from these vines contains a neurologically active *bis*-isoquinoline alkaloid known as *tubocurarine.* It is stored by the natives in gourds, clay pots, or bamboo *tubes.* Hence, tube curare was the original source of *tubo*curarine used today.

Synthetic derivatives of curare eliminate the dependence on naturally grown foreign plant products, and in addition, exhibit improved pharmacologic activity in the form of fewer side effects, greater potency, and longer duration of action. (As an added bonus, they do not have to be stored in bamboo tubes on pharmacy shelves.)

Kreig M: Green Medicine. Rand McNally, New York, 1964.
Liska K: Drugs and the Human Body: With Implications for Society. Macmillan, New York, 1981.
Modell W, Lansing A, and Editors of Time-Life Books: Drugs. Life Science Library. Time, New York, 1969.
Taylor P: Neuromuscular blocking agents. In Goodman AG et al (eds): Goodman and Gilman's The Pharmacologic Basis of Therapeutics, ed 7. Macmillan, New York, 1985.

INDICATIONS, CONTRAINDICATIONS, AND PRE-CAUTIONS. See D-tubocurarine.

PANCURONIUM (Pavulon). A common non-depolarizing blocking agent is pancuronium bromide. It has five times more potency than cu-rare, lacks ganglionic blocking effects, and does not promote histamine release. Potential adverse effects include tachycardia and hypertension.

INDICATIONS, CONTRAINDICATIONS, AND PRE-CAUTIONS. See D-tubocurarine.

VECURONIUM (Norcuron). Vecuronium bromide is similar to pancuronium, but unlike pancuronium, it lacks any significant cardiovascular system effects and rarely causes tachycardia or blood pressure changes. It does not stimulate histamine release. Vecuronium exhibits about four times the potency of atracurium.

INDICATIONS, CONTRAINDICATIONS, AND PRE-CAUTIONS. See D-tubocurarine.

GALLAMINE (Flaxedil). The lack of a hista-mine-liberating response and the absence of bronchospastic activity make gallamine triethio-dide an excellent neuromuscular blocker for use in individuals with asthma. The major disadvantage exhibited by gallamine is its potential to cause tachycardia through an atropinelike blocking action at cardioinhibitory fibers. An increase in blood pressure and cardiac output is the outcome of the circulatory side effects.

INDICATIONS, CONTRAINDICATIONS, AND PRE-CAUTIONS. See D-tubocurarine.

Depolarizing Blockers

SUCCINYLCHOLINE (Anectine). Succinyl-choline, or suxamethonium, consists basically of two ACh molecules connected together. The chemical bond linking the two choline esters is rapidly hydrolyzed by plasma cholinesterase (pseudocholinesterase). Therefore, succinylcho-line acts like an excess of ACh at the NMJ once the enzyme has acted on it. The breakdown products cause initial muscle fasciculations followed by paralysis of skeletal muscle. At therapeutic doses, succinylcholine is selective for neuromuscular sites. At higher doses, however, it begins to affect the heart and blood vessels due to an ACh-like action resulting in bradycardia and hypotension.

The onset of action is less than 1 minute and the duration of action is short (5–10 minutes) because the drug is prone to enzymatic destruction by the plasma cholinesterases. The rapid inactivation by pseudocholinesterase is sufficient for reversal of the effect. Therefore, the use of nondepolarizing blockers to bring about rever-

sal is impractical. Succinylcholine is metabolized before the nondepolarizing effect of a curarelike drug can be established.

INDICATIONS. Recognized therapeutic uses for the depolarizing group of neuromuscular blocking agents include short-duration muscle relaxation, which is invaluable in procedures such as endotracheal intubation. Short-acting muscle relaxants are also used to facilitate laryngoscopy and bronchoscopy procedures when used in combination with a general anesthetic (Taylor, 1985).

PRECAUTIONS. In an interesting example of pharmacogenetics, a genetic defect occurring in some people results in the production of faulty, or atypical, cholinesterase. When given succinyl-choline, these individuals experience prolonged apnea and are prone to respiratory muscle paralysis that may persist for several *hours* instead of a few minutes (Clark et al, 1988). They may require assisted ventilation for the duration of the neuromuscular blockade. In order to screen these patients prior to administration of suc-cinylcholine, an assessment is made of their plasma cholinesterase level through determination of a *dibucaine number*. Dibucaine is a local anesthetic that has the ability to temporarily inhibit cholinesterase. On this comparison scale, a high dibucaine number such as 80 indicates that normal levels of cholinesterase are available. In other words, a large amount of dibucaine is required to inhibit the cholinesterase found in the plasma. Low dibucaine numbers such as 22 indicate that a relatively small amount of cholinesterase is available in the plasma. Patients having a low dibucaine number are unusually susceptible to the toxic effects of drugs such as succinylcholine that are normally degraded by the cholinesterase enzyme system (Clark et al, 1988).

In other individuals, the function of plasma cholinesterase is normal, but succinylcholine triggers a desensitization (dual) block. In such a response, a nondepolarizing blockade occurs after the initial depolarizing blockade. The depolarizing block is called **Phase I**; the nondepolarizing block is called **Phase II.** In individuals exhibiting this atypical response, cholinesterase inhibitor drugs, such as neostigmine, are used to boost ACh levels to help reverse Phase II. Because of the extreme variability in response among individuals, facilities for artificial ventilation are essential. This is the only reliable antidote to prolonged apnea (Clark et al, 1988).

A summary of the pharmacologic activity of a representative group of neuromuscular blockers is presented in Table 7–1. Drug names of the

TABLE 7–1 COMPARISON OF NEUROMUSCULAR BLOCKING AGENTS*

Drug	Type of Inhibition	Reversal of Inhibition by Cholinesterase Inhibition	Hydrolysis by Plasma Cholinesterase	Ganglionic Inhibition and Release of Histamine	Duration (min)
Curare	Competitive	Yes	No	Yes	30–40
Gallamine	Competitive	Yes	No	No	25–30
Pancuronium	Competitive	Yes	No	No	15–25
Succinylchloine	Depolarize end-plate	No—inhibition increased	Yes	No	5–8

Source: From Long, 1989; with permission.

*Initial depolarization of skeletal muscle produces fasciculations (contraction of skeletal muscle), possibly increases intraocular pressure by contracting extraocular skeletal muscles, and possibly releases potassium into the systemic circulation, which on rare occasions may depress cardiac muscle.

TABLE 7–2 DRUG NAMES: NICOTINIC ANTAGONISTS

Generic Name	Trade Name
GANGLIONIC BLOCKERS	
Mecamylamine (mek-ill-a-**MĒN**)	Inversine
NONDEPOLARIZING NEUROMUSCULAR BLOCKERS	
Curare (Ka-RAIR-ā)	Turarine
Metocurine (met-ō-KYOO-rēn) iodide	Metubine
Atracurium (a-tra-KYOO-rē-um)	Tracrium
Pancuronium (pan-kyoo-**RON**-ē-um) bromide	Pavulon
Vecuronium (vek-ū-**RON**-ē-um) bromide	Norcuron
Gallamine (**GAL**-a-mēn) triethiodide	Flaxedil
DEPOLARIZING NEUROMUSCULAR BLOCKERS	
Succinylcholine (sux-sin-il-**KŌ**-lēn) or suxamethonium (**SUX**-a-meth-ōn-ē-um)	Anectine

nicotinic antagonists covered in this chapter are summarized in Table 7–2.

CHAPTER SUMMARY

This chapter introduces the drugs that interfere with ACh neurotransmission at N_1- and N_2-nicotinic sites. A discussion of the ganglionic blockers is followed by a consideration of the neuromuscular blockers. The differing mechanisms of action of neuromuscular blockers are examined, as are the means employed to reverse skeletal muscle relaxation.

BIBLIOGRAPHY

Alpern RJ: The physiologic basis of neuromuscular transmission disorders (editorial). Hosp Pract (Off Ed) 27:12–13, Jul 15, 1992.

Carola R, Harley JP, and Noback CR: Human Anatomy and Physiology, ed 2. McGraw-Hill, New York, 1992.

Clark WG, Brater DC, and Johnson AR: Goth's Medical Pharmacology, ed 12. CV Mosby, St Louis, 1988.

Horn JP: The heroic age of neurophysiology. Physiology in Medicine Series. Hosp Pract (Off Ed) 27:65–74, Jul 15, 1992.

Howder CL: Cardiopulmonary Pharmacology: A Handbook for Respiratory Practitioners and Other Allied Health Personnel. Williams and Wilkins, Baltimore, 1992.

Kaminski HJ and Ruff RL: Congenital disorders of neuromuscular transmission. Physiology in Medicine Series. Hosp Pract (Off Ed) 27:73–85, Sep 15, 1992.

Katzung BG: Cholinergic receptor antagonists. In Katzung BD (ed): Basic and Clinical Pharmacology. Lange Medical Publications, Los Altos, 1982.

Lehnert BE and Schachter EN: The Pharmacology of Respiratory Care. CV Mosby, St Louis, 1980.

Long JP: Drugs acting on the peripheral nervous system. In Conn PM and Gebhart GF (eds): Essentials of Pharmacology. FA Davis, Philadelphia, 1989.

Martin AR: Principles of neuromuscular transmission. Physiology in Medicine Series. Hosp Pract (Off Ed) 27:147–158, Aug 15, 1992.

Miller RD: Skeletal muscle relaxants. In Katzung BD (ed): Basic and Clinical Pharmacology. Lange Medical Publications, Los Altos, 1982.

Neher E and Sakmann B: The patch clamp technique. Sci Am 266:44–51, Mar 1992.

Rau JL: Respiratory Care Pharmacology, ed 3. Yearbook Medical Publishers, Chicago, 1989.

Taylor, P: Neuromuscular blocking agents. In Goodman AG (ed): Goodman and Gilman's The Pharmacologic Basis of Therapeutics, ed 7. Macmillan, New York, 1985.

Tortora GJ and Grabowski SR: Principles of Anatomy and Physiology, ed 7. HarperCollins, New York, 1993.

Unwin N: The structure of ion channels in excitable cells. Neuron 3:665–676, 1989.

CHAPTER 8

Muscarinic Antagonists

CHAPTER OUTLINE

Chapter Introduction
Muscarinic Blockers
  TERMINOLOGY
  MECHANISM OF ACTION

Pharmacologic Effects
  TERTIARY AND QUATERNARY
    AMINES
  PERIPHERAL EFFECTS

CENTRAL EFFECTS
TOXIC EFFECTS
Therapeutic Agents
Chapter Summary

CHAPTER OBJECTIVES

After studying this chapter the reader should be able to:

- Review the location of muscarinic receptors and name the neurotransmitter and catabolic enzymes found at such sites.
- Describe the mechanism of action of muscarinic antagonist drugs.
- Define the following terms:
  - Anticholinergic, antimuscarinic, belladonna alkaloid, cycloplegic, miosis, mydriasis, parasympatholytic.
- Explain the role of secondary messengers in relation to the mechanism of action of muscarinic blocking agents.
- Explain the differences between tertiary and quaternary amine antimuscarinics on the basis of structure, solubility, and ease of penetration of the blood-brain barrier.
- Describe the peripheral and central effects of muscarinic antagonist drugs.
- Describe the symptoms of atropine toxicity and outline the treatment that would help manage the toxicity.
- Describe three indications and three contraindications for use of the muscarinic antagonists and explain the rationale behind each of their uses and limitations.
- Explain the precaution regarding the use of atropinelike antimuscarinics with an asthmatic condition.
- Describe the pharmacologic activity of the following muscarinic antagonist drugs:
  - atropine, scopolamine.

KEY TERMS

antimuscarinic (muscarinic
  antagonist,
  parasympatholytic)

belladonna alkaloid
cycloplegia (sī-klō-**PLĒ**-ja)

miosis (mī-**Ō**-sis)
mydriasis (mī-**DRI**-a-sis)

CHAPTER INTRODUCTION

Anticholinergics that compete with acetylcholine at muscarinic receptors are known as **muscarinic antagonists,** or **antimuscarinics.** These drugs primarily affect postganglionic neuroeffector synapses of the parasympathetic division. They are a versatile group of drugs employed for their antonomic effects on the eye, the gastrointestinal and urinary tracts, and the respiratory system. In addition, a few members of the group exhibit prominent actions on the central nervous system (CNS).

MUSCARINIC BLOCKERS

Terminology

Drugs that interfere with muscarinic transmission are referred to as **muscarinic antagonists, antimuscarinics,** or **parasympatholytics** (see Table 5–6). In addition, the term *anticholinergic* is often used, but has a more general application because it can also refer to nicotinic blockers. The prototype muscarinic antagonist drug atropine is derived from the *Atropa belladonna* plant. Hence, muscarinic antagonists are also referred to as **belladonna alkaloids** (Box 8–1).

Mechanism of Action

The mechanism of action of muscarinic antagonist drugs and the resulting change in autonomic balance can be discussed in several ways. (Details of these mechanisms are presented in Chapter 5.) First, muscarinic antagonist drugs block parasympathetic neurotransmission. This block allows sympathetic effects to go unopposed, and results in changes such as reflex tachycardia, pupil dilation, and decreased gastrointestinal and urinary tract motility (see Fig. 5–5). Second, because of their autonomic receptor activity, antimuscarinic drugs possess affinity but lack efficacy. They exhibit competitive antagonism with acetylcholine (ACh) for available postjunctional M_3-muscarinic receptors (see Fig. 5–7). The complexes formed between the antagonist drug and muscarinic receptors are reversible. The autonomic imbalance created, however, temporarily allows norepinephrine-adrenergic receptor complexes to predominate and trigger characteristic sympathetic organ responses. Finally, the temporary blockade of muscarinic receptors inhibits guanylate cyclase, thereby reducing the amount of cGMP (cyclic guanosine-3′,5′–monophosphate) formed (see Fig. 5–14). The resulting intracellular balance of secondary messengers shifts toward AMP (cy-

---

BOX 8–1　BELLADONNA ALKALOIDS AND BEAUTY

Muscarinic antagonist compounds are some of the oldest drugs employed in medicine. Their use both as medicinal agents and as poisons adds an interesting and colorful chapter to the history of pharmacology. They are found in a variety of natural substances, mainly in plants belonging to the deadly nightshade family (*Solanaceous* plants) and in a few poisonous species of the *Amanita* genus of mushrooms (eg, *A. muscaria,* or fly agaric, and *A. phalloides,* or death cup). Two chemically similar drugs, atropine and scopolamine, are found in various members of the above-mentioned plant and fungus groups. The active substances found in these sources are alkaloids known as L-hyoscyamine and L-hyoscine. L-Hyocine is also known as scopolamine. In DL-hyoscyamine, or atropine, a racemic mixture occurs during the extraction process. Such a mixture is a 50:50 combination of two stereoisomers, or optical isomers—a D-isomer and an L-isomer. (Optical isomers have identical molecular formulas but have structural features that are mirror images of each other.) L-Hyoscyamine is approximately 20 times more potent than D-hyoscyamine.

Atropine and scopolamine are called **belladonna alkaloids** because they are found in the deadly nightshade plant (*Atropa belladonna*). Jimsonweed, also known as locoweed, thorn apple, or stinkweed (*Datura stramonium*), contains L-hyoscyamine; black henbane (*Hyoscyamus niger*) is a source of L-hyoscine.

Over several centuries, in widely scattered countries, women have added extracts of belladonna to their eyes to produce expansive pupils. Ophthalmologists still do it today. The extremely large, dark eyes that result were seen as a sign of beauty (not of the inability to focus!); hence the name *belladonna,* which means "beautiful woman."

Gerald MC: Pharmacology: An Introduction to Drugs. Prentice-Hall, Englewood Cliffs, NJ, 1981.
Lewis WH and Elvin-Lewis MPF: Medical Botany. John Wiley and Sons, New York, 1977.
Weiner N: Atropine, scopolamine, and related antimuscarinic drugs. In Goodman, AG et al (eds): Goodman and Gilman's The Pharmacologic Basis of Therapeutics, ed 7. Macmillan, New York, 1985.

clic adenosine-3′,5′-monophosphate) predominance to cause characteristic changes such as bronchodilation, increased heart rate, and decreased glandular secretions (see Table 5–1).

PHARMACOLOGIC EFFECTS
Tertiary and Quaternary Amines

The ability of antimuscarinics to produce peripheral or central nervous system effects is proportional to their transfer from the bloodstream into brain tissue. The potential of such drugs to penetrate the blood-brain barrier is a reflection of their chemical structure.

The naturally occurring antimuscarinics, atropine and scopolamine, and some synthetic derivatives, possess a nitrogen atom attached in two places to the main portion of the molecule. Such compounds also have a chemical group attached to the nitrogen, producing a nitrogen atom with three bonds in all. A molecule possessing such a chemical configuration is called a *tertiary amine compound* (Fig. 8–1). Tertiary amines are able to cross the blood-brain barrier with relative ease. Therefore, both central and peripheral effects are produced. Applied topically, tertiary amines penetrate the cornea of the eye and are valuable in ophthalmology.

Molecules that contain a nitrogen atom having four bonds are classified as *quaternary amine compounds* (Fig. 8–1). Some of these drugs have been developed to reduce the occurrence of CNS effects. Antimuscarinics of the quaternary amine type exhibit minimal ability to cross the blood-brain barrier due to their low lipid solubility. The quaternary amines are ideally suited for the production of peripheral effects in the cardiovascular, gastrointestinal, and respiratory systems. The pharmacologic activity of quaternary amines such as ipratropium (Atrovent) is examined in Chapter 11. These antimuscarinic bronchodilators are used to treat certain dysfunctions of the respiratory system.

Peripheral Effects

The belladonna alkaloids exhibit a variety of peripheral effects on smooth muscle, cardiac muscle, and glandular tissue. Although competitive antagonism with ACh is seen at all M_3-muscarinic sites, there is a difference in sensitivity of response that is dose dependent (Table 8–1). Small doses produce effects such as dry mouth and inhibition of sweating due to the antimuscarinic effect on glands. Large doses block the cardiac vagal response, thus allowing sympathetic impulses to raise the heart rate. Smooth muscle of the gastrointestinal and urinary tracts is inhibited by even larger amounts of the drug. However, the dose required to inhibit gastric secretion is so large that secondary sites such as the heart, having greater sensitivity, are blocked first. This effect somewhat limits the use of at-

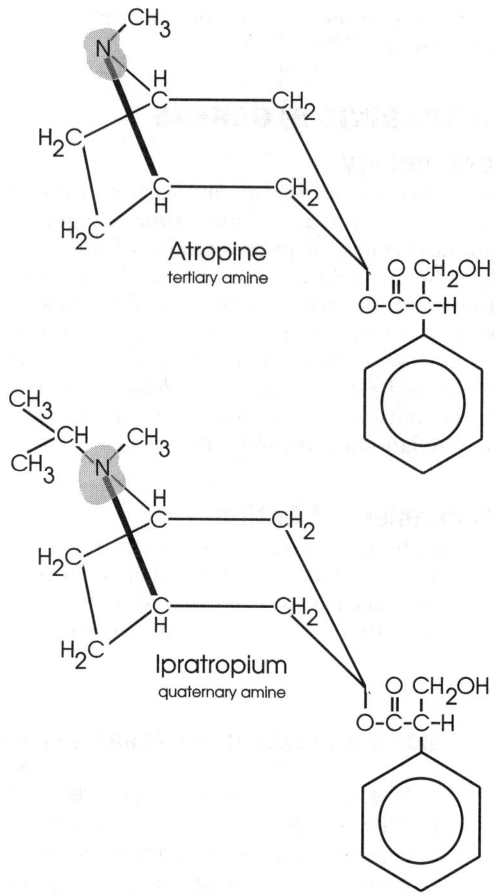

FIGURE 8–1 Muscarinic antagonists, showing tertiary and quaternary structures.

TABLE 8–1 SENSITIVITY OF RESPONSE
Peripheral Effects of Muscarinic Antagonists

Pharmacologic Effect Produced	Relative Dose Required
Inhibition of salivary and sweat glands	+++
Cardiac vagal blockade	++++
Inhibition of gastrointestinal and urinary tract smooth muscle	+++++
Inhibition of gastric secretion	++++++

ropine and scopolamine in the treatment of gastrointestinal disturbances. Some atropine derivatives, however, have been developed with more selective gastrointestinal tract activity.

Peripheral effects on smooth muscle of the eye represent a special case. Pupil diameter is controlled by the smooth muscle fibers of the iris. Concentric (circularly arranged) fibers are under parasympathetic control, and contraction results in pupil constriction, or **miosis.** Antagonistic action is provided by radially arranged fibers that contract under sympathetic control to produce pupil dilation, or **mydriasis.** The ciliary body (muscle) of the eye adjusts tension on the suspensory ligaments and the lens to change the shape of the lens. This allows the focal length of the eye to be altered (accommodation). The ciliary muscle is innervated through the parasympathetic division only. When muscarinic antagonist drugs are administered as ophthalmic solutions for eye examinations, mydriasis is produced as the sphincter (circular) muscle fibers of the iris are inhibited, allowing the effects of the radial fibers to predominate. In addition, paralysis of accommodation, or **cycloplegia,** occurs as the cholinergic effects on the ciliary muscle are inhibited.

Central Effects

As outlined above, tertiary amine muscarinic antagonists are able to cross the blood-brain barrier and enter brain tissue due to their lipid solubility. At overdose levels, the belladonna alkaloids may cause excitement and hallucinations. At therapeutic levels, however, they are used as adjuncts, or complements, to treat the symptoms of Parkinson's disease. Parkinsonism is a neuromuscular disorder characterized by tremors and muscular rigidity. Preoperative use of antimuscarinics, such as scopolamine, produces sleepiness and represents another example of central effects produced by the muscarinic antagonists.

Toxic Effects

The therapeutic use of antimuscarinic drugs causes several relatively minor, but unpleasant, side effects such as blurred vision, dry mouth, and constipation. The classic description of a person with atropine poisoning, however, is a vastly different picture, with the victim "as dry as a bone, red as a beet, and as mad as the Mad Hatter." Toxic doses lead to peripheral effects such as dilated pupils not responding to light, skin that is hot, flushed, and dry, and reflex tachycardia. Central effects include excitement, mania, and hallucinations. Management of atropine toxicity includes *sedatives* to counter the CNS stimulation, and administration of anticholinesterases such as physostigmine to provide sufficient ACh to compete with the excessive atropine levels. Some drugs belonging to the *antihistaminic* and *tranquilizer* classifications produce atropinelike side effects. These drugs may contribute to atropine toxicities.

THERAPEUTIC AGENTS

ATROPINE. Atropine is the prototype of the naturally occurring belladonna alkaloids. It contains an alkaloid known as DL-hyoscyamine. Atropine has a powerful effect on the smooth muscle of the eye, but possesses too long a duration of action to make it valuable as a mydriatic-cycloplegic drug. It is, however, the drug of choice in several other indications.

INDICATIONS. The use of antimuscarinics such as atropine prior to surgery is based on their ability to affect cardiac muscle, smooth muscle, and glands. Through blockade of muscarinic receptors, the heart is prevented from slowing in the event that the vagus nerve is mechanically stimulated during intubation. In addition, gastrointestinal and urinary tract motility are decreased, and the secretory activity of salivary, tracheobronchial, and digestive glands is reduced during surgery. These changes are desirable in the unconscious patient because clearance mechanisms such as swallowing and coughing are inoperative. Newer general anesthetics such as halothane cause minimal glandular secretion. Therefore, the need to premedicate with atropinelike drugs is reduced in comparison to some of the earliest general anesthetics such as ethyl ether.

Gastrointestinal tract disturbances such as gastric secretion and hypermotility can be treated with drugs that block parasympathetic neurotransmission. The mechanism of action allows unopposed sympathetic effects, resulting in reduced motility and cramps. Muscarinic antagonists employed for this purpose are referred to as *antispasmodics.* Although reduction in gastric secretion can be accomplished by antimuscarinics, a relatively large dose is required, and side effects such as tachycardia may be produced before control of gastric secretion occurs. Muscarinic antagonist drugs are useful given in conjunction with certain antihistamines and antacids in the treatment of gastric ulcer to delay gastric emptying and reduce acid secretion.

Reflex tachycardia occurs through the administration of antimuscarinic drugs because cardio-acceleratory (sympathetic) impulses are unopposed. This mechanism is useful in reversing an abnormally slow rhythm in the heart (bradyarrhythmia). Such conditions may result from increased vagal activity following an acute myocardial infarction (AMI). (An AMI is a sudden occlusion, or blockage, of coronary blood vessels supplying the myocardium.)

Toxic levels of cholinergic drugs can be countered by antimuscarinic drugs. Through competitive antagonism with ACh, antimuscarinics such as atropine occupy muscarinic receptors and prevent ACh or its derivatives from gaining access to the receptors (see "Management of Anticholinesterase Toxicities" in Chapter 6).

The tertiary amine antimuscarinic drugs provide a degree of relief from bronchospasm in vagally mediated asthma. This is brought about through a reduction in bronchomotor tone. Excessive secretion by tracheobronchial glands is called *bronchorrhea*. Such a condition can be effectively controlled by the tertiary amines. Newer quaternary amine derivatives exhibit minimal drying effects on tracheobronchial glands and are potent bronchodilators.

CONTRAINDICATIONS. If the smooth muscle of the gastrointestinal or urinary tract is hypoactive, introduction of a drug that blocks parasympathetic impulses would obviously prolong the condition of stasis. Lack of smooth muscle activity can lead to bowel obstruction in cases of paralytic ileus and complete urinary retention if bladder tone is significantly reduced.

Because muscarinic antagonists produce reflex tachycardia, they are contraindicated in cases of preexisting tachyarrhythmia.

Blockade of muscarinic receptors in the eye produces mydriasis. Accompanying the mydriatic response is a decrease in the anterior chamber angle as the ciliary body changes position and decreases accommodation (see Fig. 6–3). With a reduced anterior chamber angle, there is decreased drainage of aqueous humor from the anterior chamber. This decrease results in increased intraocular pressure. Because the rise in intraocular pressure worsens a condition of glaucoma, muscarinic antagonists are contraindicated. When an ophthalmologic examination is necessary in a person with glaucoma or a predisposition to glaucoma, sympathomimetic drugs can be given to produce the required mydriatic response. They do not, however, produce cycloplegia because the ciliary muscle is not innervated through the sympathetic division of the autonomic nervous system.

PRECAUTIONS. The introduction of a musca-rinic antagonist drug in a condition of bronchial asthma risks the production of inspissated (dried) secretions in the airways. The anticholinergic effect of drugs such as atropine on tracheobronchial glands may cause drying of airway secretions. As was discussed above, the use of newer agents such as ipratropium minimizes the drying effect.

As explained in Chapter 5, atropine is a non-selective antimuscarinic, blocking at M_2- and M_3-muscarinic receptors. Because prejunctional M_2-muscarinic receptors function as autoreceptors to limit ACh release, blockade may result in elevated ACh levels and increased muscarinic stimulation (see Cholinergic Receptors in Chapter 5). This effect in turn may lead to increased bronchomotor tone and airway resistance (Barnes, 1993). Newer subtype-selective anti-muscarinics are discussed in Chapter 11.

SCOPOLAMINE. Scopolamine is a naturally occurring belladonna alkaloid known as *L-hyoscine*. It has a chemical structure very similar to that of atropine. Scopolamine and atropine produce similar effects on the cardiovascular system and on the eye, but differ in the CNS effects produced at therapeutic levels. At low doses both drugs produce sedation, and at high doses both produce CNS stimulation such as excitement, restlessness, and hallucinations. At very high doses of either drug, coma, respiratory depression, and death may occur. Therapeutic doses of scopolamine, however, cause sleepiness, whereas therapeutic doses of atropine fail to produce sedation (Fig. 8–2).

INDICATIONS. The primary indications for use are the same as those described for atropine. Scopolamine has been used in the treatment of parkinsonism, but produces comparatively severe peripheral side effects relative to the symptomatic relief provided.

Scopolamine is a tertiary amine and therefore crosses the blood-brain barrier. As was described above, scopolamine at therapeutic doses produces CNS depression. The development of se-

TABLE 8-2   DRUG NAMES: NATURALLY OCCURRING ANTIMUSCARINICS

Generic Name	Trade Name
Atropine (**A**-trō-pēn) Scopolamine (skō-**PAWL**-a-mēn)	(Belladonna alkaloids are given as pure substances or as galenic preparations. Trade names are not used.)

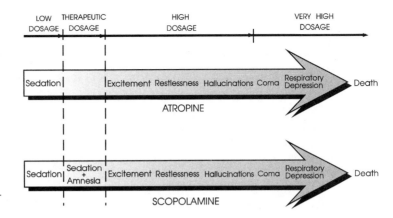

FIGURE 8–2 CNS effects of tertiary amine antimuscarinics.

dation and amnesia make scopolamine especially attractive as a preoperative medication.

The symptomatic treatment of motion sickness is also an indication for use of scopolamine because it decreases gastrointestinal motility and secretion.

CONTRAINDICATIONS AND PRECAUTIONS. See Atropine.

Generic names of the antimuscarinic drugs discussed in this chapter are listed in Table 8–2. Trade names are often not available for drugs that have been in continuous use for many years. Pharmaceutical companies market such drugs by generic name only. This unique feature applies to atropine and scopolamine, drugs that have been used for centuries. The belladonna alkaloids are used in pure form or in *galenic preparations*—standard preparations containing one or several organic substances as contrasted with pure chemical substances (Clark et al, 1988). The term originally referred to the ancient formulas of Galen (Greek physician, circa AD 130–200).

CHAPTER SUMMARY

The tertiary amine cholinergic antagonists acting at M_3-muscarinic receptors are discussed in this chapter. An examination of the mechanism of action and pharmacologic activity of the antimuscarinics is carried out through the study of atropine as the prototype drug. The chapter also covers some of the peripheral, central, and toxic effects exhibited by the group. Quaternary amine derivatives having specific pulmonary use are covered in the following unit.

BIBLIOGRAPHY

Barnes PJ: Autonomic pharmacology of the airways. In Chung KF and Barnes PJ (eds): Pharmacology of the Respiratory Tract: Experimental and Clinical Research. Marcel Dekker, New York, 1993.

Bethel AB and Irvin CG: Anticholinergic, antimuscarinic drugs (atropine sulfate, ipratropium bromide). In Cherniak RM (ed): Drugs for the Respiratory System. Grune and Stratton, Orlando, 1986.

Clark WG, Brater DC, and Johnson AR: Goth's Medical Pharmacology, ed 12. CV Mosby, St Louis, 1988.

Howder CL: Cardiopulmonary Pharmacology: A Handbook for Respiratory Practitioners and Other Allied Health Personnel. Williams and Wilkins, Baltimore, 1992.

Katzung BG: Cholinergic receptor antagonists. In Katzung BD (ed): Basic and Clinical Pharmacology. Lange Medical Publications, Los Altos, 1982.

Lehnert BE and Schachter EN: The Pharmacology of Respiratory Care. CV Mosby, St Louis, 1980.

Long JP: Drugs acting on the peripheral nervous system. In Conn PM and Gebhart GF (eds): Essentials of Pharmacology. FA Davis, Philadelphia, 1989.

Rau JL: Respiratory Care Pharmacology, ed 3. Yearbook Medical Publishers, Chicago, 1989.

Weiner N: Atropine, scopolamine, and related antimuscarinic drugs. In Goodman, AG et al (eds): Goodman and Gilman's The Pharmacologic Basis of Therapeutics, ed 7. Macmillan, New York, 1985.

DRUGS AFFECTING THE RESPIRATORY SYSTEM

UNIT INTRODUCTION

Bronchoactive drugs are used to promote bronchiolar smooth muscle relaxation, to alter the consistency of respiratory tract secretions, or to reduce the volume of such secretions. Included in this category are the various drug classifications that make up Unit 3: antiallergics, histamine receptor antagonists, antimuscarinic bronchodilators, β_2-agonists, methylxanthines, glucocorticoids, mucokinetic agents, and others. Most of these chemically dissimilar groups promote bronchodilation directly at bronchiolar smooth muscle or indirectly through the control of mediators responsible for the narrowing of air passages. Control of such mediators often controls secretions as well. Mucokinetic agents alter the viscosity and/or the volume of secretions from the exocrine glands of the airways. The bronchoactive drugs are a formidable group containing most of the therapeutic agents with which the respiratory care practitioner comes into contact.

CHAPTER 9

Allergic Mediators

CHAPTER OUTLINE

CHAPTER OBJECTIVES

After studying this chapter the reader should be able to:

- Briefly describe the mechanism of allergy, including the role of antigens, antibodies, target cells, and effector cells.
- Differentiate between primary and secondary exposure to an antigen.
- Explain the physiologic mechanism responsible for a typical wheal-and-flare allergic reaction.
- Define the following:
  - spasmogen, hapten, atopic, autacoid.
- Briefly compare the allergic responses seen in hay fever, asthma, and anaphylaxis.
- Name three different target cells and list the allergic mediators produced by each.
- Describe the role of the intracellular cAMP-cGMP system in the allergic response.
- List the physiologic effects produced by the following allergic mediators:
  - Histamine, eosinophil chemotactic factor of anaphylaxis (ECF-A), neutrophil chemotactic factor of anaphylaxis (NCF-A), platelet-activation factor (PAF), prostaglandins ($PGF_{2\alpha}$, PGD_2), leukotrienes (LTB_4, LTC_4, LTD_4, LTE_4), thromboxane (TXA_2), bradykinin.

KEY TERMS

allergic mediators
  bradykinin
  eosinophil chemotactic factor of
    anaphylaxis (ECF-A)
  histamine
  leukotrienes (LTs)
  neutrophil chemotactic factor of
    anaphylaxis (NCF-A)
  platelet activation factor (PAF)
  prostaglandins (PGs)
  thromboxane (TXA_2)
allergy
anaphylaxis (anaphylactic
  reaction)

antibody
antigen (allergen)
antigen-antibody reaction
arachidonic (a-**RACK**-i-don-ik)
  acid
atopic
autacoid
bronchial asthma (reactive
  airway disease)
challenge reaction (secondary
  exposure; shocking dose)
chemoattractant

cyclooxygenase (sī-klō-**OXY**-jen-
  ās)
eicosanoids
eosinophilia
γ-globulin (gamma globulin;
  immunoglobulin)
hapten
hay fever (allergic rhinitis;
  seasonal rhinitis)
immunoglobulin E (IgE)
lipoxygenase (lī-**POX**-i-je-nās)
primary exposure (sensitization;
  sensitizing dose)

prostanoid
resistance factors
  acquired resistance
  natural resistance
spasmogen

status asthmaticus
target cell
  basophil
  eosinophil

mast cell (tissue basophil)
neutrophil
platelet (thrombocyte)
wheal-and-flare reaction

CHAPTER INTRODUCTION

Most of the bronchoactive agents discussed in Unit 3 bring about the relaxation of airway smooth muscle and the control of airway secretions through two mechanisms. These drugs act *directly* at effector organs and *indirectly* at the specialized cells that manufacture and store mediators of the allergic response. A few bronchoactive drugs exert control through only one mechanism.

This chapter introduces the principal mediators of the allergic response. These mediators are the inflammatory compounds released as part of allergic reactions such as hay fever and asthma. Some of the compounds are **spasmogens,** or substances which induce bronchospasm. Others are **chemoattractants** that promote the accumulation of additional spasmogen-containing storage cells. Associated topics concerning the mechanism of allergy and the role of target cells are also included in the chapter.

MECHANISM OF ALLERGY

Resistance Factors

Several different lines of defense provide protection from foreign substances. Some of these **resistance factors** are present at birth, whereas others occur after exposure to foreign material. The first line of defense is made up of physical and chemical barriers such as unbroken skin, mucus membranes, tear secretion in the eyes, and acid production in the stomach. The second line of defense is a cellular defense consisting of phagocytic cells, including some of the leukocytes in the bloodstream and their derivatives, such as alveolar macrophages in the lungs. **Natural resistance** consists of the first and second lines of defense and is a nonspecific type of resistance. Such a defense is not directed at any one particular noxious substance or microorganism, but provides a general defense for the tissues. By contrast, the third line of defense is termed a *humoral defense* and is very specific. It is known as **acquired resistance,** and is not fully developed when a baby is born. Instead, it must be acquired following exposure to foreign substances.

Antigens

Foreign materials capable of stimulating the body's immune system are known as **antigens,** or **allergens.** Most of them are high molecular weight proteins and include many substances with which we come into contact daily. Some are found in the diet, others originate in plants and animals, a few are drug molecules, and many consist of substances derived from pathogenic microorganisms. Prophylactic, or protective, immunization against infective diseases is based on artificial stimulation of the immune system. This is accomplished through the introduction of modified antigenic substances of microbial origin.

Some drug molecules are too simple to act as antigens on their own, but are capable of combining with circulating plasma proteins. In this way the drug molecule gains both molecular weight and antigenic status. A drug combining in such a fashion is termed a **hapten** (Fig. 9–1). Hapten formation is responsible for many drug allergies.

Antibodies

Antigens are generally present in extremely small quantities. For example, microgram amounts are usually sufficient to trigger an immune response. The response involves production of highly specific proteins called **antibodies,** which are released by cells in lymphoid tissue. There is a lag time between introduction of the antigen and the first appearance of antibodies in the bloodstream. This latent interval is quite variable, ranging from a few days to several months. The plasma proteins that are converted into antibodies are known as **γ-globulins** (gamma-globulin), or **immunoglobulins.** The specific immunoglobulin serving as an antibody in allergic responses is **immunoglobulin E (IgE).** IgE antibodies have a three-dimensional shape that precisely matches that of a particular antigen. The exact conformation is necessary for host antibodies to bridge, or connect with, a foreign antigen to neutralize it (Fig. 9–2). Two unique features of the allergic response, therefore, are the high sensitivity and the high specificity of the reaction.

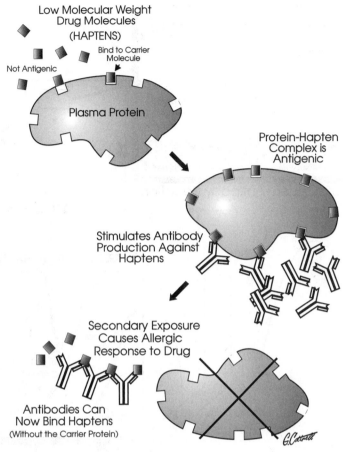

Low Molecular Weight
Drug Molecules
(HAPTENS)

Bind to Carrier
Molecule

Not Antigenic

Plasma Protein

Protein-Hapten
Complex is
Antigenic

Stimulates Antibody
Production Against
Haptens

Secondary Exposure
Causes Allergic
Response to Drug

Antibodies Can
Now Bind Haptens
(Without the Carrier Protein)

FIGURE 9–1 Haptens.

Primary Versus Secondary Exposure

Presentation of antigen to the immune system through initial exposure or as a result of repeated exposure to the same antigen may result in **sensitization.** This **primary exposure,** or **sensitizing dose,** is the antigenic stimulus that induces special cells in the immune system to produce specific antibodies. More important, it is the stimulus that causes memory cells in the immune system to retain a structural record of the specific antibody. This "blueprint" for future production of antibodies is invaluable because it enables the immune system to mount a rapid antibody response. **Secondary exposure** to an identical antigen is called the **shocking dose,** or **challenge reaction.** Such a reaction is characterized by a rapid rise in the plasma level of antibodies caused by the activity of the immune system memory cells (Fig. 9–3).

The **antigen–antibody reaction** is a neutralization reaction whereby the foreign protein is complexed by a bridging action between two antibody molecules (Fig. 9–3). The reaction takes place at the surface of target cells, which respond by releasing **allergic mediators.** The mediators in turn produce the symptoms of **allergy.** The immune reaction outlined above is termed the *humoral antibody response.*

ALLERGIC RESPONSES

Severity

Allergic responses vary considerably in severity. At one end of the spectrum is a localized and minor skin reaction to an insect bite. At the other extreme is a life-threatening anaphylactic reaction complete with widespread bronchospasm and falling blood pressure. Between the two extremes are mild dermatitis, urticaria (hives), hay fever, and some types of asthma.

Most allergic responses involve antigen-anti-

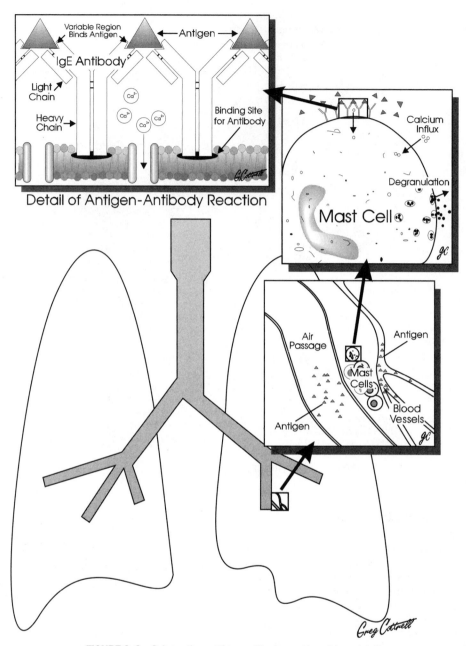

FIGURE 9–2 Schematic—antigen-antibody reaction at target cell.

body reactions and the release of inflammatory mediators. The basic differences between minor and severe inflammatory reactions depend on the *type* and *amount* of mediators released.

A typical localized inflammatory reaction can be observed with a mosquito bite or a positive allergy skin test. This characteristic tissue response is the classic **wheal-and-flare reaction.**

The signs of a raised, fluid-filled area (wheal) surrounded by a diffuse pink region (flare) are familiar to everyone and are produced by histamine, a powerful inflammatory mediator. Histamine causes an increase in capillary permeability resulting in leakage of plasma into interstitial spaces. The fluid shift causes edema and the wheal of the response. Histamine also

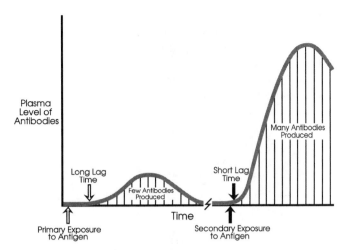

FIGURE 9-3 Graph—antibody response (primary versus secondary exposure).

causes vasodilation, which results in increased blood flow to the region and the clinical sign of redness, or erythema. This is the typical flare of the localized inflammatory response. The action of multiple inflammatory mediators operating on a massive scale in more serious allergic reactions, such as bronchial asthma, helps explain the severity and clinical symptoms of such a disorder.

Types of Allergic Reactions

As was pointed out above, allergic reactions may be mild or severe, depending on the type and amount of allergic mediator released. A minor allergic reaction is **hay fever,** characterized by nasal and sinus congestion, irritated eyes, and glandular hypersecretion. In addition, the nasal mucosa is hyperreactive, resulting in repeated bouts of sneezing as the body attempts to clear the upper respiratory passages. Many plant pollens and molds unique to different geographic regions serve as the antigenic stimuli to trigger the reaction. Because most of the allergenic substances appear seasonally, the condition is also called **seasonal rhinitis.**

Bronchial asthma, or **reactive airways disease,** is a reversible state characterized by increased reactivity of the respiratory tract to multiple stimuli. Wheezing and dyspnea are seen clinically, often accompanied by an irritating cough and airway secretions. The events that characterize an asthmatic episode are shown in Figure 9–4. Most drug therapies employed in the treatment of bronchial asthma target one or more sites in this vicious cycle. Treatments include control of mediator release, relaxation of airway smooth muscle, and inhibition of glandular secretion.

For example, *antiallergics* and *glucocorticoids* help control mediator production and release. *Antimuscarinic bronchodilators,* β_2-*agonists,* and *methylxanthines* promote bronchodilation; *mucokinetics* alter the amount and type of glandular secretions produced in the airways.

Status asthmaticus is a life-threatening condition of intense and continuous symptoms of asthma. The symptoms are intractable, or resistant, to the maximal dose of the drugs normally employed to control acute attacks.

Anaphylaxis (reversed, or altered, protection) is a very serious immune response characterized by widespread peripheral vasodilation, a dangerous fall in blood pressure, laryngospasm, and intense bronchoconstriction. The reaction is relatively rare because it involves deliberate injection of a large amount of antigen to a previously sensitized person.

Allergic reactions affecting the respiratory system are summarized in Table 9–1 with a listing of causative factors, symptoms, and treatment. The reader is encouraged to consult pathophysiology textbooks for added information regarding the classification of different types of bronchial asthma.

TARGET CELLS

Target cells function as specialized cells for the production and storage of allergic mediators (Fig. 9–7). These cells are *targets* for antigen-antibody reactions. The neutralization action that occurs at a target cell membrane between an antigen and specialized antibodies causes extracellular calcium ions to enter the cell (Fig. 9–2). Calcium ion inflow, in turn, destabilizes the target cell and causes it to degranulate. Stored al-

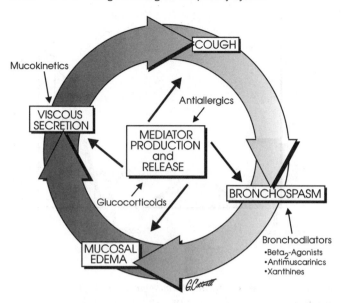

FIGURE 9–4   Schematic—bronchial asthma, showing "vicious cycle" plus sites of drug action.

TABLE 9–1   ALLERGIC REACTIONS: RESPIRATORY SYSTEM

Reaction	Causative Factors	Remarks	Drug Treatment
Hay Fever (allergic or seasonal rhinitis)	Plant pollens Molds	Seasonal	α-Mucosal vasoconstrictors H$_1$-Histamine blockers Inhaled antiallergics Inhaled glucocorticoids
Bronchial asthma (reactive airways disease)	(See subtypes below.)	Acute or chronic Reversible	Inhaled β$_2$-agonist bronchodilators Inhaled antimuscarinic bronchodilators Oral xanthine bronchodilators Inhaled antiallergics Inhaled and parenteral glucocorticoids Inhaled mucokinetics
Extrinsic asthma (allergic or atopic asthma)	IgE associated (dusts, plant pollens, foods, or drugs)	Most common in children and adolescents	(See Bronchial Asthma.)
Intrinsic asthma (idiopathic, infective, or nonatopic asthma)	Non–IgE associated (respiratory tract infections, exercise)	Most common in middle-aged adults	(See Bronchial Asthma.)
Status asthmaticus	Any of the above	Intense symptoms unrelieved by maximal doses of drugs	Parenteral β$_2$ bronchodilators (e.g., subcutaneous epinephrine) Xanthine bronchodilators (e.g., intravenous aminophylline) Glucocorticoids
Anaphylaxis (anaphylactic shock)	Large amount of antigen (insect or snake venom, blood type mismatch, drug injection in a previously sensitized person)	True anaphylaxis is uncommon (compared with hay fever or bronchial asthma)	Parenteral epinephrine (SC) (Airway maintenance and mechanical ventilation support as needed)

IgE = immunoglobulin E.

lergic mediators, such as histamine, that are in an active, preformed state bring about a rapid response in the tissues. Inactive precursors must be converted to active forms by enzymes; therefore, the tissue response is not as rapid. Some target cells are numerous and play a major role in allergic reactions, whereas less numerous target cells serve a minor function.

Basophilic leukocytes, or **basophils,** are leukocytes (white blood cells) that occasionally leave the bloodstream to reside in surrounding tissues. Here they are called **tissue basophils,** or **mast cells.** Many tissues have a resident population of mast cells, often scattered along small blood vessels and in loose connective tissue. The lungs, including the mucosal linings of small-diameter airways, are especially well endowed with such cells. Mast cells are the largest storage pool of histamine. The mediator is synthesized from inactive precursors and put into cytoplasmic storage granules. Mast cells also are the source of chemotactic factors and precursors of histaminelike allergic mediators. Such substances are released when mast cells degranulate following an antigen-antibody reaction. Such reactions are commonplace at the surface of mast cells because many binding sites exist for the attachment of **IgE** antibody.

Leukocytes such as basophils, **eosinophils,** and **neutrophils** synthesize small amounts of histamine. Such cells accumulate in areas of tissue inflammation. **Thrombocytes,** or **platelets,** synthesize thromboxane (TXA_2), another smooth muscle-contracting mediator. Leukocytes and thrombocytes are drawn to areas of inflammation by the action of chemoattractants released during the degranulation of mast cells. For example, eosinophil chemotactic factor of anaphylaxis (ECF-A) causes **eosinophilia,** or an accumulation of eosinophils in inflammatory exudate. This hematologic finding is clinically significant because eosinophilia often accompanies an allergic reaction, such as bronchial asthma. Table 9–2 lists various target cells, the allergic mediators produced by them, and the function of the allergic mediators.

MEDIATORS OF THE ALLERGIC RESPONSE

An **autacoid** is a tissue hormone. The Greek word means *self-remedy* or *self-medicinal* and refers to a group of local hormones that exert their physiologic effects at or near the site where they are synthesized. The various mediators of the allergic response are included in this autacoid classification.

Histamine

Histamine, the prototype allergic mediator, plays a protective role in the tissues when it is released in small amounts. It prevents the spread of potentially damaging material such as microorganisms by promoting edema formation in affected tissues. Histamine also carries out a protective function by causing vasodilation to bring about a local increase in blood flow. This increase delivers additional leukocytes and nutrients to the affected area. Some **atopic** individuals are extremely sensitive to the presence of antigens in the tissues and respond by releasing massive amounts of stored histamine from target cells. The result is that edema becomes widespread, bronchomotor tone increases, and peripheral vasodilation occurs, leading to systemic hypotension (Table 9–3).

Control of histamine, whether through control of its synthesis, release, or effects, goes a long way toward reducing the severity of allergic responses. Other autacoids, however, produce similar effects. Therefore, even if histamine activity is completely controlled, other allergic mediators are still free to influence effector cells. Much of the complexity of allergic responses such as bronchial asthma stems from the fact that multiple mediators are involved in the reaction.

Neutrophil Chemotactic Factor of Anaphylaxis

Chemotaxis is the mechanism responsible for causing cells to migrate to a specific area. Mast cells release **neutrophil chemotactic factor of anaphylaxis (NCF-A),** which serves as a chemoattractant to draw additional neutrophils to sensitized tissue. The total population of target cells, therefore, is expanded by the arrival of additional neutrophils. Recall that these leukocytes contain small amounts of histamine.

Eosinophil Chemotactic Factor of Anaphylaxis

Mast cells release the chemoattractant **eosinophil chemotactic factor of anaphylaxis (ECF-A),** which results in an increase in the number of eosinophils in inflammatory exudate of airways. The arrival of eosinophils expands the total population of histamine-containing cells.

Platelet Activation Factor

Platelet activation factor (PAF) is another chemical attractant released by target cells during an

TABLE 9–2 ALLERGIC MEDIATORS: SOURCES AND ACTIONS

Mediators	Actions	Comments
	MAST CELLS	
Histamine	Capillary leakage	Mast cells are largest storage pool of histamine
	Vasodilation	Mast cells (tissue basophils) are derived from
	Bronchoconstriction	circulating basophils
	Glandular secretion	Lung is well endowed with mast cells
ECF-A	Accumulation of eosinophils	Amplification effect
		Eosinophilia in airway exudate indicates allergic response
NCF-A	Accumulation of neutrophils	Amplification effect
PAF	Accumulation of thrombocytes (platelets)	Amplification effect
Arachidonic acid metabolites	Conversion to eicosanoids (histaminelike mediators)	Eicosanoids yield prostanoids through cyclooxygenase metabolism and leukotrienes through lipoxygenase metabolism
	BASOPHILS	
Histamine	Same as for mast cells.	These granulocytes (''base-loving'' cells) are stained by a basic, or alkaline, differential stain
		Make up a small fraction of total number of granulocytes
		Converted to mast cells
		Largest non–mast cell source of histamine
	EOSINOPHILS	
Histamine	Same as for mast cells	Eosinophils are attracted by ECF-A
		These granulocytes (''eosin-loving'' cells) are stained by eosin, an acidic differential stain
		Contain small amounts of histamine
		Make up a small fraction of total number of granulocytes
LTB_4	Accumulation of additional eosinophils	Amplification effect
	Accumulation of additional neutrophils	Amplification effect
		LTB_4 produced through lipoxygenase pathway
	NEUTROPHILS	
Histamine	Same as for mast cells.	Neutrophils are attracted by NCF-A
		These granulocytes (''neutral-loving'' cells) have a neutral staining reaction
		Contain small amounts of histamine but form the largest fraction of granulocytes in the blood
PAF	Same as for mast cells.	Amplification effect
	THROMBOCYTES (PLATELETS)	
Histamine	Same as for mast cells.	Attracted by PAF
		Contain small amounts of histamine
TXA_2	Histaminelike actions	TXA_2 produced through the cyclooxygenase pathway
	Accumulation of additional platelets	Amplification effect

ECF-A = eosinophil chemotactic factor of anaphylaxis; LTB_4 = leukotrine B_4; NCF-A = neutrophil chemotactic factor of anaphylaxis; PAF = platelet activity factor; TXA_2 = thromboxane A_2.

antigen-antibody reaction. PAF is especially plentiful in mast cells and neutrophils and is released along with histamine as part of the primary package of allergic mediators. This auta-coid causes histaminelike actions such as changes in vascular permeability, vasodilation, and bronchoconstriction, also causing the aggregation (accumulation) of thrombocytes in in-

TABLE 9–3   HISTAMINE EFFECTS

Tissue Effect	Outcome of Small Release of Histamine	Outcome of Large Release of Histamine
Increased capillary permeability	Localized edema to limit systemic spread of noxious substances	Widespread and severe tissue edema Migration of leukocytes into tissues
Vasodilation	Locally increased blood flow to deliver nutrients and leukocytes to the area	Hyperemia Peripheral vasodilation Systemic hypotension Accumulation of large numbers of leukocytes in inflammatory exudate leading to amplification effect
Bronchoconstriction	Increased bronchomotor tone	Intense bronchospasm Wheeze, dyspnea
Glandular secretion	Increased glandular activity	Hypersecretion of tracheobronchial glands; cough Hypersecretion of gastric acid

flammatory tissue, thereby further expanding the target cell population.

The chemotactic substances such as NCF-A, ECF-A, and PAF that are released by mast cells form a positive feedback mechanism responsible for a magnification effect seen in sensitized tissues. The effect is characterized by an expanding population of target cells, and therefore, an ex-

panding storage pool of primary mediators such as histamine.

Eicosanoids

Eicosanoids are 20-carbon compounds (Gr. *eicosa* means 20) derived from the metabolism of **arachidonic acid.** Arachidonic acid is released

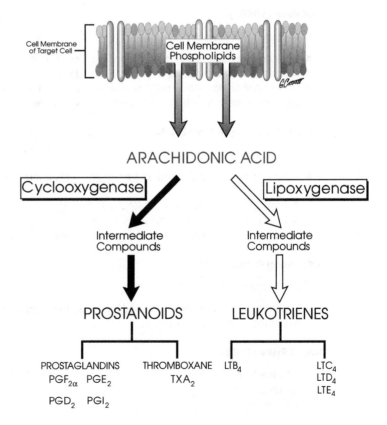

FIGURE 9–5 Arachidonic acid metabolism and the eicosanoids.

BOX 9–1   PROSTAGLANDINS: PAST, PRESENT, AND FUTURE

Prostaglandins are autacoids produced by virtually every tissue in the body and are found in most body fluids. They are implicated in a wide variety of responses. These responses range from inflammation of tissues to control of uterine contractions, and from intense bronchoconstriction to therapeutically beneficial bronchodilation. Some prostaglandins are potent vasoconstrictors; others cause blood pressure to plummet due to widespread vasodilation. Versatility is what makes the prostaglandins so intriguing. It is also the feature most difficult to control. For example, PGE relaxes smooth muscle, whereas $PGF_{2\alpha}$ produces the opposite effect. Therefore, prostaglandins have the potential to simultaneously alter ventilation-perfusion $(\dot{V}/\dot{Q})$ mismatching in the lungs. This is possible because smooth muscle in both the airways and pulmonary blood vessels can be affected by prostaglandin action. Practical clinical application, however, is not yet possible because control of the smooth muscle effect is presently lacking.

The therapeutic potential of the prostaglandins has attracted investigators for over half a century, as can be seen from the highlights listed below:

Discovery and Naming (1930s)

Ulf von Euler (Sweden)

- Seminal fluid extracts were found to contain a smooth muscle–contracting substance that was active on uterine and intestinal smooth muscle.
- Compounds were named ''prostaglandins'' by von Euler because of presumed prostate gland source.

Isolation (1940s)

Sune Bergström (Sweden)

- Isolated a fraction of the new compounds from seminal vesicles.
- Purified fractions obtained almost 10 years later.
- Designated compounds ''prostaglandins E and F,'' based on their different solvents: *e*ther and *f*osfat (Swedish for phosphate buffer).

Chemical Structure (1962–1963)

Sune Bergström

- Identified five prostaglandins in semen and a sixth found in other issues, such as lung tissue:
  - Prostaglandin E series: PGE_1, PGE_2, PGE_3
  - Prostaglandin F series: $PGF_{1\alpha}$, $PGF_{2\alpha}$, $PGF_{3\alpha}$
- Identified prostaglandins as derivatives of prostanoic acid

Additional Compounds

Bengt Samuelsson (Sweden)

- Isolated additional compounds and identified the arachidonic acid pathway responsible for their production.

Nobel Prize (1982)

John Vane (Great Britain)
Sune Bergström
Bengt Samuelsson

- Nobel Prize for Medicine or Physiology awarded to research team for elucidation of prostaglandin action.
- The mediator TXA_2 was discovered.
- Aspirin and related drugs were found to block the formation of thromboxane and prostaglandins.

Clark WG, Brater DC, and Johnson AR: Goth's Medical Pharmacology, ed. 12. CV Mosby, St. Louis, 1988.

Goldyne ME: Prostaglandins and other eicosanoids. In Katzung BD (ed): Basic and Clinical Pharmacology. Lange Medical Publications, Los Altos, 1982.

Moncada S, Flower RJ, and Vane JR: Prostaglandins, prostacyclin, thromboxane A_2, and leukotrines. In Goodman AG et al (eds): Goodman and Gillman's The Pharmacologic Basis of Therapeutics, ed. 7, Macmillan, New York, 1985.

from cell membrane phospholipids in response to autacoids such as histamine and the kinins (see below). Arachidonic acid is then converted by **cyclooxygenase** into intermediates that are changed into eicosanoids known as the **prostanoids.** Prostanoid compounds consist of the prostaglandins and TXA_2 (Fig. 9–5). Nonsteroidal drugs, such as aspirin, and steroids, such as glucocorticoids, produce their anti-inflammatory effects by blocking this cyclo-oxygenase pathway (see Fig. 9–7).

Virtually all tissues of the body possess arachidonic acid metabolites known as **prostaglandins (PGs).** These compounds were initially discovered in human seminal fluid, where it was noticed that some active substance had a uterine smooth muscle–stimulating action. Early researchers believed that the compounds were derived from the prostate gland, hence the name *prostaglandin.* The lungs are especially well supplied with several members of this versatile group of tissue hormones. Different prostaglandins are produced through the action of different enzymes in the various tissues of the body. Prostaglandin activity is linked with the intracellular cyclic nucleotide mechanism, but the role of cAMP (cyclic adenosine–3',5'–monophosphate) and cGMP (cyclic guanosine–3',5'–monophosphate) is not fully understood. The group of prostaglandins includes powerful allergic mediators known as prostaglandin $F_{2\alpha}$ ($PGF_{2\alpha}$) and prostaglandin D_2 (PGD_2). $PGF_{2\alpha}$ and PGD_2 produce histaminelike effects at gastrointestinal and airway smooth muscle to result in increased gastrointestinal tract activity and bronchoconstriction. Unlike histamine, these prostaglandins cause contraction of vascular smooth muscle.

Some prostaglandins possess actions antagonistic to those described above. For example, prostaglandin E_2 (PGE_2) causes relaxation of bronchiolar and vascular smooth muscle and suppresses the effect of histamine and acetylcholine on airways. Prostaglandin I_2 (PGI_2), also known as *prostacyclin,* works like PGE_2 to relax airway smooth muscle, and in addition aids in the suppression of a leukotriene (see below). PGI_2 also inhibits platelet aggregation and the release of histamine (see Box 9–1).

Another arachidonic acid metabolite functioning as an autacoid is **thromboxane (TXA_2).** TXA_2 causes contraction of smooth muscle in the airways, blood vessels, and gastrointestinal tract and promotes the aggregation of platelets. TXA_2 is synthesized by platelets.

Arachidonic acid derived from cell membrane phospholipids is enzymatically converted by **lipoxygenase** into intermediates that are then changed into the eicosanoids known as **leukotrienes (LTs).** Leukotriene B_4 is released by eosinophils and functions as a leukocyte chemoattractant for eosinophils and neutrophils.

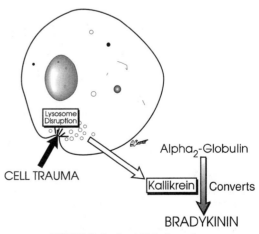

FIGURE 9–6 Bradykinin formation.

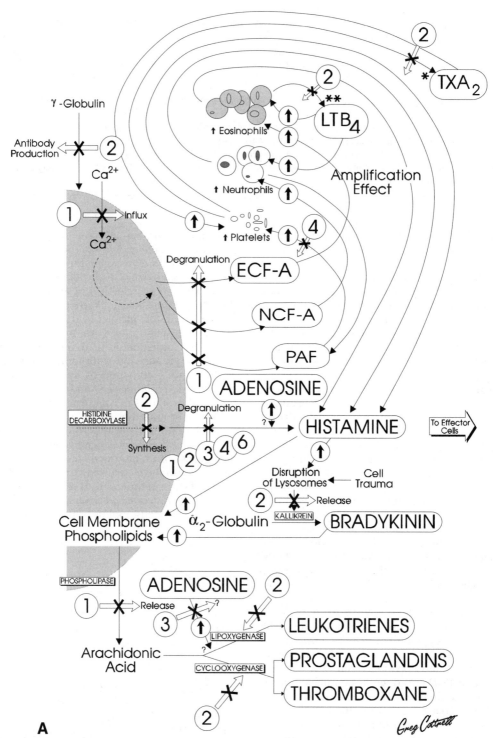

FIGURE 9–7 Bronchoactive drugs and the anti-inflammatory mechanism. (*A*) Sites of action—target cells. A variety of target cells serve as sources of allergic mediators. The mechanism by which adenosine provokes bronchoconstriction is not fully understood. The schematic pertains to the mast cell-stabilizing mechanism of action only. Some antiallergic drugs exert control over other aspects of the inflammatory reaction (e.g., neutrophils, eicosanoids, histamine receptors). See text for full explanation.

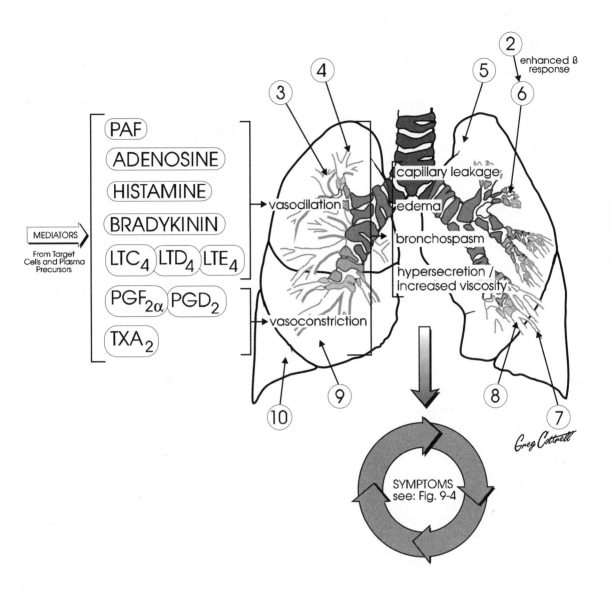

B

FIGURE 9–7 Continued. (B) Sites of action—effector cells. Many of the allergic mediators shown in (A) cause the same adverse reactions in effector cells. As a result, many of the symptoms produced by the mediators are the same. Some second-generation H_1-histamine antagonists also exhibit anti-inflammatory/antiallergic effects at target cells (see Chapter 10). Stimulation of H_2-histamine receptors in the stomach causes gastric acid secretion. (*Via the cyclooxygenase pathway. **Via the lipoxygenase pathway. †Elevated cAMP levels also retard the release of allergic mediators. ‡Some antitussives are centrally acting.)

BOX 9–2 **2001: A DRUG ODYSSEY** (with apologies to Arthur C. Clarke)

Control of **allergic mediators,** rather than airway smooth muscle, represents an alternative and promising approach to asthma therapy. Bronchodilators such as inhaled β_2-adrenergic agonists and antimuscarinics will undoubtedly be available in new and improved versions in the future. However, the respiratory care practitioner of the next decade may also see an expanding role for therapeutic agents that inhibit the formation or release of inflammatory mediators. Inhaled steroids and antiallergics such as beclomethasone and cromolyn already perform that role but may be joined by several new classes of drugs. Novel agents under investigation include prostaglandin inhibitors, leukotriene antagonists, lipoxygenase inhibitors, TXA_2 antagonists, PAF inhibitors, and bradykinin antagonists.

Mathewson HS: Asthma and bronchitis: A shift of therapeutic emphasis. Respiratory Care 35:273–277, 1990.

Leukotrienes C_4, D_4, and E_4 are derived from sensitized mast cells. These autacoids are causative agents of vasodilation, increased vascular permeability, and contraction of nonvascular smooth muscle. Prior to definitive identification, these three leukotrienes—LTC_4, LTD_4, and LTE_4—were known by the nonspecific and collective term "slow-reacting substance of anaphylaxis" or SRS-A. Drug classes such as the glucocorticoids produce some of their anti-inflammatory effects by blocking the lipoxygenase pathway summarized in Figure 9–5.

Kinins

Inhalation of noxious substances, the presence of invading microorganisms, and the occurrence of debilitating diseases can bring about tissue trauma. **Bradykinin** is a potent allergic mediator and pain-producing substance. It produces histaminelike effects at vascular and nonvascular smooth muscle and at exocrine glands but does not interact at histamine receptors. Instead, it binds at specific bradykinin receptors (see Box 25–1). Unlike histamine, bradykinin is not present in the tissues in an active form, but must be converted from an inactive precursor. Following tissue trauma, lysosomes within damaged cells undergo rupture and through a multistep mechanism release a substance called *kallikrein*. Kallikrein acts on α_2-globulin, a circulating plasma protein, and rapidly converts it to active bradykinin (Fig. 9–6). *Glucocorticoids* direct part of their anti-inflammatory action at the stabilization of lysosomal membranes, and therefore at the suppression of bradykinin formation. Kinins also can initiate the release of arachidonic acid from cell membranes. *Glucocorticoids,* therefore, are indirectly responsible for suppressing the ei-

cosanoid class of inflammatory mediators (prostaglandins, TXA_2, and leukotrienes). The sites of action of bronchoactive drugs in the inflammatory mechanism are summarized in Figure 9-7 (see also Box 9–2).

THE cAMP-cGMP SYSTEM AND THE ALLERGIC RESPONSE

The relative amounts of intracellular messengers influence the activity of target cells like mast cells. When cAMP levels are high, mast cells fail to release their primary package of mediators. Similarly, elevated cGMP levels encourage the release of mediators such as histamine from sensitized target cells. Therefore, any drug mechanism of action that promotes cAMP formation or suppresses cGMP formation has a beneficial effect in the control of allergic responses. Most of the bronchoactive drugs to be explored in Unit 3 exert at least part of their control over allergic mediators by influencing the cyclic nucleotide system. For example, *antimuscarinic bronchodilators* depress cGMP formation, whereas β_2-agonist bronchodilators elevate cAMP levels.

CHAPTER SUMMARY

Alleviation of symptoms by controlling production and release of allergic mediators is the therapeutic goal of drugs used in the treatment of allergic reactions. Allergic responses such as hay fever, allergic asthma, and anaphylaxis are triggered by complex causative factors and share a common mechanism involving the immune system, antigen stimulus, and antibody production. Such reactions are also characterized by the formation and release of various allergic mediators from diverse target cells.

Different types of storage cells, allergic mediators, and mechanisms involved in the production and release of mediators make the control of allergic symptoms difficult. Bronchoactive drugs, such as the *antiallergics* and *antihistamines,* the *antimuscarinic, sympathomimetic,* and *xanthine bronchodilators,* as well as the *glucocorticoids, antitussives,* and *mucokinetics,* all achieve varying degrees of success in regard to control of allergic symptoms.

Bibliography

Burkhalter A and Frick OL: Histamine, serotonin, and the ergot alkaloids: In Katzung BD (ed): Basic and Clinical Pharmacology. Lange Medical Publications, Los Altos, 1982.

Clark WG, Brater DC, and Johnson AR: Goth's Medical Pharmacology, ed 12. CV Mosby, St Louis, 1988.

Goldyne ME: Prostaglandins and other eicosanoids. In Katzung BD (ed): Basic and Clinical Pharmacology. Lange Medical Publications, Los Altos, 1982.

Grady D: Zeroing in on allergies. Discover 2(7):68–71, July 1981.

Hargreave FE, Dolovich J, and Newhouse MT: The assessment and treatment of asthma: A conference report. J Allergy Clin Immunol (85):1098–1111, 1990.

Holgate ST and Kay AB: Mast cells, mediators and asthma. Clinical Allergy 15:221–234, 1985.

Howder CL: Cardiopulmonary Pharmacology: A Handbook for Respiratory Practitioners and Other Allied Health Personnel. Williams and Wilkins, Baltimore, 1992.

Mathewson HS: Asthma and bronchitis: A shift of therapeutic emphasis. Respiratory Care 35:273–277, 1990.

Milavetz G and Smith JJ: Pharmacotherapy of asthma and allergic rhinitis. Primary Care 17:685–701, 1990.

Netter, FH: Respiratory system. In Divertie MB (ed): CIBA Collection of Medical Illustrations. CIBA Pharmaceutical Company, Division of CIBA-GEIGY Corporation, Summit, NJ, 1979.

Reid IA: Polypeptides. In Katzung BD (ed): Basic and Clinical Pharmacology. Lange Medical Publications, Los Altos, 1982.

Shires, TK: Anti-inflammatory drugs. In Conn PM and Gebhart GF (eds): Essentials of Pharmacology. FA Davis, Philadelphia, 1989.

Weg VB et al: Histamine, leukotriene D_4 and platelet-activating factor in guinea pig passive cutaneous anaphylaxis. Eur J Pharmacol 204:157–163, Nov 1991.

CHAPTER 10

Antiallergics and Antihistaminics

CHAPTER OUTLINE

CHAPTER OBJECTIVES

After studying this chapter the reader should be able to:

- Describe the mechanism of action of antiallergic drugs that accounts for their prophylactic activity in allergic reactions.
- List the mediators controlled by the pharmacologic activity of antiallergic drugs.
- Describe the pharmacologic activity of the following antiallergic drugs:
  - Cromolyn, ketotifen, nedocromil.
- Describe the mechanism of action of histamine receptor blockers.
- Compare the site of action of H_1- and H_2-histamine-receptor blockers.
- Describe the pharmacologic activity of the following histamine-receptor antagonists:
  - Chlorpheniramine, dimenhydrinate, promethazine, terfenadine, astemizole, loratadine, cetirizine, cimetidine.

KEY TERMS

antiallergic
antiasthmatic
antiemetic
antihistamine (antihistaminic)

antipruritic
histamine-receptor antagonist
  H_1-histamine receptor antagonist
  H_2-histamine receptor antagonist

mast cell stabilizer
nonbronchodilator antiallergic
  drug (NBAAD)
pollenosis

CHAPTER INTRODUCTION

This chapter introduces two classes of bronchoactive drugs: the **antiallergics,** which function primarily as mast cell stabilizers, and the **histamine-receptor antagonists.**

An antiallergic is a drug belonging to a class of prophylactic bronchoactive agents that control the release of various allergic mediators in the respiratory system. By contrast, classical antihistamines act directly at effector cells through pharmacologic antagonism with histamine but do not suppress histamine release. This chapter also discusses newer antihistamines that both control histamine release at target cells and antagonize histamine at effector cells.

ANTIALLERGICS

Terminology

Complex causative factors are involved in bronchial asthma. In addition, the disease can follow a variable and unpredictable course, often presenting multiple clinical facets. For these reasons, designation of a single drug entity as being an **antiasthmatic** is somewhat presumptuous. The term is used generally to describe any drug class that provides symptomatic relief of asthma. This includes *antimuscarinic bronchodilators, β₂-agonist bronchodilators, xanthine bronchodilators,* and the *glucocorticoids.* All of these drug classes produce antiasthmatic effects. The antiasthmatic drug category also includes drugs that function as mast cell stabilizers, a mechanism that limits the release of allergic mediators, such as histamine. Other target cells, including eosinophils and other allergic mediators such as bradykinin, are unaffected by this mechanism. Because asthmatic symptoms can still occur when these ''antiasthmatic'' mast cell–stabilizing drugs are administered, **antiallergic** is a more accurate description of their prophylactic mode of action.

Mechanism of Action

Drugs designated as antiallergics control allergic mediators by preventing their release from sensitized target cells. In this regard, they are most useful as asthma prophylactics or drugs used to *prevent* the onset of asthmatic symptoms. Unlike the antihistaminics, which are pharmacologic antagonists of histamine, and the β₂-sympathomimetics, which are physiologic antagonists of histamine, antiallergics such as cromolyn actually prevent the release of histamine and other mediators from sensitized mast cells. Cromolyn is a **mast cell stabilizer,** accomplishing mediator control by blocking the entry of extracellular calcium ions into the mast cell. Blockage of Ca^{2+} influx inhibits mast cell degranulation of preformed histamine and chemotactic factors, and also suppresses the release of arachidonic acid from cell membrane phospholipid. This potent antiallergic effect, therefore, prevents the release or formation of histamine, the chemotactic factors, and the eicosanoid class of mediators, which includes leukotrienes, prostaglandins, and thromboxane (see Fig. 9–7).

A bronchoactive drug that relieves the symptoms of asthma through a mechanism of action that does not directly affect bronchiolar smooth muscle is called a **nonbronchodilator antiallergic drug (NBAAD).** The following antiallergic drugs, therefore, can be referred to as NBAADs.

THERAPEUTIC ANTIALLERGIC AGENTS

CROMOLYN (Intal, Aarane^US, Fivent^CAN). Cromolyn, also known as cromolyn sodium or disodium cromoglycate, is the prototype asthma prophylactic drug. Cromolyn is the synthetic derivative of khellin, a substance found in the seeds of a Mediterranean plant known as khella (*Ammi visnaga*). Modifications to khellin to enhance its bronchodilator efficacy yielded the *bis*-chromones, a group of drugs that includes cromolyn (Fig. 10–1). Cromolyn lacks any bronchodilator activity of its own. Instead it controls the release of important autacoids from target cells. Disodium cromoglycate was introduced in Great Britain in 1968, but the natural compound, khellin, was known as an antiasthmatic for centuries in Bedouin folk medicine.

Cromolyn is poorly absorbed from the respiratory mucosa following aerosol administration by metered-dose inhaler (MDI), nebulizer solution, or dry powder inhaler (DPI). Several forms permit administration of this versatile drug through additional routes. For example, prophylaxis of seasonal rhinitis can be achieved with a nasal solution of cromolyn (Nasalcrom) or with a nasal MDI (Rynacrom^CAN), eye drops are available to treat seasonal allergic conjunctivitis (Opticrom), and oral forms are available for the relief of gastrointestinal allergic conditions. As with asthma prophylaxis, protection against seasonal rhinitis, conjunctivitis, and food allergy requires prior administration of the drug. Cromolyn must be already present to stabilize mast cells and prevent allergic symptoms from developing.

Cromolyn has no antihistaminic, anti-inflammatory, decongestant, or bronchodilator activ-

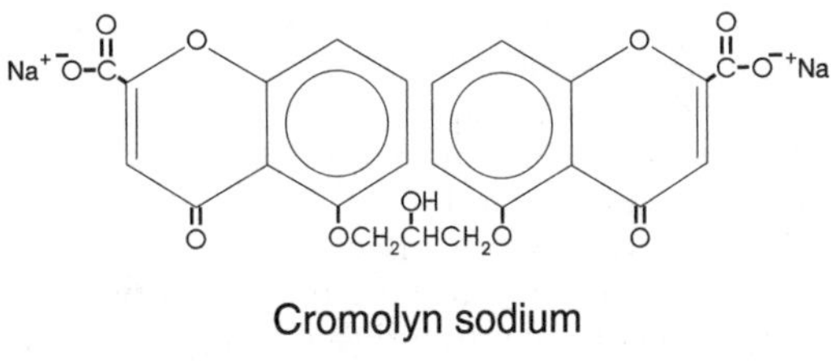

Cromolyn sodium

FIGURE 10–1 Cromolyn sodium.

ity. In addition, it is effective mainly in immediate allergic reactions. In these reactions, it suppresses the release of various spasmogens and other allergic mediators from sensitized mast cells within the mucosa and along bronchial vessels (see Fig. 9–2). It may also suppress the vagal reflex to relax bronchiolar smooth muscle tone. Development of the full prophylactic effect of cromolyn can take 6 to 12 weeks. The use of cromolyn alone may prevent asthma symptoms in children and young adults, whereas older patients may require the addition of corticosteroids to their drug regimen. On the other hand, cromolyn may be useful in reducing or eliminating corticosteroid dependence in some patients.

INDICATIONS. Cromolyn is useful in the prevention of moderately severe symptoms of extrinsic and intrinsic asthma, including cold air–induced asthma, exercise-induced bronchospasm, and hyperreactive airways. Pretreatment with cromolyn also protects against bronchospasm provoked by inhalation of industrial irritants. It is of no use in the treatment of acute bronchospasm and may in fact cause additional irritation of the bronchial mucosa. Cromolyn must be used on a continual basis to develop the maximal clinical prophylactic effect. The protective effect of cromolyn is dose dependent; therefore, physicians may need to adjust dosage of the drug to match expected asthma stimuli. For example, an increase in exercise intensity or in activity during cold weather may necessitate an increase in dosage to provide the desired asthma protection. Similarly, peak seasonal allergy challenge can be met by an increase in cromolyn dosage prior to the arrival of the pollen season.

Cromolyn delivered as a fine powder by DPI or by nebulizer solution is usually administered at a dosage of 20 mg four times daily (80 mg/d). Following stabilization of a patient after 1 to 2 months of cromolyn therapy, physicians may elect to reduce dosage to a maintenance level of 40–60 mg/d. Different delivery modes and cromolyn dosages are presented in Table 10–5 below. Variables such as patient age, inspiratory technique, breath-holding time, frequency of drug administration, and portability of the aerosol device all contribute to the selection of a proper method of delivery. These factors have been discussed in Chapter 1. Advantages and disadvantages of different aerosol generators are summarized in Table 1–5.

CONTRAINDICATIONS. Because cromolyn requires several weeks to develop its full prophylactic effect, it is contraindicated in patients experiencing acute asthma attacks and in conditions of status asthmaticus. In addition, it is contraindicated in patients exhibiting hypersensitivity to cromolyn.

PRECAUTIONS. If oral corticosteroids are to be discontinued in a patient when cromolyn therapy is initiated, gradual or tapered withdrawal of the steroids is required. Gradual withdrawal is especially important in steroid-dependent patients. This caution is necessary because cromolyn requires several weeks to develop maximal protective effect and has no activity of its own on the adrenal cortex. Resumption of normal adrenocortical function must be allowed to occur gradually over a period of weeks. (The problem of adrenocortical suppression with steroid drug therapy is fully discussed in Chapter 14.)

The inhalational capsules (Spincaps) used in the single dose Spinhaler DPI must not be taken orally. They are designed to be pierced by the device so that their powder contents can be inhaled by the patient (see Fig. 1–6A). Oral administration of cromolyn for asthma prophylaxis is ineffective.

Because cromolyn must be used several times a day and requires an extended period of therapy to establish its prophylactic effect, poor patient compliance may limit its effectiveness.

Finally, cromolyn must not be mixed with certain inhalation solutions of ipratropium, a common antimuscarinic bronchodilator (see Chapter 11). Inhalation solutions of ipratropium from multidose bottles contain the preservatives benzalkonium chloride and EDTA disodium. Benzalkonium chloride forms a precipitate with cromolyn; therefore, cromolyn must be given with preservative-free ipratropium to those patients requiring both of these drugs in combination (Boehringer Ingelheim, 1993). Preservative-free ipratropium inhalation solutions are available in unit dose vials (see Chapter 11).

ADVERSE REACTIONS. The most common complaints with the DPI form of cromolyn are throat irritation or dryness, hoarseness, coughing, and wheezing. In addition, bronchospasm may be caused by the irritating effect of the powder. Prior use of β_2-agonist bronchodilators may minimize this reaction. Additional adverse reactions include nasal congestion, rash, urticaria, and central nervous system (CNS) effects such as dizziness and headache.

KETOTIFEN (Zaditen[CAN]). The prophylactic agent ketotifen is an NBAAD that has been studied for several years in the United States but has not yet been released for general clinical use because it is classified as an investigational drug. In Canada it is currently approved as a pediatric asthma prophylactic–antiallergic agent. Ketotifen exhibits a dual action in allergic conditions because it has pronounced antiallergic *and* antihistaminic activity. These properties are especially useful in atopic individuals because ketotifen, unlike inhaled cromolyn, can relieve symptoms of asthma, rhinitis, and dermatitis when they are found together in the same patient.

The dual effects of ketotifen are reflected in its mechanism of action. It is a mast cell–stabilizing agent that prevents release of primary allergic mediators, such as histamine, platelet activating factor (PAF), and leukotrienes C_4, D_4, and E_4 (formerly known as SRS-A). It also has a powerful antihistaminic action at effector cells. Antihistamines exhibit pharmacologic antagonism at histamine receptors designated H_1-histamine receptors. Ketotifen, therefore, competes with histamine at bronchiolar smooth muscle H_1-receptors and exerts a powerful, sustained histamine-blocking action.

The full asthma prophylactic effect of ketotifen can take 6 to 12 weeks to develop. After this lengthy "run-in period," asthma symptoms and attacks may be reduced in frequency, severity, and duration. In addition, daily requirements of other antiasthmatic medications, such as *methylxanthines* and β_2-*agonists,* may be reduced. Ketotifen is administered through the oral route.

INDICATIONS. Ketotifen is indicated in the chronic treatment of mild allergic (atopic) asthma in children and is used prophylactically on a continual basis.

CONTRAINDICATIONS. Ketotifen is not effective in the treatment of acute asthmatic attack because several weeks are required for establishment of maximal clinical effect.

PRECAUTIONS. General precautions concerning antiasthmatic drugs already in use apply. For example, drugs such as methylxanthines, β_2-agonists, cromolyn, and corticosteroids cannot be immediately withdrawn when ketotifen therapy is initiated because of the extended period required for the prophylactic effect to develop. Ketotifen can produce sedative effects that potentiate those of sedatives, alcohol, and some antihistaminics.

NEDOCROMIL (Tilade). Nedocromil is another investigational antiallergic agent being studied in the United States for use in asthma therapy. It is currently available in Canada for use as a bronchial anti-inflammatory agent. Nedocromil is applied topically to the bronchi with an MDI device. At these sites it exerts a powerful anti-inflammatory effect on various cell types found in the lumen and in the mucosal lining of the tracheobronchial tree. Nedocromil suppresses the arachidonic acid pathway to block the generation of leukotriene and prostanoid allergic mediators. It may suppress the production of neutrophil-derived histamine-releasing activity (HRA-N), a substance that triggers the release of histamine from mast cells (White et al, 1991). This blockade of production of mediators is an anti-inflammatory effect not exhibited by the other anti-allergics. Cromolyn and ketotifen merely suppress the release of allergic mediators (Table 10–1).

The use of other antiasthmatics, such as inhaled *corticosteroids* and β_2-*agonists,* can generally be reduced with the introduction of nedocromil. Therapeutic benefits are seen in most patients within the first week of treatment.

INDICATIONS. Nedocromil is useful as an adjunct in the management of symptoms associated with mild to moderate chronic reversible obstructive airways disease, including bronchial asthma and bronchitis. It is especially effective in asthmatic conditions in which airway inflammation and bronchial hyperreactivity are present. Nedocromil is also valuable for prevention of bronchospasm provoked by stimuli such as in-

TABLE 10–1 MECHANISMS OF ACTION OF ANTIALLERGIC DRUGS

	Cromolyn	Ketotifen	Nedocromil
Antiallergic mechanism	Blocks Ca^{2+} entry and stabilizes mast cells	Stabilizes mast cells	Prevents release of histamine
Antihistaminic mechanism	No effect	Competes with histamine at H_1-histamine receptors	No effect
Anti-inflammatory mechanism	No effect	No effect	Prevents formation of eicosanoids (blocks arachidonic acid metabolism)

haled allergens, cold air, exercise, and pollutants.

CONTRAINDICATIONS. Nedocromil is not used for the relief of acute asthma attack, nor as a replacement for frontline bronchodilators.

Contraindications include known sensitivity to nedocromil, fluorocarbon propellants, or sorbitan trioleate, a substance used as a surfactant in the aerosol product to facilitate spread of the medication in the airways (see Table 1–2).

PRECAUTIONS. Nedocromil is not used as an alternative to bronchodilator therapy. However, the need for concurrent antiasthmatic medication may be reduced over time. Reduction of concomitant antiasthmatic drugs must be done slowly under close supervision.

In addition, patients must understand the need to take nedocromil regularly as prescribed for the full anti-inflammatory effect of the drug to develop. Nedocromil cannot be used as rescue therapy in the event of acute bronchospasm. As with all MDI aerosol medications, nedocromil must be administered properly. In addition, patients must be cautioned concerning the potential risks of fluorocarbon propellant toxicity if the product is intentionally abused (see Chapter 1).

ADVERSE REACTIONS. Some patients taking nedocromil may experience mild effects such as unpleasant taste, headache, and nausea.

For a summary of the mechanisms of action exhibited by the antiallergic drugs, see Table 10–1.

HISTAMINE-RECEPTOR ANTAGONISTS

Types of Histamine Receptors

Reactive sites for histamine are found on several effector cells in the body. Histamine can interact equally well at two different classes of receptors: **H₂-histamine receptors,** located on parietal cells in the gastric mucosa, and **H₁-histamine receptors,** found at all other histamine receptor locations. The important H₁-receptors of the respiratory system are found on the epithelial cells that line the nasal cavity and conducting passages, and on airway smooth muscle and glands. A specific antagonist of H₁-receptors is called an antihistamine, or antihistaminic, whereas a **histamine-receptor antagonist** is a drug that competes pharmacologically with histamine at an H₁- or an H₂-receptor. Because nearly all the histamine-receptor antagonists of respiratory importance are H₁-blocking agents, this section stresses the antihistaminics. A brief discussion of

H₂-receptor antagonists is included at the end of the chapter.

H₁-Histamine Receptor Antagonists

If histamine were the major spasmogen implicated in bronchial asthma, administration of a specific H₁-receptor antagonist (antihistamine) should abolish asthmatic symptoms. In practice, the introduction of such a drug does not completely control the symptoms. Most of the traditional H₁-blockers can aggravate a condition of asthma through their anticholinergic action, which has the potential to dry airway secretions. In addition, H₁-blockers are ineffective in the control of other autacoids functioning as allergic mediators. Kinins, and spasmogens such as leukotrienes, are unaffected, as are leukocyte chemoattractants such as eosinophil and neutrophil chemotactic factors of anaphylaxis (see Fig. 9–7).

The classic antihistamines were developed in the 1940s. Chemically they are similar to parasympatholytics and tranquilizers and therefore exhibit some overlap of pharmacologic effect. Most of the traditional H₁-blockers exhibit weak histamine antagonism in addition to anticholinergic side effects and sedation. Some possess an **antiemetic** effect useful in anti–motion sickness therapy, and a local anesthetic effect that makes them valuable as **antipruritics** for relief of itching associated with cutaneous allergic conditions. Members of the group produce varying amounts of sedation. In fact, drowsiness is one of the more common adverse reactions caused by the original group of H₁-blockers which includes chlorpheniramine and promethazine.

A newer group of nonsedating second-generation H₁-blockers is exemplified by terfenadine. These newer derivatives do not penetrate the blood-brain barrier readily and possess far fewer sedative effects than the traditional antihistamines. The second-generation antihistamines are also more potent than the original group and can be delivered at dosages that permit virtually complete H₁-histamine receptor blockade. This potent, more selective peripheral effect aids in suppressing symptoms of allergic asthma. By contrast, the doses necessary to bring about complete H₁-histamine block using a traditional H₁-receptor antagonist result in undesirable anticholinergic and CNS sedative side effects.

Antihistamines of the first- or second-generation type compete with histamine for H₁-histamine receptors and therefore block histamine effects such as increased capillary leakage, edema, and vasodilation (see Table 9–3). Antihistamines, however, possess no effects of their own and are unable to repair damage already inflicted on the tissues during the allergic reaction. Reversal of the tissue damage requires the administration of a *physiologic* antagonist of histamine, such as a β_2-agonist drug. *β_2-Sympathomimetics* functionally oppose histamine effects by promoting changes such as bronchodilation. Traditional first-generation antihistamines are not capable of such action.

THERAPEUTIC HISTAMINE-RECEPTOR ANTAGONISTS

First-Generation, Sedating H_1-Histamine Receptor Blockers

CHLORPHENIRAMINE (Chlor-Trimeton). Chlorpheniramine has relatively weak atropine-like and sedative properties compared with other traditional H_1-histamine receptor blockers.

INDICATIONS. In general, the antihistaminics are most effective in treating symptoms of immediate allergic reactions such as urticaria (hives) and hay fever. Chlorpheniramine is a typical antihistamine employed in over-the-counter (OTC) common cold remedies and cough medications because of its weak ability to relieve congestion.

PRECAUTIONS. All of the original H_1-receptor antagonists produce sedation, which can potentiate the effect of depressants such as tranquilizers, barbiturates, and alcohol.

The anticholinergic component useful for reducing the secretions that accompany the common cold can also reduce secretions in the airways and potentially aggravate bronchial asthma.

DIMENHYDRINATE (Dramamine, Gravol). Dimenhydrinate is another typical H_1-blocker belonging to the classic group of antihistamines.

INDICATIONS. The clinical uses are generally the same as those outlined for chlorpheniramine, but dimenhydrinate exhibits a potent anticholinergic effect, which makes it valuable as an antiemetic useful in the prevention and treatment of motion sickness.

PRECAUTIONS. See Chlorpheniramine.

PROMETHAZINE (Phenergan). Because of its close chemical similarity to tranquilizers of the phenothiazine type, promethazine exhibits relatively high sedative properties. It is available in various dosage forms, including oral, topical, and parenteral formulations.

INDICATIONS. Allergic reactions such as hay fever and urticaria respond to promethazine, as do nausea and motion sickness. Its powerful sedative component is useful in conditions of insomnia, nervousness, and anxiety. Its local anesthetic action is valuable for the relief of pruritus and mild burns.

CONTRAINDICATIONS. Known hypersensitivity to the phenothiazines is a contraindication to the use of promethazine.

PRECAUTIONS. Pronounced CNS depression can greatly potentiate the sedative effects of *barbiturates, tranquilizers, narcotics,* and *general anesthetics.* Therefore, the dosage of these agents is reduced when they are used in combination with promethazine. The atropinelike activity of promethazine can lead to unpleasant side effects such as dry mouth and blurred vision.

Second-Generation, Nonsedating H_1-Histamine Receptor Blockers

TERFENADINE (Seldane). Terfenadine represents a new class of H_1-histamine receptor blocker that lacks significant anticholinergic and CNS sedative effects. It is well tolerated and well absorbed orally and does not potentiate the CNS depression produced by tranquilizers or alcohol. Terfenadine can reduce the severity of symptoms associated with some types of allergic asthma by inhibiting bronchoconstriction and decreasing cough and wheeze. The use of concomitant bronchodilator drugs can be reduced but not completely eliminated.

INDICATIONS. Symptomatic relief of acute **pollenosis** is the recognized indication for use of terfenadine. Pollenosis includes seasonal rhinitis, hay fever, and allergic dermatoses, including urticaria.

CONTRAINDICATIONS. Known hypersensitivity to terfenadine is a contraindication for its use.

PRECAUTIONS. In certain patients, elevated drug levels of terfenadine may cause signs of cardiac toxicity such as prolonged QT intervals or ventricular arrhythmias (Monahan et al, 1990). For example, patients with preexisting cardiovascular disease, such as ischemic heart disease or depressed plasma potassium levels (hypokalemia), may already have a prolonged QT interval that can be aggravated by terfenadine. Terfenadine is extensively metabolized in the liver; therefore, patients with impaired liver function are at increased risk. For example, patients with cirrhosis or hepatitis may exhibit elevated blood levels of terfenadine and signs of cardiac toxicity.

Concurrent use of terfenadine with ketoco-

TABLE 10–2 COMPARISON OF SECOND-GENERATION ANTIHISTAMINES

Efficacy (from most to least effective)*	Absorption (time to reach peak plasma levels)†	Onset of Action (time to relief of symptoms)†
Cetirizine	Rapid (2–5 h)	Peak: 4–10 h
Terfenadine	Rapid (2–5 h)	Peak: 3–4 h
Loratadine	Rapid (2–5 h)	Peak: 4–6 h
Astemizole	Slow (2–3 d)	Initial: 2 d
		Peak: 9–12 d

*Data from Simons et al, 1991.
†Data from Woodward, 1990.

nazole (an antifungal agent) or macrolide antibiotics such as erythromycin or troleandomycin (TAO) may also result in toxicity. These medications inhibit hepatic microsomal enzymes, thereby increasing the blood level of terfenadine and the risk of cardiac toxicity.

ASTEMIZOLE (Hismanal). Another member of the group of nonsedating antihistamines is astemizole. It is a potent, long-acting peripheral H_1-histamine antagonist that inhibits the bronchial reaction to inhaled histamine and other allergens in asthmatic patients. Unlike terfenadine, which is rapidly absorbed in a matter of hours, peak plasma levels of astemizole are not reached for 2 to 3 days after administration. Development of maximal effect can take as long as 9 to 12 days.

INDICATIONS. Indications for use of astemizole include allergic rhinitis, allergic conjunctivitis, and chronic urticaria.

PRECAUTIONS. Like terfenadine, astemizole in toxic amounts can cause a prolonged QT interval, a sign of cardiac toxicity.

LORATADINE (Claritin). Loratadine is an investigational drug currently being studied by the US Food and Drug Administration (USFDA). It is available in Canada for the treatment of symptoms associated with allergic rhinitis. Loratadine is a long-acting antihistamine with selective H_1-histamine receptor activity. Like the other second-generation antihistamines, loratadine exhibits little CNS sedation and seems to be well tolerated by patients. The onset of action of loratadine is very rapid, usually occurring within the first hour following oral administration. Potential use of loratadine in the oral treatment of

TABLE 10–3 PHARMACOLOGIC ACTIVITY OF HISTAMINE RECEPTOR ANTAGONISTS

Drug	H_1-block	H_2-block	Central Nervous System Sedation	Anticholinergic Effects	Antiallergic Effects
FIRST-GENERATION H_1 BLOCKERS					
Chlorpheniramine	+	−	+	+	−
Dimenhydrinate	+	−	+	+	−
Promethazine	+	−	+++	+	−
SECOND-GENERATION H_1-BLOCKERS					
Terfenadine	+	−	Low	Low	−
Astemizole	+	−	Low	Low	−
Loratadine	+	−	Low	Low	↓ Histamine ↓ PGD_2
Cetirizine	+	−	Low	Low	↓ Histamine ↓ Eosinophils ↓ LTC_4
Sch 37370 (investigational)	+	−	Low	Low	↓ PAF ↓ Eosinophils
H_2-BLOCKERS					
Cimetidine	−	+	−	−	−
Ranitidine	−	+	−	−	−

+—effect; −—no effect; ↓ —decrease; LTC_4—leukotriene C_4; PAF—platelet-activating factor; PGD_2—prostaglandin D_2.

asthma is promising (Howarth, 1990). This is because the drug produces both a potent H_1-blockade and decreases the recovery of histamine and prostaglandin D_2 from the nasal cavity following allergen challenge. These findings indicate mast cell stabilization (Howarth, 1990).

INDICATIONS. Currently, the recognized indications for use of loratadine include symptomatic treatment of allergic rhinitis, sneezing, nasal discharge, and pruritis.

CETIRIZINE (Reactine[CAN]). Cetirizine, an antihistamine with highly selective peripheral H_1-histamine blocking effects plus antiallergic effects, is under review by the USFDA. The drug is currently available in Canada. Controlled clinical trials of cetirizine indicate that the drug is effective in the treatment of rhinitis and that it may have a future role in the treatment of allergic asthma. Cetirizine exhibits H_1-receptor antagonism and inhibits histamine release and eosinophil chemotaxis (Howarth, 1990; Sheffer and Samuels, 1990). It also decreases vascular permeability and blocks the generation of leukotriene C_4 (Naclerio, 1991).

Cetirizine, like other second-generation nonsedating H_1-receptor antagonists, is well tolerated and shows little penetration of the blood-brain barrier.

INDICATIONS. Cetirizine is effective in the treatment of seasonal and perennial allergic rhinitis. Its antiallergic component may prove valuable in the oral treatment of allergic asthma (Howarth, 1990).

Sch 37370. A promising new *dual* antagonist of PAF and histamine is Sch 37370. This investigational drug's novel action against two different mediators is especially effective because of the multifactorial nature of many allergic and inflammatory disorders. *In vitro* studies of Sch 37370 demonstrate both inhibition of platelet aggregation and blockade of histamine receptors (Billah et al, 1991). Animal studies of the drug reveal blockade of bronchospasm, hypotension, cutaneous edema, and lung eosinophilia.

A comparison of the pharmacologic activity of the newer second-generation antihistamines is presented in Table 10–2.

Recall that histamine-receptor antagonists include the H_1-histamine receptor blockers, or antihistaminics, and the H_2-histamine receptor blockers. The H_1-receptor blockers are more versatile than the H_2-receptor blockers because H_1-receptors are more widely distributed in the body. H_2-Receptors, however, play a key role in gastric secretion, as outlined below.

H_2-Histamine Receptor Blockers

CIMETIDINE (Tagamet). H_2-Histamine receptors are located on parietal cells in the gastric mucosa. The receptors are distinct from the more common H_1-histamine variety found on effectors such as bronchiolar smooth muscle. H_2-Receptor antagonist drugs were introduced in the 1970s. Cimetidine (Tagamet) is a histamine antagonist that blocks H_2-receptors and prevents parietal cells from secreting hydrochloric acid (HCl). HCl normally activates pepsinogen in the stomach, converting the precursor to the enzyme pepsin. Pepsin in turn initiates protein digestion. Therefore, H_2-receptor antagonists, such as cimetidine and ranitidine (Zantac), are useful in the control of acid production and protein digestion in the stomach.

The site and mechanism of action described above seem far removed from the tracheobron-

TABLE 10–4 DRUG NAMES: ANTIALLERGICS AND ANTIHISTAMINICS

Generic Name	Trade Name
ANTIALLERGICS	
Cromolyn (**KRŌ**-mo-lin), or disodium cromoglycate (krō-mō-**GLI**-kāt)	Intal, Aarane[US], Fivent[CAN], Nasalcrom (nasal solution), Opticrom (ophthalmic solution)
Ketotifen (ke-**TŌ**-ti-fin)	Zaditen[CAN]
Nedocromil (ne-**DŌ**-krō-mil)	Tilade[CAN]
H_1-RECEPTOR BLOCKERS	
Chlorpheniramine (kloor-**FE**-near-a-mēn)	Chlor-Trimeton
Dimenhydrinate (dī-men-**HI**-dri-nāt)	Dramamine, Gravol
Promethazine (prō-**METH**-a-zēn)	Phenergan
Terfenadine (ter-**FIN**-a-dēn)	Seldane
Astemizole (a-**STEM**-i-zol)	Hismanal
Loratadine (lōr-**AT**-i-dēn)	Claritin[CAN]
Cetirizine (se-**TEER**-a-zēn)	Reactine[CAN]
Sch 37370 (investigational)	
H_2-RECEPTOR BLOCKERS	
Cimetidine (si-**MET**-i-dēn)	Tagamet
Ranitidine (ra-**NIT**-i-dēn)	Zantac

chial tree and bronchoactive drugs familiar to the respiratory care practitioner. Intensive care unit (ICU) patients, however, are often part of the practitioner's responsibility. Some ICU patients receiving hyperalimentation therapy (intravenous nutrients) are maintained on H_2-blockers to reduce gastric activity. Other patients with various hypersecretion disorders are routinely given H_2-receptor antagonists. For these reasons, the respiratory care practitioner should at least be aware of this group of histamine antagonists because a respiratory patient may be receiving such drugs concomitantly with traditional bronchoactive drugs.

A high incidence of nonallergic asthma is seen with a gastrointestinal disorder known as *gastroesophageal reflux* (GER), which is characterized by the entry of acidic stomach contents into the lower end of the esophagus. Cimetidine improves the respiratory symptoms and pulmonary function of patients with nonallergic asthma and GER by blocking H_2-receptors on gastric parietal cells, thereby decreasing stomach acidity (Larrain et al, 1991).

INDICATIONS. Recognized indications for use of cimetidine include hyperalimentation therapy, pathologic hypersecretion, GER, and duodenal ulcer.

Table 10–3 reviews the pharmacologic activity of histamine receptor antagonists, whereas Table 10–4 lists the generic and trade names of drugs discussed in this chapter. Dosages for selected agents are given in Table 10–5.

CHAPTER SUMMARY

Antiasthmatics are drugs that control the symptoms of asthma. Antimuscarinic bronchodilators, sympathomimetic bronchodilators, and methylxanthine bronchodilators are such agents, along with corticosteroids and antiallergic drugs. Antiallergics are therapeutic agents such as cromolyn that control the release or formation of allergic mediators. Antiallergic drugs are routinely employed prophylactically in asthma therapy but do not directly produce bronchodilation. Therefore, they are called *nonbronchodilator antiallergic drugs* (NBAADs).

Histamine-receptor antagonist drugs are of two types, and exhibit pharmacologic antagonism by competing at two different subtypes of histamine receptors. H_1-Receptor blockers, or antihistamines, such as terfenadine, and H_2-receptor blockers, such as cimetidine, are discussed in this chapter. Antihistamines are most often employed in the symptomatic treatment of allergic rhinitis, although some of the newer agents exhibit a degree of antiallergic activity at the bronchial mucosa.

TABLE 10–5 DRUG DOSAGES: INHALATION AGENTS*

Drug	Availability	Dosage

Cromolyn	DPI inhalation capsules
	  20 mg/dry powder capsule
		Inhalation—adults and children
		  >5 yrs:
		  20 mg 4 times per day (80 mg/d)

	Inhalation solution
	  20 mg/2 mL liquid ampule
		20 mg 4 times per day
		  (80 mg/d)

	MDI 800 μg/inhalation	2 inhalations per day

	Nasal solution
	  40 mg/mL (4% solution)
		1 spray delivers 5.2 mg
		  1 spray in each nostril 3–6 times per day

Nedocromil	MDI
	  2 mg/inhalation
	  (17-mL canister with a
	  minimum 112 actuations)
		Inhalation—adults and children
		  >12 yrs:
		  2 actuations or 4 mg four times daily (16 mg/d)

Source: Data from Boushey and Holtzman, 1982, Deglin and Vallerand, 1993, Howder, 1992, Krogh, 1993, and Rau, 1989.

*The dosage information contained in the above table is presented as a brief outline and summary of acceptable dosages. It is *not* meant to replace the detailed information available from manufacturers of these drugs. Package inserts provide the most current dosage information from pharmaceutical manufacturers. Guidelines describing the preparation and delivery of the drug, dose strengths, dosage schedules, shelf life, and storage requirements are also included in the package inserts. In addition, precautions and adverse reactions are described in detail. The respiratory care practitioner is strongly urged to read this information supplied by the pharamaceutical manufacturer to provide safe and effective drug therapy.

BIBLIOGRAPHY

Aalbers R et al: The effect of nedocromil sodium on the early and late reaction and allergen-induced bronchial hyperresponsiveness. J Allergy Clin Immunol 87:993–1001, 1991.

Billah MM et al: Sch 37370: A new drug combining antagonism of platelet-activating factor (PAF) with antagonism of histamine. Agents Actions Suppl 34:313–321, 1991.

Boehringer Ingelheim (Canada) Ltd: Product Monograph: Atrovent Inhalation Solution. Boehringer Ingelheim (Canada) Ltd, Burlington, ON, 1991.

Boushey HA and Holtzman MJ: Bronchodilators and other agents used in the treatment of asthma. In Katzung BD (ed): Basic and Clinical Pharmacology. Lange Medical Publications, Los Altos, 1982.

Busse W: Asthma in the 1990s: A new approach to therapy. Postgrad Med 92:183–186; 189–190, 1992.

Campoli-Richards DM, Buckley MM, and Fitton A: Cetirizine: A review of its pharmacological properties and clinical potential in allergic rhinitis, pollen-induced asthma, and chronic urticaria. Drugs 40:762–781, 1990.

Clark WG, Brater DC, and Johnson AR: Goth's Medical Pharmacology, ed 12. CV Mosby, St Louis, 1988.

Deglin JH and Vallerand AH: Davis's Drug Guide for Nurses, ed 3. FA Davis, Philadelphia, 1993.

Douglas WW: Histamine and 5-hydroxytryptamine (serotonin) and their antagonists. In Goodman AG et al (eds): Goodman and Gilman's The Pharmacologic Basis of Therapeutics, ed 7. Macmillan, New York, 1985.

Grant SM et al: Ketotifen: A review of its pharmacodynamic and pharmacokinetic properties, and therapeutic use in asthma and allergic disorders. Drugs 40:412–448, 1990.

Hoag JE and McFadden ER: Long-term effect of cromolyn sodium on nonspecific bronchial hyperresponsiveness: A review. Ann Allergy 66:53–63, 1991.

Hoppu K et al: Accidental astemizole overdose in young children. Lancet 338:538–540, 1991.

Howarth PH: Histamine and asthma: An appraisal based on specific H_1-receptor antagonism. Clin Exp Allergy 20 (Suppl 2): 31–41, 1990.

Howder CL: Cardiopulmonary Pharmacology: A Handbook for Respiratory Practitioners and Other Allied Health Personnel. Williams and Wilkins, Baltimore, 1992.

Krogh CM (ed): Compendium of Pharmaceuticals and Specialties, ed. 28. Canadian Pharmaceutical Association, Ottawa, 1993.

Larrain A et al: Medical and surgical treatment of nonallergic asthma associated with gastroesophageal reflux. Chest 99:1321–1324, 1991.

Lewis WH and Elvin-Lewis MPF: Medical Botany. John Wiley and Sons, New York, 1977.

Marshall LM: Cromolyn sodium and other mast-cell–stabilizers. In Cherniak RM (ed): Drugs for the Respiratory System. Grune and Stratton, Orlando, 1986.

Monahan BP et al: *Torsades de pointes* occurring in association with terfenadine use. JAMA 264:2788–2790, 1990.

Naclerio RM: Additional properties of cetirizine, a new H_1-antagonist. Allergy Proc 12:187–191, 1991.

Putnam PE, Ricker DH, and Orenstein SR: Gastroesophageal reflux. In Beckerman RC, Brouillette RT, and Hunt CE (eds): Respiratory Control Disorders in Infants and Children. Williams and Wilkins, Baltimore, 1992.

Rafferty P: Antihistamines in the treatment of clinical asthma. J Allergy Clin Immunol 86(4 Pt 2):647–650, 1990.

Rafferty P et al: Terfenadine, a potent histamine H_1-receptor antagonist in the treatment of grass pollen sensitive asthma. Br J Clin Pharmacol 30:229–235, 1990.

Rau JL: Respiratory Care Pharmacology, ed 3. Yearbook Medical Publishers, Chicago, 1989.

Ricci AR et al: The effect of chlorpheniramine on asthma. Allergy Proc 11:229–233, 1990.

Sheffer AL and Samuels LL: Cetirizine: Antiallergic therapy beyond traditional H_1-antihistamines. J Allergy Clin Immunol 86(6 Pt 2):1040–1046, Dec 1990.

Simons FE: New H_1-receptor antagonists: Clinical pharmacology. Clin Exp Allergy. 20(Suppl 2):19–24, 1990.

Simons FE, McMillan JL, and Simons KJ: A double-blind, single-dose, crossover comparison of cetirizine, terfenadine, loratadine, astemizole, and chlorpheniramine versus placebo: Suppressive effects on histamine-induced wheals and flares during 24 hours in normal subjects. J Allergy Clin Immunol 86(4 Pt 1):540–547, 1990.

White MV, Phillips RL, and Kaliner MA: Neutrophils and mast cells: Nedocromil sodium inhibits the generation of neutrophil-derived histamine-releasing activity (HRA-N). J Allergy Clin Immunol 87:812–820, 1991.

Woodward JK: Pharmacology of antihistamines. J Allergy Clin Immunol 86(4 Pt 2):606–612, 1990.

CHAPTER 11

Antimuscarinic Bronchodilators

CHAPTER OUTLINE

CHAPTER OBJECTIVES

After studying this chapter the reader should be able to:

- Differentiate between the conducting portion and the respiratory portion of the respiratory system.
- Briefly outline the structure and function of the conducting portion of the respiratory system.
- List the sources of respiratory tract secretions.
- Explain the operation of the mucociliary escalator as a clearance mechanism.
- Describe the microscopic structure of bronchioles and terminal bronchioles and explain how such passages can change airway resistance.
- Describe the operation of the bronchoconstriction reflex in protection of small airways and explain how its effects can become detrimental to respiratory function.
- Outline the mechanism of action of parasympatholytic drugs in the respiratory system.
- List the disadvantages of the use of belladonna alkaloids in the respiratory system.
- State one indication and one contraindication for use of the quaternary amine antimuscarinics in the respiratory system and explain the rationale behind their use and limitation.
- Describe the pharmacologic activity of the following quaternary amine antimuscarinics:
  - Ipratropium, glycopyrrolate, oxitropium.

KEY TERMS

antimuscarinic
bronchoconstriction reflex
  (irritant reflex)
conducting portion (conducting
  zone; conductive zone)

quaternary amine
respiratory portion (respiratory
  zone)

tracheobronchial tree
  (respiratory tree)

CHAPTER INTRODUCTION

The use of tertiary amine antimuscarinics, such as the belladonna alkaloids, in the treatment of bronchial asthma has several disadvantages and precautions. The parent compounds reduce contraction of airway smooth muscle to relieve bronchospasm but have the potential to inhibit glandular secretion. Development of quaternary amine antimuscarinics has reduced the drawbacks while retaining the excellent bronchodilating qualities of the original compounds.

This chapter discusses the linings, glands, and smooth muscle of the airways and the associated topics of airway resistance, clearance mechanisms, and protective reflexes. This discussion serves as an introduction to the antimuscarinic bronchodilators that target bronchiolar smooth muscle cells and tracheobronchial glands.

CONDUCTING PASSAGES

The respiratory system is subdivided into the **conducting portion,** or **conducting (conductive) zone,** composed of all the passageways that conduct air and the **respiratory portion,** or **respiratory zone,** which is made up of microscopic alveoli involved in gas exchange between the air and blood. In terms of the pharmacologic effects of bronchoactive drugs, only certain elements of the conducting zone are considered—namely, the linings of airways, including any associated glands, and the smooth muscle located in the wall of such airways.

Cartilaginous Airways

The posterior part of the nasal cavity is called the nasopharynx. It blends into the laryngopharynx, which opens into the larynx. The larynx is composed of several flexible cartilages, which enclose and protect the vocal cords. Mucus-secreting cells are scattered among the ciliated epithelial lining cells of the larynx.

The trachea is a large-diameter (about 2 cm) air passage that continues inferiorly from the larynx. Because of its cartilaginous structure, the trachea is highly flexible, extensible, and yet able to retain its patency. Mucus-secreting goblet cells are found as part of the tracheal lining, whereas submucosal tracheal glands are located beneath the lining cells. These exocrine glands open to the luminal surface of the trachea and produce both a watery secretion and mucus, which is added to the mucus output from the goblet cells. The use of drugs to control the production and consistency of mucus is covered in Chapter 15.

At the bifurcation, or branching, of the trachea, two large-diameter branches, called the right and left primary bronchi or main stem bronchi, separate to enter the respective lungs. The incomplete ("C-shaped") cartilages characteristic of the trachea continue through the primary bronchi. There is, however, a steady decline in the percentage of cartilage in the wall of air passages and a gradual increase in the amount of smooth muscle. This subtle transition is seen from proximal to distal portions of the **respiratory tree,** or **tracheobronchial tree** (Fig. 11–1). A mixed secretion consisting of a serous (watery) and mucous discharge is produced by the submucosal bronchial glands lying beneath the lining of epithelial cells (see Fig. 15–1). Like the tracheal glands, bronchial glands are under parasympathetic control. Therefore, they are sensitive to the action of antimuscarinic drugs. Primary bronchi split into secondary, or lobar, bronchi to supply lobes within each lung. The rings of cartilage change to smaller plates of cartilage that become even thinner in the most distal segments. The secondary bronchi branch into several tertiary, or segmental, bronchi to supply bronchopulmonary segments within each lobe (Fig. 11–1). A further reduction in cartilage content and a corresponding increase in the amount of smooth muscle occurs in small-diameter branches of the segmental bronchi called subsegmental bronchi.

Noncartilaginous Airways

Subsegmental bronchi give off innumerable branches known as *bronchioles.* The lining of the small-diameter (less than 1 mm) bronchioles changes to a single layer of ciliated cuboidal cells. Submucosal glands are absent and the mucous cells become less numerous. The bronchioles have a high percentage of smooth muscle in their relatively thin walls. The smooth muscle of the bronchioles is typically arranged in a spiral fashion resembling an elastic band loosely wrapped at intervals around a soft, collapsible tube (Fig. 11–2). Such a spiral muscle fiber arrangement efficiently constricts and shortens a hollow structure when the muscle contracts. When bronchiolar smooth muscle undergoes spasm (as in bronchial asthma), the diameter of the airways decreases dramatically because there is no supportive cartilage to keep the tubes patent.

The bronchioles give off extremely small diameter (approximately 0.5 mm) branches called terminal bronchioles. The lining undergoes transition from simple cuboidal to simple squa-

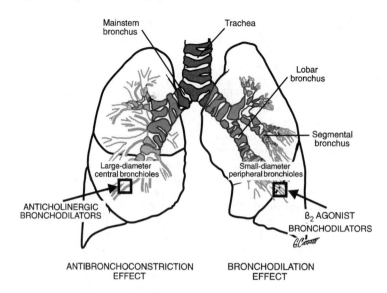

FIGURE 11–1 Tracheobronchial tree.

mous epithelium and the cilia gradually disappear, along with the goblet cell population. Spirally arranged smooth muscle continues around the thin walls of this class of noncartilaginous airway. Therefore, loss of patency occurs easily as a result of smooth muscle spasm. Terminal bronchioles represent the last elements of the conducting portion of the respiratory system.

Airway Resistance and Bronchiolar Smooth Muscle

The total cross-sectional area of the bronchiolar system is substantial—many times greater than that of the trachea. Bronchioles and terminal bronchioles play a key role in the control of airway resistance which is inversely proportional to the fourth power of the radius (r^4) of the air passages:

$$\text{Resistance varies } \frac{1}{r^4}$$

As can be seen by this inverse relationship derived from Poiseuille's Law (Box 11–1), a single small-diameter airway offers far more resistance to laminar flow than a single large-diameter airway. There are, however, a large number of small-diameter (less than 2 mm) peripheral bronchioles (see Fig. 1–11). Because of their large *total* cross-sectional area, such airways account for a relatively small fraction of total air-

way resistance in a normal lung. By contrast, the less numerous but larger-diameter central bronchioles present a small total cross-sectional area and are responsible for much of the total airway resistance in the lung (Des Jardins, 1994). A small change in muscle tension of collapsible, noncartilaginous airways translates into immediate alteration of bronchiolar diameter and resistance to airflow.

The respiratory zone of the lung has an even larger total cross-sectional area than the terminal portions of the conducting zone (Des Jardins, 1994). The alveolar components of the respiratory zone, however, lack smooth muscle in their walls and are incapable of actively changing resistance to flow. (Respiratory bronchioles possess a few smooth muscle fibers in their walls but do not change their diameters significantly.)

Hyperreactive airways usually exhibit both bronchoconstriction and increased exocrine gland activity. When the lumen-restricting effect of accumulated secretions is added to bronchiolar smooth muscle contraction, the overall reduction in airway diameter is substantial. Decreasing the radius of a bronchiole by one half results in a *16-fold increase* in resistance to airflow (Fig. 11–2). Considering the increase in resistance triggered by narrowing of airways, it is little wonder that clinical signs of wheezing and dyspnea appear nearly instantaneously when bronchiolar smooth muscle contracts and tra-

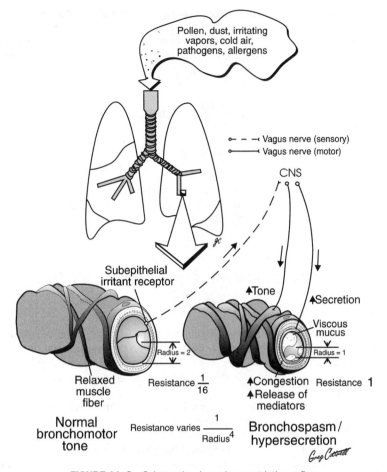

FIGURE 11–2 Schematic—bronchoconstriction reflex.

cheobronchial glands begin to oversecrete (Box 11–1).

Bronchoconstriction Reflex

Bronchoconstriction is not always undesirable. On a frosty winter day, cold air inhaled through the mouth, rather than through the nose, is not warmed sufficiently for entry into the lungs. When the chilled air reaches the upper airways, it stimulates the protective **bronchoconstriction reflex,** or **irritant reflex.** The response is characterized by a reflex spasm of bronchiolar smooth muscle. This change rapidly restricts luminal diameters and prevents entry of potentially damaging cold air to the delicate and vulnerable respiratory portions of the lung. Similarly, the entry of inhaled pollutants, irritating chemical vapors, allergic substances (allergens), or pathogenic microorganisms (patho-

gens) activates subepithelial irritant receptors. The reflex arc includes a sensory branch of the vagus nerve that transmits afferent impulses into the central nervous system (CNS), and a motor branch of the vagus that sends efferent impulses through parasympathetic fibers to bronchiolar smooth muscle, mucous glands, and target cells containing stored histamine (Fig. 11–2). The motor activity results in bronchoconstriction, glandular secretion, and possible release of histamine from storage sites. The mechanism of action of antimuscarinic bronchodilators is directed at suppression of these events.

Stimuli such as allergens and pathogens often cause the release of allergic mediators, especially in individuals with predisposition to allergic reactions. Histamine induces bronchoconstriction and tracheobronchial gland activity, thereby decreasing airway diameter (see Table 9–3). At the point where wheezing, coughing, and dyspnea

BOX 11–1 BRONCHIOLES, BRONCHODILATORS, AND POISEUILLE'S LAW

The remarkable change in airway resistance that occurs when airway radius is altered is revealed by the Hagen-Poiseuille Law, which describes laminar flow. The relationship of the flow rate of a gas, pressure gradient, radius of the airway, viscosity of the gas, and length of the airway is shown below:

$$\dot{V} = \frac{\pi \Delta P r^4}{8 \eta l}, \text{ where}$$

$\dot{V}$ = flowrate of the gas   r = radius
π = mathematical constant (pi) η = viscosity (eta)
ΔP = pressure gradient   l = length

Conductance is a measure of the ability of a substance to pass through a tube, and in this relationship, where $\dot{V}$ = flowrate and ΔP = pressure gradient, the remainder of the equation represents conductance (C); therefore:

$$C = \frac{\pi r^4}{8 \eta l}$$

Conductance (C) is the reciprocal of resistance (R); therefore,

$$R = \frac{8 \eta l}{\pi r^4}$$

Resistance to laminar flow is directly proportional to the viscosity (η) of the gas and the length (l) of the airway, but it is inversely proportional to the fourth power of the radius (r^4) of the airway. Assuming both a constant length of conducting passages and a constant viscosity of gas, a small change in the radius of an airway produces a sizable change in airway resistance.

Factors that promote bronchoconstriction include parasympathetic nervous activity, muscarinic cholinergic drugs, and allergic mediators, such as histamine. These factors cause profound changes in bronchiolar diameter because the small passages lack cartilage and are relatively collapsible. Similarly, drugs employed to promote relaxation of bronchiolar smooth muscle often produce dramatic results—alleviating clinical signs of respiratory distress because of the same *inverse relationship* between the radii of airways and resistance to airflow.

Dupuis YG: Ventilators: Theory and Clinical Application, ed 2. Mosby–Year Book, St Louis, 1992.
Guyton AC: Textbook of Medical Physiology, ed 7. WB Saunders, Philadelphia, 1986.

appear clinically, the protective nature of the bronchoconstriction reflex has given way to an undesirable response.

MUSCARINIC ANTAGONISTS AND THE RESPIRATORY SYSTEM

Mechanism of Action

Aerosol derivatives of the classic belladonna alkaloids possess the same nonspecific mechanism of action as the parent compounds, namely, competitive antagonism of acetylcholine (ACh) at M_2– and M_3–muscarinic receptors (see Fig. 5–9). Through the blockade of postjunctional M_3–

muscarinic sites, guanylate cyclase is inhibited and cGMP (cyclic guanosine-3′,5′-monophosphate) levels are suppressed. Decreased cGMP, in turn, prevents contraction of airway smooth muscle, inhibits glandular secretion, and blocks the release of histamine. Figure 9–7 shows the site of action of antimuscarinic bronchodilators and other bronchoactive drugs.

Limitations of Belladonna Alkaloids

Relief of bronchospasm and control of airway secretions are often the goals of pulmonary drug therapy. Antimuscarinics, such as atropine, block ACh neurotransmission and unmask sympathetic activity to cause relaxation of airway smooth muscle. A drawback, however, to the use of belladonna alkaloids is their potential drying effect on secretions and their lack of selectivity at muscarinic receptor subtypes (see Chapter 8). A moderate amount of muscarinic blockade and suppression of exocrine gland activity is desirable in hyperreactive airways and in vagally mediated asthma. Atropine and its close derivatives, however, can reduce glandular secretion to such an extent that inspissated (dried) mucus secretions may accumulate in the small-bore passages. In addition, antimuscarinics such as atropine and scopolamine are tertiary amines and therefore can cross the blood-brain barrier to produce unwanted central nervous system effects. CNS depression occurs at low dosages; CNS stimulation is seen at high dosages. Atropine and scopolamine, however, exhibit differences in CNS effect at therapeutic dosages (see Fig. 8–2).

Despite these shortcomings, tertiary amine atropinelike drugs may be beneficial in the treatment of bronchoconstriction caused by vagal activity. For most asthmatic patients, however, the risk of mucus plug formation often overshadows the widespread use of tertiary amine antimuscarinics.

Quaternary Amine Derivatives of Atropine

With the limitations of the prototype belladonna alkaloids in mind, researchers have developed **quaternary amine** derivatives that exhibit more selective peripheral activity (see Fig. 8–1). These agents deliver adequate bronchodilation but do not cause the degree of glandular inhibition seen with atropine and scopolamine. In addition, the quaternary amine derivatives are slow to cross the blood-brain barrier due to their low lipid solubility and therefore have less severe CNS side effects.

THERAPEUTIC AGENTS

IPRATROPIUM (Atrovent). In the 1960s, the pharmacologic results produced by a quaternary amine antimuscarinic showed promise. The experimental parasympatholytic bronchodilator codenamed Sch 1000 was released nearly 20 years later as ipratropium bromide (Atrovent) an aerosol antimuscarinic for bronchodilator use. Ipratropium applied topically by inhalation fulfills the requirements that had been sought by researchers: (1) it possesses potent bronchodilating activity and (2) it does not cause the profound drying effect on secretions characteristic of atropine. In addition, the drug has minimal ocular (mydriatic-cycloplegic) and CNS activity. Desirable peripheral effects at bronchiolar smooth muscle and exocrine glands make ipratropium valuable in the treatment of respiratory disorders.

Ipratropium is applied topically when given as an inhalational aerosol. Therefore, absorption of the drug is reduced and unwanted systemic effects are minimized. The bronchodilator is most effective on large-diameter central airways, whereas smaller-diameter peripheral airways respond well to β_2-adrenergic agonists. Ipratropium administered in conjunction with a β_2-sympathomimetic drug produces an enhanced bronchodilation response that is maintained over time. This occurs because the two drugs produce selective effects at different classes of airways. The antimuscarinic drug opposes bronchoconstriction caused by parasympathetic activity, and the β_2-agonist drug stimulates β_2-receptors to produce bronchodilation. Combination products containing both ipratropium and a β_2-agonist are showing promise as effective bronchodilators in asthma therapy. For example, Boehringer Ingelheim is marketing Duovent (ipratropium and fenoterol) in the United Kingdom and is currently testing Combivent (ipratropium and salbutamol[CAN] [albuterol[US]]) for future clinical use in North America. These compounds are discussed further in the following chapter.

INDICATIONS. Quaternary amine antimuscarinics are useful in alleviating the symptoms of bronchial asthma when inhibition of parasympathetic activity is desirable. The larger-diameter upper airways are affected more than the small-diameter lower airways by aerosol antimuscarinics such as ipratropium. Airway resistance is lowered, mucus plug formation is minimized, and the work of breathing is lessened with the quaternary amine derivatives of atropine.

Antimuscarinics such as ipratropium are effective in some patients with chronic obstructive pulmonary disease such as emphysema and chronic bronchitis. The aerosol antimuscarinics often dilate airways better and exhibit a longer duration of action than β_2-adrenergic agonists administered for the same indications.

CONTRAINDICATIONS. Known hypersensitivity to ipratropium or related belladonna alkaloid drugs is a contraindication to use of the drug. In addition, known hypersensitivity to chlorofluorocarbon propellants is a contraindication to ipratropium administration by metered-dose inhaler (MDI).

PRECAUTIONS. Because of its ability to suppress

cholinergic activity, ipratropium must be used cautiously in patients with gastrointestinal and urinary tract hypomotility and in patients with glaucoma (see ''Atropine'' in Chapter 8).

Ipratropium has a slow onset of action compared with β₂-adrenergic agonists. Therefore, it should not be used alone to treat an acute asthma attack. Ipratropium is always used concurrently with an inhaled β₂-agonist to treat acute severe asthma.

Inhalation solutions (0.025%) of ipratropium contain preservatives that may trigger bronchoconstriction in some patients with hyperreactive airways. These preservatives include benzalkonium chloride and edetate disodium. Benzalkonium chloride may form a precipitate with cromolyn if ipratropium and cromolyn are mixed together. Cromolyn must be given separately (see Chapter 10).

Propellant toxicity is a precaution with the MDI form of ipratropium. The toxicity, caused by trichlorofluoromethane (Freon 11), dichlorodifluoromethane (Freon 12), and cryofluorane (Freon 114) is discussed in Chapter 1.

ADVERSE REACTIONS. Typical anticholinergic adverse effects include dry mouth, blurred vision, nausea, gastrointestinal tract irritation, and palpitations. In addition, cough and bronchospasm may be induced by ipratropium administered by inhalation. Cholinesterase inhibitors are used in the management of serious anticholinergic toxicities (Box 11–2).

GLYCOPYRROLATE (Robinul). Glycopyrrolate is another quaternary amine derivative of atropine classified as an antimuscarinic bronchodilator. It is available in injectable form and as an aerosol solution. Peripheral effects at the airways predominate to produce smooth muscle relax-

---

BOX 11-2 ''. . . SMOKE TWO OF THESE AND CALL ME IN THE MORNING.''

Interest in the use of modern aerosol antimuscarinic drugs increased with better understanding of the role of the parasympathetic division in the mediation of the bronchoconstriction reflex. Inhaled antimuscarinics were found to diminish the effect of vagal influences on both bronchiolar smooth muscle and airway secretions.

Of course, these facts were not known to practitioners of Ayurvedic medicine (folk remedies) in India when they treated asthma symptoms many centuries ago. Several North American Indian tribes routinely used a medicinal herb to relieve respiratory ailments. Yet these widely separated cultures recognized the therapeutic benefits derived from inhaling fumes derived from burning the leaves of certain local plants. Often the roots of folk medicine are grounded in superstition and ritual, false hopes, and a dash of quackery. But in the case of some very early asthma remedies, they were (and are) valid.

Datura stramonium is known as jimsonweed, Jamestown weed, thorn apple, or Devil's apple and is widely distributed in North America and on other continents. The plant thrives in pastures, cultivated fields, and waste areas and can be found along roadsides. It contains the belladonna alkaloids scopolamine (L-hyoscine) and small amounts of atropine (DL-hyoscyamine). Leaves from the plant were burned and the fumes inhaled as a popular asthma treatment in the first half of the 19th century. Stramonium was the active ingredient in Asthmador cigarettes and was available as an asthma remedy in several brands of cigars and cigarettes. The Spanish Cigarette Company of London and New York marketed Spanish Herbal Cigarettes and advertised that ''. . . the fumes of this plant afford instantaneous relief from afflictions of the respiratory system . . . and in cases of Coughs, Colds, Bronchitis, Asthma, and Pulmonary Complaints, generally they will be found of the greatest value and benefit.''

Pulmonary physicians no longer prescribe stramonium cigarettes to be smoked by their asthmatic patients, but they do prescribe ipratropium delivered by aerosol. Both compounds provide symptomatic relief through the same mechanism of action; both are administered through inhalation. They are just separated by half a century of pharmaceutical progress.

Gerald MC: Pharmacology: An Introduction to Drugs. Prentice-Hall, Englewood Cliffs, 1981.
Lewis WH and Elvin-Lewis MPF: Medical Botany. John Wiley and Sons, New York, 1977.

ation with minimal glandular suppression. Blood-brain barrier penetration and CNS activity are minimal due to the quaternary amine structure of the drug. Such a structure remains ionized and therefore lacks suitable lipid solubility for entry into nervous tissue.

Like other antimuscarinics, glycopyrrolate may be employed to inhibit cholinergic stimulation at muscarinic sites. It possesses fewer ocular and central nervous system effects than atropine when used as such a blocking agent. Glycopyrrolate is also used preoperatively to produce a vagolytic (blocking) effect at the heart. In addition, it inhibits gastrointestinal and urinary tract motility without the CNS or ocular effects of atropine.

INDICATIONS, CONTRAINDICATIONS, PRECAUTIONS, AND ADVERSE REACTIONS. See Ipratropium Bromide.

OXITROPIUM BROMIDE (Ba 253). Oxitropium is an experimental quaternary amine derivative of scopolamine. It is classified as an aerosol antimuscarinic bronchodilator.

INDICATIONS, CONTRAINDICATIONS, PRECAUTIONS, AND ADVERSE REACTIONS. See Ipratropium Bromide.

NEWER ANTIMUSCARINICS

Atropine, ipratropium, and oxitropium are nonselective muscarinic antagonists that block both at prejunctional M_2- and postjunctional M_3-muscarinic receptors. An alternative may prove to be the *selective* blockade of muscarinic receptor subtypes (see Fig. 5–9). Ideally, such a mechanism would permit systemic administration and produce bronchodilation without anticholinergic or sedative side effects.

Animal and human studies of methacholine-induced airway spasm have shown that the contraction can be blocked by specific muscarinic antagonists (Doods, 1991; Mahesh et al, 1992; Barnes, 1993). Such drugs may have a future role as bronchoactive agents. Many of the experimental subtype-selective blockers have curious names such as pirenzepine (M_1), 4-DAMP (M_3), AF-DX 116 (M_2), AQ-RA 721 (M_1, M_3), and even hexahydrosiladifenidol (HHSiD) (M_3)! The reader should not be discouraged by these cryptic names and acronyms for chemical compounds—the names are usually simplified by the time the drugs become available clinically. Recall that ipratropium, although familiar now by its generic name, was originally investigated in the 1960s and 1970s as Sch 1000.

Table 11–1 lists the generic and trade names of the antimuscarinic bronchodilators discussed

in this chapter. Dosages for selected agents are given in Table 11–2.

TABLE 11–1 DRUG NAMES: ANTIMUSCARINIC BRONCHODILATORS

Generic Name	Trade Name
Ipratropium (ip-ra-**TRŌP**-ē-um)	Atrovent
Glycopyrrolate (glī-kō-**PĪ**-rō-lāt)	Robinul
Oxitropium (oks-i-**TRŌP**-ē-um)	*(Investigational) Ba253

*Oxivent in Europe.

CHAPTER SUMMARY

The distal portions of the tracheobronchial tree possess little or no cartilage, but have a high percentage of smooth muscle in their walls. Shortening of the muscle fibers in response to cholinergic nerve impulses, cholinergic drugs, or irritants such as dusts and pollen greatly reduces the diameter of small-diameter airways. This reduction causes a substantial increase in airway resistance. Blockade of M_3–muscarinic receptors at bronchiolar smooth muscle membranes by the antimuscarinic bronchodilators provides effective symptomatic treatment of asthma, especially in conjunction with inhaled β_2-adrenergic agonists.

We have seen that tertiary amine antimuscarinics, such as the prototype belladonna alkaloids, relax bronchiolar smooth muscle but have the potential to suppress glandular secretions. Quaternary amine derivatives retain the smooth muscle–relaxing properties of atropine but produce less inhibition of glandular secretion and produce less CNS sedation. A novel approach being investigated to control bronchospasm involves the systemic administration of drugs that exhibit selective blockade of muscarinic receptor subtypes.

BIBLIOGRAPHY

Avital A, Sanchez I, and Chernick V: Efficacy of salbutamol and ipratropium bromide in decreasing bronchial hyperreactivity in children with cystic fibrosis. Pediatr Pulmonol 13:34–37, 1992.

Barnes PJ: Autonomic pharmacology of the airways. In Chung KF and Barnes PJ (eds): Pharmacology of the Respiratory Tract: Experimental and Clinical Research. Marcel Dekker, New York, 1993.

Bethel RA and Irvin CG: Anticholinergic, antimuscarinic drugs (atropine sulfate, ipratropium bromide). In Cherniak RM (ed): Drugs for the Respiratory System. Grune and Stratton, Orlando, 1986.

TABLE 11-2   DRUG DOSAGES: INHALATION AGENTS*

Drug	Availability	Dosage
Ipratropium[a]	**ATROVENT INHALATION SOLUTION**	
	20 mL MULTI-USE BOTTLE Contains 250 µg/mL (0.025%) in normal saline (0.9% sodium chloride solution) preserved with benzalkonium chloride and EDTA-disodium (see "Precautions") **2 mL** UNIT DOSE VIAL (UDV) Single-use ampules in normal saline (0.9% sodium chloride solution) Preservative free Available in two UDVs: 2 mL vial: 250 µg/mL contains 250 µg/mL (0.025%) ipratropium bromide; 1 single-use vial contains 500 µg of ipratropium bromide 2 mL vial: 125 µg/mL contains 125 µg/mL (0.0125%) ipratropium; 1 single-use vial contains 250 µg of ipratropium bromide	**ADULTS** Average single dose is 1–2 mL (250–500 µg) of Atrovent (ipratropium) solution **CHILDREN 5–12 YEARS** Recommended dose is 0.5–1 mL (125–250 µg) **DOSE** Should be diluted to 3–5 mL with preservative-free sterile normal saline (sodium chloride inhalation solution, USP 0.9%) or with a bacteriostatic sodium chloride solution, 0.9% preserved with benzalkonium chloride **NEBULIZER** Gas flow (oxygen or compressed air) of 6–10 L/min with solution inspired over 10–15 min Treatment repeated every 4–6 h as necessary
	ATROVENT INHALATION AEROSOL	
	METERED-DOSE INHALER Supplied as a pressurized metal canister containing 140 or 200 doses of Atrovent Each valve depression (actuation) delivers 20 µg of Atrovent (as a micronized powder)	**OPTIMAL MAINTENANCE DOSE** Must be individually determined Recommended dosage is 2 metered doses (40 µg) 3 or 4 times daily Some patients may need up to 4 actuations (80 µg) at a time to obtain maximum benefit during early treatment Maximal daily dosage should not exceed 8 metered doses (160 µg); minimum interval between doses should not be less than 4 h
Glycopyrrolate[b]	**INHALATION SOLUTION**	
	0.2 mg/mL (0.02%) (injectable solution)	**ADULTS** 5 mL (1 mg) 3 or 4 times daily
Oxitropium[b]	**INHALATION AEROSOL**	
	METERED-DOSE INHALER Each valve depression (actuation) delivers 0.1 mg of oxitropium	**ADULTS** 2 metered doses (0.2 mg) 2 or 3 times daily

Source: [a]Data from Boehringer Ingelheim (Canada) Ltd, 1990, 1991, 1993.
      [b]Data from Howder, 1993.
*The dosage information contained in this table is presented as a brief outline and summary of acceptable dosages. It is *not* meant to replace the detailed information available from manufacturers of these drugs. Package inserts provide the most current dosing information from pharmaceutical manufacturers. Guidelines describing the preparation and delivery of the drug, dose strengths and dosage schedules, shelf life, and storage requirements are also included in the package inserts. In addition, precautions and adverse reactions are described in detail. The respiratory care practitioner is strongly urged to read this information supplied by the pharmaceutical manufacturer to provide safe and effective drug therapy.
USP—US Pharmacopeia.

Boehringer Ingelheim (Canada) Ltd: Product Monograph: Atrovent Inhaler. Boehringer Ingelheim (Canada) Ltd, Burlington, ON, 1990.

Boehringer Ingelheim (Canada) Ltd: Product Monograph: Atrovent Inhalation Solution. Boehringer Ingelheim (Canada) Ltd, Burlington, ON, 1991.

Boehringer Ingelheim (Canada) Ltd: Product Monograph: Atrovent Inhalation Solution. Boehringer Ingelheim (Canada) Ltd, Burlington, ON, 1993.

Boushey HA and Holtzman MJ: Bronchodilators and other agents used in the treatment of asthma. In Katzung BD (ed): Basic and Clinical Pharmacology. Lange Medical Publications, Los Altos, 1982.

Braun SR et al: A comparison of the effect of ipratropium and albuterol in the treatment of chronic obstructive airway disease. Arch Intern Med 149:544–547, 1989.

Carola R, Harley JP, and Noback CR: Human Anatomy and Physiology, ed 2. McGraw-Hill, New York, 1992.

Chapman KR: The role of anticholinergic bronchodilators in adult asthma and chronic obstructive pulmonary disease. Lung (Suppl):295–303, 1990.

Des Jardins TR: Cardiopulmonary Anatomy and Physiology, ed 2. Delmar, Albany, 1994.

Doods HN: Selective muscarinic antagonists as bronchodilators. Agents Actions Suppl 34:117–130, 1991.

Dupuis YG: Ventilators: Theory and Clinical Application, ed 2. Mosby–Year Book, St Louis, 1992.

Gerald MC: Pharmacology: An Introduction to Drugs. Prentice-Hall, Englewood Cliffs, 1981.

Hargreave FE, Dolovich J, and Newhouse MT: The assessment and treatment of asthma: A conference report. J Allergy Clin Immunol 85:1098–1111, 1990.

Howder CL: Cardiopulmonary Pharmacology: A Handbook for Respiratory Practitioners and Other Allied Health Personnel. Williams and Wilkins, Baltimore, 1992.

Howder CL: Antimuscarinic and β_2-adrenoreceptor bronchodilators in obstructive airways disease. Respiratory Care 38:1364–1388, 1993.

Katzung BG: Cholinergic receptor antagonists. In Katzung BD (ed): Basic and Clinical Pharmacology. Lange Medical Publications, Los Altos, 1982.

Lehnert BE and Schachter EN: The Pharmacology of Respiratory Care. CV Mosby, St Louis, 1980.

Lewis WH and Elvin-Lewis MPF: Medical Botany. John Wiley and Sons, New York, 1977.

Magnussen H, Nowak D, and Wiebicke W: Effect of inhaled ipratropium bromide on the airway response to methacholine, histamine, and exercise in patients with mild bronchial asthma. Respiration 59:42–47, 1992.

Mahesh VK et al: A minority of muscarinic receptors mediate rabbit tracheal smooth muscle contraction. Am J Respir Cell Mol Biol 6:279–286, 1992.

Mathewson HS: Asthma and bronchitis: A shift of therapeutic emphasis. Respiratory Care 35:273–277, 1990.

Mathewson HS: Combined drug therapy in asthma (editorial). Respiratory Care 38:1340, 1993.

Netter FH: Respiratory system. In Divertie MB (ed): Ciba Collection of Medical Illustrations. CIBA Pharmaceutical Company, Division of CIBA-Geigy Corporation, Summit, NJ, 1979.

O'Driscoll BR et al: Nebulised salbutamol with and without ipratropium bromide in acute airflow obstruction. Lancet i:1418–1420, 1989.

Polosa R et al: The effect of inhaled ipratropium bromide alone and in combination with oral terfenadine on bronchoconstriction provoked by adenosine 5'-monophosphate and histamine in asthma. J Allergy Clin Immunol 87:939–947, 1991.

Rau JL: Respiratory Care Pharmacology, ed 3. Yearbook Medical Publishers, Chicago, 1989.

Roffel AF, Elzinga CR, and Zaagsma J: Muscarinic M_3 receptors mediate contraction of human central and peripheral airway smooth muscle. Pulm Pharmacol 3:47–51, 1990.

Simon PM and Statz EM: Drug treatment of COPD: Controversies about agents and how to deliver them. Postgrad Med 91:473–479, 1992.

Tortora GJ and Grabowski SR: Principles of Anatomy and Physiology, ed 7. HarperCollins, New York, 1993.

van Schayck CP et al: Bronchodilator treatment in moderate asthma or chronic bronchitis: Continuous or on demand? A randomised controlled study. BMJ 303 (6815):1426–1431, 1991.

CHAPTER 12

Adrenergic Agonists

CHAPTER OUTLINE

CHAPTER OBJECTIVES

After studying this chapter the reader should be able to:

- Describe the biosynthesis of catecholamines.
- Briefly explain the action of MAO and COMT enzymes in the metabolism of catecholamines.
- Explain how changes in the catechol nucleus and the ethylamine side chain of a catecholamine molecule can alter its duration of action and its adrenergic receptor specificity.
- Explain the role of cyclic AMP in adrenergic neurotransmission.
- Contrast the mechanism of action of indirect-acting, direct-acting, and mixed-action sympathomimetic drugs.
- List two precautions and two adverse effects of the sympathomimetics used as bronchodilators and mucosal vasoconstrictors.
- Describe the effect that the route of administration (parenteral, aerosol, oral) has on the plasma levels and pharmacologic action of a sympathomimetic bronchodilator.
- Describe the pharmacologic activity of the following bronchodilators:
  - Ephedrine, epinephrine, racemic epinephrine, ethylnorepinephrine, isoproterenol, isoetharine, bitolterol, metaproterenol, terbutaline, fenoterol, albuterol[US] (salbutamol[CAN]), pirbuterol, procaterol.
- Describe the pharmacologic activity of the following mucosal vasoconstrictors:
  - Ephedrine, epinephrine, phenylephrine.

KEY TERMS

adrenochrome
biogenic amine
bronchodilator
catecholamine

catechol nucleus
ethylamine side chain
mucosal vasoconstrictor

racemic compound
resorcinol (re-**SORS**-si-nol)
saligenin (sa-**LIJ**-i-nin)

CHAPTER INTRODUCTION

Details of norepinephrine activity, adrenergic receptors, and catabolic enzymes were introduced with autonomic pharmacology in Chapter 5. Drugs that simulate, or mimic, adrenergic transmission are the frontline drugs administered in the treatment of bronchial asthma, circulatory shock, and cardiac arrest. Some are employed in minor roles as nasal decongestants, cold remedies, and appetite suppressants. Potent effects on the cardiopulmonary system place the adrenergic agonists at the forefront of the therapeutic drugs with which the respiratory care practitioner is involved.

CATECHOLAMINES AND THEIR DERIVATIVES

The pharmacologic uses of adrenergic agonists are focused in three major body systems:

- The respiratory system (bronchodilators and nasal decongestants)
- The cardiovascular system (cardiac stimulants and vasopressors)
- The central nervous system (CNS) (adrenergic drugs with CNS stimulant activity)

The adrenergic drugs to be introduced in this chapter are catecholamines and catecholamine derivatives affecting the respiratory system. Most of these *sympathomimetics* are **bronchodilators** affecting β_2-adrenoceptors on airway smooth muscle, primarily in small-diameter peripheral bronchioles (Howder, 1993). Other sympathomimetics acting as **mucosal vasoconstrictors** stimulate α_1-adrenoceptors on blood vessels in the nasal mucosa.

Catecholamines belong to a larger group of compounds known as the **biogenic amines.** This larger group of amines includes serotonin, which serves as a neurotransmitter in the CNS, and the catecholamines dopamine, norepinephrine, and epinephrine. Catecholamines serve as chemical messengers (neurohormones) of adrenergic nerves and of the adrenal medulla. Norepinephrine (or levarterenol) is the neurotransmitter released from adrenergic nerve endings. Norepinephrine and epinephrine are the hormones secreted by the adrenal medulla. Dopamine serves as a neurotransmitter in the CNS and as a precursor in catecholamine synthesis.

Biosynthesis

The synthesis of catecholamines takes place in adrenergic nerve terminals and in adrenomed-

ullary cells. Norepinephrine is the final product of catecholamine synthesis in adrenergic nerve terminals but is converted into epinephrine in the adrenal medulla. The rate of synthesis increases with adrenergic neuronal firing and adrenomedullary secretion to keep pace with the demand. The availability of tyrosine hydroxylase is the rate-limiting enzyme step in catecholamine synthesis (Fig. 12–1).

Metabolism

Metabolism of the catecholamines is carried out mainly by monoamine oxidase (MAO) intraneuronally and by MAO and catechol-O-methyltransferase (COMT) acting in tissues such as the liver and kidneys. Following the release of norepinephrine into a synapse, 50%–60% of the transmitter reenters the adrenergic nerve terminal through the uptake-1 mechanism (see Fig. 5–10). MAO within the prejunctional neuron then degrades norepinephrine by oxidative deamination to an intermediate product. Norepinephrine is inactivated by COMT in nonneuronal tissues to an intermediate metabolite that is excreted (see Fig. 12–1). Because norepinephrine and epinephrine can be acted on by MAO, COMT, or both, a variety of catecholamines and their metabolic byproducts appear in the plasma and urine. This effect can occur as a result of catecholamine drug administration, repeated adrenergic neuronal firing, or excessive adrenomedullary secretion. Sensitive biochemical assays of urine can detect metabolites such as 3-methoxy-4-hydroxy mandelic acid. This substance is generally referred to as *vanillylmandelic acid* (VMA) and is the endproduct of both MAO and COMT metabolism of catecholamines (see Fig. 12–1). Urine assays of VMA and other key metabolites are useful diagnostic tools in identifying disorders such as tumors of the adrenal medulla (pheochromocytoma).

Structure-Activity Relationships

A catecholamine consists of two parts: a **catechol nucleus** and an **ethylamine side chain** (Fig. 12–2). The six-carbon ring (benzene) has two hydroxide groups (–OH) attached at adjacent carbon positions 3 and 4, while the side chain is attached at carbon position 1. In addition, a hydroxide group is attached to the β-carbon atom, the connection between side chain and catechol nucleus. This β-hydroxide group is essential for β-adrenergic receptor activity. (The "beta" designation, as in β-hydroxide, is coincidental and does not refer to β-receptors.)

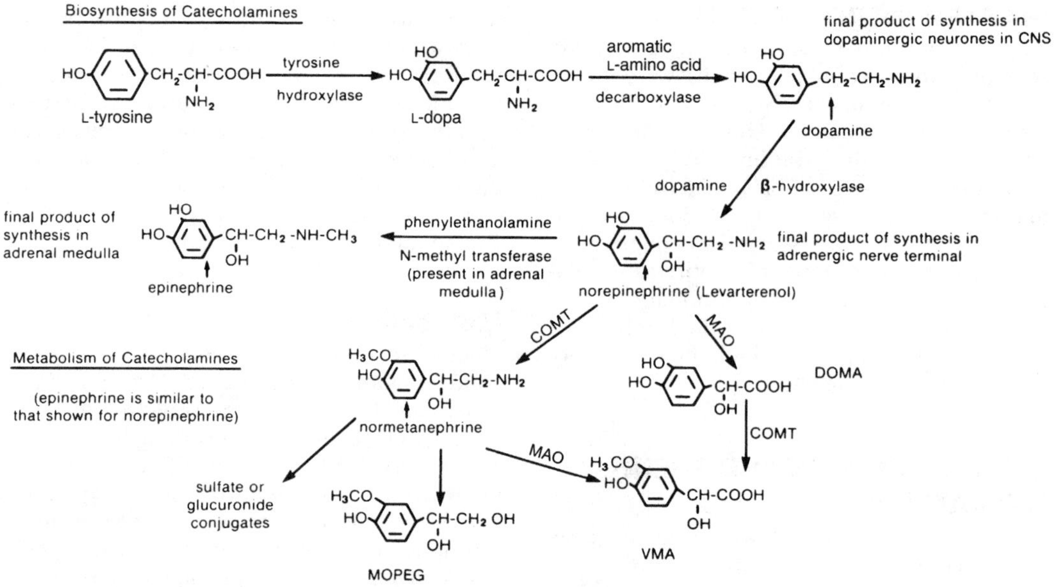

Biosynthesis of Catecholamines

final product of synthesis in dopaminergic neurones in CNS

L-tyrosine → tyrosine hydroxylase → L-dopa → aromatic L-amino acid decarboxylase → dopamine

dopamine / β-hydroxylase

final product of synthesis in adrenal medulla — epinephrine ← phenylethanolamine N-methyl transferase (present in adrenal medulla) ← norepinephrine (Levarterenol) final product of synthesis in adrenergic nerve terminal

Metabolism of Catecholamines

(epinephrine is similar to that shown for norepinephrine)

COMT → normetanephrine

MAO → DOMA

COMT → VMA

MAO → MOPEG

sulfate or glucuronide conjugates

FIGURE 12–1 Biosynthesis and metabolism of catecholamines. Most compounds that are not branched on the α carbon undergo deamination and oxidation through MAO activity. COMT transfers a -CH_3 group and therefore methylates the 3-OH of catecholamines. MAO = monoamine oxidase; COMT = catechol-O-methyltransferase; DOMA = 3,4-dihydroxymandelic acid; VMA = 3-methyoxy-4-hydromandelic acid; MOPEG = 3-methyoxy-4-hydroxyphenylethylglycol. (Modified from Conn PM and Gebhart GF (eds): Essentials of Pharmacology. FA Davis Co, Philadephia, 1989, p. 93.)

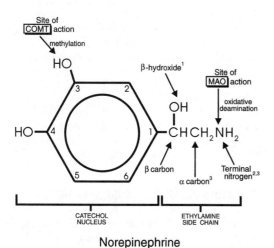

Site of COMT action / methylation

β-hydroxide[1]

Site of MAO action / oxidative deamination

β carbon

α carbon[3]

Terminal nitrogen[2,3]

CATECHOL NUCLEUS

ETHYLAMINE SIDE CHAIN

Norepinephrine

FIGURE 12–2 Structural features of a catecholamine. ([1]The beta-hydroxide group is required for beta-adrenoceptor activity in the molecule. [2]Adrenergic activity shifts from alpha to beta effects as chemical groupings are added to the terminal amine. [3]The addition of more groups on the alpha-carbon and the terminal amine increases the adrenergic specificity of the molecule, shifting it from beta$_1$ to increased beta$_2$ activity.)

All catecholamines are prone to rapid enzymatic degradation by COMT, especially within liver and kidney cells. Catechol-O-methyl*transfer*ase (COMT) catalyzes the *transfer* of a methyl group (methylation) to the hydroxide grouping at carbon-3 on the catechol nucleus, thus inactivating the molecule (Fig. 12–1). Because COMT and MAO are also found in the gut and liver, orally administered catecholamines are subject to methylation by COMT and oxidative deamination by MAO (Fig. 12–1). Lack of efficacy when administered by the oral route and a short duration of action when administered by parenteral or aerosol routes limit the therapeutic usefulness of catecholamines.

Alterations in the type and location of substituted groups on the benzene ring have led to the development of more selective sympathomimetics that resist enzymatic breakdown. Such catecholamine derivatives are long acting and orally active. For example, the inclusion of hydroxide groups at carbon-3 and carbon-5 (rather than carbon-3 and carbon-4) produces a noncatecholamine known as a **resorcinol** (Fig. 12–3). Bronchodilators such as metaproterenol, terbutaline, and fenoterol are classified as resorcinols. Substitution of a chemical grouping other than hydroxide at carbon-3 produces a nonca-

CATECHOLAMINE (3-OH; 4-OH)

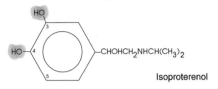

Isoproterenol

RESORCINOL (3-OH; 5-OH)

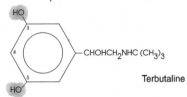

Terbutaline

SALIGENIN (3-not OH; 4-OH)

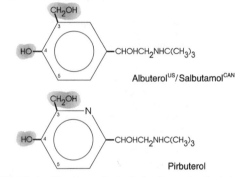

Albuterol^{US}/Salbutamol^{CAN}

Pirbuterol

FIGURE 12–3 Structure of catecholamine and catecholamine derivatives (resorcinols and saligenins).

techolamine known as a **saligenin** (see Fig. 12–3). The bronchodilator known as albuterol in the United States and as salbutamol in Canada is classified as a saligenin. Alteration of the benzene ring itself with the incorporation of nitrogen in place of a carbon atom yields an analog of albuterol^{US} known as pirbuterol. The resulting structure of pirbuterol is extremely enzyme resistant (Fig. 12–3).

Variation in adrenergic receptor activity is caused by the nature of the side chain attached to the catechol nucleus. The uncomplicated linear chain (–CHOH–CH$_2$–NH$_2$) and terminal nitrogen of norepinephrine result in more α- than β-adrenergic activity (Fig. 12–3). (*Nor*, as in norepinephrine, stands for *Nitrogen ohne Radikal*. This is a German chemical technology term meaning "nitrogen without a radical," or chemical grouping attached [Clark et al, 1988]). As more chemical groupings are added to the terminal nitrogen, however, receptor activity shifts

away from α-stimulation toward β-stimulation. For example, a single methyl group (–CH$_3$) on the nitrogen atom causes epinephrine (adrenalin) to have α-effects roughly equal to β-effects. The addition of an isopropyl group (CH$_3$–CH–CH$_3$) to the terminal nitrogen yields the synthetic catecholamine isoproterenol, a β-agonist almost totally devoid of α-activity (see Fig. 3–4). Loading the side chain further, at the midpoint carbon (or α-carbon), confers even greater adrenergic specificity. For example, the synthetic catecholamine isoetharine exhibits more β$_2$- than β$_1$-activity.

Catecholamine derivatives such as metaproterenol, terbutaline, salbutamol^{CAN} (albuterol^{US}), and fenoterol possess ethylamine side chains that are loaded with various chemical substituents. They are described as being "bulky." As with the synthetic catecholamines described above, the synthetic noncatecholamines gain β$_2$-adrenoceptor specificity when their side chains possess multiple chemical groupings. Enhanced β$_2$-specificity is attributed to this bulk, presumably allowing the sympathomimetic to conform more closely to the β$_2$-receptor on airway smooth muscle and combine with it to activate the secondary messenger system. Another benefit of the complex side chains on sympathomimetic bronchodilators is that the chain is less susceptible to enzymatic breakdown by MAO. Catecholamine derivatives such as fenoterol have extremely bulky side chains and are more persistent than native catecholamines. Such bronchodilators exhibit relatively long durations of action.

Receptor specificity, potency, and duration of action of the bronchodilators discussed above are summarized in Table 12–1. The site of action of the β$_2$-agonists can be seen in Figure 9–7.

Adrenergic Stimulation and Secondary Messengers

The role of secondary messengers in adrenergic stimulation has been previously outlined. As briefly stated, the intracellular mechanism of action of β-adrenergic stimulants such as isoproterenol is one of adenylate cyclase induction and a subsequent rise in intracellular cAMP (cyclic adenosine–3′,5′-monophosphate) (see Table 5–6). Cyclic AMP in turn activates protein kinases intracellularly to trigger characteristic β$_2$ effects such as bronchiolar smooth muscle relaxation, inhibition of allergic mediator release, and facilitated mucociliary transport (see Fig.

TABLE 12-1 PHARMACOLOGIC ACTIVITY OF COMMON BRONCHODILATORS

Drug*	Receptors Stimulated†	Duration of Action‡	Comments
Ephedrine (Ephed II[US], Fedrine[CAN])	α_1, β_1, β_2	++	Mixed sympathomimetic Not classified as a catecholamine, resorcinol, or saligenin
CATECHOLAMINES			
L-Epinephrine (Adrenalin)	α_1, β_1, β_2	+	High potency Invaluable for the treatment of allergic emergencies
D,L-Epinephrine (Vaponefrin)	α_1, β_1, β_2	+	Racemic mixture is less potent than the L-form
Ethylnorepinephrine (Bronkephrine[US])	(α_1), β_1, β_2	++	Low glycogenolytic activity Weak α-activity
Isoproterenol (Isuprel)	(α_1), β_1, β_2	++	One of the first synthetic bronchodilators produced Nonspecific β-agonist High potency
Isoetharine (Bronkosol[US])	(β_1), β_2	++	One of the first bronchodilators with some β_2-specificity
Bitolterol (Tornalate[US])	β_2	+++	Inactive prodrug converted to colterol (catecholamine) Very high potency
RESORCINOLS			
Metaproterenol (Alupent)	(β_1), β_2	++	Low potency
Terbutaline (Bricanyl)	β_2	+++	High selectivity β_2 High potency
Fenoterol (Berotec[CAN])	β_2	+++	Derivative of metaproterenol High potency
SALIGENINS			
Albuterol[US] (salbutamol[CAN]) (Ventolin)	β_2	+++	Low potency
Pirbuterol (Maxair[US])	β_2	+++	Albuterol derivative Unique N-containing ring Low potency
OTHER AGENTS			
Procaterol (Pro-Air[CAN])	β_2	++++	Unique double ring with nitrogen No hydroxide (OH) groups
NEWER DRUGS			
Formoterol (investigational)	β_2	++++++	Unique complex structure Very high β_2-specificity
Salmeterol (investigational)			Very high potency Ultra-long-acting

*Additional trade names are listed in Table 12-4.
†It should be noted that the relatively selective β_2 agonists also exhibit a very small degree of cardiac (β_1) stimulation.
‡Durations of action are determined, in part, by the COMT- and MAO-resistance exhibited by the drug. In general, catecholamines possess short durations of action (ca. 1 h), whereas noncatecholamines (resorcinols, saligenins) exhibit longer durations of action (ca. 4 to 6 h) (Rau, 1989).
+—duration of action (short, moderate, etc); (/)—slight action.

5–12). β_1 effects include cardiac muscle contraction.

α-Adrenergic stimulants, such as phenylephrine, acting at postjunctional α_1-receptors cause a membrane change that permits rapid influx of calcium ions. Calcium ions activate the enzyme calmodulin, which then mobilizes intracellular protein kinases (see Fig. 5–16). The kinases in turn bring about a characteristic effector response, such as vasoconstriction (α_1 effect).

Mechanism of Action

Drugs such as the synthetic catecholamines and their derivatives are chemically similar to the neurotransmitter norepinephrine. These *direct-acting sympathomimetics* combine at various adrenergic receptors to mimic adrenergic transmission (see Fig. 5–10). Through receptor complexing they can accelerate the heart, relax airway smooth muscle, or cause vascular changes.

Indirect-acting sympathomimetics promote the accumulation of norepinephrine at the synapse to bring about adrenergic stimulation of the postsynaptic cell. These drugs are nonspecific in regard to adrenoceptor activity. Mechanisms of action that result in indirect stimulation of adrenergic receptors include MAO inhibition, increased norepinephrine release, and inhibition of the norepinephrine uptake-1 mechanism at prejunctional neurons (see Fig. 5–10).

Mixed-action sympathomimetics, such as ephedrine, act indirectly by promoting the release of norepinephrine at adrenergic sites, and directly by stimulating α- and β-adrenergic receptors.

Precautions

Several precautions apply generally to the sympathomimetics and are summarized in Table 12–2. These include the production of cardiac arrhythmias and the development of tolerance. Paradoxic bronchospasm may occur in some susceptible individuals after repeated excessive use of sympathomimetic inhalers. The response may be due to allergic reactions precipitated by chlorofluorocarbon (CFC) propellants used in metered-dose inhalers (MDI). Allergic responses in patients with hyperreactive airways are also linked to various drug preservatives used in some aerosol inhalation solutions. These preservatives include sulfites, edetate disodium, and benzalkonium chloride. Drug additives such as propellants and preservatives are discussed in Chapter 1 and summarized in Table 1–2.

Routes of Administration

Direct delivery of relatively high drug concentrations to the adrenoceptors on target tissue, and the rapid onset of action, contribute to the efficacy of aerosolized β_2-adrenergic agonists. Sympathomimetic bronchodilators introduced through the oral, subcutaneous, or intravenous routes are delivered to airway smooth muscle through the circulatory system. The higher dosages required to produce adequate bronchodilation by these nonaerosol routes are more likely to cause undesirable side effects, such as cardiac palpitations. The development of tachycardia is the dose-limiting response of bronchodilators, such as isoproterenol, delivered by the parenteral route. Development of skeletal muscle tremor limits the maximal dose of noncatecholamines, such as metaproterenol, introduced through the oral route. Adverse reactions are listed in Table 12–3.

THERAPEUTIC AGENTS: BRONCHODILATORS

EPHEDRINE (Ephed II[US], Fedrine[CAN]). Ephedrine is the oldest therapeutic drug currently in use for the treatment of asthma. Its history can be traced to Chinese medicine, where the herb Ma Huang (*Ephedra* spp.) has been used medicinally for more than 2000 years to relieve symptoms of cough and fever and to improve circulation. Ephedrine, the active ingredient in the plant, was introduced into Western medicine in the mid-1920s as a drug for asthma therapy. Ephedrine possesses bronchodilating (β_2) and nasal decongestant (α_1) effects due to its mixed sympathomimetic action. Ephedrine stimulates the release of norepinephrine and inhibits MAO to potentiate the amount of epinephrine and norepinephrine at adrenergic synapses. It also directly stimulates α_1-, β_1-, and β_2-adrenoceptors. It is a weak, orally active drug that can cross the blood-brain barrier to produce mild CNS stimulation. D-Pseudoephedrine is a related stereoisomer that is less potent than ephedrine. (Stereoisomers are discussed with epinephrine.) Pseudoephedrine is frequently combined with antihistamines in oral over-the-counter "common cold" medications such as Sudafed and Actifed. These compounds are used for the symptomatic relief of sinus and nasal congestion and for mild bronchoconstriction.

The structure of ephedrine differs significantly from that of the catecholamines, resorcinols, and saligenins. Ephedrine resists COMT and MAO action and can be given orally. Compared with epinephrine, ephedrine lacks potency and adrenoceptor specificity. These disadvantages and the development of tachyphylaxis following repeated use have resulted in ephedrine being displaced in asthma therapy by the newer selective β_2-agonists.

TABLE 12–2 PRECAUTIONS WITH ADRENERGIC AGONISTS

RESPIRATORY SYSTEM

Repeated excessive use may result in tolerance, tachyphylaxis, and loss of bronchodilator efficacy.

β_2-Agonists should not be used on a regular basis or in high amounts without appropriate concurrent antiallergic medication to control airway inflammation.

Repeated use may cause paradoxic bronchospasm in some susceptible individuals. (The cause of the refractory state is not fully understood but may be caused by allergic reactions triggered by CFC propellants, such as trichlorofluoromethane (Freon 11), dichlorodifluoromethane (Freon 12), or cryofluorane (Freon 114). Allergic responses are also linked to sulfite preservatives such as sodium metabisulfite used in the MDI device, or preservatives such as EDTA-disodium used in some inhalation solutions [see Table 1–2 in Chapter 1].)

CARDIOVASCULAR SYSTEM

Patients with a history of cardiac disease such as hypertension, coronary insufficiency (anginal attacks), and cardiac arrhythmias (electrical abnormalities in heart muscle) warrant special mention because of the β_1-adrenoceptor stimulation caused by less specific β-agonists.

METABOLIC EFFECTS

Diabetes mellitus can be worsened by the administration of the sympathomimetic amines because the drugs normally bring about a rise in blood glucose level (glycogenolytic effect). This reversible metabolic effect is most pronounced during infusions of the drug.

Development of hypokalemia during β_2-agonist therapy may increase the susceptibility of digitalis-treated patients to cardiac arrhythmias. In acute severe asthma, hypokalemia may be potentiated by concurrent therapy with xanthines, steroids, and diuretics. Patients may need to be monitored to determine their serum K^{1+} levels.

OTHER EFFECTS

β_2-Agonists may reduce preterm labor contractions by decreasing the force of uterine contractions.

Exposure of a catecholamine to light, heat, air, or an alkaline solution may cause it to be oxidized to a pigmented, unstable metabolite known as adrenochrome. A catecholamine that has become discolored through these changes should not be administered to a patient.

DRUG INTERACTIONS

Interaction with MAO-inhibitor or TCA drugs may boost catecholamine levels in a patient and lead to greater incidence of hypertensive crises such as CVA or stroke.

The concurrent administration of a nonspecific β-blocking agent such as propranolol may reduce the activity of a β-agonist drug and lead to bradycardia and bronchoconstriction. (Each drug inhibits the effect of the other.) If a patient's condition requires β-blocker therapy, a cardioselective β-blocker such as metoprolol or atenolol is used.

Sympathomimetics such as ephedrine and epinephrine possess α- and β-adrenergic activity. Therefore, an α-blocker given at the same time allows β-effects to go unopposed resulting in vasodilation and hypotension. Similarly, the concurrent administration of a β- blocker allows unopposed α-affects to produce vasoconstriction and a rise in blood pressure.

Concurrent administration of other β-adrenergic agonists, anticholinergic bronchodilators, xanthine derivatives, or corticosteroids may enhance the effects of β_2-agonists used as inhalation agents and add to the development of unwanted side effects.

CFC—chlorofluorcarbon; CVA—cerebral vascular accident; MDI—metered-dose inhaler; TCA—tricyclic antidepressant.

INDICATIONS. Indications for use of ephedrine include the oral treatment of mild bronchospasm, sinus congestion, and nasal congestion. Pseudoephedrine is most often found in proprietary compounds marketed for the relief of nasal and sinus congestion symptoms.

CONTRAINDICATIONS Because ephedrine lacks significant adrenoceptor specificity, vasopressor effects (α) and cardiac stimulation (β_1) can worsen preexisting conditions of hypertension or cardiac disease. Ephedrine can cross the blood-brain barrier and produce mild CNS stimulation to aggravate conditions such as insomnia, nervousness, or agitation.

Catecholamine Bronchodilators

EPINEPHRINE (Adrenalin [Nebulization 1:100 epinephrine solution; injection 1:1000 epinephrine solution, 1:10,000 epinephrine solution]; AsthmaHaler[US]; Medihaler-Epi[US]; DysneInhal[CAN]; and Bronkaid [aerosol preparations]). As is the case with nearly all biological molecules, the L-isomer of epinephrine (L-epinephrine) is the physiologically active stereoisomer. Stereoisomers are molecules of the same substance that are identical in every way except the orientation of their substituent groups. The isomers are mirror images of each other and, therefore, exhibit significantly different receptor activity and pharmacologic action.

TABLE 12–3 ADVERSE REACTIONS TO ADRENERGIC AGONISTS

RESPIRATORY SYSTEM

Paradoxic bronchospasm in certain patients (exact cause unknown)
Cough

CARDIOVASCULAR SYSTEM

Palpitations, tachycardia, and hypertension due to β_1-adrenergic stimulation. (The more specific β_2-stimulants, such as albuterol[US] [salbutamol[CAN]] produce less severe cardiovascular effects.)

CENTRAL NERVOUS SYSTEM

Headache, dizziness, and nervousness (some bronchodilators can penetrate the blood-brain barrier)

METABOLIC EFFECTS

Hyperglycemia (glycogenolytic effect)
Hypokalemia (potentially serious)

OTHER EFFECTS

Skeletal muscle tremor (due to the stimulating action of β_2-agonist drugs at β_2-receptors located on skeletal muscle)

Epinephrine is a nonspecific adrenergic stimulant, exhibiting both α-adrenergic effects and β_1- and β_2-effects. For these reasons, epinephrine is valuable for its vasopressor and cardiostimulatory effects in addition to its use in the management of bronchospasm.

Epinephrine is a native catecholamine that is rapidly inactivated through both the COMT and MAO metabolic pathways; therefore, its duration of action is predictably short (Table 12–1). The catecholamine structure of epinephrine also renders the drug unsuitable for oral administration because of rapid inactivation by COMT in the gut and liver. However, aerosol and parenteral forms of epinephrine are available. The use of epinephrine in the daily *management* of bronchospasm has decreased since the development of more selective β_2-agonists, such as albuterol[US] (salbutamol[CAN]), but epinephrine is still an invaluable catecholamine in clinical emergencies such as acute asthmatic episodes, anaphylactic shock, and cardiac arrest.

INDICATIONS. Epinephrine is a potent catecholamine, making it ideal for the treatment of acute asthma and hypersensitivity reactions. It is available in inhalational solutions (1:100) and parenteral solutions (1:1000 and 1:10,000). All personnel must take the utmost care to ensure that the more potent inhalational solution is not accidentally given by injection—the outcome could be *FATAL.*

Subcutaneous injection of epinephrine is indicated in the treatment of acute hypersensitivity reactions to insect venoms, drugs, or immunizations (see Table 9–1). (Prophylactic immunization often introduces animal serum products,

which may trigger a violent anaphylactic reaction in some individuals.)

Nonpulmonary indications for use of epinephrine include topical application to wound surfaces to constrict blood vessels (α_1-effect) and slow the blood loss; administration in conjunction with a local anesthetic to promote vasoconstriction (α_1-effect) and thereby increase the duration of effect and limit the systemic spread of the local anesthetic; and the emergency treatment of hypoglycemia (a β_2-effect promotes the conversion of glycogen to glucose in the liver).

CONTRAINDICATIONS. Preexisting cardiac arrhythmias can be made worse by epinephrine because it possesses potent (β_1) cardiostimulating activity. Digitalis is a cardiac drug that increases the force of contraction but is very irritating to the myocardium. Concomitant administration of epinephrine must be avoided because the sympathomimetic can further disrupt electrical patterns in the heart.

PRECAUTIONS. Exposure of a catecholamine drug such as epinephrine to light, heat, air, or an alkaline solution causes the drug to be oxidized to a pink, unstable metabolite known as **adrenochrome.** Adrenochrome may then be polymerized to a brown pigment. A catecholamine that has undergone such change should not be administered to a patient. Additional precautions concerning catecholamine use are summarized in Table 12–2.

RACEMIC EPINEPHRINE (D,L-EPINEPHRINE) (Micronefrin[US], Vaponefrin). Racemic epinephrine is delivered as an inhalational solution. It produces roughly equivalent α- and β-adrenergic activity, and like epinephrine lacks selectivity for β-receptor subtypes. Racemic compounds are 50:50 mixtures of D- and L-isomers. Because L-epinephrine is the biologically active isomer, the overall physiologic effects of racemic epinephrine are less than those of epinephrine. Consequently, racemic mixtures are given in higher solution strengths or in higher dosages.

INDICATIONS. Racemic epinephrine is indicated for the symptomatic relief of bronchospasm and mucous secretions associated with bronchial asthma, hay fever, chronic bronchitis, and pulmonary emphysema.

CONTRAINDICATIONS. See Epinephrine.

ETHYLNOREPINEPHRINE (Brokephrine[US]). In spite of its relatively simple terminal amine structure, ethylnorepinephrine is primarily a β-adrenergic stimulant, acting at β_1- and β_2-adrenoceptors. It also has a degree of α-agonist activity, which causes local vasoconstriction and aids in the relief of pulmonary congestion. Ethylnorepinephrine has a relatively slow onset of action and a characteristically short duration of action due to rapid inactivation by COMT (Table 12–1).

The mechanism of action, precautions, adverse reactions, and drug interactions pertaining to ethylnorepinephrine are the same as those described generally for the sympathomimetic amines.

INDICATIONS. Ethylnorepinephrine is administered intramuscularly or subcutaneously to treat bronchospasm and is well suited for use in children because of a low incidence of adverse side effects. (It is not available in aerosol form.) Due to its relatively weak α-adrenergic agonist vasopressor activity, ethylnorepinephrine is safer than epinephrine in patients with hypertension. It also exhibits less tendency than epinephrine to stimulate the conversion of glycogen to glucose (glycogenolytic action). Therefore, ethylnorepinephrine is ideal as a bronchodilator for asthmatics who also have a diabetic condition.

CONTRAINDICATIONS. See Epinephrine.

ISOPROTERENOL, ISOPRENALINE (Isuprel, Medihaler-Iso, Vapo-Iso). One of the earliest synthetic bronchodilators developed was isoproterenol. The drug is a primary catecholamine and is enzymatically degraded by COMT. Isoproterenol is not affected by the uptake-1 mechanism as readily as epinephrine and norepinephrine; therefore, it has a longer duration of action (Table 12–1).

The structure of isoproterenol differs enough from that of epinephrine to render isoproterenol relatively selective for β-adrenergic receptors (Fig. 12–3). (It possesses virtually no α-adrenoceptor activity.) The debut of isoproterenol represented the first step in the development of synthetic, receptor-specific compounds suitable for asthma therapy. Although deficient by today's bronchodilator standards, isoproterenol marked a significant advance in the management of acute and chronic bronchospasm. For example, of the drugs available when isoproterenol was released, norepinephrine was a poor bronchodilator due to extremely weak β_2-activity. Ephedrine produced mild bronchodilation but lacked potency and receptor specificity. Epinephrine, although a reasonably effective bronchodilator, lacked receptor specificity and was an extremely potent vasopressor and cardiac stimulant.

Isoproterenol exhibits vigorous β_2-adrenoceptor stimulation and has excellent airway muscle–relaxing capabilities. In addition, it inhibits antigen-induced release of histamine, a feature also found in the newer, β_2-selective sympathomimetics, such as albuterol[US] (salbutamol[CAN]). Isoproterenol is nonselective in its β-adrenergic actions, producing equally powerful β_1 stimulation of the heart. Increasingly selective β_2-agonists have been developed over the past few decades. The pharmacologic activity of such drugs is often compared with that of isoproterenol, the prototype of the first-generation bronchodilators.

INDICATIONS. The main indication for use of isoproterenol is in the relief of acute or chronic bronchospasm in asthma. The drug is available in a variety of dosage forms: MDI devices, nebulizer solutions, powder inhalers, and parenteral solutions. (Oral and sublingual forms of isoproterenol are available but are generally unreliable.)

CONTRAINDICATIONS. Preexisting heart disease such as congestive heart failure, hypertension, or coronary artery disease can be worsened by the administration of isoproterenol.

ISOETHARINE. (Bronkosol[US] [nebulizer solution], Bronkometer[US] [oral MDI]). Isoetharine is classified as a catecholamine and was one of the first sympathomimetic amines developed with a demonstrated degree of β_2-adrenoceptor specificity. Isoetharine exhibits relatively little β_1-activity and produces fewer cardiac side effects than epinephrine or isoproterenol. The duration of action of isoetharine is longer than that of isoproterenol (Table 12–1). Resistance to MAO occurs as a result of substitution on the α-carbon. The α-adrenergic activity of the drug is negligible. Isoetharine possesses less β_2-selectivity than either metaproterenol or albuterol[US] (salbutamol[CAN]) (see below).

INDICATIONS. Isoetharine is available as an aerosol and is indicated in the symptomatic relief of reversible bronchospasm associated with bronchial asthma, bronchitis, and emphysema.

CONTRAINDICATIONS. The current sympathomimetic bronchodilators are far more β_2-adrenoceptor selective than the isoproterenol prototype, but they are not "pure" β_2-agonists because a degree of β_1 cardiac stimulation exists. Consequently, contraindications such as preexisting congestive heart failure, hypertension, or coronary artery disease that apply to isoproterenol also pertain to the "second-generation" bronchodilators. The extent of cardiac involvement, however, is much less than that seen with isoproterenol.

BITOLTEROL (Tornalate^{US}). The search for noncatecholamine bronchodilators with longer durations of action took an innovative turn in the mid-1980s with the development of bitolterol (Tornalate^{US}). The metabolism of bitolterol represents a radical departure from the pharmacokinetics of β_2-sympathomimetic amines discussed thus far. Bitolterol, as it is delivered to the airways from an MDI, is present as a precursor substance, or prodrug. It is inactive at β_2-adrenoceptors in its initial form. Due to enzyme action in the tissues, however, it becomes progressively available as large aromatic (cyclic, or carbonring) groupings are split off carbons at positions 3 and 4 on the catechol nucleus (Fig. 12–4). The resulting active drug is a catecholamine known as colterol. Colterol is a selective β_2-stimulant with bronchodilating properties greater than those of isoproterenol. Like the primary catecholamines, colterol is metabolized normally through the COMT and MAO pathways (Fig. 12–1).

The unique chemical structure of bitolterol makes it COMT resistant because of the large atypical groups at carbons 3 and 4. In addition, the bulky terminal nitrogen with its four-carbon butyl group is similar to that of terbutaline and renders colterol highly β_2 selective. As a consequence of these chemical modifications and the gradual conversion of inactive prodrug to active colterol in the lungs, bitolterol exhibits a relatively long duration of action (Table 12–1).

INDICATIONS AND CONTRAINDICATIONS. See Isoetharine.

Resorcinol Bronchodilators

METAPROTERENOL (Alupent, Metaprel^{US}). In the mid-1960s, early pharmaceutical manipulation of the basic catecholamine structure resulted in the synthesis of a resorcinol known as metaproterenol, or orciprenaline (Alupent, Metaprel^{US}). The hydroxide group at the 5-C po-

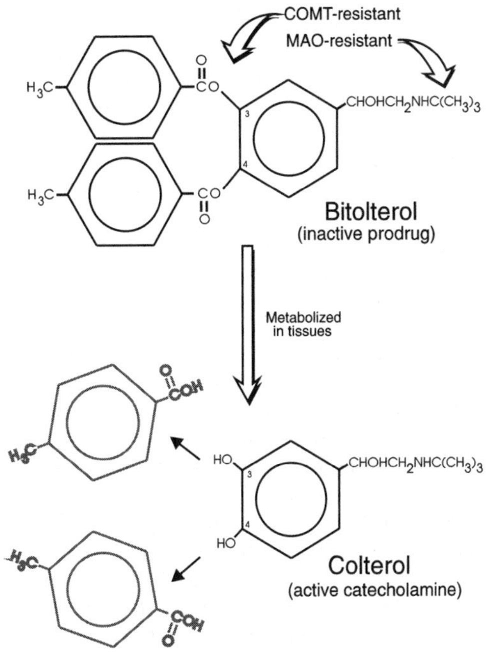

FIGURE 12–4 Bitolterol conversion.

sition rather than at the 4-C position slows enzymatic destruction, increases the β_2-selectivity of the drug, and permits oral administration. Metaproterenol is prone to MAO metabolism, however, and has a shorter duration of action than other selective β_2-agonists, such as terbutaline and albuterol^{US} (salbutamol^{CAN}) (Table 12–1). In general, bronchial and cardiovascular effects of metaproterenol are similar to those of isoproterenol, although metaproterenol is considerably less potent.

INDICATIONS. Primary indications for use of metaproterenol include symptomatic treatment of bronchial asthma and for reversible bronchospasm seen with bronchitis and emphysema. It is available as an MDI, inhalational solution for nebulization, and in several oral forms.

CONTRAINDICATIONS. see: Isoetharine.

TERBUTALINE (Bricanyl^{CAN} Oral, DPI; Bricanyl^{US} Oral; Brethaire^{US} MDI; Brethine^{US} Injection). Pharmaceutical research in the mid-1970s concerning the metabolism of catecholamine derivatives resulted in the addition of a bulky terminal *N*-butyl group on the ethylamine side chain of the molecule (Fig. 12–3). As a result, terbutaline demonstrates relatively selective β_2-adrenergic activity. Its bronchodilator potency is greater than that of metaproterenol, as is its duration of action (Table 12–1). The resorcinol nucleus of terbutaline, like that of metaproterenol, resists methylation by COMT. Terbutaline is available for aerosol delivery by MDI or a ready-to-use 50- or 200-dose dry powder inhaler (DPI) marketed in Canada as Bricanyl[CAN] Turbuhaler® (see Fig. 1–6D). Terbutaline resists enzymatic activity in the gastrointestinal tract and is, therefore, suitable for oral administration.

INDICATIONS. Terbutaline, like the other β_2-adrenergic agonists discussed so far, is valuable in the symptomatic treatment of reversible bronchospastic conditions associated with bronchial asthma, chronic bronchitis, and pulmonary emphysema. In addition, the subcutaneous form of terbutaline provides an alternative means of introducing the drug. The subcutaneous route is especially valuable in patients with coexisting hypertension or cardiac disease in whom the vasopressor effects of epinephrine would be undesirable. Cardiac effects similar to those produced by isoproterenol occur and are indicative of the decreased β_2-selectivity when terbutaline is administered subcutaneously.

CONTRAINDICATIONS. See Isoetharine.

FENOTEROL[US] (Berotec[CAN]). Fenoterol became available for use as an aerosol bronchodilator in the late 1970s in Canada. It is a derivative of metaproterenol and belongs to the resorcinol group of bronchodilators, which also includes terbutaline. The addition of a very bulky carbon–ring substituent on the terminal nitrogen of fenoterol renders the drug highly selective for β_2-adrenoceptors. The resorcinol configuration permits oral administration and results in pronounced COMT resistance and a prolonged duration of action (Table 12–1). The potency of fenoterol is comparable with that of terbutaline but several times greater than that of albuterol[US] (salbutamol[CAN]). A combination product consisting of fenoterol and the antimuscarinic bronchodilator ipratropium bromide is marketed in the United Kingdom as Duovent. At present there are no plans to market this combination aerosol MDI in North America. In addition, there is a growing trend away from regular use of high-potency β_2-agonists toward less frequent administration of lower-potency β_2-agonists (Table 12–5).

INDICATIONS. The oral form of fenoterol (tablets) and MDI routes of administration provide symptomatic relief of bronchospasm associated with bronchial asthma, chronic bronchitis, and pulmonary emphysema. The nebulizer form is indicated for acute severe bronchospasm, as is seen with exaggeration of the symptoms of bronchial asthma or severe chronic bronchitis.

CONTRAINDICATIONS. See Isoetharine.

Saligenin Bronchodilators

ALBUTEROL[US] OR SALBUTAMOL[CAN] (Ventolin, Proventil[US]). The β_2-adrenergic stimulant known as albuterol in the United States and salbutamol in Canada is a highly selective β_2-bronchodilator with less potency than other β_2-agonists, such as fenoterol. Albuterol belongs to the saligenin group of noncatecholamine bronchodilators and, like terbutaline, resists COMT, has a long duration of action, and can be given by mouth (Table 12–1). In addition, the loaded terminal nitrogen of the drug confers a high degree of β_2-specificity.

A variety of dosage forms, including oral preparations, nebulizer solutions, MDIs, and DPIs, such as Beclovent Diskhaler and Rotohaler, are available in both countries. Injectable solutions of salbutamol are available in Canada from Allen and Hansburys (Glaxo Canada). As a general trend in the pharmaceutical industry, there is increasing interest in the development of dry powder formulations. This is a result of continuing controversy concerning the potential toxicity of aerosol propellants in MDIs, and more recently, goals and guidelines concerning the use of CFCs and their release into the atmosphere. In line with these trends, Boehringer Ingelheim of Canada has developed and is testing Combivent, a dry powder combination product containing salbutamol and ipratropium for the symptomatic relief of asthma.

INDICATIONS. Albuterol[US] (salbutamol[CAN]) is valuable in the symptomatic relief of bronchospasm that accompanies bronchial asthma, chronic bronchitis, and pulmonary emphysema. Parenteral salbutamol[CAN] is also indicated in cases of acute *severe* bronchospasm and in conditions of status asthmaticus.

CONTRAINDICATIONS. See Isoetharine (Box 12–1).

PIRBUTEROL (Maxair). Pirbuterol is an aerosol (MDI) β_2-selective agonist with pharmacologic activity similar to that of albuterol. Like albuterol from which it is derived, pirbuterol belongs to the saligenin group of catecholamine derivatives and therefore resists COMT-inactivation. It also has a bulky terminal nitrogen butyl group, which renders it β_2-selective, and a modified ring structure that includes a nitrogen atom. This unique pyridine ring structure contributes to the relatively long duration of action exhibited by pirbuterol (Table 12–1). The drug is available for delivery by the novel breath-actuated MDI called Autohaler (see Fig. 1–5C).

INDICATIONS AND CONTRAINDICATIONS. See Isoetharine.

BOX 12–1 METERED-DOSE INHALERS, CHLOROFLUOROCARBONS, AND OZONE DEPLETION (. . . or *something else to worry about* . . .)

Chlorofluorocarbons (CFCs) have been produced in large quantities for industrial use. A sizable consumer of CFCs has been the refrigeration industry, where tons of the compounds are used in automobile, home, office, and commercial air conditioners. CFCs have also been used as inert propellants in a variety of aerosol products (e.g., spray paint) but have been gradually phased out over the past few years.

Chlorofluorocarbon propellants such as trichlorofluoromethane, dichlorodifluoromethane, and dichlorotetrafluoroethane (CFCs 11, 12, and 114, respectively) are used in extremely small amounts by the pharmaceutical industry to power the MDI. For example, pharmaceutical aerosols account for only about 0.4%–0.5% of the total CFCs produced worldwide (American Association for Respiratory Care, 1991). MDIs are valuable in pulmonary medicine because they deliver precise doses to the airways and yet are simple enough to be operated properly by most patients. Concern over ozone layer damage has led to development of the Montreal Protocol on Substances That Deplete the Ozone Layer. The Montreal Protocol, first drawn up in 1987 and revised several times, is an international agreement on a phased withdrawal of CFC-containing products. In 1991, a total ban on CFC use was projected for the year 2000 (Kacmarek and Hess, 1991). However, in November 1992, the phase-out deadline was moved forward to January 1, 1996. Countries of the European Union have voluntarily moved the date forward again, to January 1, 1995 (3M Pharmaceuticals, 1994).

Although the pharmaceutical industry consumes a very small fraction of the CFCs produced worldwide, it is bound by the same international accord to replace CFC-containing products, such as MDIs. Development and testing of alternative delivery techniques that use clinically effective and safe propellants could conceivably take 5 to 10 years. An extension on the ban for pharmaceutical use of CFCs has been granted, but ultimately, all MDIs will have to be CFC-free.

In the meantime, researchers are developing alternative compounds as replacement refrigerants in air conditioners and as propellants for use in pharmaceutical aerosols. Hydrofluorocarbons (HFCs), also known as hydrofluoroalkanes (HFAs), such as HFC-134a (1,1,1,2-tetrafluoroethane) do not liberate ozone-destroying chlorine molecules as they break down in the upper atmosphere. Similarly, the hydrochlorofluorocarbon (HCFC), known as HCFC-123 (2,2-dichloro-1,1,1-trifluoroethane), does not have the same ozone-depleting properties of CFCs. For example, the lifetime of HFAs and HCFCs in the upper atmosphere is between 1 and 50 years compared to 50 to 500 years for CFC propellants (3M Pharmaceuticals, 1994).

The effects in humans have not been fully determined for the CFC propellant substitutes. Animal studies of HFC-134a show it to have relatively little toxic potential (Olson and Surbrook, 1991). However, HCFC-123 has produced immunologically mediated hepatitis similar to that produced by the general anesthetic halothane, a structurally related compound (Harris et al, 1991). HFC-134a propellant does not liberate chlorine molecules during degradation and is being used to power the Airomir system that is undergoing testing in Europe. This CFC-free MDI as well as several types of DPIs are fully discussed in Chapter 1 as alternative "ozone-friendly" devices for the delivery of drugs to the airways.

Balmes JR: Propellant gases in metered dose inhalers: Their impact on the global environment. Respiratory Care 36:1037–1044, 1991.

Faculty and Writing Committee, American Association for Respiratory Care. Aerosol Consensus Statement, 1991. Respiratory Care 36:916–921, 1991.

Harris JW et al: Tissue acylation by the chlorofluorocarbon substitute 2,2-dichloro-1,1,1-trifluoroethane. Proc Natl Acad Sci USA 88:1407–1410, 1991.

Kacmarek RM and Hess D: The interface between patient and aerosol generator. Respiratory Care 36:952–976, 1991.

Olson HJ and Surbrook SE: Defluorination of the CFC-substitute 1,1,1,2-tetrafluoroethane: Comparison in human, rat and rabbit hepatic microsomes. Toxicol Lett. 59:89–99, 1991.

3M Pharmaceuticals: The big issue: CFCs and the destruction of the ozone layer. Background Information (Airomir). 3M Pharmaceuticals, St Paul, 1994.

Other Bronchodilators

PROCATEROL (Pro-Air[CAN]). Procaterol is an aerosol (MDI) β_2-selective sympathomimetic amine useful in the symptomatic treatment of bronchospasm. The chemical ring structure of procaterol is quite different from that of other β_2-agonists. It consists of a *double* ring with a nitrogen atom incorporated into one of the rings and no attached hydroxide groups. This configuration renders the ring portion of the drug molecule virtually immune to the methylation action of COMT. Procaterol also has a substituted group on its α-carbon; therefore, the drug is very resistant to oxidation by MAO. Procaterol exhibits pronounced enzyme resistance and a long duration of action (Table 12–1).

INDICATIONS. Procaterol is useful in the symptomatic relief of bronchospasm primarily in instances of bronchial asthma and chronic bronchitis.

CONTRAINDICATIONS. See Isoetharine.

Newer Bronchodilators

A group of ultra–long-acting sympathomimetic bronchodilators is currently being investigated for future use in asthma therapy (Lofdahl and Chung, 1991; Patessio et al, 1991). The mid-1990s may mark the release of formoterol and salmeterol (Serevent) for general clinical use in several European countries. Approval for their use in North America could follow at a later date. The structures of the drugs differ significantly from those of primary catecholamine bronchodilators, such as isoproterenol. For example, a stereoisomer of formoterol has atypical groupings on its main carbon ring and ethylamine side chain. These characteristics contribute to substantial COMT resistance and a long duration of action (Table 12–1). The extremely bulky nature of the terminal nitrogen substituent group on formoterol results in a high degree of β_2-adrenoceptor specificity.

Formoterol and salmeterol are similar in their long durations of action, preferential adrenergic receptor stimulation, and bronchodilating capabilities. Inhaled formoterol (MDI) and salmeterol (MDI, DPI) have produced no unexpected side effects, nor has their use resulted in development of tachyphylaxis. Comparison studies with albuterol[US] (salbutamol[CAN]) (MDI) have shown the new longer-acting agents to possess remarkable activity, producing equivalent bronchodilation at less than one quarter the dosage of albuterol[US] (Gongora et al, 1991; Kesten et al, 1991). The high potency of these agents is reflected in the dosing disks used in the salmeterol

Diskhaler DPI. Such disks contain only 4 doses of salmeterol compared with the customary 8 doses contained in the Ventolin Diskhaler (see Fig. 1–6C).

THERAPEUTIC AGENTS: MUCOSAL VASOCONSTRICTORS

Sympathomimetics such as ephedrine and epinephrine have mixed α_1-adrenergic and β-adrenergic effects. They are useful for promoting bronchodilation (β_2) in the airways and vasoconstriction (α_1) of blood vessels. Vasopressor effects have already been discussed with the decongestant action of ephedrine and the topical hemostatic action of epinephrine. α-Adrenergic stimulants that are basically devoid of β-activity have also been developed. These specific α_1-adrenergic agonists are discussed below.

PHENYLEPHRINE (Neo-Synephrine). Phenylephrine is a powerful α_1-adrenoceptor stimulant which lacks appreciable cardiac (β_1) and bronchodilator (β_2) effects. The predominant effects of phenylephrine are directed at peripheral arterioles, where it produces potent vasoconstriction. The structure of phenylephrine differs only slightly from that of epinephrine. This subtle chemical difference is responsible for the selective α-activity of phenylephrine.

INDICATIONS. Various dosage forms of phenylephrine are available: oral, parenteral, nasal, and ophthalmic solutions. In addition, phenylephrine is combined with isoproterenol as an aerosol known as Duo-Medihaler. Such combination products provide relief of pulmonary congestion (α_1-effect) in addition to relaxation of airway smooth muscle (β_2-effect). The vasopressor effects of phenylephrine also offset the vasodilator (β_2) effects of isoproterenol. (Recall that isoproterenol lacks any appreciable α-activity.)

Phenylephrine is also employed as a pressor agent in cases of hypotension and as a mydriatic agent to promote pupil dilation. Like epinephrine, phenylephrine can be combined in solutions of local anesthetics to produce vasoconstriction, minimize systemic distribution, and prolong the action of the local anesthetic.

Nasal solutions (sprays, drops) of phenylephrine and similar drugs such as xylometazoline (Otrivin) and oxymetazoline (Afrin) are effective when used alone as decongestants. However, their use may be followed by an increase in nasal congestion. Vasoconstrictors such as tetrahydrozoline (Visine) are available as ophthalmic solutions.

CONTRAINDICATIONS. Preexisting conditions of hypertension can be worsened by α-adrenergic receptor stimulants having pronounced vasopressor effects.

PRECAUTIONS. Because of the presence of a small number of α_1-adrenergic receptors on airway smooth muscle, there is a slight risk of inducing bronchoconstriction with the administration of an α_1-agonist.

The concurrent administration of an α-antagonist drug such as phentolamine (Regitine) may diminish the pharmacologic action of α-agonists such as phenylephrine.

Table 12–4 lists the generic and trade names for the adrenergic agonists discussed in this chapter. Dosages for selected agents are given in Table 12–5.

CHAPTER SUMMARY

Adrenergic agonists mimic sympathetic neuronal transmission. These sympathomimetics are employed as bronchodilators for the symptomatic treatment of reversible bronchospasm associated with bronchial asthma, chronic bronchitis, and pulmonary edema. They are also used as mucosal vasoconstrictors in the treatment of vascular congestion seen with nasal and pulmonary congestion.

Early sympathomimetics, such as ephedrine, lacked adrenergic receptor specificity. However, increased understanding of structure-activity relationships and the development of more sophisticated synthesis techniques made it possible to create drugs with preferential action at adrenoceptors. Relatively pure β-stimulants, such as

TABLE 12–4 DRUG NAMES: ADRENERGIC AGONISTS

Generic Name	Trade Name
Ephedrine	Ephed II[US], Fedrine[CAN]
CATECHOLAMINE BRONCHODILATORS	
Epinephrine (adrenalin)	Adrenalin: nebulizer, injection AsthmaHaler[US]: aerosol Medihaler-Epi[US]: aerosol Dysne-Inhal[CAN]: aerosol Bronkaid: aerosol
Racemic epinephrine (D,L-epinephrine)	MicroNefrin[US], Vaponefrin
Ethylnorepinephrine	Bronkephrine[US]
Isoproterenol (isoprenaline)	Isuprel, Medihaler-Iso, Vapo-Iso
Isoetharine	Bronkosol[US]: nebulizer Bronkometer[US]: MDI
Bitolterol	Tornalate[US]
RESORCINOL BRONCHODILATORS	
Metaproterenol (orciprenaline)	Alupent, Metaprel[US]
Terbutaline	Bricanyl[CAN]: oral, DPI Bricanyl[US]: oral Brethaire[US]: MDI Brethine[US]: injection
Fenoterol	Berotec[CAN]
SALIGENIN BRONCHODILATORS	
Albuterol[US] (salbutamol[CAN])	Ventolin, Proventil[US]
Pirbuterol	Maxair
OTHER BRONCHODILATORS	
Procaterol	Pro-Air[CAN]
NEWER BRONCHODILATORS	
Formoterol	(investigational)
Salmeterol	(investigational); Serevent in Europe
MUCOSAL VASOCONSTRICTORS	
Phenylephrine	Neo-Synephrine

DPI—dry powder inhaler; MDI—metered-dose inhaler.

TABLE 12–5   DRUG DOSAGES FOR INHALATION AGENTS*

Drug	Availability	Dosage
Ephedrine	Not available as an inhalation agent	
L-Epinephrine	Inhalation aerosol: MDI: 300 μg/ inhalation	Individualized dosage†
D,L-Epinephrine	Inhalation solutions: 1.25%, 2.25%	0.25–0.5 mL diluted with 3–5 mL of NS every 1–2 h†
Ethylnorepinephrine	Not available as an inhalation agent	
Isoproterenol	Inhalation aerosols: MDI: 80 μg/inhalation 131 μg/inhalation	1 or 2 inhalations; may be repeated every 3–4 h†
	Inhalation solutions: 0.25% (1:400), 0.5% (1:200), 1% (1:100)	0.25–0.5 mL 1:200 solution diluted with 2–2.5 mL NS (concentration of 1:800–1:1000) given up to 5 times daily by nebulization†
	Inhalation solutions: UD: 0.031% (in 4 mL) 0.062% (in 4 mL)	1 vial per treatment†
Isoetharine	Inhalation aerosol: MDI: 340 μg/ inhalation (0.61%)	1 or 2 inhalations every 4 h or individualized†‡
	Inhalation solutions: 1%, 0.5%	Adults and children >12 y:†‡ 0.5% solution: 0.5 mL diluted 1:3 with NS given every 3–4 h by nebulization 1% solution: 0.25–0.5 mL diluted 1:3 with NS given every 3–4 h or individualized
	Inhalation solutions: UD: 0.062% to 0.25% in 2–4-mL vials	1 vial per treatment†
Bitolterol	Inhalation aerosol: MDI: 370 μg/ inhalation (0.8%)	Adults and children >12 y:‡ 2 inhalations every 4–6 h
Metaproterenol (orciprenaline)	Inhalation aerosol MDI: 0.75 mg/inhalation 15 mL MDI canister contains 300 metered doses	Single dose of 1 or 2 puffs (0.75–1.5 mg) usually provides control for up to 5 h or longer; patients should not exceed 12 inhalations per day§
	Inhalation solution: Each 10-mL bottle contains 50 mg/mL (5%) orciprenaline	Hand nebulizer: 5–15 inhalations of 50 mg/mL (5%) solution administered up to 3 times daily§ IPPV: 0.5–1 mL of 50 mg/mL (5%) solution diluted if desired and administered over about 20 min§
Terbutaline	Inhalation aerosol: MDI: 200 μg/ inhalation	Adults and children >12 yrs:¶ 1–2 inhalations every 4–6 h
	Multiple-dose DPI (Bricanyl^CAN Turbuhaler) DPI: 0.5 mg/ inhalation: 50-dose DPI, 200-dose DPI	Individualize dosage; recommended dosage is 1 inhalation 4 times daily; not more than 6 doses in 24 h**
Fenoterol	Inhalation aerosols MDI: 100 μg/inhalation 200 μg/inhalation MDI canister delivers at least 200 metered doses of fenoterol as a micronized powder	Adults and children >12 y:§ individualize dosage; single dose of 1–2 inhalations If required, this dose of 1–2 inhalations may be repeated up to 3 times daily
	Inhalation solution: 20-mL bottle contains 1 mg/mL (0.1%)	Adults and children >12 y:§ Nebulizer and IPPV average single dose 0.5–1 mL of 1 mg/mL Berotec solution (containing 0.5–1 mg) Should be diluted to 5 mL with NS and total volume nebulized over 10–15 minutes
Albuterol^US (salbutamol^CAN)	Inhalation aerosol: MDI: 90 μg/ inhalation	Adults and children >12 y:‡¶ 2 inhalations, repeated every 4–6 h or 2 inhalations prior to exercise
	Inhalation solution: 0.5% (5 mg/ mL)	Adults and children >5 y:‡¶ nebulizer or IPPV: 2.5 mg (0.5 mL) diluted with 2.5 mL NS given every 3–4 h by nebulization
	Inhalation solution: UD: 0.083% in 3 mL	1 vial per treatment†

TABLE 12–5 DRUG DOSAGES FOR INHALATION AGENTS (*Continued*)

Drug	Availability	Dosage
Pirbuterol	Inhalation aerosol: MDI: 200 μg/inhalation	Adults and children >12 y:¶ 1–2 inhalations every 4–6 h; not to exceed 12 inhalations in 24 h
Procaterol	Inhalation aerosol: MDI: 10 μg/inhalation; MDI canister delivers 200 doses of procaterol	Adults and children >12 y:** Individualized or 1–2 inhalations (10–20 μg) 3 times daily

*The dosage information contained in this table is presented as a brief outline and summary of acceptable dosages. It is not meant to replace the detailed information available from manufacturers of these drugs. Package inserts and product monographs provide the most current dosage information from pharmaceutical manufacturers. Guidelines describing drug preparation and delivery, dosage strengths and schedules, shelf life, and storage requirements are also included in the package inserts. In addition, precautions and adverse reactions are described in detail. The respiratory care practitioner is strongly urged to read this information supplied by the pharmaceutical manufacturer to provide safe and effective drug therapy.

†Rau, 1989

‡Howder, 1992

§Aladin, 1992

¶Deglin and Vallerand, 1993

**Krogh, 1993

DPI—dry powder inhaler; IPPV—intermittent positive pressure ventilation; MDI:—metered-dose inhaler; NS—normal saline, or preservative-free, sterile sodium chloride inhalation solution, US Pharmacopeia 0.9%; UD—unit dose (vial or ampule).

isoproterenol, and equally selective α-stimulants, such as phenylephrine, became available as a result of these breakthroughs. The next logical step in drug design was the development of even more selective β-agonists. This included the release of the second-generation β_2-bronchodilators, such as albuterol[US] (salbutamol[CAN]).

Research into the adrenergic agonists is focused on the development of bronchodilators that are β_2 selective, long acting, effective at low dosages, versatile in regard to the mode of delivery, and devoid of undesirable side effects.

BIBLIOGRAPHY

Aladin F: Personal Communication. Boehringer Ingelheim (Canada) Ltd, Respiratory Products, Feb 1992.

Ahlquist RP: A study of the adrenotropic receptors. Am J Physiol 153:586–600, 1948.

Avital A, Sanchez I, and Chernick V: Efficacy of salbutamol and ipratropium bromide in decreasing bronchial hyperreactivity in children with cystic fibrosis. Pediatr Pulmonol 13:34–37, 1992.

Balmes JR: Propellant gases in metered dose inhalers: Their impact on the global environment. Respiratory Care 36:1037–1044, 1991.

Barnes PJ: Autonomic pharmacology of the airways. In Chung KF and Barnes PJ: Pharmacology of the Respiratory Tract: Experimental and Clinical Research. Marcel Dekker, New York, 1993.

Braun SR et al: A comparison of the effect of ipratropium and albuterol in the treatment of chronic obstructive airway disease. Arch Intern Med 149:544–547, 1989.

Budavari S (ed): The Merck Index: An Encyclopedia of Chemicals, Drugs, and Biologicals. Merck and Company, Rahway, NJ, 1989.

Clark WG, Brater DC, and Johnson AR: Goth's Medical Pharmacology, ed 12. CV Mosby, St Louis, 1988.

Deglin JH and Vallerand AH: Davis's Drug Guide for Nurses, ed 3. FA Davis, Philadelphia, 1993.

Executive Committee of the American Academy of Allergy and Immunology. Position statement: Inhaled β_2-adrenergic agonists in asthma. J Allergy Clin Immunol 91:1234–1237, 1993.

Fanta CH: Emergency management of acute, severe asthma. Respiratory Care 37:551–560, 1992.

Fernandez E and Cherniak RM: β_2 Agonists. In Cherniak RM (ed): Drugs for the Respiratory System. Grune and Stratton, Orlando, 1986.

Goldie RG, Paterson JW, and Lulich KM: Adrenoceptors in airway smooth muscle. Pharmacol Ther 48:295–322, 1990.

Gongora HC, Wisniewski AF, and Tattersfield AE: A single-dose comparison of inhaled albuterol and two formulations of salmeterol on airway reactivity in asthmatic subjects. Am Rev Respir Dis 144(3 Pt 1):626–629, 1991.

Gustafsson B and Persson CG: Effect of different bronchodilators on airway smooth muscle responsiveness to contractile agents. Thorax 46:360–365, 1991.

Hargreave FE, Dolovich J, and Newhouse MT: The assessment and treatment of asthma: A conference report. J Allergy Clin Immunol 85:1098–1111, 1990.

Hoffman BB: Adrenergic receptor–activating drugs. In Katzung BD (ed): Basic and Clinical Pharmacology. Lange Medical Publications, Los Altos, 1982.

Howder CL: Cardiopulmonary Pharmacology: A Handbook for Respiratory Practitioners and Other Allied Health Personnel. Williams and Wilkins, Baltimore, 1992.

Howder CL: Antimuscarinic and β_2-Adrenoreceptor

Bronchodilators in obstructive airways disease. Respiratory Care 38:1364–1388, 1993.

Kesten S et al: A three-month comparison of twice daily inhaled formoterol versus four times daily inhaled albuterol in the management of stable asthma. Am Rev Respir Dis 144 (3 Pt 1):622–625, 1991.

Krogh CM (ed): Compendium of Pharmaceuticals and Specialties, ed 28. Canadian Pharmaceutical Association, Ottawa, 1993.

Liippo K, Silvasti M, and Tukiainen H: Inhaled procaterol versus salbutamol in bronchial asthma. Eur J Clin Pharmacol 40:417–418, 1991.

Lofdahl CG and Chung KF: Long-acting beta 2–adrenoceptor agonists: A new perspective in the treatment of asthma. Eur J Clin Pharmacol 4:218–226, 1991.

Long JP: Drugs acting on the peripheral nervous system. In Conn PM and Gebhart GF (eds): Essentials of Pharmacology. FA Davis, Philadelphia, 1989.

Long JW: The Essential Guide to Prescription Drugs. Harper and Row, New York, 1990.

Mathewson HS: Adrenergic bronchodilators: Trends in drug design. Respiratory Care 36:861–863, 1991.

McAlpine LG and Thomson NC: Prophylaxis of exercise-induced asthma with formoterol, a long-acting beta 2–adrenergic agonist. Respir Med 84:293–295, 1990.

National Heart, Lung, and Blood Institute. National Asthma Education Program Expert Panel Report.

Guidelines for the diagnosis and management of asthma. J Allergy Clin Immunol 88(3 Part 2):425–534, 1991.

Newman SP: Aerosol physiology, deposition, and metered dose inhalers. Allergy Proc 12:41–45, 1991.

O'Driscoll BR et al: Nebulised salbutamol with and without ipratropium bromide in acute airflow obstruction. Lancet i:1418–1420, 1989.

Patessio A et al: Protective effect and duration of action of formoterol aerosol on exercise-induced asthma. Eur Respir J 4:296–300, 1991.

Rau JL: Respiratory Care Pharmacology, ed 3. Yearbook Medical Publishers, Chicago, 1989.

Simon PM and Statz EM: Drug treatment of COPD: Controversies about agents and how to deliver them. Postgrad Med 91:473–479, 1992.

Spitzer WO et al: The use of beta-agonists and the risk of death and near death from asthma. N Engl J Med 326:501–506, 1992.

van Schayck CP et al: Bronchodilator treatment in moderate asthma or chronic bronchitis: Continuous or on demand? A randomised controlled study. BMJ 303(6815):1426–1431, 1991.

Weiner N: Norepinephrine, epinephrine, and the sympathomimetic Amines: In Goodman, AG et al (eds): Goodman and Gilman's The Pharmacologic Basis of Therapeutics, ed 7. Macmillan, New York, 1985.

CHAPTER 13

Xanthine Bronchodilators

CHAPTER OUTLINE

CHAPTER OBJECTIVES

After studying this chapter the reader should be able to:
- Describe the mechanism of action of the methylxanthines.
- Describe three pharmacologic actions of the methylxanthines other than their effect on bronchiolar smooth muscle.
- Define loading dose and maintenance dose in relation to theophylline blood levels and explain why monitoring of serum blood levels is critical in xanthine bronchodilator therapy.
- Describe how theophylline blood levels are affected by age, drug interactions, and environmental factors and state how theophylline dosage levels must be adjusted to compensate for these variables.
- State two indications and two contraindications for use of the methylxanthines in treating dysfunctions of the respiratory system and explain the rationale behind each of their uses and limitations.
- Compare the pharmacologic activity of the following drugs:
  - Theophylline, aminophylline, dyphylline, oxtriphylline.
- Describe the rationale for the use of products containing a combination of methylxanthines, sympathomimetics, central nervous system depressants, and expectorants in the treatment of certain respiratory disorders.

KEY TERMS

loading dose
maintenance dose
methylxanthine (meth-il-**ZAN**-thēn)
purine receptors (purinoceptors)

CHAPTER INTRODUCTION

The xanthine derivatives are not easily described in terms of traditional pharmacologic classifications. They are mild stimulants of the central nervous system (CNS), but they also possess distinct autonomic effects. Their arousal effects on the cerebral cortex are enjoyed by millions of people daily in the form of caffeine in cola, coffee and tea, theophylline in tea, and theobromine in cacao. The autonomic effects of the methylxanthines on airway smooth muscle and glands of the respiratory tract confer significant therapeutic value to this otherwise common group of drugs.

MECHANISM OF ACTION

Xanthine bronchodilators such as the **methyl-xanthines** can promote relaxation of airway smooth muscle even in individuals who no longer respond to β_2-adrenergic stimulants. Such persons are said to have *epinephrine-fast asthma,* an asthmatic condition unresponsive to normal aerosol drug therapy with β_2-agonists.

Several mechanisms, such as interaction with prostaglandins, calcium, or protein kinases, have been proposed to explain the action of methylxanthines. The most promising explanation involves the pharmacologic antagonism of membrane receptors by methylxanthines such as theophylline. Such agents block A_1- and A_2-adenosine receptors on airway smooth muscle. Adenosine receptors belong to a group called the **purine receptors,** or **purinoceptors.** In experimental studies, chemically induced asthma can be evoked by methacholine, histamine, adenosine, or adenosine analogues introduced into the airways. Although it is not fully understood how adenosine produces its effects, it is known to cause a powerful bronchoconstriction response (see Fig. 9–7). Adenosine seems to act as an autacoid in the tissues and functions indirectly by promoting the release of leukotrienes and histamine from mast cells (Bjorck et al, 1992; Ng et al, 1990). The adenosine receptor–blocking action of theophylline has been demonstrated with both *in vivo* and *in vitro* studies. However, it has also been found that enprofylline, a drug closely related to theophylline, is a potent bronchodilator but does not antagonize adenosine receptors (Clark et al, 1988). This finding has shed some doubt on the receptor-blocking theory of methylxanthine action.

The classic description of the mechanism of action of the methylxanthines is cAMP (cyclic adenosine-3′,5′-monophosphate) phosphodiesterase (PDE) inhibition, which potentiates intracellular cAMP levels, promotes relaxation of airway smooth muscle, and inhibits the release of histamine from sensitized target cells. Unfortunately, this explanation of the mechanism of theophylline is valid only *in vitro.* It has not been demonstrated *in vivo* using therapeutic dosages. At the drug levels necessary to cause PDE inhibition, adverse reactions such as cardiotoxicity occur. Animal studies of bronchodilation, however, have shown that theophylline inhibits cAMP PDE *and* blocks adenosine receptors both *in vitro* and *in vivo.* Final clarification of methylxanthine action on the human airway response awaits further study.

PHARMOCOLOGIC EFFECTS

Respiratory Effects

Asthmatics who fail to respond to or cannot be given the β_2-adrenergic drugs can still be treated for bronchoconstriction with the xanthine bronchodilators. The methylxanthines are useful in refractory cases of asthma because they relax airway smooth muscle and inhibit glandular secretion through a mechanism of action independent of that exhibited by the sympathomimetic amines (see Fig. 9–7). In addition, the xanthine bronchodilators offer a measure of prophylaxis because they retard the release of allergic mediators, such as histamine and leukotrienes C_4, D_4, and E_4, from sensitized target cells (see Chapter 9).

Respiratory effects may be produced by the action of the methylxanthines on other body systems. These effects include an increase in alveolar ventilation caused by an increase in carbon dioxide sensitivity of the medullary respiratory centers, and an increase in diaphragmatic contractility. Chapter 28 discusses the stimulatory effects of methylxanthines on ventilatory drive.

Extrapulmonary Effects

Because the mechanism of action of the methylxanthines is nonspecific, many body systems other than the respiratory system can be affected. For example, methylxanthine administration causes a dramatic increase in cardiac output by increasing both the strength and the rate of contraction. A variety of vascular effects are produced by the methylxanthines, which thus affect pulmonary, coronary, renal, and cerebral blood flow. In addition, stimulation of the central nervous system, skeletal muscle, and gastrointestinal tract may occur. These extrapulmonary effects of the methylxanthines are summarized in Table 13–1.

Serum Theophylline Levels

The appearance of therapeutic and toxic effects of the methylxanthines is directly related to the serum concentration of drug. Monitoring of blood theophylline levels and rational adjustment of dosage minimizes extrapulmonary effects. However, patients exhibit considerable variation in drug response because the blood level of drug is affected by distribution, metabolism, and clearance. Numerous precautions related to theophylline therapy exist because of

TABLE 13–1   EXTRAPULMONARY EFFECTS OF THE METHYLXANTHINES

CARDIAC EFFECTS

Positive inotropic effect (increased strength of contraction)
Positive chronotropic effect (increased rate of contraction)
Increased myocardial oxygen demand (as the cardiac output increases)
Cardiac arrhythmias

VASCULAR EFFECTS

Methylxanthine effects at vascular smooth muscle result in a mixture of vasodilation and vasoconstriction:
Dilation of the pulmonary vascular bed, producing increased flow of blood through the lungs
Dilation of coronary vessels, allowing an increased volume of blood to reach the myocardium (offsetting the increased
     oxygen demand that accompanies cardiac stimulation)
Dilation of renal vessels, resulting in improved circulation through the kidneys and potentiation of the action of
     diuretics
Constriction of vessels associated with cerebral circulation, elevating the pressure of blood going to the brain but
     decreasing cerebral blood flow

BLOOD PRESSURE EFFECTS

The net effect of the methylxanthines on blood pressure is difficult to predict because the drugs possess varied
     pharmacologic activities. As a general rule, blood pressure is increased slightly in most cases, but considerable
     variation among individuals is seen:
     Hypotension due to stimulation of the cardioinhibitory center of the medulla, and direct action on vascular smooth
          muscle, causing vasodilation
     Hypertension due to stimulation of the vasomotor center of the medulla, which produces vasoconstriction, and
          increased cardiac activity due to positive inotropic and chronotropic effects

OTHER EFFECTS

Mild CNS stimulation, including stimulation of the cerebral cortex (improvement in reaction times, mental
     concentration, and the ability to perform difficult tasks)
Stimulation of ventilatory, cardiac, and vasomotor centers of the brainstem
Skeletal muscle stimulation (increased irritability can cause fine tremors or fasciculations of skeletal muscle fibers)
Indirect diuretic effect on the kidneys through increased renal perfusion due to improved cardiac output, and
     vasodilation of blood vessels in the kidneys
Increased glandular secretion and increased motility of gastrointestinal tract smooth muscle

CNS—central nervous system.

theophylline's relatively narrow therapeutic margin and highly variable pharmacokinetics.

Pulmonary function generally improves in most patients at a serum theophylline concentration in the range of 10–20 μg/mL (Boushey and Holtzman, 1982; Clark et al, 1988; Howder, 1992). Mild toxicity signs of nausea, vomiting, and abdominal discomfort begin in some patients at serum levels around 15 μg/mL and become common at concentrations above 20 μg/mL. Extremely serious toxicity signs, such as seizures and cardiac arrhythmias, occur at serum theophylline concentrations in excess of 40 μg/mL (Boushey and Holtzman, 1982; Clark et al, 1988; Howder, 1992). Although pharmacokinetic variables affect all drugs, the rate of theophylline metabolism and clearance is especially important in view of the close relationship between therapeutic and toxic dosages.

Theophylline is predominantly metabolized by hepatic microsomal enzymes. Therefore, conditions such as cigarette smoking that induce these enzymes enhance the clearance, decrease the half-life ($t_{1/2}$), and decrease the action of theophylline. Conditions such as cirrhosis or congestive heart failure decrease hepatic blood flow and decrease the clearance of theophylline. This increased half-life, in turn, prolongs the action of theophylline and increases the risk of toxic accumulation of drug even at relatively low dosages. Table 13–2 lists some of the common drug interactions and other factors that change theophylline serum levels and necessitate dosage adjustments.

The therapeutic target range (10–20 μg/mL) for serum theophylline levels is achieved through the administration of a **loading dose** and a **maintenance dose.** The loading dose is determined by the volume of distribution (V_d) of the drug. The maintenance dose of theophylline is determined by its rate of plasma clearance (Boushey and Holtzman, 1982). This dose is nec-

TABLE 13–2 HEPATIC METABOLISM OF THEOPHYLLINE AND RELATED COMPOUNDS*

Drugs	Factors
INHIBITING DRUGS AND FACTORS†	
Ca²⁺ channel blockers (eg, verapamil, diltiazem, nifedipine)	Alcoholism
Cimetidine	Congestive heart failure
Erythromycin	Liver disease
Furosemide	
Oral contraceptives	
Troleandomycin	
Vaccinations (BCG, influenza)	
INDUCING DRUGS AND FACTORS‡	
Activated charcoal	Cigarette smoking
Benzodiazepine	
Some corticosteroids	
Isoproterenol	
Phenobarbital	
Phenytoin	
Rifampin	
Terbutaline	

Source: Data from Clark et al., 1988; Houston, 1982; Howder, 1992; Upton, 1991.
*Only some studies can substantiate an influence, which may highlight the sensitivity of some interactions to particular experimental or clinical conditions.
†Enhanced plasma concentration and half-life; decreased clearance.
‡Decreased plasma concentration and half-life; increased clearance.

essary to produce a continuous pharmacologic effect. The loading dose of theophylline is distributed throughout the plasma and can be calculated using the volume of distribution for theophylline ($V_d = 0.5$ L/kg). Therefore, to achieve a therapeutic plasma concentration of 10 µg/mL:

$$\text{Loading Dose} = \frac{10\ \cancel{\mu g}}{1\cancel{mL}} \times \frac{1000\ \cancel{mL}}{1\ \cancel{L}}$$
$$\times \frac{1\ \cancel{g}}{1000000\ \cancel{\mu g}} \times \frac{1000\ mg}{1\ \cancel{g}} \times \frac{0.5\ \cancel{L}}{1\ kg}$$
$$= 5\ mg/kg$$

(Refer to Appendix A for practice with pharmaceutical calculations and the unit conversion method.) Loading and maintenance doses of various theophylline preparations are given at the end of the chapter in Table 13–7. As can be seen with the therapeutic agents below, some calculations must be corrected because certain theophylline preparations contain less than 100% theophylline.

THERAPEUTIC AGENTS

Xanthine bronchodilators used as therapeutic agents are administered through oral, rectal, and intravenous routes. Intramuscular administration is painful and lacks efficacy. Aerosols lack the ability to penetrate the mucus blanket of the respiratory tract and are generally ineffective in treating bronchoconstriction.

THEOPHYLLINE (Aerolate[US], Elixophyllin, Slo-phyllin[US], Theo-dur, Theolair, Quibron-T[CAN]). The naturally occurring xanthine derivatives, such as theophylline, caffeine, and theobromine, all have similar pharmacologic action, but only theophylline has any practical therapeutic value in the treatment of bronchial asthma. (Caffeine produces marked CNS stimulation, whereas theobromine virtually lacks therapeutic potency.) Theophylline is the prototype drug of the xanthine class of bronchodilators. The pharmacologic activity of other methylxanthines, used alone and in combination with other products, is generally compared with that of theophylline. Dozens of trade names exist for theophylline.

INDICATIONS. Oral sustained-release preparations of theophylline, such as Aerolate[US] and Theo-dur, are well suited for infrequent administration and are especially useful for controlling asthma symptoms such as nocturnal dyspnea (Minotti et al, 1992).

Reversible bronchoconstriction associated with chronic obstructive pulmonary disease such as emphysema and chronic bronchitis, responds to bronchiolar smooth muscle relaxation and histamine inhibition caused by the xanthine bronchodilators.

CONTRAINDICATIONS. Because methylxanthines have the potential to cause gastrointestinal tract secretion, a preexisting condition of gastric or peptic ulcer can be worsened by administration of the drugs, especially by the oral route. Hypermotility, hypersecretion, and bleeding can result from methylxanthine administration.

The potent cardiac effects of the methylxanthines result in increased metabolism of myocardial cells and a rise in oxygen demand. If a pathologic condition causing narrowing of coronary arteries already exists in such vessels, the relative lack of oxygen in the myocardium supplied by the vessels becomes pronounced.

The levels of endogenous catecholamines, such as norepinephrine, are increased when an individual is given drugs that inhibit monoamine oxidase. Elevated catecholamine levels, in turn, induce adenylate cyclase and increase intracel-

TABLE 13-3 PRECAUTIONS RELATING TO THEOPHYLLINE

Impaired hepatic metabolism results in toxic accumulations of the drug even at the normal therapeutic dosage range (10–20 μg/mL).

Concurrent use of theophylline and drugs that reduce its clearance, increase its plasma half-life and potential toxicity. (The mechanism is unclear, but the interaction is thought to be due to inhibition of hepatic microsomal enzymes by certain drugs. See Table 13–2.)

Plasma half-life of methylxanthines in adults is greater than in children, making dosage calculations difficult.

Methylxanthines administered rapidly have the potential to cause widespread vasodilation resulting in hypotension.

When administered concurrently with diuretics, methylxanthines have the potential to cause electrolyte imbalances due to an increased diuretic effect.

Drugs such as digitalis that increase the activity of the heart are potentiated by the action of methylxanthines.

Myocardial ischemia (relative oxygen deficiency) can occur because the methylxanthines promote an increase in cardiac output

Methylxanthines can increase production of cardiac arrhythmias.

---

lular cAMP levels. Methylxanthines can exaggerate the effects and contribute to increased cardiac output, hypertension, and risk for stroke.

PRECAUTIONS. Therapeutic use of the methylxanthines is not without considerable risk. For example, rapid administration can cause widespread vasodilation and hypotension. Therefore, factors that delay the clearance of theophylline add to the therapeutic risk. Many of these factors are listed in Table 13–2. For example, impaired hepatic metabolism can increase the half-life of theophylline and delay its clearance. Drug interactions with macrolide antibiotics, histamine antagonists, or digitalis can also add to the therapeutic risk (Kamada et al, 1992; Upton, 1991). Precautions concerning theophylline therapy are summarized in Table 13–3.

ADVERSE REACTIONS. Symptoms such as nausea, vomiting, and gastric bleeding are indicative of the toxic effects that may be produced by methylxanthine administration. Table 13–4 lists some of the adverse reactions associated with theophylline therapy. Such adverse effects contribute to the low safety margin of the methylxanthines and reflect the serum theophylline levels.

AMINOPHYLLINE (THEOPHYLLINE ETHYLENEDIAMINE) (Aminophyllin, Somophyllin, Corophyllin[CAN]). The methylxanthine found in aminophylline is theophylline. The bronchodilator is dissolved in a solvent called ethylenediamine. In this form, theophylline is extremely water soluble and suitable for intravenous injection. Because aminophylline is composed of approximately 85% theophylline, its pharmacologic activity on bronchiolar smooth muscle is correspondingly less than that of pure theophylline. For this reason, aminophylline is usually administered at a slightly higher dosage to ensure theophylline equivalence.

INDICATIONS. Aminophylline (theophylline ethylenediamine) is ideal for the intravenous administration of relatively large volumes of theophylline. Determining serum levels of theophylline allows administration of the optimal dosage to maintain the therapeutic range of 10–20 μg/mL (Table 13–7).

Cheyne-Stokes respiration is characterized by periods of apnea followed by periods of increasing depth of ventilation (hyperpnea). This type of ventilation cycle is sometimes seen in premature infants, patients with head trauma, or instances of narcotic overdose, congestive heart failure, or impending death. Decreased carbon dioxide

TABLE 13-4 ADVERSE REACTIONS TO THEOPHYLLINE*

MILD TO MODERATE TOXICITY (dosage range 20–30 μg/mL)

Respiratory System
  Tachypnea
Cardiovascular system
  Hypotension
  Palpitations, tachycardia
Gastrointestinal tract
  Hypermotility and hypersecretion
  Nausea, vomiting, abdominal discomfort, gastric
    bleeding (effects are most pronounced with oral
    administration of theophylline preparations)
Central nervous system
  Headache, dizziness
  Nervousness, agitation, insomnia

SEVERE TOXICITY (dosage range >40 μg/mL)

  Marked reaction to one or more of the above
    symptoms
  Seizures
  Arrhythmias

Source: Data from Boushey and Holtzman, 1982; Howder, 1992.

*These adverse reactions "may not be preceded by gastrointestinal or neurological warning symptoms." (Boushey and Holtzman, 1982)

sensitivity in medullary chemoreceptors is responsible for the ventilatory pattern. As was discussed earlier, theophylline can stimulate these central control centers. In addition, the ethylenediamine component of aminophylline can stimulate ventilation. This dual action of aminophylline makes it especially valuable in the treatment of Cheyne-Stokes breathing.

CONTRAINDICATIONS, PRECAUTIONS, AND ADVERSE REACTIONS. See Theophylline.

OXTRIPHYLLINE (Choledyl, Chophylline[CAN]). The concentration of theophylline found in oxtriphylline, or choline theophyllinate, is approximately 64%. Choline theophyllinate, and other therapeutic agents having decreased percentages of theophylline, have similar pharmacologic activities but lack the potency of pure theophylline products.

INDICATIONS, CONTRAINDICATIONS, PRECAUTIONS AND ADVERSE REACTIONS. See Theophylline.

DYPHYLLINE (Aerophylline, Dilor[US], Protophylline). Dyphylline is usually assigned a "theophylline equivalence" of 70%, although it is chemically distinct from theophylline and is not converted to theophylline following administration. It lacks the bronchodilator efficacy of theophylline but is useful in the control of mild bronchoconstriction.

INDICATIONS, CONTRAINDICATIONS, PRECAUTIONS AND ADVERSE REACTIONS. See Theophylline.

METHYLXANTHINE COMBINATION PRODUCTS. The pharmacologic activity of combination products usually reflects that of the individual drugs composing the mixture, although in some cases drug synergism is seen. The rationale of using combination products is to produce a pharmacologic effect with the minimum amount of drug, a strategy that reduces the risk of untoward side effects. Fixed-dosage combination products, however, lack the versatility of dosage adjustment allowed by the administration of single agents. Methylxanthine-containing products include various combinations of the following components:

- Theophylline relaxes bronchial smooth muscle and retards histamine release. Some combination products contain theophylline in the form of aminophylline, oxtriphylline, or dyphylline, but most contain pure theophylline.
- Ephedrine, by means of its β_2-adrenergic activity, induces adenylate cyclase, which raises cAMP levels. This in turn relaxes bronchial smooth muscle and retards histamine release. In addition, ephedrine possesses α_1-adrenergic activity, which produces a decongestant effect due to vasoconstriction of mucosal blood vessels.
- CNS depressants are used as sedatives to induce a state of calmness that stabilizes breathing patterns. The depressant effect on the brain also tends to offset the CNS stimulation action of methylxanthines, such as theophylline. In some combination products, intermediate-acting barbiturates such as amobarbital or butabarbital are employed, whereas others use long-acting barbiturates such as phenobarbital. A few combination products possess hydroxyzine, a major tranquilizer related to the antihistamines.
- Expectorants are used to mobilize secretions in the respiratory tract by promoting fluid movement from cells lining the tract. This fluid movement thins tenacious secretions and decreases their viscosity, thus pro-

TABLE 13-5 METHYLXANTHINE COMBINATION PRODUCTS

Trade Name	Methylxanthine	Sympathomimetic	Central Nervous System Depressant	Expectorant
Asbron[US]	Theophylline			Guaifenesin
Choledyl Expectorant	Oxtriphylline			Guaifenesin
Elixophyllin−KI[CAN]	Theophylline			Potassium iodide
Protophylline+KI[CAN]	Dyphylline			Potassium iodide
Quibron-T/SR	Theophylline			Guaifenesin
Amesec[CAN]	Aminophylline	Ephedrine	Amobarbital	
Marax	Theophylline	Ephedrine	Hydroxyzine	
Tedral	Theophylline	Ephedrine	Phenobarbital	
Bronkotabs[US]	Theophylline	Ephedrine	Phenobarbital	Guaifenesin
Duovent[US]	Theophylline	Ephedrine	Phenobarbital	Guaifenesin
Quibron Plus[US]	Theophylline	Ephedrine	Butabarbital	Guaifenesin

Source: Data from Deglin and Vallerand, 1993; Krogh, 1993.

TABLE 13–6 DRUG NAMES: XANTHINE BRONCHODILATORS
Theophylline and Related Drugs Having Theophylline Equivalence

Generic Name	Trade Name
Theophylline (thē-**OFF**-fi-lin) anhydrous (100%)*	Aerolate[US], Elixophyllin, Slo-phyllin[US], Somophyllin-T, Theo-Dur, Theolair, Quibron-T[CAN]
Aminophylline (a-mē-**NOF**-i-lin) (theophylline ethylenediamine) (78%–86%)*	Amyphylline[US], Corophyllin, Somophyllin
Dyphylline (**DĪ**-fi-lin) (70%)*†	Aerophylline, Dilor[US], Protophylline
Oxtriphylline (**OKS**-tri-fi-lin) (64%)*	Choledyl, Chophylline[CAN]
Combination products	See Table 13–5

*Number in parentheses is the approximate theophylline equivalence.
†Dyphylline is not metabolized to free theophylline and cannot be measured by normal serum theophylline assays. It is equivalent to approximately 70% theophylline by weight. (Hirnle, 1990)

ducing a state of bronchorrhea. In addition, expectorants are usually mildly irritating to the oropharynx and capable of triggering the cough reflex. The most common expectorant found in theophylline combination products is guaifenesin (glycerol guaiacolate). A few combination products contain potassium iodide as the expectorant.

Dozens of methylxanthine-containing products are available in nearly any conceivable combination of the above components. A representative sample of such combination products is presented in Table 13–5. Box 13–1 discusses the newer bronchodilators.

Table 13–6 gives the generic and trade names of the xanthine bronchodilators discussed in this chapter. Dosing guidelines for aminophylline are listed in Table 13–7.

CHAPTER SUMMARY
Methylxanthines produce bronchodilator and anti-inflammatory effects through a nonspecific mechanism independent of that exhibited by

TABLE 13–7 DOSING GUIDELINES FOR AMINOPHYLLINE§

Group	Loading Dose	Maintenance Dose for Next 12 h	Maintenance Dose Beyond 12 h†
Patients with congestive heart failure, liver disease	6 mg/kg*(5)	0.5 mg/kg/h*(0.4)	0.1–0.2 mg/kg/h*(0.1)
Older patients and patients with cor pulmonale	6 mg/kg*(5)	0.6 mg/kg/h*(0.5)	0.3 mg/kg/h*(0.26)
Otherwise healthy nonsmoking adults	6 mg/kg*(5)	0.7 mg/kg/h*(0.6)	0.5 mg/kg/h*(0.43)
Children 9–16 y and young adult smokers	6 mg/kg*(5)	1.0 mg/kg/h*(0.85)	0.8 mg/kg/h*(0.7)
Children 6 mo–9 y	6 mg/kg*(5)	1.2 mg/kg/h*(1.0)	1.0 mg/kg/h*(0.85)
Preterm infants <40 weeks postconception		1 mg/kg/q 12 h	‡
Term infants		1–2 mg/kg/q 12 h	‡
Infants 4–8 wk		1–2 mg/kg/q 8 h	‡
Infants 8 wk–6 mo		1–3 mg/kg/q 6 h	‡

Source: Data from Hirnle, 1990.
*Based on estimated lean (ideal) body weight. Equivalent anhydrous theophylline dose indicated in parentheses.
†If theophylline levels are not available, the maintenance infusion rate beyond 12 hours needs to be reduced so that adverse effects associated with drug accumulation may be minimized.
‡These dosages are based upon clinical reports; because of widely variant theophylline clearance in infants, theophylline is not recommended for use in children less than 6 months of age. If used, serum theophylline levels must be monitored scrupulously.
§The dosage information contained in this table is presented as a brief outline and summary of acceptable dosages. It is *not* meant to replace the detailed information available from manufacturers of these drugs. Package inserts provide the most current dosage information from pharmaceutical manufacturers. Guidelines describing the preparation and delivery of the drug, dosage strengths, dosage schedules, shelf life, and storage requirements are also included in the package inserts. In addition, precautions and adverse reactions are described in detail. The respiratory care practitioner is strongly urged to read this information supplied by the pharmaceutical manufacturer to provide safe and effective drug therapy.

BOX 13–1 NONTRADITIONAL BRONCHODILATORS

Because a few α_1-adrenergic receptors are located on bronchiolar smooth muscle, administration of α_1-adrenergic antagonists, such as phentolamine (Regitine), has the potential to produce mild inhibition of bronchoconstriction. It is not yet known whether such a mechanism will be clinically useful. The development of undesirable side effects, such as hypotension due to inhibition of sympathetic vasoconstriction, remains a persistent problem with the α-blockers.

The promise of relief from bronchospasm is inherent in the smooth muscle–relaxing properties of prostaglandin E_2 (PGE_2). Unfortunately, PGE_2 also relaxes vascular smooth muscle to lower blood pressure. Prostaglandin I_2 (PGI_2), or prostacyclin, causes bronchodilation, vasodilation, and decreased histamine release. In addition, PGI_2 blocks the formation of leukotriene C_4. One of the derivatives of prostacyclin currently being studied as an antithrombotic agent is designated KP-10614. The finding that PGI_2 derivatives can halt the aggregation of platelets could have beneficial effects in the control of allergic mediators because platelets function as target cells in many allergic reactions.

A novel class of drugs called K^{1+} channel activators, or K^{1+} channel openers is currently under investigation. Potential clinical uses include the treatment of hypertension and alleviation of the symptoms of asthma. The mechanism of action is not clearly defined nor is the precise site of action identified. These drugs have a high affinity for potassium ion channels on smooth muscle membranes, where they open or activate the channel to allow K^{1+} to move to the extracellular fluid. The K^{1+} outflow causes hyperpolarization of the cell membrane, promotes relaxation, and inhibits contraction induced by agonists such as histamine and carbachol. Drugs currently being studied in this class include cromakalim and lemakalim (BRL 38227).

Bronchoconstriction is a calcium-mediated process; therefore, Ca^{2+} channel–blocking agents could conceivably have some future respiratory value. By inhibiting the inflow of Ca^{2+} into muscle cells, calcium channel blockers such as verapamil (Pronestyl) are useful in the treatment of some cardiac dysfunctions. Verapamil, however, has yet fulfilled its promise as an effective drug in the management of asthma symptoms.

Drugs such as aspirin and ibuprofen (Nuprin and others) are classified as nonsteroidal anti-inflammatory drugs (NSAIDs) and may prove to be beneficial in the control of asthma symptoms, especially when inflammation is one of the causative factors in the allergic reaction. NSAIDs are inhibitors of the cyclooxygenase pathway of arachidonic acid metabolism. Such drugs suppress the formation of the prostanoids (prostaglandins and thromboxane) and therefore have the potential to control some of the symptoms of the allergic reaction.

Experimental compounds such as DAMGO and BW 443C are classified as μ-opioid agonists. These promising drugs appear to block prejunctional μ-opioid receptors and suppress release of acetylcholine from nerve cells. Animal studies indicate that these novel receptor-selective agents may be able to reduce cholinergic neurotransmission at airway smooth muscle to bring about relaxation.

Belvisi MG et al: Inhibition of cholinergic neurotransmission in human airways by opioids. J Appl Physiol 72:1096–1100, Mar 1992.

Black JL et al: The action of a potassium channel activator, BRL 38227 (lemakalim), on human airway smooth muscle. Am Rev Respir Dis 142:1384–1389, 1990.

Harman E et al: Inhaled verapamil–induced bronchoconstriction in mild asthma. Chest 100:17–22, 1991.

Kanayama T et al: Antithrombotic effects of KP-10614, a novel and stable prostacyclin (PGI_2) analog. J Pharmacol Exp Ther 255:1210–1217, 1990.

Mathewson HS: Asthma and bronchitis: A shift of therapeutic emphasis. Respiratory Care 35:273–277, 1990.

Sandhaus RA: Newer agents. In Cherniak RM (ed): Drugs for the Respiratory System. Grune and Stratton, Orlando, 1986.

the β_2-agonist bronchodilators. This unique property makes the xanthine bronchodilators, exemplified by theophylline, important therapeutic alternatives in the treatment of reversible bronchospasm associated with asthma and with chronic obstructive pulmonary disease. In addition, methylxanthines in the form of water-soluble aminophylline solutions are ideally suited for rapid intravenous administration. Several theophylline preparations containing different percentages of active ingredient are available to the physician prescribing this versatile group of bronchodilators.

BIBLIOGRAPHY

Bierman CW and Shapiro GG: Clinical expression of bronchial hyperreactivity in children. Clin Rev Allergy 7:301–320, Fall 1989.

Bjorck T, Gustafsson LE, and Dahlen SE: Isolated bronchi from asthmatics are hyperresponsive to adenosine, which apparently acts indirectly by liberation of leukotrienes and histamine. Am Rev Respir Dis 145:1087–1091, 1992.

Boushey HA and Holtzman MJ: Bronchodilators and other agents used in the treatment of asthma. In Katzung BD (ed): Basic and Clinical Pharmacology. Lange Medical Publications, Los Altos, 1982.

Clark WG, Brater DC, and Johnson AR: Goth's Medical Pharmacology, ed 12. CV Mosby, St Louis, 1988.

Deglin JH and Vallerand AH: Davis's Drug Guide for Nurses, ed 3. FA Davis, Philadelphia, 1993.

Hausten PD: Important drug interactions. In Katzung BD (ed): Basic and Clinical Pharmacology. Lange Medical Publications, Los Altos, 1982.

Hirnle RW: Agents used to treat bronchial obstruction. In Kuhn MM (ed): Pharmacotherapeutics: A Nursing Process Approach, ed 2. FA Davis, Philadelphia, 1990.

Howder CL: Cardiopulmonary Pharmacology: A Handbook for Respiratory Practitioners and Other Allied Health Personnel. Williams and Wilkins, Baltimore, 1992.

Kamada AK et al: Effect of low-dose troleandomycin on theophylline clearance: Implications for therapeutic drug monitoring. Pharmacotherapy 12:98–102, 1992.

Krogh CM (ed): Compendium of Pharmaceuticals and Specialists, ed 28. Canadian Pharmaceutical Association, Ottawa, 1993.

Mathewson HS: Asthma and bronchitis: A shift of therapeutic emphasis. Respiratory Care 35:273–277, 1990.

Mathewson HS: Theophylline: A continuing enigma. Respiratory Care. 36(3): 218–221, Mar 1991.

Minotti DA et al: Once-a-day dosing with theophylline: A comparison of four sustained-release products. Ann Allergy 68:500–506, 1992.

Ng WH, Polosa R, and Church MK: Adenosine bronchoconstriction in asthma: Investigations into its possible mechanism of action. Br J Clin Pharmacol 30 (Suppl 1):89S–98S, 1990.

Polosa R, Holgate ST, and Church MK: Adenosine as a proinflammatory mediator in asthma. Pulm Pharmacol 2:21–26, 1989.

Szefler SJ: Theophylline and other methylxanthine derivatives. In Cherniak RM (ed): Drugs for the Respiratory System. Grune and Stratton, Orlando, 1986.

Upton RA: Pharmacokinetic interactions between theophylline and other medication (Part I). Clin Pharmacokinet 20:66–80, 1991.

Williamson HE: Allergy and asthma drugs. In Conn PM and Gebhart GF (eds): Essentials of Pharmacology. FA Davis, Philadelphia, 1989.

CHAPTER 14

Glucocorticoids

CHAPTER OUTLINE

CHAPTER OBJECTIVES

After studying this chapter the reader should be able to:

- State the site of production and the control and target areas for corticotropin-releasing factor (CRF) and adrenocorticotropic hormone (ACTH), or corticotropin.
- Describe the physiology of the adrenal cortex, with particular emphasis on the area responsible for glucocorticoid production.
- List the targets for cortisone and cortisol, and describe the hormonal action produced at each site.
- Define Cushing's syndrome, Addison's syndrome, cushingoid, addisonian crisis.
- Explain hypothalamic-pituitary-adrenal (HPA) axis suppression.
- State the differences between systemic and nonsystemic corticosteroids.
- State four cushingoid effects caused by chronic corticosteroid therapy and explain the mechanisms responsible for the effects.
- Describe circadian rhythms and alternate-day therapy as they pertain to corticosteroid drugs.
- State three precautions and adverse reactions in regard to chronic corticosteroid therapy.
- Name three indications and three contraindications for use of the corticosteroids and explain the rationale behind each of their uses and limitations.
- Compare the pharmacologic activity of the following glucocorticoids with respect to the respiratory system:
    - Hydrocortisone, cortisone, methylprednisolone, prednisolone, prednisone, triamcinolone, betamethasone, dexamethasone, paramethasone, beclomethasone, flunisolide, budesonide.

KEY TERMS

adenohypophysis (a-den-nō-hī-
    PO-fi-sis)

adrenocorticotropic hormone
    (ACTH) (corticotropin)

addisonian crisis
addisonian effects

Addison's syndrome
alternate-day therapy
circadian (sir-**KĀ**-dē-an) rhythm
diurnal variation
corticosteroid
corticotropin-releasing factor
    (CRF) (corticotropin-releasing
    hormone)
cushingism (cushingoid
    symptoms)

Cushing's syndrome
glucocorticoid (glū-kō-**KOR**-ti-
    kōyd)
gluconeogenesis (glū-kō-nē-ō-
    JEN-e-sis)
hypothalamic-hypophyseal
    portal system (pituitary portal
    system)

hypothalamic-pituitary-adrenal
    (HPA) axis suppression
hypothalamus
systemic and nonsystemic
    glucocorticoids
zona fasciculata (fa-sik-ū-**LA**-ta)

CHAPTER INTRODUCTION

Glucocorticoids are a subtype of **corticosteroid** hormone and are produced by the adrenal cortex. To better understand the indications for and the potentially dangerous side effects of glucocorticoids when they are used as therapeutic agents, this chapter first outlines the physiologic control mechanisms, normal functions, and consequences of over- and underproduction of these naturally occurring substances. The therapeutic benefits of this powerful class of compounds are substantial, but drug intervention often disrupts intricate control mechanisms and produces a corresponding increase in detrimental effects.

CONTROL OF THE ADRENAL CORTEX

Role of the Hypothalamus and Adenohypophysis

The **hypothalamus** is located on the inferior surface of the brain, just posterior to the nasal cavity (Fig. 14–1). As part of the brain, it receives incoming sensory impulses and coordinates these afferent signals with chemical information arriving continually through the blood supply. In addition, the hypothalamus is capable of producing chemical messengers of its own and releasing them into the bloodstream. Glands such as the hypothalamus lack secretory ducts and are referred to as *endocrine glands*. Hormones, the products of such glands, are regulatory substances secreted into general circulation and carried to target areas. Hormones have the ability to alter a preexisting reaction, usually by enhancing it in some way. Most hormones are composed of proteins or modified amino acids, but a few possess a complex ring structure and are referred to as *steroid hormones*. This unique structural configuration is shared by cholesterol, testosterone, progesterone, and the adrenal corticosteroids, and can be seen in Figure 14–5.

Hypothalamic nuclei consist of distinct cell populations, each of which synthesizes a specific hormone. The posterior portion of the hypothalamus is responsible, in part, for the maintenance of fluid levels in the body through the production of antidiuretic hormone. The anterior part controls the glandular portion of the pituitary gland, which is known as the **adenohypophysis,** or anterior pituitary (Fig. 14–1). Various hypothalamic hormones stimulate or inhibit the secretion of anterior pituitary hormones. Anterior pituitary hormones in turn control other endocrine glands.

Various physiologic stress factors, or stressors, such as infection or debilitating disease, trauma, emotional stress, exercise, surgery, or thermal changes, can stimulate the hypothalamus to secrete a controlling hormone called **corticotropin releasing factor (CRF).** This hormone enters a vascular network called the **pituitary portal system,** or **hypothalamic-hypophyseal portal system,** and is transported a short distance to the adenohypophysis. CRF selectively stimulates corticotropic cells in the anterior pituitary, causing them to synthesize and release **corticotropin,** or **adrenocorticotropic hormone (ACTH).** ACTH then enters the bloodstream, where it reaches the adrenal cortex and controls much of its activity (Fig. 14–2).

Corticosteroids and Negative Feedback

Adrenocortical release of hormones is primarily under adenohypophyseal control, although the renin-angiotensin mechanism is responsible for secretion of one class of hormone that includes aldosterone. (This mechanism is discussed in Chapter 21.) The control of steroid hormone release is accomplished through a hormonal pathway, or sequence, with each hormone triggering the release of another to maintain homeostasis. General circulation carries ACTH from the anterior pituitary throughout the body, but target

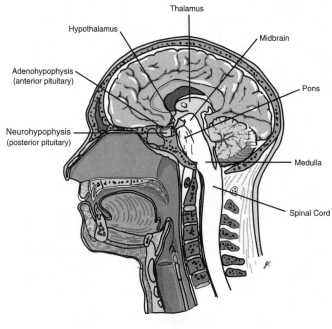

Brain
sagittal view

FIGURE 14–1 Location of hypothalamus and adenohypophysis.

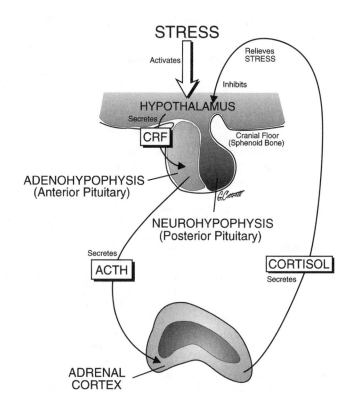

FIGURE 14–2 Schematic—hypothalamic-pituitary-adrenal (HPA) axis, sagittal view. Elevated plasma cortisol levels inhibit the hypothalamus through a negative feedback loop. (CRF = Corticotropin-releasing factor or hormone; ACTH = adrenocorticotropic hormone or corticotropin.)

cell populations located in the middle and deep layers of the adrenal cortex gland recognize the hormonal message and respond to it. These cells possess membrane receptors that bind with ACTH. The resulting ACTH-receptor complex activates adenylate cyclase, which brings about the conversion of ATP (adenosine triphosphate) to cAMP (cyclic adenosine 3', 5'-monophosphate). Elevated intracellular cAMP levels stimulate the synthesis of corticosteroid hormones by the adrenocortical cells, which then release the hormones into circulation.

The adrenocortical hormones are carried throughout the body, where they perform two basic functions: (1) restorating homeostasis by minimizing the effects of the original stressor and (2) inhibiting the hypothalamus to reduce the output of additional CRF (Fig. 14–2). This sequential suppression of endocrine function is termed **hypothalamic-pituitary-adrenal (HPA) axis suppression.** If the physiologic stress persists, the suppression of the hypothalamus by adrenocortical hormones is incomplete and another round of hormonal release is initiated. The cyclic nature of this sensitive hormonal control is a classic example of a negative feedback loop that culminates in the restoration of homeostasis.

PHYSIOLOGY OF THE ADRENAL CORTEX

When corticosteroids are employed as therapeutic agents, their pharmacologic effects mimic those produced by the native corticosteroids. In addition, many corticosteroid drugs have the ability to influence the HPA axis control mechanism. For these reasons, the normal functions of adrenocortical hormones are discussed below.

The adrenal, or suprarenal, glands are small, vascularized glands located on the superior aspect of the kidneys (Fig. 14–3). Within a single gland, two distinct endocrine glands are found. They share a blood supply but little else. Their embryologic origins, cell populations, hormone chemical types, physiologic controls, and functions differ significantly. They are as separate as two glands can be, yet they appear grossly as one organ approximately 5 cm long, 3 cm wide and

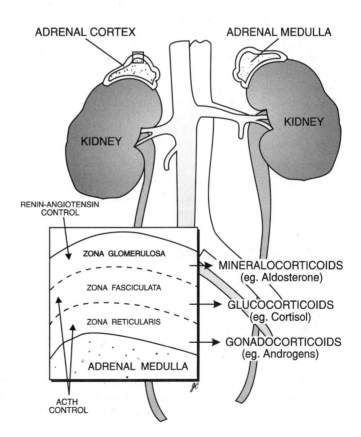

FIGURE 14–3 Adrenal glands and kidneys, anterior view (adrenals are shown in coronal section to reveal internal detail).

only 1 cm thick. The outer portion, or adrenal cortex, is present as a relatively thin layer over the catecholamine-producing adrenal medulla. The adrenal cortex possesses three histologically distinct secretory cell populations, each located in a separate layer of the cortex and each responsible for the synthesis of a different class of corticosteroid hormone (Fig. 14–3).

Steroid Hormones and Overlapping Functions

The steroid hormones synthesized in the three layers of the adrenal cortex are described in functional terms. One group helps regulate plasma electrolytes, another is involved in the maintenance of blood glucose levels, and a third promotes protein synthesis. The relatively complex chemical structure of the steroid nucleus is common to all the adrenocortical hormones. They differ in the location and type of substituted groups on the nucleus. These slight structural variations account for the observed differences in activity of the hormones. However, the differences are better viewed as differences in *potency.*

The ability of one class of corticosteroids to influence body functions usually regulated by another is the cause of many side effects seen with steroid drug therapy. These recognized side effects are simply exaggerations of body functions normally controlled by the adrenocortical hormones. The overlapping effects of various steroid compounds are due to their close chemical similarity. For example, steroid hormones that have gained notability for their potent anabolic effects on the muscular system also produce unwanted side effects. These undesirable effects include salt and water retention because the structure of the anabolic steroids is similar to that of the steroids that promote electrolyte and fluid shifts.

Glucocorticoids: Targets and Functions

The middle layer of the adrenal cortex, or **zona fasciculata,** synthesizes hormones that are especially potent in their ability to increase blood glucose levels. Consequently, they are called sugar-active steroids, or **glucocorticoids.** Two naturally occurring corticosteriods from this layer of the adrenal cortex are cortisone and cortisol (Fig. 14–5). They are released in response to ACTH liberated by the adenohypophysis and are capable of influencing a variety of target areas

and functions in the body, including targets normally associated with corticosteroids released from other layers of the adrenal cortex.

The ability of the glucocorticoids to raise blood glucose levels is due to a biochemical mechanism called **gluconeogenesis.** This mechanism is responsible for the production of glucose from sources other than carbohydrates. Noncarbohydrate sources such as fats and proteins provide energy for the body should carbohydrates be deprived or an unusually severe stress situation persist. These substances enter the gluconeogenesis pathway to be converted to glucose. The increase in blood glucose level offsets the hypoglycemia that may have initiated the adrenocortical release of cortisone. Overall, the mechanism diverts resources from dispensable tissues, such as muscle and adipose tissue. These resources are then converted to glucose for use by indispensable tissues, such as the brain and heart.

Glucocorticoids such as cortisone and cortisol are especially potent in regard to anti-inflammatory and immunosuppressive activity. This action is due to several mechanisms that are detailed below.

- Substances such as collagen and mucoproteins are associated with the inflammatory reaction in tissue. The level of such inflammatory products is reduced when they are mobilized to serve as noncarbohydrate sources of glucose. In addition, glucocorticoids suppress the activity of common connective tissue cells known as *fibroblasts.* These cells normally respond to tissue trauma by producing collagen.
- Lymphoid tissue is a site of antibody production and of glucocorticoid action. Proteins in lymphoid tissue are shunted into the gluconeogenesis pathway causing a reduction in the level of circulating antibodies. Glucocorticoids suppress plasma γ-globulin, the material from which antibodies are made. With decreased antibody levels, the severity of inflammatory reactions is reduced.
- Glucocorticoids inhibit the synthesis and release of histamine from target cells.
- Glucocorticoids also reduce the severity of the inflammatory response by stabilizing lysosomal membranes, preventing kallikrein release, and blocking the conversion of plasma α_2-globulin to bradykinin.
- The release of arachidonic acid from membrane lipids is blocked by glucocorticoids; therefore, the formation of allergic media-

tors, such as prostaglandins, thromboxane, and the leukotrienes, is inhibited. (Figure 9–7 shows the sites of action of major classes of bronchoactive drugs, including the glucocorticoids.)

▪ β-Adrenoceptor responsiveness to β$_2$-agonist drugs during acute episodes of asthma can be enhanced by the glucocorticoids. Steroids increase the number of β-receptors on cell membranes (upregulation), increase the affinity of the receptors for the β-agonists, and inhibit the extraneuronal uptake (uptake-2 mechanism) of circulating catecholamines (see Fig. 5–10).

The other classes of adrenal corticosteroids lack appreciable anti-inflammatory potency and are not discussed in detail. Briefly, the outer layer, or *zona glomerulosa*, of the adrenal cortex produces mineralocorticoids such as aldosterone. These salt-active steroids are under control of the renin-angiotensin pathway. Aldosterone promotes sodium and water recovery in the kidney to help regulate plasma volume. The innermost layer of the cortex is under ACTH control and is called the *zona reticularis*. It is the site of production of the gonadocorticoids, or androgens. The androgenic steroids display an impressive protein anabolic effect necessary for the normal maintenance and repair of muscle tissue.

Dysfunctions

A discussion of the pathophysiology of the adrenal cortex—hormonal excesses and deficiencies—aids in the understanding of the potential benefits and limitations of exogenous corticosteroids when they are administered therapeutically.

Hypersecretion

Hyperactivity in regard to mineralocorticoids results in edema formation and elevated sodium (Na^{1+}) blood levels. The compensatory excretion of potassium (K^{1+}) results in hypokalemia, or a low plasma level of potassium. Occasionally, an individual's appearance changes as fluid accumulates. Alternations in facial features produce an edematous condition known as "moon face."

Hypersecretion of glucocorticoids results in an elevated blood glucose level, which can be a predisposing factor in adrenocortical diabetes. (Conditions capable of causing diabetes are referred to as *diabetogenic factors*.) Mobilization of adipose tissue as fat enters the gluconeogenesis

pathway causes a shift of the body's fat storage depots, sometimes causing visible changes in the overall appearance of the body. For example, fluid accumulation and deposition of adipose tissue between the scapulae results in the appearance of "buffalo hump." Excess protein use in the gluconeogenesis pathway can result in immunosuppression and increased incidence of infection due to decreased blood levels of circulating antibodies. In addition, many people experience a general weight gain through increased dietary intake as the body attempts to replace the protein being mobilized.

The result of excess production of adrenocortical sex hormones is most visible in women. General masculinizing effects, such as the appearance of facial hair, increased muscle mass, and voice change, are noted in addition to disruption of the menstrual cycle. In men the effects of hypersecretion are masked to some extent, but greatly increased muscle anabolism can be seen.

A condition characterized by elevated plasma ACTH levels and hyperplasia (enlargement) of the adrenal cortex with hyperactivity of the gland is known as **Cushing's syndrome.** In this syndrome the individual exhibits the hypersecretory symptoms described above (Table 14–1).

Hyposecretion

Depressed levels of aldosterone represent the most serious deficiency condition of the adrenal cortex. This mineralocorticoid is crucial in the regulation of the body's fluid levels as well as Na^{1+} and K^{1+} levels in the blood. Sodium ions are eliminated rapidly by the kidney when aldosterone levels are deficient. This rapid excretion rate has two important consequences. First,

TABLE 14–1   ADRENOCORTICAL DYSFUNCTIONS

Symptoms of Adrenocortical Hypersecretion (Cushingoid Effects)	Symptoms of Adrenocortical Hyposecretion (Addisonian Effects)
Edema	Diuresis, fluid loss, hypovolemia
Hypertension	Hypotension
Hypernatremia	Hyponatremia
Hypokalemia	Hyperkalemia
Hyperglycemia	Hypoglycemia
Adrenocortical diabetes	Renal suppression
Immunosuppression	Decreased resistance to stress
Masculinization	Muscle weakness
Weight gain	Weight loss

the high concentration of Na^{1+} exerts an osmotic effect, which causes water to follow passively and urine output to be increased. The diuretic effect due to Na^{1+} loss results in a potentially fatal condition of renal suppression as the plasma volume decreases. Without adequate volume, blood pressure falls and the filtration step of urine formation fails to occur. Prolonged suppression of kidney function culminates in the retention of toxic materials. Second, the excretion of Na^{1+} is accompanied by a compensatory retention of K^{1+} that results in hyperkalemia. If the plasma concentration of K^{1+} exceeds the homeostatic range, death can occur.

Depressed levels of glucocorticoids can cause blood glucose levels to fall if noncarbohydrate sources of glucose are not shunted into the gluconeogenesis pathway. The potential hypoglycemia is not as serious as the mineralocorticoid deficiency discussed above, primarily because the body has several alternative mechanisms, such as adrenalin release, for restoring the optimum blood glucose level. Diminished output of glucocorticoids from the zona fasciculata can result in decreased ability to resist physiologic stress because these hormones normally are released from the adrenal cortex in response to stressors.

The most striking response to deficient production of the sex hormones is muscular weakness, because the androgens normally are involved with protein anabolism and the maintenance of muscle tissue.

The adrenocortical deficiency known as **Addison's syndrome** involves insufficient hormone production by all three layers of the adrenal cortex. The symptoms of this condition mirror those described above for hyposecretion in each of the three layers of the adrenal cortex (Table 14–1).

The overlapping functions and differing potencies that exist with the corticosteroids can present an obscured view of the exact location of a lesion or dysfunction. It is common to refer to **addisonian effects, cushingoid symptoms,** or **cushingism** in the absence of definitive diagnostic tests. Effects resembling Cushing's or Addison's syndrome can be produced by dysfunctions that do not originate in the adrenal cortex, but arise elsewhere in the hormonal pathway. For example, overproduction of CRF in the hypothalamus can ultimately stimulate the adrenal cortex and cause cushingoid symptoms. Similarly, hyposecretion of ACTH by the corticotroph cells of the adenohypophysis can produce addisonian effects. (There is no significant change in aldosterone secretion because this hormone is controlled via the renin-angiotensin pathway.)

SYSTEMIC GLUCOCORTICOID DRUGS

The naturally occurring corticosteroids, such as cortisone and cortisol, and their close synthetic derivatives such as prednisone, are called **systemic glucocorticoids.** They possess widespread activity not restricted to a specific organ or region and cause generalized rather than specific changes. In addition, they suppress the physiologic mechanisms that normally control hormonal secretion. (As a general rule, the systemic agents delivered as aerosols produce less severe systemic effects.) In spite of these limitations, systemic corticosteroids are valuable therapeutic agents, especially for the symptomatic treatment of inflammatory conditions (Box 14–1). The chronicity of disorders such as asthma adds to the treatment problem because the above-mentioned limitations are magnified over a longer treatment interval.

Suppression of Endocrine Glands

Corticosteroids administered as therapeutic agents alter the physiology of the body by suppressing the mechanism that normally controls the release of endogenous steroids. Systemic agents, whether natural or exogenous in origin, act as an excess of corticosteroid hormone. The elevated blood level produces the chemical and physiologic equivalent of hyperactivity of the adrenal cortex and triggers a response in the negative feedback loop:

- Elevated plasma concentration of corticosteroids inhibits the hypothalamus, which responds by decreasing its output of CRF.
- Depressed levels of CRF fail to stimulate the corticotroph cells of the adenohypophysis; therefore, the release of adrenocorticotropic hormone (ACTH) is curtailed.
- Without sufficient levels of ACTH, the zona fasciculata of the adrenal cortex is suppressed and the blood levels of endogenous hormones such as cortisone and cortisol decrease.

Suppression of the HPA axis by exogenous systemic corticosteroid drugs results in physiologic dependency. The body becomes increasingly dependent on corticosteroid levels artificially maintained by exogenous hormones, while the

---

BOX 14–1 LET THE PAINS BEGIN: WEAKENED WARRIORS

Golf, tennis, cycling, and jogging often attract the out-of-shape but zealous "weekend warrior" every time the weather turns warm. The results of the overindulgence and undertraining can be measured in tubes of liniment and bottles of aspirin. The aches and pains, however, began long ago.

During the preseason, gladiators training for ancient games undoubtedly suffered the occasional overuse injury as well—sprains, strains, dislocations, or the odd spear wound. Inflammation (L. *inflammare,* to flame within) certainly followed and was recognized in the first century AD by Aulus Cornelius Celsus. Celsus was a famous Roman medical author who wrote the medical classic *De medicina.* He described the familiar signs of inflammation as *rubor et tumor cum calor et dolor.* It would seem that redness and swelling with heat and pain have been with us for some time.

The New Encyclopædia Britannica, Vol 3. Micropædia, ed 15. Encyclopædia Britannica, Chicago, 1991.
Thomas CL (ed): Taber's Cyclopedic Medical Dictionary, ed 16. FA Davis, Philadelphia, 1989.
Weissmann G: The actions of NSAIDs. Hosp Pract (Off Ed) 26:60–76, 1991.

---

levels of native hormones gradually decrease. Systemic steroid drugs administered for their therapeutic benefit, by acting through the negative feedback mechanism, transform the adrenal cortex, anterior pituitary, and hypothalamus into functionally dependent glands. These endocrine glands enter a state of physiologic dormancy and only slowly emerge from the suppressed state when the exogenous source of hormones is cautiously withdrawn.

CUSHINGOID EFFECTS

The pharmacologic effects of the systemic corticosteroids mirror the physiologic effects of hypersecretion by the adrenal cortex and are called cushingoid symptoms, or cushingoid effects. The condition is called cushingism. Because the systemic corticosteroid drugs owe their pharmacologic activity to the basic chemical configuration they share with the natural steroid hormones, drug therapy mimics the physiologic changes normally caused by hyperactivity of any layer of the adrenal cortex. Pharmacologic effects covering the entire spectrum of cushingoid symptoms are commonplace. The severity of the cushingoid response varies somewhat with the potency of the corticosteroid drug, but nevertheless mimics adrenocortical hypersecretion. For example, cortisone possesses a potency only 1/500 that of aldosterone in regard to mineralocorticoid activity. However, in spite of this low potency, cortisone is potentially capable of causing Na^{1+} and fluid retention, high blood pressure, and K^{1+} loss. Hyperglycemia leading to adrenocortical diabetes and anabolic effects can occur if cortisone is used for a prolonged period. Cushingoid effects caused by extended therapeutic use of systemic corticosteroids are, in fact, exaggerations of the normal functions of the adrenal cortex (Table 14–2).

Withdrawal and Addisonian Crisis

When a patient receives systemic corticosteroid drugs for an extended period, two undesirable

TABLE 14–2 EFFECTS OF PROLONGED SYSTEMIC CORTICOSTEROID USE

GENERAL EFFECTS

Hypothalamic suppression
Adenohypophyseal suppression
Adrenocortical suppression

MINERALOCORTICOID EFFECTS

Hypernatremia (increased plasma levels of Na^{1+})
Edema
Hypertension
Hypokalemia (decreased plasma levels of K^{1+})

GLUCOCORTICOID EFFECTS

Fat and protein mobilization
Immunosuppression
Connective tissue destruction
Hyperglycemia
Adrenocortical diabetes
Glaucoma

GONADOCORTICOID EFFECTS

Protein anabolism
Masculinization

responses can develop: cushingoid effects and hypothalamic suppression. A third response, **addisonian crisis,** can occur in steroid-dependent patients who experience sudden withdrawal of exogenous systemic steroids.

An artificial and precarious hormonal balance is created when the body is continually supplied with steroid hormones in the form of therapeutic agents. In the absence of the stimulus provided by ACTH, most of the adrenal cortex reduces its activity. Adrenocortical suppression is a manageable side effect if the plasma hormone levels are monitored closely and cushingoid symptoms are not too severe. If the administration of exogenous hormones is abruptly terminated, however, a life-threatening condition resembling Addison's disease can be precipitated. The symptoms include any and all of the dysfunctions described in Table 14–1 for hyposecretion of the adrenal cortex. The inability to respond to stress, added to suppression of kidney function and K^{1+} retention, represent the greatest threat if the condition is not reversed by the reintroduction of corticosteroid drugs.

When systemic steroid therapy is no longer indicated in a patient, withdrawal of the drugs is carried out very slowly to allow gradual restoration of normal hormonal activity. Such weaning procedures can take weeks or months before the physiologic dependency of the adrenal cortex, anterior pituitary, and hypothalamus fades enough to reduce the threat of addisonian crisis.

Circadian Rhythms and Alternate-Day Therapy

The secretion of corticosteroids and ACTH increases and decreases in a predictable manner during the course of a day. A biologic pattern that is repeated every 24 hours is referred to as a **circadian rhythm** or a **diurnal variation.** Plasma hormone levels rise and fall in a cyclic manner, with changes in ACTH levels preceding those in corticosteroid levels. If a daily activity–nighttime sleep pattern is maintained, ACTH plasma levels peak in the very early morning, stimulating the adrenocortical output of steroids (especially glucocorticoids) sufficiently to elevate blood glucose levels. The rise in plasma glucocorticoid levels lags about 4 hours behind the rise in ACTH. Therefore, peak plasma levels of cortisol occur around 8:00 AM to meet the physiologic stress of "starting a new day." The concentration of the two hormones in the blood declines gradually during the day, with ACTH reaching a low in the early evening and cortisol around midnight (Fig. 14–4).

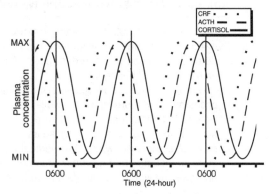

· **FIGURE 14–4**   Circadian rhythm.

If there is no major change to upset the intricate biologic pattern, diurnal variation quietly functions to provide the body with optimal levels of the hormones required to respond to various physiologic stressors. However, if the cyclic nature is upset, as occurs with the administration of corticosteroid drugs or with day-night activity patterns that are drastically altered, plasma levels of hormones can be disrupted. For example, shift-work necessitates changes in sleeping, eating, and working patterns. These changes severely upset the circadian rhythm of corticosteroid secretion for most people. Passing through several time zones produces the common complaint of "jet lag," caused by disruption of the circadian rhythm of the corticosteroid hormones. Restoration of the biologic clocks that govern some body functions can take several days.

Judicious administration of glucocorticoid drugs can minimize the risk of disruption of circadian rhythms. If an individual is active in the day, sleeps at night, and requires corticosteroid drugs on a chronic basis, **alternate-day therapy** is used. Corticosteroids are administered in the morning when natural corticosteroid levels are already at their peak, thus imitating the suppression of the hypothalamus, adenohypophysis, and adrenal cortex that occurs normally at this time of day. Suitable corticosteroids such as methylprednisolone, prednisolone, or prednisone have durations of action of approximately 24 hours. Such agents are used in the morning and withheld on the following day (Baxter, 1992). This alternate-day therapy allows plasma corticosteroid levels to fall normally on the "off day." The technique minimizes the cushingoid effects and HPA axis suppression characteristic of chronic systemic corticosteroid therapy.

THERAPEUTIC SYSTEMIC AGENTS

The drugs that follow have been selected because their pharmacologic activity (primarily glucocorticoid) includes *respiratory system effects.* Some trade names of these generic compounds have been omitted because their primary therapeutic use involves the treatment of electrolyte disturbances, severe arthritis, or dermatologic conditions. The following list represents a very small sample of the systemic corticosteroid drugs currently available.

Short-Acting Glucocorticoids (8–12 Hours)

HYDROCORTISONE (CORTISOL [Solu-Cortef, S-Cortilean]) and CORTISONE (Cortone). Hydrocortisone (cortisol) and cortisone are used in several therapeutic compounds, many of which are administered topically. The oral and parenteral (intramuscular) forms are used in the symptomatic treatment of a wide variety of diseases but are extremely limited in the treatment of *chronic* respiratory disorders. This is because the drugs exhibit significant mineralocorticoid activity, causing sodium retention. In addition, they are degraded rapidly and must be administered more frequently than the intermediate- and long-acting corticosteroids. In spite of these limitations, they are considered as prototype drugs in the following discussion of systemic glucocorticoids.

INDICATIONS. In general, the potent anti-inflammatory action of the glucocorticoids may be useful in reducing the inflammatory reaction of asthma and other inflammatory conditions, such as rheumatoid arthritis and bursitis. This effect is due, in part, to the ability of glucocorticoids to control the production and release of histamine and bradykinin.

Glucocorticoids are also useful in conjunction with tissue transplantation because the drugs reduce the rejection phenomenon. They are also used as replacement hormones in patients with adrenal insufficiency.

CONTRAINDICATIONS. Because corticosteroids cause retention of fluid through the renal mechanism of Na^{1+} retention, they can contribute to hypertension. Preexisting conditions of heart disease or hypertension with congestive heart failure can be worsened by the resulting accumulation of fluid. Fluid retention can also elevate intraocular pressure to aggravate glaucoma.

The body's third line of defense against infections, acquired resistance, is based on the production of specific antibodies. Plasma antibody levels, however, are reduced by the immunosuppressive action of the glucocorticoids. Therefore, glucocorticoids are contraindicated in serious infections because the drug therapy may worsen the patient's condition.

Because glucocorticoids elevate blood glucose levels through the gluconeogenesis pathway, they have the potential to overload the glucose-processing ability of individuals with diabetic conditions.

Finally, acute psychoses, such as behavioral disturbances, may occur in some patients on corticosteroid therapy. Diverse central nervous system effects can be manifested as euphoria, insomnia, and wide fluctuations in mood, including severe depression.

PRECAUTIONS. As was outlined previously, gradual withdrawal of systemic corticosteroids in steroid-dependent patients must be carried out in minimize addisonian crisis.

Drug-drug interactions may occur with barbiturates or phenytoin because these drugs induce hepatic microsomal enzymes, which then increase the metabolism of the corticosteroid and decrease its effect.

Corticosteroids must be used cautiously in patients with preexisting infections because steroid effects may mask fever and inflammation.

ADVERSE REACTIONS. As was explained above with the general description of systemic glucocorticoid drugs, suppression of endocrine glands (HPA axis suppression) and development of cushingoid signs are adverse reactions produced by systemic agents such as cortisol and cortisone.

Note: The indications, contraindications, precautions, and adverse reactions for the following systemic corticosteroids are the same as those described for hydrocortisone and cortisone unless it is stated otherwise.

Intermediate-Acting Glucocorticoids (12–36 Hours)

METHYLPREDNISOLONE (Medrol [Oral]; Solu-Medrol [Intravenous]; Depo-Medrol[CAN] [Intramuscular]). The relative glucocorticoid potency of methylprednisolone is approximately five times that of the native glucocorticoids. Therefore, methylprednisolone is of some value in treating allergic conditions. It is nearly devoid of mineralocorticoid side effects. Hepatic metabolism of the drug is slowed by the macrolide antibiotic troleandomycin when they are given together. Troleandomycin decreases methylprednisolone elimination and increases the plasma half-life of the steroid to improve pulmonary function in certain asthmatics (Barnes, 1989). Troleandomycin given concurrently reduces steroid use in patients with steroid-dependent asthma and chronic obstructive pulmonary disease (Shivaram and Cash, 1991).

Depo-Medrol^{CAN} is administered intramuscularly for asthma prophylaxis; Medrol is given orally for the same indication. In conditions of status asthmaticus, intravenous administration of Solu-Medrol may provide the necessary control of airway obstruction.

PREDNISOLONE (Delta-Cortef^{US}). Prednisolone is classified as an intermediate-acting corticosteroid with systemic effects. Its glucocorticoid activity is several times greater than that of cortisone or cortisol and its mineralocorticoid activity is slightly less.

PREDNISONE (Colisone, Deltasone, Winpred). The therapeutic usefulness of prednisone is limited somewhat by its intermediate duration of action. Its glucocorticoid potency, however, is four to five times that of cortisol. It is an orally administered preparation and exhibits systemic absorption. Its pharmacologic activity is virtually the same as that of prednisolone.

Because the systemic glucocorticoids have a delayed onset and action, they are given early in a severe asthma attack. Depending on the severity of the inflammatory reaction, several hours or days may be required for the anti-inflammatory effect of the drugs to control the edema and cellular infiltration of severe asthma. The action of the systemic steroids gradually clears the airways of cellular debris and secretions. Oral forms of methylprednisolone or prednisone may also reduce the risk of recurrent severe attacks in some patients (Fanta, 1992).

TRIAMCINOLONE. (Azmacort [Oral MDI]; Aristocort [Oral, intramuscular]; Kenacort [Oral]). Triamcinolone is an intermediate-acting synthetic corticosteroid similar in activity to prednisone. Its relative glucocorticoid potency is about five times that of the native glucocorticoids, but it lacks any appreciable mineralocorticoid activity. Systemic side effects are seen with orally administered triamcinolone preparations, such as Aristocort and Kenacort. Aerosol (metered-dose inhaler [MDI]) administration of systemic agents, such as Azmacort reduces the occurrence of systemic side effects.

Long-Acting Glucocorticoids (36–72 Hours)

BETAMETHASONE (Celestone [Intramuscular]; Betnelan^{CAN} [Oral]; Betnesol^{CAN} [Oral]). Many of the available betamethasone preparations are topical corticosteroids, but several long-acting betamethasone drugs are useful in the treatment of allergic conditions involving the respiratory tract. Intramuscular injections of betamethasone have relatively slow onset but long duration of action. The efficacy of betamethasone in the treatment of allergic conditions is related to its glucocorticoid potency, which is many times greater than that of the native glucocorticoids. Like the native glucocorticoids, orally administered betamethasone exhibits systemic effects, such as HPA axis suppression.

Betnelan^{CAN} and Betnesol^{CAN} are available as oral compounds. Celestone is administered intramuscularly for the treatment of bronchial asthma, allergic bronchitis, hay fever, and allergic rhinitis.

DEXAMETHASONE (Decadron [Oral, intramuscular, intravenous, nasal MDI]; Hexadrol [Oral, intramuscular, intravenous]; Dexasone [Oral]). Dexamethasone is a synthetic corticosteroid that is chemically similar to hydrocortisone but differs from it in pharmacologic activity. For example, dexamethasone exhibits a long duration of action, extremely potent glucocorticoid activity, and virtually no mineralocorticoid activity. Dexasone is available orally; Hexadrol is provided in oral, intramuscular, and intravenous formulations. Regardless of the route of administration, including aerosol delivery, dexamethasone exhibits the pharmacologic activity characteristic of systemic corticosteroids and must be used with caution in individuals requiring chronic therapy.

Decadron is available as an intravenous or an intramuscular preparation, in tablet form for oral administration, and as an aerosol nasal spray (Turbinaire Decadron) for allergic or inflammatory nasal conditions. The injectable form is valuable for the control of allergic conditions such as seasonal allergic rhinitis, bronchial asthma, and status asthmaticus.

FLUPREDNISOLONE (Alphadrol^{US}). Fluprednisolone is classified as a long-acting systemic corticosteroid. Its glucocorticoid activity, although much greater than that of cortisone or hydrocortisone, is approximately half that of other long-acting corticosteroids, such as betamethasone and dexamethasone. Fluprednisolone exhibits marked glucocorticoid activity but relatively few mineralocorticoid effects.

PARAMETHASONE (Haldrone^{US}). The pharmacologic activity of paramethasone is virtually identical to that described for fluprednisolone—a potent, long-lasting glucocorticoid with relatively few mineralocorticoid effects. Systemic side effects, however, include any of the corticosteroid effects previously described.

Figure 14–5 compares the relative potency of the systemic glucocorticoids discussed above.

NONSYSTEMIC GLUCOCORTICOID DRUGS

In striking contrast to the corticosteroids exhibiting systemic effects such as cushingism and HPA axis suppression are the **nonsystemic glucocorticoids.** The nonsystemic steroid drugs are virtually devoid of systemic effects, as is evidenced by the reduced severity of cushingoid effects and the lack of adrenocortical suppression. The body's normal output of hypothalamic, adenohypophyseal, and adrenocortical hormones is largely unaffected by the nonsystemic corticosteroid drugs. In addition, the circadian rhythms are still operative, even in the presence of exogenous steroids. At therapeutic dosages, nonsystemic corticosteroids produce a localized anti-inflammatory effect in the airways, whereas systemic agents produce generalized effects such as hyperglycemia.

THERAPEUTIC NONSYSTEMIC AGENTS

BECLOMETHASONE (Beclovent, Vanceril [Oral MDI]; Beclovent Becloforte[CAN] [Oral MDI]; Beclovent Beclodisk/Diskhaler [Oral DPI]; Beclovent Rotacaps/Rotahaler [Oral DPI]; Beconase, Vancenase [Nasal MDI]). Beclomethasone is a synthetic glucocorticoid that has potent anti-inflammatory activity and is long acting. It is delivered by aerosol and does not exhibit signs of systemic absorption or immunosuppression even at therapeutic doses. Therefore, cushingoid effects are minimal and HPA axis suppression is lacking. Beclomethasone is available in several dry powder formulations delivered by breath-activated devices. Like other dry powder inhalers, only the active ingredient is present, with a carrier such as lactose. These dry powder inhaler (DPI) devices are ideal for certain patients who are hypersensitive to chlorofluorocarbon (CFC) propellants used in metered-dose inhalers (MDI) (see Chapter 1).

INDICATIONS. Inhaled glucocorticoids are used in the chronic symptomatic treatment of steroid-responsive bronchial asthma. Aerosol steroids have been traditionally used in patients having chronic asthma that is unresponsive to normal drug therapy. In other words, if bron-choactive drugs such as β_2-adrenergic agonists, antimuscarinics, methylxanthines, or antiallergics fail to provide the necessary control, inhaled glucocorticoids are the next choice. This approach to asthma therapy is being reassessed and is gradually changing. For example, newer high-dose steroids, such as Beclovent Becloforte[CAN], deliver 250 μg per inhalation in an MDI form versus only 42–50 μg per inhalation for the regular formulation of Beclovent. These high-dose formulations are generally used in patients with steroid-responsive asthma requiring inhaled steroid drug therapy in the range of 500–1000 μg per day (Krogh, 1993). They exhibit the same efficacy as the regular dose formulations and produce better patient compliance since a less-frequent dosing schedule is required (Barnes, 1989). Use of inhaled steroids as front-line bronchoactive agents rather than third-choice agents (after β_2-agonists and theophylline) in the control of asthma symptoms makes therapeutic sense (Executive Committee of the American Academy of Allergy and Immunology, 1993). This is especially true in light of the increased awareness of the role of inflammation in triggering symptoms of bronchial asthma (Barnes, 1989; Barnes, 1993; Toogoode, 1991).

The normal course of steroid therapy in bronchial asthma employs low-dose aerosol nonsystemic glucocorticoids followed by high-dose inhaled steroids if required. This regimen is followed by alternate-day therapy, and then by oral daily therapy with the systemic glucocorticoids if the inhaled agents do not improve the patient's condition. The systemic steroids, if needed, are given at the lowest possible dose to control symptoms (Barnes, 1989).

Inhaled nonsystemic glucocorticoids are also indicated in patients in whom reduction of systemic side effects is desirable.

Nasal forms of the inhaled steroids are also used in the treatment of nasal polyps, perennial and seasonal rhinitis, and allergic or inflammatory nasal conditions.

CONTRAINDICATIONS. Aerosol corticosteroids with nonsystemic effects are contraindicated in status asthmaticus. They are not used as primary therapeutic agents in the treatment of acute asthmatic episodes because they have no bronchodilating effect and require a period of time to develop their anti-inflammatory effect. In cases of severe acute asthma or in patients with status asthmaticus, inhaled β_2-adrenergic agonists are administered with systemic glucocorticoids. Steroids are given early in the emergency treatment. This allows the drugs to begin clear-

Natural Adrenocortical Steroids	Relative Anti-inflam. Potency	Relative Na⁺ Retaining potency	Biological Half-life
Cortisol (hydrocortisone)	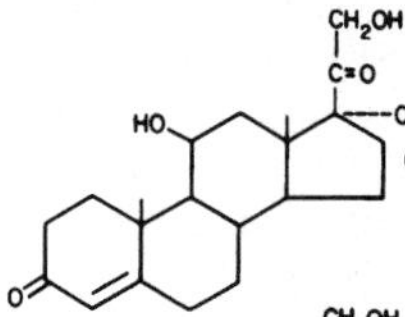 1	1	8-12 hrs.
Cortisone	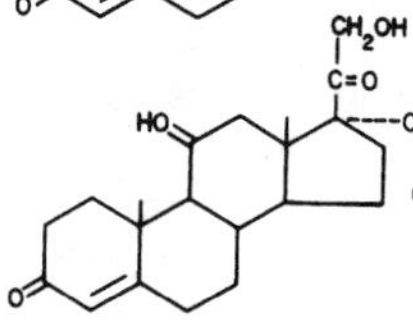 0.8	0.8	

Synthetic Steroids

	Relative Anti-inflam. Potency	Relative Na⁺ Retaining potency	Biological Half-life
Prednisone	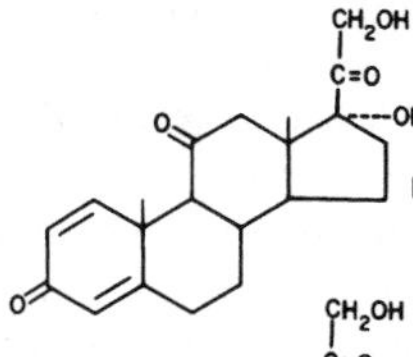 4	0.8	12-36 hrs.
Prednisolone	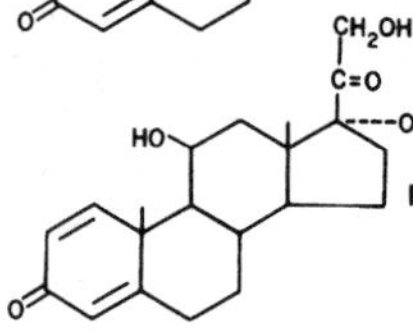 4	0.8	
Methyl-prednisolone	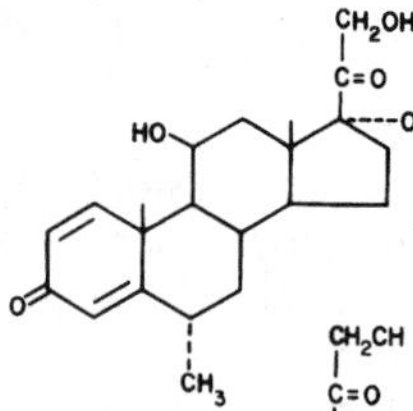 5	0.5	
Triamcinolone	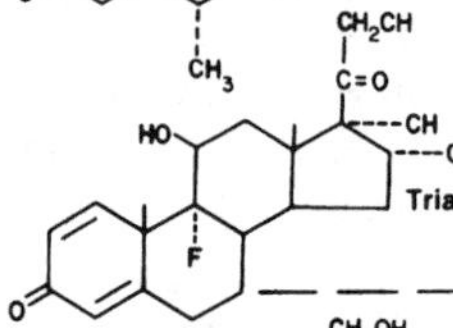 5	0	
Paramethasone	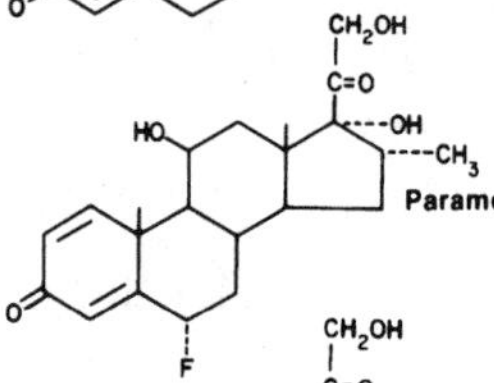 10	0	36-72 hrs.
Betamethasone	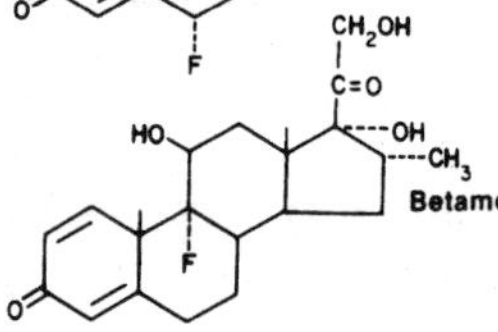 25	0	
Dexamethasone	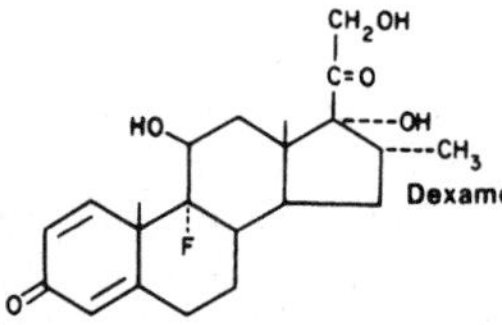 25	0	

FIGURE 14–5 Natural and synthetic anti-inflammatory steroids. (From Shires, TK: Anti-inflammatory drugs. In Conn PM and Gebhart GF (eds): Essentials of Pharmacology. FA Davis Co, Philadelphia, 1989, p. 311, with permission.)

ing the inflammatory exudate that commonly accumulates in the airways during an acute asthma attack (Fanta, 1992). Additional oral dosages are administered as needed to maintain airway patency.

Aerosol corticosteroids delivered by MDI are contraindicated in patients who are hypersensitive to CFC propellants.

PRECAUTIONS. Abrupt withdrawal of a systemic corticosteroid from a patient who is steroid dependent, and replacement with a nonsystemic glucocorticoid, can induce a state of adrenal insufficiency (addisonian crisis). Termination of systemic glucocorticoid therapy must be gradual over several weeks. This weaning procedure allows resumption of normal endocrine function.

Chronic administration of nonsystemic corticosteroids at dosages above the recommended level may lead to HPA axis suppression. With dosages in the normal therapeutic range, however, this risk is minimal because of low systemic absorption, relatively low dosage, and a pronounced local effect.

Acute asthma attacks require the intravenous administration of systemic glucocorticoids because the nonsystemic aerosol steroids do not provide the needed control of airway obstruction. Similarly, during periods of acute stress such as a severe infection, the nonsystemic agents do not provide the systemic steroid that is needed to meet the physiologic emergency. In these instances, systemic corticosteroids, such as prednisone, must be administered until the physiologic stress subsides.

The use of aerosol steroids may promote oral fungal infections in susceptible individuals. The most common etiologic (causative) agent is the yeastlike fungus *Candida albicans* (see Chapter 17). Rinsing the mouth and gargling after MDI therapy with aerosol steroids minimizes the occurrence of candidiasis (Toogoode, 1991).

ADVERSE REACTIONS. Wheezing and bronchospasm may occur following aerosol administration of steroids. In addition, throat irritation, dry mouth, and coughing may be observed in some patients. A surfactant called oleic acid is present in MDI preparations of beclomethasone and may cause airway irritation in some patients (Toogoode, 1991).

Pharyngeal and laryngeal fungal infections following inhalation of steroids may develop. Proper oral hygiene following MDI use, as described above, minimizes the occurrence. In some patients, however, antifungal drug therapy may have to be initiated or use of the inhaled steroid discontinued.

Nasal forms of nonsystemic glucocorticoids may produce sneezing and nasal irritation or burning.

Note: The indications, contraindications, precautions, and adverse reactions for the following nonsystemic corticosteroids are the same as those described for beclomethasone unless stated otherwise.

FLUNISOLIDE (Bronalide [Oral MDI]; AeroBid [Oral MDI]; Nasalide[US] [Nasal spray]; Rhinalar[CAN] [Nasal spray]). Flunisolide is very similar in pharmacologic activity to beclomethasone. It is classified as a nonsystemic corticosteroid, and therefore, produces minimal cushingoid effects and HPA axis suppression. It has pronounced local anti-inflammatory effects on the airways. High-concentration forms such as AeroBid or AeroBid-M, a mint-flavored formulation, deliver 250 μg per puff and are useful for patients in whom control of inflammation and reduction of β$_2$-adrenergic agonist overuse is desirable.

BUDESONIDE (Pulmicort[CAN] [Oral MDI];

TABLE 14-3 DRUG NAMES: GLUCOCORTICOIDS

Generic Name	Trade Name
SYSTEMIC GLUCOCORTICOIDS	
SHORT-ACTING (8–12 h)	
Hydrocortisone	Solu-Cortef, S-Cortilean
Cortisone	Cortone
INTERMEDIATE-ACTING (12–36 h)	
Methylprednisolone	Medrol, Depo-Medrol[CAN], Solu-Medrol
Prednisolone	Delta-Cortef[US]
Prednisone	Colisone, Deltasone, Winpred
Triamcinolone	Azmacort, Aristocort, Kenacort
LONG-ACTING (36–72 h)	
Betamethasone	Betnelan, Betnesol, Celestone
Dexamethasone	Decadron, Dexasone, Hexadrol
Paramethasone	Haldrone[US]
NONSYSTEMIC GLUCOCORTICOIDS	
Beclomethasone	Beclovent, Vanceril, Beconase, Vancensase
Flunisolide	Bronalide, AeroBid, Rhinalar
Budesonide	Pulmicort[CAN], Rhinocort[CAN]

TABLE 14-4 DRUG DOSAGES: INHALATIONAL AGENTS*

Drug	Availability	Dosage
Triamcinolone	Oral MDI: 100 μg/inhalation	Adults: 2 inhalations 3 to 4 times per day; not to exceed 16 inhalations per day Children 6–12 y: 1 to 2 inhalations 3 to 4 times per day; not to exceed 12 inhalations per day
	Nasal MDI: 55 μg/spray	2 sprays in each nostril once daily (safety has not been established for intranasal administration in children < 12 y)
Dexamethasone	Oral MDI: Respihaler 84 μg/inhalation	Adults: 3 inhalations 3 to 4 times daily (up to 12 inhalations/d) Children: 2 inhalations 3 to 4 times daily (up to 8 inhalations/d)
	Nasal MDI: Turbinaire 200 μg/spray	Adults: 2 sprays in each nostril 2 to 3 times daily (not to exceed 1200 μg/d) Children 6–12 y: 1 to 2 sprays in each nostril 2 times daily (not to exceed 800 μg/d)
Beclomethasone	Oral MDI: 42 μg/inhalation[US] 50 μg/inhalation[CAN] 80- and 200-dose MDI canisters	Adults: 2 inhalations 3 to 4 times daily; not to exceed 20 inhalations/d ($\approx$1 mg) Children 6–12 y: 1 to 2 inhalations 3 or 4 times daily; not to exceed 10 inhalations/d
	250 μg/inhalation Becloforte[CAN] 80- and 200-dose MDI canisters	Adults and children >16 y: 1 inhalation 2 to 4 times daily. "Some patients may do well with 2 inhalations (500 μg) twice daily."† Note: Becloforte Inhaler is used only when the required total daily dosage of beclomethasone is in the range of 500–1000 μg.
	Oral DPI: Rotacaps—each contains 100 μg or 200 μg	Same as oral MDI: total daily dose should not exceed 1 mg or 5 200-μg Rotacaps
	Beclodisk—each disk contains 100 μg or 200 μg	200 μg 3–4 times daily; total daily dose should not exceed 1 mg
	Beconase nasal MDI: 50 μg/spray 200-dose MDI canisters	Usual dosage: 2 applications (100 μg) into each nostril 3 or 4 times daily; maximum daily dosage should not exceed 12 sprays (600 μg) in adults and 8 sprays (400 μg) in children
	Beconase Aq. nasal spray: 50 μg/spray 80- and 200-dose glass bottles with a metering atomizing pump and a nasal applicator	Note: "When Beconase or Beconase Aq. nasal spray is used concurrently with Beclovent, the combined total daily dosage should not exceed the maximum daily recommended dosage of beclomethasone dipropionate (1000 μg)."†
Flunisolide	Oral MDI: 250 μg/inhalation	Adults: 2 inhalations 2 times daily; not to exceed 4 inhalations 2 times daily Children 4–15 y: 2 inhalations 2 times daily; not to exceed 2 inhalations 2 times daily
	Nasal MDI: 25 μg/spray	Adults: 2 sprays in each nostril 2 times daily (not to exceed 8 sprays in each nostril daily) Children 4–14 y 1 spray in each nostril 3 times daily or 2 sprays in each nostril 2 times daily; not to exceed 4 sprays in each nostril
Budesonide	Oral MDI: 50 μg/inhalation 200-dose canister 200 μg/inhalation 100- and 200-dose MDI canisters	Adults and children >12 y: Initial dose: 400 to 2400 μg in 1–4 administrations/d Maintenance dose usually 200–400 μg 2 times daily Children 6–12 y: 200–400 μg daily; 2 times daily at 100 to 200 μg/inhalation
	Oral DPI: Turbuhaler 100 μg—200 doses 200 μg—200 and 100 doses 400 μg: 200 and 50 doses	Same as oral MDI

TABLE 14-4   DRUG DOSAGES: INHALATIONAL AGENTS (*Continued*)

Drug	Availability	Dosage
	Inhalation solution unit dose: Nebuamp 0.25 mg/mL 0.5 mg/mL (UD of 2 mL)	Adults: 0.5–1 mg 2 times daily Children 3 mo to 12 y: 0.5–1 mg 2 times daily 2–4-mL volume fill for most nebulizers; gas flow 6–10 L/min nebulized over 10–15 min

Source: Data from Deglin and Vallerand, 1993; Howder, 1992; Krogh, 1993; Rau, 1989.

*The dosage information contained in this table is presented as a brief outline and summary of acceptable dosages. It is *not* meant to replace the detailed information available from manufacturers of these drugs. Package inserts provide the most current dosage information from pharmaceutical manufacturers. Guidelines describing the preparation and delivery of the drug, dosage strengths, dosage schedules, shelf life, and storage requirements are also included in the package inserts. In addition, precautions and adverse reactions are described in detail. The respiratory care practitioner is strongly urged to read this information supplied by the pharmaceutical manufacturer to provide safe and effective drug therapy.

†Krogh, 1993

DPI—dry powder inhaler; MDI—metered-dose inhaler; UD—unit dose (vial or ampule)

Pulmicort[CAN] Turbuhaler [Oral DPI]; Rhinocort[CAN] [Nasal DPI]). Budesonide is a very potent, topically active synthetic glucocorticoid. It exhibits strong topical and weak systemic effects. Budesonide has strong affinity for glucocorticoid receptors, undergoes rapid liver biotransformation, and exhibits a relatively short plasma half-life.

Table 14–3 lists the generic and trade names of the glucocorticoids discussed in this chapter. Dosages for selected agents are given in Table 14–4.

CHAPTER SUMMARY

The corticosteroid hormones have similar structures and exhibit similar physiologic effects, differing mainly in potency. When systemic anti-inflammatory glucocorticoids are used as therapeutic agents, they can produce unwanted side effects such as electrolyte imbalances and hyperglycemia. Most of these effects are exaggerations of normal physiologic processes and resemble hypersecretion of steroid hormones by the adrenal cortex. Anti-inflammatory effects are produced by both systemic and nonsystemic glucocorticoids—both have their place in pulmonary medicine. The inhalational nonsystemic glucocorticoids, however, lack appreciable cushingoid effects and HPA axis suppression. Glucocorticoids can be referred to as *nonbronchodilator antiallergic drugs*.

BIBLIOGRAPHY

Ball BD et al: Effect of low-dose troleandomycin on glucocorticoid pharmacokinetics and airway hyperrespon-

siveness in severely asthmatic children. Ann Allergy 65:37–45, 1990.

Barnes PJ: A new approach to the treatment of asthma. N Engl J Med 321:1517–1527, 1989.

Barnes PJ: Autonomic pharmacology of the airways. In Chung KF and Barnes PJ: Pharmacology of the Respiratory Tract: Experimental and Clinical Research. Marcel Dekker, New York, 1993.

Baxter, JD: The effects of glucocorticoid therapy. Hosp Pract (Off Ed) 27:111–134, Sep 1992.

Chang S and King TE: Corticosteroids. In Cherniak RM (ed): Drugs for the Respiratory System. Grune and Stratton, Orlando, 1986.

Clark WG, Brater DC, and Johnson AR: Goth's Medical Pharmacology, ed 12. CV Mosby, St Louis, 1988.

Cockcroft DW and Murdock KY: Comparative effects of inhaled salbutamol, sodium cromoglycate, and beclomethasone dipropionate on allergen-induced early asthmatic responses, late asthmatic responses, and increased bronchial responsiveness to histamine. J Allergy Clin Immunol 79:734–740, 1987.

Conn PM: Endocrine Drugs. In Conn PM and Gebhart GF (eds): Essentials of Pharmacology. FA Davis, Philadelphia, 1989.

Deglin JH and Vallerand AH: Davis's Drug Guide for Nurses, ed 3. FA Davis, Philadelphia, 1993.

Dutoit JI, Salome CM, and Woolcock AJ: Inhaled corticosteroids reduce the severity of bronchial hyperresponsiveness in asthma but oral theophylline does not. Am Rev Respir Dis 136:1174–1178, 1987.

Executive Committee of the American Academy of Allergy and Immunology: Position statement: Inhaled β₂-adrenergic agonists in asthma. J Allergy Clin Immunol 91:1234–1237, 1993.

Fanta CH: Emergency management of acute, severe asthma. Respiratory Care 37:551–563, 1992.

Flotte TR and Loughlin GM: Benefits and complications of troleandomycin (TAO) in young children with steroid-dependent asthma. Pediatr Pulmonol 10:178–82, 1991.

Fuller RW, Choudry NB, and Eriksson G: Action of budesonide on asthmatic bronchial hyperresponsiveness:

Effects on directly and indirectly acting bronchoconstrictors. Chest 100:670–674, 1991.

Goldfien A: Adrenocorticosteroids and adrenocortical antagonists. In Katzung BD (ed): Basic and Clinical Pharmacology. Lange Medical Publications, Los Altos, 1982.

Haahtela T et al: Comparison of a beta-2 agonist, terbutaline, with an inhaled corticosteroid, budesonide, in newly-detected asthma. N Engl J Med 325:388–392, 1991.

Harper GD et al: A comparison of inhaled beclomethasone dipropionate and nedocromil sodium as additional therapy in asthma. Respir Med 84:463–460, 1990.

Howder CL: Cardiopulmonary Pharmacology: A Handbook for Respiratory Practitioners and Other Allied Health Personnel. Williams and Wilkins, Baltimore, 1992.

Kerrebijn KF, van Essen-Zandvliet EE, and Neijens HJ: Effect of long-term treatment with inhaled corticosteroids and beta-agonists on the bronchial hyperresponsiveness in children with asthma. J Allergy Clin Immunol 79:653–659, 1987.

Krogh CM (ed): Compendium of Pharmaceuticals and Specialties, ed 28. Canadian Pharmaceutical Association, Ottawa, 1993.

Mathewson H: Asthma and bronchitis: A shift of therapeutic emphasis. Respiratory Care 35:273–277, 1990.

National Heart, Lung, and Blood Institute: Executive Summary: Guidelines for the Diagnosis and Management of Asthma. Publication NIH 91-3042-A. US Department of Health and Human Services, Bethesda, MD, 1991.

Ratto D et al: Are intravenous corticosteroids required in status asthmaticus? JAMA 262:1772–1773, 1989.

Rau JL: Respiratory Care Pharmacology, ed 3. Yearbook Medical Publishers, Chicago, 1989.

Shires TK: Anti-inflammatory drugs. In Conn PM and Gebhart GF (eds): Essentials of Pharmacology. FA Davis, Philadelphia, 1989.

Shivaram U and Cash M: Use of troleandomycin as a steroid-sparing agent in both asthma and chronic obstructive pulmonary disease. J Assoc Acad Minor Phys 2:131–133, 1991.

Toogoode JH: Inhaled steroids for chronic asthma. Hosp Pract (Off Ed) 26:15–26, 1991.

Wempe JB et al: Separate and combined effects of corticosteroids and bronchodilators on airflow obstruction and airway hyperresponsiveness in asthma. J Allergy Clin Immunol 89:679–687, 1992.

CHAPTER 15

Mucokinetic, Surface-Active, and Antitussive Agents

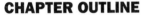

CHAPTER OUTLINE

CHAPTER OBJECTIVES

After studying this chapter the reader should be able to:

- Name the glandular sources of respiratory tract secretions and the stimuli which cause release of such secretions.
- Define sol, gel, rheology, viscosity, and elasticity.
- Describe three conditions that can alter the viscoelasticity of bronchial mucus.
- Describe the mucociliary escalator as a clearance mechanism.
- List three mechanisms by which mucokinetic agents can alter the characteristics of mucus.
- Describe the pharmacologic activity of the following mucokinetic and expectorant agents:
  - *N*-Acetylcysteine, carbocysteine, propylene glycol, sodium bicarbonate, proteases, saline solutions, iodides, guaifenesin.
- Describe the role of surface tension in pulmonary edema secretions and in alveolar diameter.
- Describe the pharmacologic activity of the following surface-active agents:
  - Alcohol, exogenous surfactant.
- Describe the cough reflex as a respiratory tract clearance mechanism.
- Explain the difference between productive and nonproductive cough and the difference between peripheral and central mechanisms of action of antitussive agents.
- Describe the pharmacologic activity of the following antitussive agents:
  - Local anesthetics, codeine, hydrocodone, dextromethorphan, diphenhydramine.

KEY TERMS

adult respiratory distress
   syndrome (ARDS)
antioxidant (free-radical
   scavenger)
antitussive agent
elasticity
expectorant
hyaline membrane disease
   (HMD) (respiratory distress

syndrome of infants [IRDS],
   surfactant deficiency disease
   [SDD])
mucoactive agent (mucokinetic
   agent, mucoregulatory agent,
   mucus-controlling agent)
mucociliary escalator (ciliary
   transport system)
mucus: gel and sol phases

pulmonary surfactant
rheology
sputum
surface-active agent
surface tension
vagal gastric reflex
   (gastropulmonary vagal reflex)
viscosity

CHAPTER INTRODUCTION

The preceding chapters in this unit have discussed the principal therapeutic agents employed in respiratory care to control the release or synthesis of allergic mediators, and the drugs used to relax airway smooth muscle and control tracheobronchial gland secretions. Bronchoactive drugs that alter the consistency or volume of airway secretions (mucokinetic agents) are introduced in this chapter along with drugs that decrease the surface tension of bubbles and alveoli (surface-active agents) and drugs that control cough (antitussive agents). Many of the following drugs are valuable adjuncts to bronchodilator therapy because they generally improve the clearance of respiratory tract secretions.

RESPIRATORY TRACT SECRETIONS

Source

Pseudostratified ciliated columnar epithelial cells make up most of the lining cells found in the airways, but scattered among them are distinctive cup-shaped cells called goblet cells (Fig. 15–1). Thousands of goblet cells release mucus at the luminal surface of the conducting passages. Mucus entraps inhaled particulate matter, such as smoke and dust, provides a relatively impervious layer at the epithelial cells, and contains antioxidants. Oxidant-induced injury in the lung can be lessened by such antioxidants. Goblet cells are found from the nasal cavity to the terminal bronchioles, whereas passages distal to the terminal bronchioles are devoid of mucus-secreting cells. Irritants such as smoke, dust, and chemicals stimulate the production of mucus from the goblet cells of the surface epithelium.

Exocrine glands located below the mucosal surface of the airways are called submucosal glands. Tracheal and bronchial glands are subtypes of such glands. Both possess secretory cell types known as mucous cells and serous cells (Fig. 15–1). The mucous cells produce a thick secretion, whereas the serous cells release a thin, watery secretion. The resulting fluid is secreted at the luminal surface of the airways through small-diameter ciliated ducts. Total secretion from the submucosal glands is far in excess of the mucus output from the combined goblet cell population. Profuse secretions from the submucosal glands result when the glands are stimulated by parasympathetic nerve impulses (vagus nerve) or by cholinergic drugs, such as bethanechol. The secretion can be blocked by muscarinic antagonists, such as atropine or its derivatives.

Mucus

Characteristics

Mucus is a complex fluid created by the combined action of the tracheobronchial secretory cells described above. It is *not* the same as sputum. Sputum is the term used by most patients to describe any material coughed up (expectorated) by them and collected in the mouth. A *sputum* sample does indeed contain mucus from the conducting passages, but it can also include material of oropharyngeal and nasopharyngeal origin, such as saliva, food particles, cellular debris, and microflora. Sputum is composed of two separate secretions from exocrine glands: saliva from salivary glands and mucus from tracheobronchial glands.

Mucus is composed of about 95% water, with the balance made up of glycoproteins, carbohydrates, lipids, DNA, and cellular debris. Glycoproteins are macromolecules consisting of long chains of amino acids (proteins) with shorter attached side chains of carbohydrates (sugars) (Fig. 15–2). The resulting long mucus strands

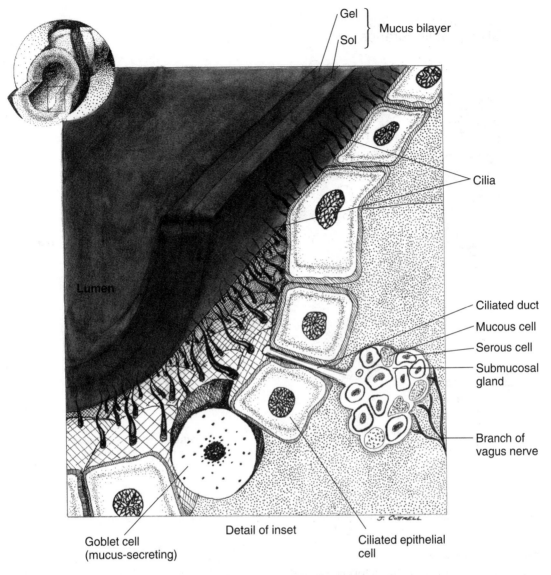

Gel ⎤
Sol ⎦ Mucus bilayer

Cilia

Lumen

Ciliated duct

Mucous cell

Serous cell

Submucosal gland

Branch of vagus nerve

Goblet cell (mucus-secreting)

Detail of inset

Ciliated epithelial cell

Note that the cilia project into the sol layer of mucus. Rhythmic ciliary action propels the "cylinder" of protective mucus toward the oral cavity.

FIGURE 15-1 Cells producing tracheobronchial secretions.

possess a variety of chemical bonds. These include intramolecular and intermolecular bonds. The intramolecular bonds are called dipeptide links. These connect adjacent amino acid groups. Intermolecular bonds, such as disulfide bonds and hydrogen bonds, cross-link adjacent macromolecules. The interlocking bond arrangement of mucus results in distinctive physiochemical properties. These properties impart a unique character to this complex fluid because it behaves as both a liquid and a solid. For example, mucus is present as a two-phase blanket of material resting on the ciliated epithelial lining of the airways. This mucous blanket is part of the mucociliary escalator (discussed below) and is composed of two distinct layers. The **gel phase** is relatively viscous and elastic and is present at the luminal surface of the passageway. The

Two Interconnected Glycoprotein Strands

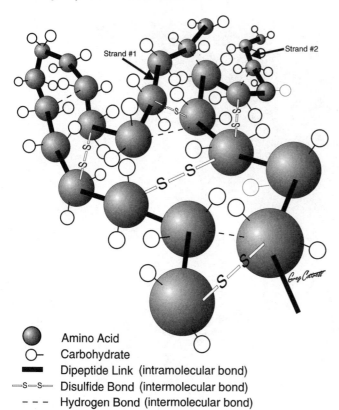

● Amino Acid
○– Carbohydrate
▬ Dipeptide Link (intramolecular bond)
—S—S— Disulfide Bond (intermolecular bond)
– – – Hydrogen Bond (intermolecular bond)

FIGURE 15–2 Schematic—glycoprotein macromolecule of mucus.

less viscous **sol phase** contacts the beating cilia of the surface epithelial cells (see Fig. 15–1).

Rheologic Properties

Rheology is the study of the deformation and flow of matter when forces are applied and removed. As is outlined above, the intricate chemical bonding of the gel phase of mucus gives it the physical properties of a liquid and a solid.

Elasticity is a property of solids whereby a solid deforms, or changes shape, when a force is applied. An "ideal elastic solid" stores the energy of deformation and returns to its normal shape when the force is removed (Fig. 15–3A). This rheologic character is seen in mucus gel when it is stretched—it tends to flow and return to its original shape once a force is removed. The propulsive force is delivered by the rhythmic action of millions of cilia beating at the airway surface. Maintenance of a certain degree of mucus elasticity is absolutely essential to allow the ciliary

transport system to clear respiratory tract secretions.

Viscosity is a property of liquids and measures the resistance of a fluid to flow when a force is applied (Fig. 15–3B). The more viscous the fluid, the greater is its resistance to flow. In other words, a greater force must be applied to move a liquid with high viscosity.

An ideal mechanical model to show the flow characteristics of bronchial mucus involves a coil spring and a shock absorber as shown in Figure 15–4. The coil spring represents elasticity and is *connected in series* with a shock absorber representing viscosity. In other words, one end of the spring is fastened to the movable piston of a shock absorber and the other end of the shock absorber is anchored in place. In this way, movement in the spring affects the piston. If a constant force is applied to the free end of the coil spring, the spring elongates proportionally. As it does so, it stores the energy of the deformation.

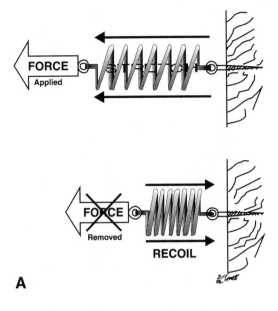

A

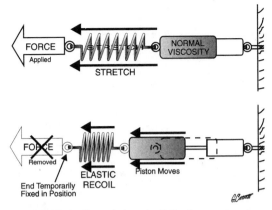

FIGURE 15–4 Normal viscoelasticity of mucus (mechanical model).

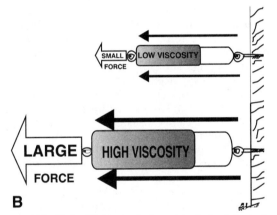

B

FIGURE 15–3 (A) Mechanical model of elasticity (coil spring). (B) Mechanical model of viscosity (shock absorber).

If the force is removed when the spring is fully extended, the piston moves continuously toward the spring, using the stored energy of the spring to overcome the resistance of the piston in the shock absorber. This linear piston movement continues until the spring reaches its original unextended length and is totally relaxed.

In mucus, a similar sequence of events occurs. The constant force is provided by the beating cilia at the gel surface. This force causes the chemical bonds of mucus to be stretched. The stretching action of the bonds temporarily stores energy, as in the stretching of the mechanical spring. At the end of the power stroke of a cil-

ium, the force is briefly removed. This allows the elastic recoil of the mucus strands to overcome the viscosity of the mucus gel, just as the viscosity of the shock absorber is overcome by the recoil of the spring. As a result of its viscoelastic properties, the mucus blanket is propelled forward.

In mucus having high viscosity, as in sputum samples from individuals with bronchitis, the elastic recoil of the gel is insufficient to overcome its viscosity. The ciliary beat frequency determines the duration of the applied force and the amount of stretch of the mucus strands. The viscosity of bronchitic mucus, however, is so great that the mucus blanket only moves a short distance before the power stroke of the cilia is exhausted and the mucus strands relax again. The situation involving transport of viscous mucus is analogous to a mismatched spring and shock absorber model in which a weak spring is attached to a large shock absorber (Fig. 15–5). When the spring is stretched and then relaxed, very little movement of the shock absorber's piston occurs. This is because the force required to extend the piston is almost as great as the maximum force that can be applied by the recoiling spring.

Physiologically normal mucus has a relatively low viscosity but a sufficiently high elasticity to flow in response to the forward propulsion provided by the beating cilia. Propulsion occurs as small clawlike structures on the distal ends of the cilia contact the gel layer on their forward power stroke and cause the gel layer to deform. The elastic recovery of the gel layer overcomes the resistance to flow inherent in the viscous nature of the gel, propelling the layer forward. The combined rheologic properties of the gel phase

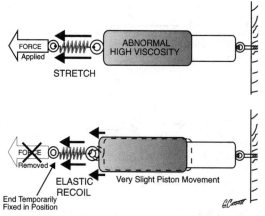

FIGURE 15–5 Abnormal high-viscosity mucus (mechanical model).

of mucus constitute the steps involved in the mucociliary transport system.

Conditions Affecting Viscoelasticity

The volume and the viscoelasticity of mucus can be adversely affected by certain drugs and by various pathophysiologic conditions. As was previously discussed, cholinergic nerve impulses and cholinergic drugs can stimulate the submucosal glands. Antimuscarinic drugs can reduce the secretory activity by blocking the vagal impulses going to the glands. Adequate hydration, or intake of water, is absolutely essential to maintain the mobility of respiratory tract secretions. Water is necessary for the production of mucus with normal viscoelastic properties, but relatively little water can be incorporated into the mucus gel once it has been formed. Conditions such as chronic bronchitis (without infection) and bronchial asthma cause an increase in the viscosity of mucus gel. The presence of concurrent respiratory tract infections greatly increases the viscosity of secretions because of the presence of cellular debris, bacteria, and DNA derived from phagocytic leukocytes.

The currently available mucoactive agents, such as *N*-acetylcysteine, operate by lowering both the viscosity and the elasticity of mucus. This approach to control of mucus consistency is not necessarily the best for every clinical application. As can be seen from the preceding discussion regarding the physiochemical properties of mucus gel, a substantial reduction in elasticity could actually *reduce* the efficacy of respiratory tract clearance. This effect can come about if secretions are liquefied to such an extent that sufficient elastic recoil is lost. Cilia churning away

uselessly in a watery solution would not effectively move the layer. The development of specific therapeutic agents that alter mucus consistency—viscosity, elasticity, or both—will greatly add to the versatility and effectiveness of mucokinetic drug therapy.

Mucociliary Escalator

The clearance, or removal, of potentially harmful substances such as smoke and dust particles from the airways is accomplished through the combined action of the cough reflex and the **mucociliary escalator,** or **ciliary transport system.**

The rheologic characteristics of mucus have already been discussed. These viscoelastic properties enable mucus to flow upward, carrying embedded particulate matter toward the oropharynx, where the mucus is either swallowed or expectorated.

Cilia found on the free border of epithelial cells of the respiratory tract move rhythmically to propel mucus. The ciliary movement provides the propulsive force to deform the mucus gel. This force allows elastic recoil to pull the mucus blanket along. The propulsive force also overcomes the resistance to flow inherent in the viscosity of the mucus gel. This viscoelastic nature of mucus draws the mucus coating along the surface epithelial cells. Cilia contact the bottom surface of the mucus gel and move very rapidly in the low-viscosity, watery sol layer of mucus (Fig. 15–1). Ciliary beat frequency and the rheologic properties of mucus determine the transport rate and therefore the rate of mucociliary clearance. Factors such as the administration of antimuscarinic and general anesthetic drugs, advancing age, cigarette smoking, and atmospheric pollutants such as sulfur dioxide and ozone can slow the ciliary beat frequency (Pedersen, 1990).

Under normal physiologic conditions, cilia are exposed to a wide range of viscous loadings due to the varying rheologic properties of mucus. As the viscosity of mucus increases, the activity of cilia would be expected to decrease. However, respiratory ciliated cells autoregulate their activity to maintain normal mucus transport rates even as the viscosity of bronchial mucus increases. There is little change in beat frequency, but the force generated by the cilia increases (Johnson et al, 1991). There are, of course, physiologic limits to this mechanical reserve. For example, cystic fibrosis is a pulmonary disorder characterized by production of extremely viscous mucus and decreased ciliary action. As a result, mucus transport is severely impaired (Lethem et al, 1990). Similarly, some respiratory tract infections, especially those that are purulent, result in the production of mucus that may be too viscous to be transported effectively by the increased mechanical output of respiratory cell cilia.

MUCOKINETIC AGENTS
Mechanisms of Mucokinesis
Mobilization, or movement, of airway secretions is termed *mucokinesis* and can be attained through the administration of specific drugs called **mucokinetic agents.** The pharmacologic action of such drugs is directed at altering the chemical makeup of mucus, which in turn changes its physical characteristics to optimize mucociliary clearance. Mechanisms of action include:

- Weakening of the intermolecular forces binding adjacent glycoprotein chains together by splitting disulfide (–S–S–) bonds and replacing them with sulfhydryl (–SH) groups (example: N-acetylcysteine)
- Rupture of hydrogen bonds to weaken the intermolecular binding of adjacent macromolecules (example: propylene glycol)
- Alteration of pH to weaken the saccharide (sugar) side chains of glycoproteins (example: sodium bicarbonate)
- Destruction of protein contained in the glycoprotein core of macromolecules through the action of proteolytic enzymes (example: seaprose)
- Transfer of extracellular fluid to the bronchial lumen to thin the secretions (example: hypertonic saline solutions, iodides)

Most of the mechanisms outlined above accomplish a reduction in mucus gel viscosity by splitting, or *lysing,* the secretions in some way. For example, N-acetylcysteine is technically a *mucolytic.* However, because future pharmacologic development may result in the introduction of mucokinetic drugs that exhibit mechanisms of action other than mucolysis, descriptive terms such as **mucoregulatory, mucoactive,** or **mucus-controlling** are preferable to *mucolytic* when used as a generalized classification.

THERAPEUTIC MUCOKINETIC AGENTS
ACETYLCYSTEINE (Mucomyst, Mucosol[US], Airbron[CAN]). Mucus viscosity and elasticity are both decreased by the local mucolytic activity of N-acetylcysteine on bronchial mucus. N-Acetylcysteine is known chemically as N-acetyl-L-cysteine and is a derivative of the naturally occurring amino acid L-cysteine. The drug is also a *thiol* derivative because it is a sulfur-containing compound. N-Acetylcysteine possesses a free sulfhydryl (–SH) group that replaces the disulfide (–S–S–) bond found between mucus glycoprotein molecules (Fig. 15–6). As was explained above, disulfide bonds normally strengthen the tangled meshwork of glycoprotein macromolecules in mucus. Therefore, the architecture of mucus is weakened by N-acetylcysteine action. This causes a significant reduction in mucus viscosity. In addition, the mucolytic activity of the drug increases with increasing pH. Solution strengths of 10% and 20% N-acetylcysteine are available for aerosol administration and direct instillation into the respiratory system. Common dosages are listed in Table 15–2.

INDICATIONS. Pulmonary indications for use include conditions that are accompanied by the presence of tenacious, high-viscosity mucus. These pathophysiologic conditions include bronchitis, emphysema, pneumonia, cystic fibrosis, and bronchial asthma with abnormally viscid sputum. In addition, therapeutic bronchoscopy and pulmonary complications associated with surgery and tracheostomy care are indications for N-acetylcysteine use when mucus viscosity is high.

An important nonpulmonary use for N-acetylcysteine is its use as a **free-radical scavenger,** or **antioxidant,** in the treatment of acetaminophen (also called paracetamol) toxicities. (The pharmacologic activity of acetaminophen [Tylenol] is covered in Chapter 25.) Free radicals are toxic substances known to cause cellular and tissue damage. Free-radical scavengers neutralize these cell-damaging toxins. Most of an acetaminophen dose is metabolized in the liver, with a small portion of the drug being converted to a reactive metabolite that can cause oxidative hepatorenal damage. The harmful metabolite is normally detoxified when it combines with reduced glutathione within hepatic cells before being excreted in the urine (Fig. 15–7). In excessive quantities, however, there is simply not enough glutathione available to inactivate the metabolite and prevent hepatic tissue damage. N-Acetylcysteine and glutathione both possess free–SH groups to inactivate the toxic metabolite; however, glutathione cannot cross hepatic cell membranes, whereas N-acetylcysteine can. Oral or intravenous N-acetylcysteine given within 10 hours of acetaminophen overdose prevents major he-

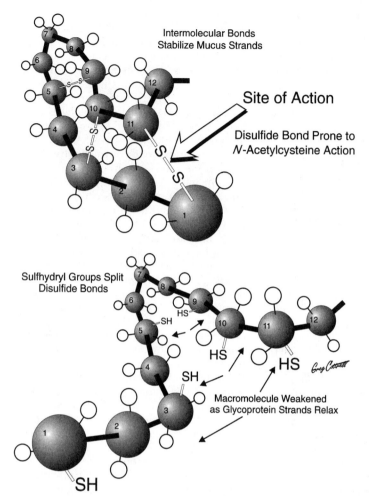

Intermolecular Bonds
Stabilize Mucus Strands

Site of Action

Disulfide Bond Prone to
N-Acetylcysteine Action

Sulfhydryl Groups Split
Disulfide Bonds

Macromolecule Weakened
as Glycoprotein Strands Relax

FIGURE 15–6 Rupture of disulfide bonds in mucus macromolecules.

patic damage (Flanagan and Meredith, 1991; Smilkstein et al, 1991). It should be noted that *in vivo* acetylcysteine forms L-cysteine, L-methionine, glutathione, and other products, and that L-methionine also forms L-cysteine and glutathione. The tissue protection afforded by N-acetylcysteine and its metabolites, therefore, is substantial (see Fig. 15–7).

CONTRAINDICATIONS. Contraindications to use include hypersensitivity to N-acetylcysteine or its metabolic products.

ADVERSE EFFECTS AND PRECAUTIONS. Induction of bronchospasm is sometimes seen with the administration of N-acetylcysteine. For this reason, an aerosol bronchodilator is often administered prophylactically prior to or in conjunction with the mucoregulatory agent. A combination product containing 10% N-acetylcysteine and 0.05% isoproterenol is also available. Additional undesirable pulmonary effects include irritation of the oral and tracheal mucosa resulting in cough.

The efficacy of N-acetylcysteine action on bronchial mucus is such that a large volume of low-viscosity mucus can be formed. Because the volume may be in excess of the patient's ability to clear the secretions, tracheal suctioning of the profuse secretions may be required.

Because the mechanism of action of N-acetylcysteine involves the liberation of –SH groups, hydrogen sulfide (H_2S) can be formed to create a characteristic "rotten egg" odor and taste. These sensations are extremely unpleasant to many patients; therefore, nausea and vomiting may occur.

N-Acetylcysteine is capable of inactivating several antimicrobials, such as penicillins (ampicillin, oxacillin, methicillin), erythromycin, and amphotericin B when it is physically combined with them. Topical administration of N-acetyl-

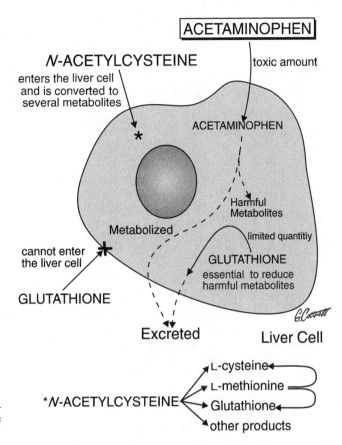

FIGURE 15–7 Schematic—hepatic metabolism of acetaminophen and the metabolic products of *N*-acetylcysteine.

cysteine in the airways with concurrent administration of antimicrobials by alternate routes does not result in the incompatibilities noted.

Finally, because *N*-acetylcysteine is a reducing agent, it is reactive with oxidizing agents and is inactivated. It is also reactive with rubber, iron, and copper and is delivered with a chelating agent, EDTA-disodium, to prevent the interaction with some metals.

In spite of the formidable list of adverse reactions and precautions outlined above, *N*-acetylcysteine has very low toxicity and a reasonable margin of safety as a mucokinetic agent.

CARBOCYSTEINE (Viscorex^CAN). Carbocysteine is a thiol substance known chemically as *S*-(carboxymethyl)-L-cysteine, or simply *S*-carboxymethylcysteine. (It is marketed as Mucodyne in Great Britain.) It is a cysteine derivative with mucolytic activity similar to that of *N*-acetylcysteine. Carbocysteine splits disulfide links between glycoprotein chains to weaken the intermolecular structure of viscid mucus.

INDICATIONS. Reduction of mucus viscosity in cases of chronic bronchitis is the major indication for use of carbocysteine. Decreased mucus viscosity is seen *in vitro,* but the clinical benefits of mucolysis following oral administration of carbocysteine are not consistent in all patients.

CONTRAINDICATIONS. Hypersensitivity to carbocysteine or its metabolites are general contraindications to its use.

Researchers are investigating several promising mucokinetic agents that are thiol derivatives. The mucolytic effects of nesosteine, a cysteine derivative, have been studied in animal models and in human patients with chronic bronchitis (Braga et al, 1989). The drug improves the rheologic properties of bronchial mucus, resulting in improved viscoelasticity and increased mucociliary clearance.

The rheologic characteristics of mucus are also improved with the administration of erdosteine, another new cysteine derivative (Marchioni et al, 1990). Like the drugs discussed so far, erdosteine is a thiol derivative able to reduce mucus viscosity. The new drug, like *N*-acetylcysteine, exhibits free-radical–scavenging properties in addition to mucolytic action.

PROPYLENE GLYCOL. Hydrogen bonds are intermolecular bonds that stabilize the structure of mucus by linking adjacent macromolecules. Propylene glycol is a hygroscopic agent that absorbs moisture and ruptures the hydrogen bonds of mucus, thus lowering its viscosity.

INDICATIONS. Indications for use include reduction of mucus viscosity and stabilization of aerosol particles because it slows evaporation and allows deeper penetration of an aerosol into the tracheobronchial tree.

CONTRAINDICATIONS. Propylene glycol is bacteriostatic against the tubercle bacillus (*Mycobacterium tuberculosis*). Therefore, this mucoregulatory drug must not be used in a patient in whom tuberculosis is suspected (Chapter 16).

SODIUM BICARBONATE. Sodium bicarbonate ($NaHCO_3$) is the salt of a weak acid and functions as a weak base, with a pH of 7.4–8.5. It produces a topical pH change at the bronchial mucosal cells that weakens the saccharide side chains on the glycoprotein molecules. This action in turn reduces mucus viscoelasticity and aids in mucociliary clearance.

An additional use of sodium bicarbonate, unrelated to its mucoregulatory activity, is the alkalinization of urine in certain types of drug overdose (see "Absorption" in Chapter 2). For example, an alkaline urine promotes the excretion of weak acids, such as phenobarbital and the salicylates (Chapters 24 and 25).

PROTEASES. Historically, proteases, or proteolytic enzymes, have been investigated and abandoned as mucolytic agents in the respiratory system. Such enzymes included desoxyribonuclease, also known as pancreatic dornase (Dornavac), and trypsin (Tryptar). Adverse reactions such as irritation of the airways, bronchospasm, and allergic responses were common. These reactions suggest that the mechanism of action is very nonspecific, affecting the protein of mucus strands as well as that of underlying tissues. These adverse effects resulted in rejection of mucolytic therapy with the original proteolytic enzymes.

A new protease called seaprose (Flaminase, Puropharma) is being investigated in Europe. On the basis of early *in vitro* studies, it shows promise as a mucolytic drug (Braga et al, 1990). The enzyme is derived from *Aspergillus melleus* and works on the polymeric structure of macromolecules such as glycoproteins and DNA to reduce the chain length and thereby reduce mucus viscosity. The effect of seaprose on mucus elasticity is not yet known.

THERAPEUTIC EXPECTORANT AGENTS

Mucus consistency and mucokinesis can be improved by the administration of **expectorants.** In general, these drugs promote the transfer of fluid into the bronchial lumen to thin secretions. Most of them are mildly irritating to the oropharynx and therefore trigger the cough reflex to aid in clearance. Aerosol and orally active expectorants are available.

AEROSOL SOLUTIONS The greater the osmotic pressure difference between an inhaled solution and the mucosal cells, the greater the fluid transfer and the greater the irritation of tissues. The normal osmotic makeup of tissue fluid is approximately 0.85% sodium chloride.

PHYSIOLOGIC SALINE. Administration of 0.9% saline solution to the airways delivers a fluid that is physiologically compatible, or isotonic, with tissue fluid. As a result, there is no net fluid transfer across cell membranes. Irritation of the tracheobronchial tree is minimal with the use of physiologic, or "normal," saline. The major use of such a solution is in the dilution of aerosol bronchodilators.

STERILE DISTILLED WATER. Aerosolized sterile water is hypotonic compared with tissue fluid. Therefore, some water moves into the mucosal cells and some enters bronchial secretions, thinning the secretions and promoting expectoration. Humidification of inspired gases is the primary indication for use of sterile, distilled water.

HYPERTONIC SALINE. Inhalation of saline solution in excess of 0.9% sodium chloride promotes fluid movement out of bronchial mucosal cells. As a result, the mucosal cells tend to dehydrate and the bronchial lumen receives additional water to produce a state of bronchorrhea. High-concentration saline solutions tend to be very irritating to the airways and can induce bronchospasm. The main indication for use is to induce a sputum sample for expectoration and to stimulate cough.

In general, adverse reactions are seen most often with hypertonic solutions of inhaled saline. Bronchospasm, coughing, edema, and fluid overload are the most common responses. Patients with coexisting congestive heart failure are at greatest risk because edema and fluid overload are already present.

HYPOTONIC SALINE. Solutions consisting of 0.45% saline cause fluid to pass from the bronchial lumen into cells because of an osmotic pressure gradient. Hypotonic saline solutions do not cause much irritation of mucosal lining cells. Patients who cannot tolerate high sodium intake are candidates for inhalation of "half-normal" saline aerosols.

IODIDES. Despite more than fifty years' therapeutic use of iodides as expectorants in respiratory care, agreement on their mode of action and clinical efficacy is lacking. Various mechanisms of action have been proposed to explain the pharmacologic action of iodides such as potassium iodide (Saturated Solution of Potassium Iodide, SSKI), and hydriodic acid. They include the following.

DIRECT ACTION

- An *in vitro* mucolytic effect on sputum is exhibited by the iodides, resulting in decreased mucus viscosity.
- Iodides can directly stimulate salivary, nasal, and bronchial glands, causing them to produce a lower-viscosity secretion.

INDIRECT ACTION

- Orally administered iodides, at higher dosages, are capable of stimulating sensory receptors in the gastric mucosa, which then relay afferent impulses via the vagus nerve to the central nervous system (CNS). The efferent component of the reflex arc is transmitted through the vagus nerve to the tracheobronchial glands, which respond by secreting. This reflex is called the **gastropulmonary vagal reflex,** or **vagal gastric reflex.** Iodide drug dosages necessary to evoke the reflex, however, are in excess of recommended oral dosages.

The lack of agreement on the mechanisms of action of iodides is typical of the entire group of expectorants. There simply is a lack of convincing studies concerning mechanisms, rationale for use, and clinical efficacy.

INDICATIONS. Iodides are useful in conditions of asthma and chronic bronchitis to decrease mucus viscoelasticity and improve mucociliary clearance.

PRECAUTIONS. Hypersensitivity reactions such as urticaria are seen in some patients. Long-term administration of iodides may cause increased salivation, headache, and gastric irritation. In addition, the presence of adverse reactions and the lack of clear proof of clinical usefulness dictate that the iodides be used only in patients in whom other expectorants have failed to produce desirable effects.

CONTRAINDICATIONS. Use of iodides in preg-

nancy, breastfeeding, and adolescents is contraindicated due to a relatively low therapeutic index.

GUAIFENESIN (Robitussin, Glycotuss[US]). One of the most widely used expectorants in respiratory care is guaifenesin, also known as glyceryl guaiacolate. It is commonly found in both prescription and nonprescription cough medications. However, like the other expectorants, guiafenesin lacks clear proof of clinical efficacy. At high dosages, guaifenesin stimulates bronchial gland secretion through direct action at the glands and indirectly through the gastropulmonary vagal reflex. At recommended oral dosages, however, mucokinetic effects are minimal or lacking.

INDICATIONS. Oral guaifenesin is indicated in conditions of chronic bronchitis and is found in innumerable over-the-counter patent cold remedies, in which it is used for the relief of dry, nonproductive coughs. The rationale for the administration of an expectorant is the thinning of respiratory tract secretions to render the cough more productive (see the following discussion on Antitussive Agents).

PRECAUTIONS. Nausea and vomiting are occasional side effects seen with guaifenesin administration.

SURFACE-ACTIVE AGENTS

Surface Tension

Cohesion refers to the attraction between similar molecules. Cohesive forces bind glycoprotein molecules together to produce the flexible mucus blanket already discussed. Cohesive forces are also responsible for producing the characteristic spherical shape of a common soap bubble. In such a structure, the monolayer of soap molecules assumes the most compact, efficient shape, which equally distributes the forces acting at the film interface.

Surface tension (ST) is the force that holds the liquid surface intact at the liquid-gas interface. In a bubble completely submerged in a liquid there is only one liquid-gas interface. The relationship between the pressure required to keep the bubble open (the *distending pressure*) and the surface tension is given by LaPlace's law:

$$\text{pressure} = \frac{2 \times \text{surface tension}}{\text{radius}}$$

When two liquid-gas interfaces are present (as in a soap bubble being blown from a tube or in an alveolus), a factor of four is used in LaPlace's law, therefore:

$$pressure = \frac{4 \times surface\ tension}{radius}$$

From the relationship it is clear that the distending pressure varies directly with surface tension and is inversely proportional to the radius of a sphere.

At a constant surface tension, the distending pressure of a sphere with radius of 1 cm is double that of a sphere with radius 2 cm. As the radius decreases, the distending pressure necessary to hold the bubble open increases.

Drugs called **surface-active agents,** such as ethyl alcohol and surfactants, lower surface tension and the pressure required to expand a sphere. Therefore, spherical structures such as bubbles and alveoli expand in size and thus dissipate the lower forces. Terms such as "antifoamant," "dispersant," and "wetting agent" are occasionally used, but they are relevant only within the context of reducing the surface tension of bubbles. *Surface-active agent* is the preferred term because it can apply to drugs that act on alveoli as well as bubbles.

Respiratory Distress Syndrome

In the alveolus, two major cell types are seen in addition to phagocytic alveolar macrophages. Type 1 alveolar epithelial cells form the lining of alveoli; type 2 alveolar epithelial cells synthesize and secrete a protein-phospholipid complex called **pulmonary surfactant.** The most important component of pulmonary surfactant is a phospholipid called 1,2-dipalmitoylphosphatidylcholine.

Pulmonary surfactant reduces surface tension at the air-liquid interface within alveoli and decreases the force required for their expansion. This effect is most important in stabilizing the alveoli to prevent collapse at end-expiration, when they are at their smallest. Without surfactant, forces are uneven in alveoli of slightly different size. If these structures are interconnected, as is the case with alveolar sacs, the sphere with the higher pressure (smaller radius) simply inflates the low-pressure adjacent sphere (larger radius). As a result, effective ventilation cannot occur. With a surfactant layer in place, however, the alveoli become stable, surface tension decreases, and lung compliance increases. Therefore, less effort is required to expand the lungs.

The amount of surfactant in the alveolar lining is constant as the alveoli change volume. In a small-diameter alveolus the surface tension is low because there is an increased ratio of surfactant to alveolar surface area. As the alveolus enlarges, the surface tension progressively increases because the surfactant-to-alveolar surface area decreases.

Type 2 alveolar epithelial cells become prominent after 34 weeks' gestation. At this stage of fetal development, they are able to secrete sufficient quantities of pulmonary surfactant to bring about the changes that will be necessary for ventilation in extrauterine life. In preterm infants, however, surfactant production is deficient, surface tension is high, and the work required to expand the alveoli is substantial. Infants with this biochemical deficiency are diagnosed with **respiratory distress syndrome of infants (IRDS),** also known as **surfactant deficiency disease (SDD)** or **hyaline membrane disease (HMD).** *Hyaline* (Greek *hyalos,* glass) refers to the smooth, glassy appearance of the alveolar membranes on histologic examination. The hyaline membranes are produced when proteinaceous material and cellular debris are deposited within alveoli.

Acute lung injury associated with major trauma and with aspiration of gastric contents or water, as in near-drowning, can result in a condition known as **adult respiratory distress syndrome (ARDS).** In this condition there is damage to the alveolar-capillary membrane and increased pulmonary vascular permeability. These phenomena result in interstitial and alveolar edema and impaired gas exchange. In ARDS there is also loss of surfactant function.

Therapeutic Surface-Active Agents

EXOGENOUS SURFACTANT. Surfactant from an external source, or exogenous surfactant replacements, have been investigated for many years using synthetic derivatives and biologically derived extracts from animal and human (amnionic fluid) sources. Early concerns involving microbial contamination of the extracts and allergic responses to the replacements seem to be ungrounded. Exogenous surfactant recently became available for clinical use in neonatology after exhaustive investigational new drug studies.

The synthetic version of pulmonary surfactant is a protein-free compound containing colfosceril palmitate, cetyl alcohol, and tyloxapol (Exosurf Neonatal). Colfosceril palmitate (1,2-dipalmitoylphosphatidylcholine) is the phospholipid functioning as the surface-active agent. Cetyl alcohol (hexadecanol) and tyloxapol, acting as wetting agents, facilitate rapid spreading of the surface-active agent at the air-alveolar interface to lower surface tension. (Tyloxapol was available several years ago in a mucoactive combination product marketed as Alevaire. The combination product is no longer used.)

The surfactant animal source available clinically is a modified extract called beractant (Survanta) purified from bovine lungs. Like Exosurf discussed above, beractant contains 1,2-dipalmitoylphosphatidylcholine (colfosceril palmitate) as the major surface-active component.

Clinical efficacy, indications, precautions, and other pharmacologic features have been established for both of these exogenous surfactant preparations. Early studies comparing the clinical efficacy of artificial surfactant with that of surfactant of human origin reveal very few significant differences. More extensive comparison studies of treatment protocols, routes of administration, and specific surfactant-replacement drugs will undoubtedly follow (Dechant and Faulds, 1991).

INDICATIONS. Exogenous surfactant via intratracheal administration is indicated in the prophylactic treatment of premature infants of low birth weight (1250–1350 g) who are at risk of developing IRDS (Liechty et al, 1991; Long et al, 1992). Larger babies (birth weight greater than 1250 g) who have evidence (radiographic confirmation) of lung immaturity are also prophylactically treated with surfactant replacements (Long et al, 1991b). In addition, exogenous surfactant is indicated in the rescue treatment of infants who have developed IRDS.

The use of surfactant replacement therapy in ARDS and the most effective means of drug administration in adults is currently under investigation.

CONTRAINDICATIONS. There are no known contraindications to surfactant replacement therapy in infants.

WARNINGS. An adult requires large volumes of surfactant compared with a neonate. This need increases the chance of an adverse allergic reaction, especially with biologically derived surfactant. Aerosol delivery may prove to be the most effective means of administering surfactant in ARDS (Lewis et al, 1991b).

In cases of IRDS in infants, exogenous surfactants are administered only by instillation into the trachea. However, animal studies investigating aerosol administration are currently being conducted (Lewis et al, 1991a). Clinical expertise in regard to neonatal intubation, monitoring, and ventilatory support is absolutely essential for administering exogenous surfactants.

Surface-active agents, such as Exosurf and Survanta, can change alveolar surface tension *rapidly* to cause acute clinical signs such as improvement in lung compliance and oxygenation. As a result, respiratory care practitioners must be able to quickly make appropriate ventilator adjustments to prevent complications perinatally (Wellcome Medical Division, 1991).

The use of biologically derived and synthetic surfactant may cause apnea and pulmonary hemorrhage in infants. Apnea may occur because surfactant-treated babies showing an improvement in their clinical condition are usually extubated and taken off ventilatory support early (Dechant and Faulds, 1991). The incidence of pulmonary bleeding is related to the improvement in ventilation, which leads to decreased pulmonary vascular resistance.

ALCOHOL (ETHYL ALCOHOL, ETHANOL). Reducing surface tension of frothy, small-diameter bubbles in the airways results in the production of fewer but larger-diameter bubbles that have a tendency to coalesce, or liquefy. The liquid secretions are more easily cleared (expectoration or suctioning) than with foamy bubbles in the airways.

INDICATIONS. In conditions of pulmonary edema, plasma exudes, or transfers, across the respiratory membrane (alveolar-capillary membrane). This transfer of fluid fills alveoli and small airways with frothy bubbles that are very difficult to clear. Ethyl alcohol, also known as ethanol, delivered to the airways lowers surface tension of the bubbles to allow easier clearance.

ADVERSE REACTIONS. Ethyl alcohol delivered by aerosol or instilled directly into the lungs is highly irritating to the airways and may induce bronchospasm. In addition, alcohol depresses the CNS to cause sedation and decrease central ventilatory drive. For these reasons, even in the short-term treatment of acute pulmonary edema, alcohol is very rarely used. Instead, drugs such as digitalis to improve cardiac output, and diuretics to stimulate urine production and unload excess fluid from the circulatory system are used to prevent the symptoms of pulmonary edema.

ANTITUSSIVE AGENTS
Cough As a Clearance Mechanism
The clearance mechanism of coughing, like the mucociliary escalator discussed earlier in the chapter, is a nonspecific defense mechanism.

Along with the cellular defense provided by phagocytic leukocytes, these clearance mechanisms make up the body's first line of defense. Under normal physiologic conditions, cough does not occur very frequently, owing to the effectiveness of the mucociliary escalator in clearing the airways. However, if respiratory tract secretions begin to overwhelm ciliary transport (as occurs in bronchitis) or the transport system itself is damaged (as occurs in the airways of cigarette smokers), coughing becomes more frequent. An effective cough can expel airway secretions with great force. Ineffective coughs can lead to retention of secretions, which may trigger a cyclical bout of coughing.

Most **antitussive agents** provide symptomatic relief of cough while the underlying causative condition is unaltered. In many cases, however, controlling the cause controls the symptom of coughing. For example, bronchodilators used in asthma therapy relax airway smooth muscle and break the vicious cycle of bronchial asthma, which can include episodes of coughing (see Fig. 9–4). Similarly, lowering mucus viscosity with N-acetylcysteine can remove the cough stimulus produced by tenacious mucus. The following section deals with antitussives administered symptomatically to control nonspecific cough.

The Cough Reflex

The mechanism of coughing involves a classic reflex loop consisting of:

- Sensory cells
- Sensory nervous pathway
- Central processing center
- Motor nervous pathway
- Effector cells

Irritant receptors located in the larynx, trachea, and bronchi have been discussed in Chapter 11 as part of the bronchoconstriction reflex (see Fig. 11–2). These receptors respond to chemical and mechanical stimuli such as inhaled smoke or noxious chemicals. The sensory component of the reflex arc consists of an afferent pathway in the vagus, glossopharyngeal, or trigeminal nerve. Functional groupings of neurons in the medulla and pons of the hindbrain act as a cough control center. These cell groups relay motor impulses via the vagus nerve to the muscles of ventilation acting as effectors in the reflex arc. Muscles trigger the mechanical cough with an abrupt inspiratory phase, a compression phase as intra-alveolar pressures rise markedly,

and an explosive expiratory phase that generates sufficient velocity to clear the airways. Ineffective cough occurs when an insufficient force is generated by the respiratory muscles. Insufficiency may be caused by neuromuscular blockers such as pancuronium or conditions such as bronchial asthma, chronic obstructive pulmonary disease, spinal cord trauma, surgical pain, or neuromuscular disease such as myasthenia gravis.

Nonproductive Cough Versus Productive Cough

The rationale for cough suppression with antitussive drugs is concerned with control of coughs that are nonproductive. In such a cough, stimulation of airway irritant receptors, as occurs with mucosal drying, triggers the cough reflex although tracheobronchial glands are producing few secretions. The result is a dry, hacking cough that does not clear any secretions. In addition, it becomes self-destructive because mucosal linings become more and more inflamed. The cough cycle becomes more violent and the patient is unable to rest. Under these circumstances, cough suppression makes good therapeutic sense. Antitussive therapy directed at a productive cough, however, makes considerably less sense because the cough is fulfilling its clearance role in getting rid of secretions. Inhibiting the mechanism causes retention of secretions. Many proprietary cold remedies are combination products of questionable therapeutic value. These compounds often contain an expectorant, which mobilizes secretions, and an antitussive, which suppresses clearance of the secretions.

THERAPEUTIC ANTITUSSIVE AGENTS

Antitussive mechanisms of action are directed at components of the cough reflex arc: peripherally acting drugs suppress the sensory irritant receptors on the mucosal linings while centrally acting drugs control the medullary cough center.

Drugs with local anesthetic action are useful for reducing the action of peripheral irritant receptors in the airways. Many of these agents such as benzocaine and phenol are found in OTC cough lozenges. Benzonatate (Tessalon) is an orally administered antitussive drug that has peripheral effects on irritant receptors.

INDICATIONS. Cough suppression is a recognized indication for use of these antitussives.

CODEINE. Codeine is the least potent of the opiate (narcotic) analgesics and is used primarily in the relief of moderate to severe pain (Chapter 25). It is also useful in the suppression of the medullary cough control center.

In terms of its antitussive effects, codeine is presently considered a centrally acting cough suppressant. However, recent animal studies (Karlsson et al, 1990) with codeine have revealed a peripheral (local) effect at certain opioid receptors in the airways. At these sites, codeine exerts both a rapid antitussive effect and suppression of bronchoconstriction (an anti-bronchoconstriction effect). It does this without first being metabolized to morphine. It remains to be seen whether studies of human airways will show the same response.

The dosage of codeine required to produce an antitussive effect is substantially less than that needed to produce analgesia. As a consequence, euphoric feelings and undesirable effects such as physical and psychologic dependency are minimal. In addition, ventilatory depression is slight compared with that produced by powerful narcotic analgesics, such as morphine. In fact, low-potency, codeine-containing pain relievers and cough suppressants such as Benilyn-C[CAN] are controlled but available in Canada without prescription. In the United States, however, codeine products can only be obtained through prescription.

INDICATIONS. See general information above.

ADVERSE EFFECTS. Because codeine is a CNS depressant, repeated dosing can result in sedation and potentiation of other CNS depressants, such as general anesthetics, tranquilizers, and ethyl alcohol. Nausea, vomiting, and constipation, and respiratory system effects such as inhibition of mucociliary clearance and reduced ventilation, may be seen in some patients.

HYDROCODONE (Triaminic DH). Hydrocodone is a derivative of codeine with essentially the same antitussive and adverse effects as codeine. It is marketed under many trade names.

DEXTROMETHORPHAN. Dozens of cough suppressant medications such as Triaminicol, Robitussin-DM, and Triaminic-DM are currently marketed as dextromethorphan products. These drugs *usually* have the initials "DM" following the trade name. Dextromethorphan hydrobromide is classified as a centrally acting nonopioid antitussive. It is the dextro-isomer of a narcotic analgesic known as levorphanol. Dextromethorphan, however, lacks the analgesic and addictive properties typically seen with the opioid group of drugs. In addition to its central effects, dextromethorphan is a pharmacologic antagonist of an excitatory amino acid neurotransmitter called NMDA (N-methyl-D-aspartate). NMDA receptors may be involved in the regulation of the cough reflex. Therefore, NMDA-blocking activity may contribute to a peripheral antitussive effect exhibited by dextromethorphan (Kamei et al, 1989; Tortella et al, 1989).

INDICATIONS. Dextromethorphan is indicated in the suppression of nonproductive cough.

PRECAUTIONS. Side effects such as nausea, dizziness, and drowsiness are occasionally noted with dextromethorphan, but the incidence and severity is much less than is seen with codeine. A mild anticholinergic action is noted; therefore, preexisting conditions such as glaucoma, paralytic ileus, and urinary retention may be worsened by the administration of dextromethorphan.

Several other centrally acting nonnarcotic antitussives are available. These drugs exhibit pharmacologic activity similar to that of dextromethorphan in regard to cough suppression and side effects such as anticholinergic activity. The group includes caramiphen, carbetapentane, and noscapine.

DIPHENHYDRAMINE (Benadryl). The H_1-histamine receptor blocker known as diphenhydramine belongs to the group of first-generation antihistaminics (Chapter 10). It exhibits an antitussive effect in addition to its histamine antagonist activity. However, the precise mechanism of action of cough suppression is not fully understood.

INDICATIONS. See Local anesthetics.

PRECAUTIONS. First-generation H_1-receptor blockers cause sedation, which can be additive with other CNS depressants, such as tranquilizers and barbiturates. In addition, diphenhydramine and related compounds possess anticholinergic activity and can therefore produce drying of secretions, blurred vision, and constipation. They should be used with caution in patients with glaucoma, gastrointestinal tract stasis, or urinary retention.

Table 15–1 lists generic and trade names of the drugs presented in this chapter. Drug dosages for selected agents are given in Table 15–2.

CHAPTER SUMMARY

Respiratory tract secretions generally serve a protective function in the body. Foreign material found in such secretions is continually removed

TABLE 15–1 DRUG NAMES: MUCOKINETIC, SURFACE-ACTIVE, AND ANTITUSSIVE AGENTS

Generic Name	Trade Name
MUCOKINETIC AGENTS	
N-Acetylcysteine (a-sē-til-**SIS**-ti-ēn)	Mucomyst, Mucosol[US], Airbron[CAN]
Propylene glycol	
Sodium bicarbonate (NaHCO₃)	
EXPECTORANTS	
Aerosol solutions	
Physiologic saline (0.9% NaCl)	
Sterile distilled water	
Hypertonic saline (>0.9% NaCl)	
Hypotonic saline (0.45% NaCl)	
Iodides	
Potassium iodide (KI)	
Saturated solution of potassium iodide (SSKI)	
Hydriodic acid (HI)	
Guaifenesin (gwaf-i-**NES**-in)	Robitussin, Glycotuss[US]
(or glyceryl guaiacolate) (**GLIS**-sir-il gwī-**AK**-ō-lāt)	
SURFACE-ACTIVE AGENTS	
Exogenous surfactant	Exosurf Neonatal
Colfosceril palmitate, cetyl alcohol, and tyloxapol	
Beractant	Survanta
Ethyl alcohol (ethanol)	
ANTITUSSIVE AGENTS	
Local anesthetics	
Benzocaine	
Phenol	
Benzonatate	Tessalon
Codeine	Benilyn-C[CAN]
Hydrocodone	Triaminic DH
Dextromethorphan (deks-trō-me-**THŌR**-fan)	Triaminicol, Robitussin-DM, Triaminic-DM
Diphenhydramine	Benadryl
NEWER AGENTS	
Mucokinetic agents	
Thiol derivations	
Nesosteine (ne-**SŌS**-ti-ēn)	
Erdosteine (er-**DŌS**-ti-ēn)	
Proteases	
seaprose	Flaminase, Puropharma
Nonnarcotic antitussives	
Caramiphen	
Carbetapentane	
Noscapine	

NaCl—sodium chloride.

by clearance mechanisms such as cough and mucociliary transport. Occasionally the amount or consistency of the secretions changes so dramatically as to overwhelm these normal clearance mechanisms. This chapter shows us that mucoregulatory agents, such as *N*-acetylcysteine, and expectorants, such as guaifenesin, are employed in respiratory care to facilitate the clearance of secretions from the airways. The limited use of surface-active agents, such as ethyl alcohol, to aid clearance is also discussed, as is the special use of exogenous surfactant to treat infant respiratory distress syndrome of the infant. Finally, the use of antitussives, such as dextromethorphan, to control cough is outlined.

TABLE 15–2   DRUG DOSAGES: INHALATION AGENTS*

Inhalation Agent	Availability	Dosage
N-Acetylcysteine	10% and 20% solutions When 25% of medication remains in nebulizer, dilute with an equal amount of 0.9% NaCl or sterile water Because the production of liquified secretions may increase, suction equipment should be available for patients unable to clear airways	Inhalation: 3–5 mL of 20% solution equally diluted with sterile water for injection or inhalation (USP) or with normal saline (0.9% NaCl) for injection or inhalation (USP) given 3–4 times daily via nebulization 6–10 mL of 10% solution (undiluted) 3–4 times daily via nebulization Direct instillation into lungs of an intubated patient: 1–2 mL of 10% or 20% solution Diagnostic bronchograms: 1–2 mL of 20% solution or 2–4 mL of 10% solution given before or during the procedure Acetaminophen overdose: Loading dose—140 mg/kg Maintenance dose—70 mg/kg for a total of 17 doses (total: 1330 mg/kg)
Propylene glycol	2% inhalation solution	1–2 mL of 2% solution nebulized concurrently with a bronchodilator or another mucokinetic agent
Sodium bicarbonate	Inhalation solutions: 1.4%, 5%, 7.5% (Recommended strength for less irritating effects is equal dilution of the 5% solution, producing a 2.5% solution)	Nebulization: 2–5 mL every 4–8 h Intratracheal instillation: 5–10 mL as needed
Physiologic saline (normal saline)	0.9% NaCl	As needed for dilution of bronchodilators
Sterile distilled water		As needed for humidification of inspired gases
Hypertonic saline	>0.9% NaCl	As needed for sputum induction
Hypotonic saline (half-normal saline)	0.45% NaCl	As needed in patients who cannot tolerate high Na^{1+} intake for dilution, humidification, or sputum induction

Colfosceril palmitate (exogenous surfactant)	Exosurf Neonatal
	10 mL vial (108 mg/vial)
	Each vial should be reconstituted immediately before use with 8 mL of preservative-free sterile water for injection [USP] (do *not* use bacteriostatic water for injection [USP])
		For intratracheal instillation only
		Prophylactic treatment:
		   "The first dose of Exosurf Neonatal should be administered as a single 5 mL/kg dose as soon as possible after birth. Second and third doses should be administered approximately 12 and 24 hours later to all infants who remain on mechanical ventilation at those times."†
		Rescue treatment:
		   "Exosurf Neonatal should be administered in two 5 mL/kg doses. The initial dose should be administered as soon as possible after the diagnosis of RDS is confirmed. The second dose should be administered approximately 12 hours following the first dose, provided the infant remains on mechanical ventilation."†
		Note: "Each Exosurf Neonatal dose is administered in two 2.5 mL/kg half-doses. Each half-dose is instilled slowly over a minimum of 1 to 2 minutes. . ."†

Ethyl alcohol	30–50% solution	Nebulization: 5–15 mL

Source: Data from Deglin and Vallerand, 1993; Howder, 1992; Wellcome Medical Division, 1991.

*Note The dosage information contained in this table is presented as a brief outline and summary of acceptable dosages. It is *not* meant to replace the detailed information available from manufacturers of these drugs. Package inserts provide the most current dosage information from pharmaceutical manufacturers. Guidelines describing the preparation and delivery of the drug, dosage strengths, dosage schedules, shelf life, and storage requirements are also included in the package inserts. In addition, precautions and adverse reactions are described in detail. The respiratory care practitioner is strongly urged to read this information supplied by the pharmaceutical manufacturer to provide safe and effective drug therapy.

†Wellcome Medical Division, 1991.

NaCl—sodium chloride; USP—US Pharmacopeia.

BIBLIOGRAPHY

Allegra L, Moavero NE, and Rampoldi C: Ozone-induced impairment of mucociliary transport and its prevention with *N*-acetylcysteine. Am J Med 91:67S–71S, 1991.

Avery ME: Twenty-five years of progress in hyaline membrane disease. Respiratory Care 36:283–287, 1991.

Bernard GR: *N*-Acetylcysteine in experimental and clinical acute lung injury. Am J Med 91:54S–59S, 1991.

Braga PC et al: In vitro rheological assessment of mucolytic activity induced by seaprose. Pharmacol Res 22:611–617, Sep–Oct 1990.

Braga PC et al: Rheological profile of nesoteine: A new mucoactive agent. Int J Clin Pharmacol Res 9:77–83, 1989.

Cominiti SP and Young SL: The pulmonary surfactant system. Hosp Pract (Off Ed) 26:87–100, 1991.

Clarke SW: Rationale of airway clearance. Eur Respir J (Suppl) 7:599s–603s, 1989.

Corbet AJ et al: Reduced mortality in small premature infants treated at birth with a single dose of synthetic surfactant. J Paediatr Child Health 27:245–249, 1991.

Cott GR: Drug therapy in the management of cough. In Cherniak RM (ed): Drugs for the Respiratory System. Grune and Stratton, Orlando, 1986.

Dechant KL and Faulds D: Colfosceril palmitate: A review of the therapeutic efficacy and clinical tolerability of a synthetic surfactant preparation (Exosurf Neonatal) in neonatal respiratory distress syndrome. Drugs 42:877–894, 1991.

Deglin JH and Vallerand AH: Davis's Drug Guide for Nurses, ed 3. FA Davis, Philadelphia, 1993.

Des Jardins TR: Cardiopulmonary Anatomy and Physiology. Delmar Publishers, Albany, 1988.

Fiascone JM, Vreeland PN, and Frantz ID: Neonatal lung disease and respiratory care. In Burton GC, Hodgkin JE and Ward JJ (eds): Respiratory Care: A Guide to Clinical Practice, ed 3. JB Lippincott, Philadelphia, 1991.

Flanagan RJ and Meredith TJ: Use of *N*-acetylcysteine in clinical toxicology. Am J Med 91:131S–139S, 1991.

Hoekstra RE et al: Improved neonatal survival following multiple doses of bovine surfactant in very premature neonates at risk for respiratory distress syndrome. Pediatrics 88:10–18, 1991.

Howder CL: Cardiopulmonary Pharmacology: A Handbook for Respiratory Practitioners and Other Allied Health Personnel. Williams and Wilkins, Baltimore, 1992.

Jobe AH: The role of surfactant therapy in neonatal respiratory distress. Respiratory Care 36:695–704, 1991.

Johnson NT et al: Autoregulation of beat frequency in respiratory ciliated cells: Demonstration by viscous loading. Am Rev Respir Dis 144:1091–1094, 1991.

Johnson PA and Malinowski C: Respiratory distress syndrome in the newborn. In Wilkins RL and Dexter JR (eds): Respiratory Disease: Principles of Patient Care. FA Davis, Philadelphia, 1993.

Kakuta Y, Sasaki H, and Takishima T: Effect of artificial surfactant on ciliary beat frequency in guinea pig trachea. Respir Physiol 83:313–321, 1991.

Kamei J et al: Effects of *N*-methyl-D-aspartate antagonists on the cough reflex. Eur J Pharmacol 168:153–158, 1989.

Karlsson JA, Lanner AS, and Persson CG: Airway opioid receptors mediate inhibition of cough and reflex bronchoconstriction in guinea pigs. J Pharmacol Exp Ther 252:863–868, 1990.

Lehnert BE and Schachter EN: The Pharmacology of Respiratory Care. CV Mosby St Louis, 1980.

Lethem MI, James SL, and Marriot C: The role of mucous glycoproteins in the rheologic properties of cystic fibrosis sputum. Am Rev Respir Dis 142:1053–1058, 1990.

Levine D, Edwards DK and Merrit TA: Synthetic vs human surfactants in the treatment of respiratory distress syndrome: Radiographic findings. AJR Am J Roentgenol 157:371–374, 1991.

Lewis JF et al: Aerosolized surfactant treatment of preterm lambs. J Appl Physiol 70:869–876, 1991a.

Lewis JF et al: Nebulized vs instilled exogenous surfactant in an adult lung injury model. J Appl Physiol 71:1270–1276, 1991b.

Liechty EA et al: Reduction of neonatal mortality after multiple doses of bovine surfactant in low birth weight neonates with respiratory distress syndrome. Pediatrics 88:19–28, 1991.

Long W et al: Retrospective search for bleeding diathesis among premature newborn infants with pulmonary hemorrhage after synthetic surfactant treatment. The American Exosurf Neonatal Study Group I, and the Canadian Exosurf Neonatal Study Group. J Pediatr 120:S45–S48, 1992.

Long W et al: A controlled trial of synthetic surfactant in infants weighing 1250 g or more with respiratory distress syndrome. The American Exosurf Neonatal Study Group I, and the Canadian Exosurf Neonatal Study Group. N Engl J Med 325:1696–1703, 1991.

Marchioni CF et al: Effects of erdosteine on sputum biochemical and rheologic properties: Pharmacokinetics in chronic obstructive lung disease. Lung 168:285–293, 1990.

Majima Y et al: Effects of orally administered drugs on dynamic viscoelasticity of human nasal mucus. Am Rev Respir Dis 141:79–83, 1990.

Maunder RJ and Hudson LD: Pharmacologic strategies for treating the adult respiratory distress syndrome. Respiratory Care 35:241–246, 1990.

McCarty KD: Adult respiratory distress syndrome. In Wilkins RL and Dexter JR (eds): Respiratory Disease: Principles of Patient Care. FA Davis, Philadelphia, 1993.

Pedersen M: Ciliary activity and pollution. Lung 168 (Suppl):368–376, 1990.

Phibbs RH et al: Initial clinical trial of Exosurf, a protein-free synthetic surfactant, for the prophylaxis and early treatment of hyaline membrane disease. Pediatrics 88:1–9, 1991.

Rau JL: Respiratory Care Pharmacology, ed 3. Yearbook Medical Publishers, Chicago, 1989.

Smilkstein MJ et al: Acetaminophen overdose: A 48-hour intravenous *N*-acetylcysteine treatment protocol. Ann Emerg Med. 20:1058–63, Oct 1991.

Soll, RF et al: Multicenter trial of single-dose modified bovine surfactant extract (Survanta) for prevention of respiratory distress syndrome. Ross Collaborative Surfactant Prevention Study Group. Pediatrics. 85:1092–102, Jun 1990.

Stevenson, D et al: Controlled trial of a single dose of synthetic surfactant at birth in premature infants weighing 500 to 699 grams. The American Exosurf Neonatal Study Group I. J Pediatr 120:S3–S12, 1992.

Taylor AE et al: Clinical Respiratory Physiology. WB Saunders, Philadelphia, 1989.

Tortella FC, Pellicano M, and Bowery NG: Dextromethorphan and neuromodulation: Old drug coughs up new activities. Trends Pharmacol Sci 10:501–507, 1989.

Wellcome Medical Division: Exosurf NEONATAL (Colfosceril Palmitate for Suspension) Product Monograph. Burroughs Wellcome, Inc., Kirkland, QUÉ, 1991.

Whitsett JA, Hull WM, and Luse S: Failure to detect surfactant protein-specific antibodies in sera of premature infants treated with survanta, a modified bovine surfactant. Pediatrics 87:505–510, 1991.

Ziment I: History of the treatment of chronic bronchitis. Respiration 58 (Suppl 1):37–42, 1991.

Ziment I: Pharmacologic therapy of obstructive airway disease. Clin Chest Med 11:461–486, 1990.

CHAPTER 16

Antibacterials

CHAPTER OUTLINE

CHAPTER OBJECTIVES

After studying this chapter the reader should be able to:

- Define the following terms:
  - Pathogenic, nosocomial infection, epidemiology.
- Discuss respiratory tract infections in terms of:
  - Portal of entry, respiratory care procedures, host susceptibility, resistant microorganisms.
- Explain how differential staining techniques are used in the identification of microorganisms and name two such stains.
- Explain the difference between a bactericidal and a bacteriostatic mechanism of action.
- Describe the pharmacologic activity of the following antibacterials used to treat respiratory tract infections:
  - β-Lactams (penicillins, cephalosporins, monobactams, carbapenems), aminoglycosides, antituberculosis drugs, miscellaneous antibacterials, and sulfonamides.

KEY TERMS

antibiotic
antibiotic resistance
bactericidal
bacteriostatic

differential stain
epidemiology
eucaryote (yoo-**KARY**-ot)
nosocomial infection

pathogenic
penicillinase (a β-lactamase)
procaryote (prō-**KARY**-ot)

CHAPTER INTRODUCTION

In terms of sheer numbers, versatility, and reproductive potential, microorganisms dominate the planet. They are hardy, adaptable life forms that have the capability to overwhelm our best defenses. A classic example of this dynamic potential is the development of penicillin resistance in certain strains of bacteria, an adaptation that rendered the first antibiotic "wonder drug" virtually useless against certain microorganisms a few years after its introduction.

Antimicrobials are drugs administered to con-

220

trol populations of microorganisms. Other means of control exist, such as physical methods (heat and sterilization) and chemical methods (detergents and disinfectants), but the administration of antimicrobial drugs remains our most effective way of preventing and treating microbial disease. This chapter introduces the major antibacterial drugs with which the respiratory care practitioner comes into contact, and briefly examines those microorganisms that present an *airborne* threat to the body.

MEDICAL MICROBIOLOGY

Scope

Microorganisms as a group exhibit amazing adaptation qualities. They have been recovered from high-temperature sulfur springs and from bone-numbing glacial meltwater. Some thrive in deep-ocean trenches under extreme pressures, and others are found in lofty air currents above the earth. By contrast, the human environment presents a comparatively mild set of conditions for microbial invasion or colonization.

The study of the relationships between humankind and microbes is found in the field of medical microbiology. As can be seen in Table 16–1, some relationships are beneficial, whereas others are detrimental.

Microorganisms include fungi, bacteria, viruses, protozoa, and algae. Fortunately, a small fraction of the total microbial population is even capable of living in or on humans. More important, an even smaller percentage is potentially **pathogenic** to humans. Pathogenic microbes have the potential to overwhelm host defenses and produce the structural and functional changes we associate with disease. Unfortunately, this relatively small group of microbes is responsible for a great deal of human misery and suffering. Upsets range from minor stomach discomfort to worldwide influenza outbreaks to deadly plagues.

Microbiology and Respiratory Care

A discussion of the antimicrobial drugs and associated topics in the field of microbiology can easily exceed the scope of an introductory pharmacology textbook. The respiratory care practitioner, however, needs a fundamental understanding of microbiologic control methods and the antimicrobial drugs routinely used in pulmonary medicine.

Some potential pathogens are airborne microorganisms, capable of entering the body through the respiratory system. Aerosols containing microbes can be produced by coughs and sneezes and by mechanical nebulizers. Distribution in the respiratory tract largely depends on the size of the aerosol, although inspiratory flow and the nature of the particle play a role in determining the site of deposition. In general, the largest droplets deposit in the nasopharynx while the smallest impact in the alveoli.

Many common respiratory care techniques and equipment, such as endotracheal tubes, nebulizers, and tracheostomies, effectively bypass normal host defense mechanisms, which include mucociliary transport, coughing, and the unbroken skin. Once the first lines of defense have been bridged, microorganisms need only overcome cellular and humoral (antibody) defenses to establish an infection in the host.

Many respiratory patients are compromised in some way and have either reduced defenses or none at all. A timely example is the patient with AIDS (acquired immunodeficiency syndrome) who succumbs to an overwhelming respiratory infection. Increased susceptibility to infection may occur as a result of the respiratory care procedures discussed above, but it also occurs in response to pathophysiologic conditions that impair basic defense mechanisms. For example, an ineffective cough, as occurs in cases of emphysema, does not adequately clear tracheobronchial secretions. In addition, patients maintained on immunosuppressive drugs, such as the corticosteroids, are unable to mount an effective

TABLE 16–1 MICROBIAL RELATIONSHIPS

Relationship	Effect on Microorganism	Effect on Host
Commensalism*	Beneficial	None
Mutualism*	Beneficial	Beneficial
Parasitism†	Beneficial	Detrimental

*Opportunistic microbes such as mutuals or commensals may cause infection in a susceptible host.
†Caused by pathogenic microbes (microbes capable of overwhelming host defenses and establishing an infection).

antibody defense in response to microbial invasion. Clearly, persons with bypassed, ineffective, or suppressed defenses are at greater risk for infection than most.

Resistant Microorganisms

Some microorganisms are resistant to commonly employed antimicrobial drugs such as the **antibiotics** (*antibiosis*—against life). An antibiotic, in the classic definition, is a substance of microbial origin that in small amounts has the ability to suppress the growth of other microbes. Because some drugs used to control microorganisms are of synthetic origin, the terms *antimicrobial* and *anti-infective* agent are more inclusive than *antibiotic.*

Continuous low-level exposure to an adverse condition, such as the widespread use of antibiotics in a hospital, may encourage the development of very small numbers of mutant microorganisms. These surviving microbes exhibit **antibiotic resistance** and some are able to pass that survival capability on when reproducing. In general, antibiotic resistance is directly proportional to indiscriminate use of the antibiotic. Strains that possess antibiotic resistance are more virulent. In other words, they have a greater potential to establish infection because they are inherently more difficult to treat.

Some patients admitted to a hospital develop a pulmonary infection that they did not have prior to admission. These occurrences are called **nosocomial infections** (Greek *nosos*—disease—

and *komeion*—to care for; pertaining to a hospital). **Epidemiology** is the study of common causes of disease and health. Epidemiologic or infection control studies in a hospital can implicate a respiratory care procedure such as an aerosol treatment, an item of equipment such as a nebulizer, an individual practitioner, or an entire department. The easy accessibility of the respiratory tract and invasive nature of many respiratory care procedures permit airborne microbial invasion. When this infective potential is combined with the vulnerability of compromised respiratory patients and the virulence of some respiratory pathogens, a basic understanding of microbiologic topics becomes a necessity for the respiratory care practitioner. Table 16–2 summarizes the airborne bacteria causing upper respiratory infections; those causing lower respiratory infections are summarized in Table 16–3.

AIRBORNE BACTERIAL INFECTIONS

Bacterial Characteristics

Bacteria belong to a relatively primitive group of cells known as the **procaryotes.** Procaryotic cells differ substantially from more complex **eucaryotes,** such as human cells (Table 16–4). Differences in cellular complexity have an important bearing on the mechanism of action of many antimicrobial drugs. For example, the antimicrobial activity of the penicillins is directed against

TABLE 16–2 AIRBORNE BACTERIA CAUSING UPPER RESPIRATORY INFECTIONS (URI)

Causative Agent	Disease	Antibacterial	Comments
Streptococcus pyogenes (strep-tō-**KA**-kus pī-**OJ**-i-nēs)	Pharyngitis Pneumonia Pleuritis	Penicillin Benzyl penicillin Penicillin V Erythromycin	Bacteriostatic drugs such as sulfonamides and tetracyclines are not used Poststreptococcal complications include rheumatic fever and glomerulonephritis
Bordetella pertussis (bōrd-i-**TEL**-a per-**TUS**-sis)	Pertussis (whooping cough)	Erythromycin (Chloramphenicol and tetracyclines have been used)	Catarrhal, spasmodic, and convalescent stages Prophylactic immunization in childhood (DPTP vaccine)
Corynebacterium diphtheriae (kō-**RĪ**-nē-bak-**TEER**-ē-um dif-**THEER**-ē-ī)	Diphtheria Acute pharyngitis	Penicillin Erythromycin (with diphtheria antitoxin)	Fibrous pseudomembrane develops in response to exotoxin; may occlude trachea Prophylactic immunization in childhood (DPTP vaccine)
Haemophilus influenzae (hē-**MOF**-i-lus in-flū-**IN**-zī)	Acute bacterial meningitis Acute epiglottitis in children	Chloramphenicol Penicillin Streptomycin Tetracycline Erythromycin	Chloramphenicol readily crosses the blood-brain barrier

DPTP—diphtheria, pertussis, tetanus, poliomyelitis.

TABLE 16-3 AIRBORNE BACTERIA CAUSING LOWER RESPIRATORY INFECTIONS (LRI)

Causative Agent	Disease	Antibacterial	Comments
Mycoplasma pneumoniae (mī-kō-**PLAZ**-ma nyoo-**MŌN**-ē-ī)	Bronchitis Primary atypical pneumonia	Streptomycin Erythromycin Tetracyclines	Very small, cell wall deficient Transmission in crowded conditions Pneumonia debilitating but rarely fatal
Legionella pneumophila (lē-ja-**NEL**-a nyoo-mō-**FĒL**-ya)	Legionellosis (Legionnaires' disease)	Erythromycin	Multiplication within alveolar macrophages Transmission through inhalation of aerosol containing a high density of microbes
Streptococcus pneumoniae (strep-tō-**KA**-kus nyoo-**MŌN**-ē-ī)	Bronchitis Pneumococcal pneumonia	Penicillin Tetracyclines Ampicillin and/or co-trimoxazole	Originally known as the "pneumococcus" or "diplococcus" Lobar pneumonia common in the elderly population Healthy asymptomatic carriers harbor microbes in upper respiratory tract and can spread infection
Staphylococcus aureus (staf-i-lō-**KA**-kus **OR**-ē-us)	Suppurative infections (bronchopneumonia, necrotizing pneumonia)	Benzyl penicillin (many strains are resistant) Modified penicillins (eg, cloxacillin) Cephalosporins Clindamycin Gentamicin	Virulent hospital strains carried in the nasopharynx Penicillinase-producing strains are prevalent Methicillin-resistant strains are emerging
Klebsiella pneumoniae (kleb-sē-**EL**-a nyoo-**MŌN**-ē-ī)	Friedländer's pneumonia (a rare form of lobar pneumonia)	Newer aminoglycosides (gentamicin, tobramycin, amikacin)	Low incidence, high mortality Serious Gram-negative infection Asymptomatic nasal carriers Alcoholic, elderly, or debilitated persons at highest risk Antibiotic-resistant strains are prevalent
Haemophilus influenzae (hē-**MOF**-i-lus in-flū-**IN**-zī)	Bacterial pneumonia Chronic bronchitis	Most commonly administered antibacterials ampicillin	Secondary invader in influenza outbreaks
Pseudomonas aeruginosa (syoo-dō-**MŌN**-as a-rūj-i-**NŌ**-sa)	Pneumonia (especially in lungs of children with cystic fibrosis)	Carbenicillin Aztreonam Gentamicin Tobramycin	Resistant to most commonly administered antibiotics Opportunistic gram-negative microorganisms
Mycobacterium tuberculosis (mī-kō-bak-**TEER**-ē-um too-ber-kyoo-**LŌ**-sis)	Tuberculosis	Combination therapy (see Table 16–9)	*M. bovis* from infected beef or milk may cause tuberculosis HIV infection contributes to increased risk for tuberculosis *M. avium-intracellulare* complex of microorganisms may invade in late stages of HIV infection
Neisseria meningitidis (nī-**SEER**-ē-a men-in-**JI**-ti-dis)	Acute bacterial meningitis (adults)	Penicillin (benzyl penicillin or ampicillin) Sulfonamides (rapidly cross the blood-brain barrier) Erythromycin or chloramphenicol in penicillin-sensitive patients	Airborne transmission; no respiratory disease Spreads from nasopharynx to cranial meninges

TABLE 16-3 AIRBORNE BACTERIA CAUSING LOWER RESPIRATORY INFECTIONS (LRI)
(Continued)

Causative Agent	Disease	Antibacterial	Comments
Chlamydia psittaci (kla-**MID**-ē-a si-**TAS**-ē)	Psittacosis (ornithosis)	Tetracyclines	Very small, obligate, parasitic, intracellular bacteria Inhalation of dried particles from caged birds (parakeets, parrots, turkeys)
Chlamydia pneumoniae (kla-**MID**-ē-a nyoo-**MŌN**-ē-ī)	Chlamydial pneumonia (similar to mycoplasma pneumonia)	Tetracyclines	Acute, mild, relatively common respiratory illness
Coxiella burnetii (**KOK**-sē-el-a bur-**NET**-ē-ē)	Q fever (a type of pneumonia)	Tetracyclines	"Q" (query) originally referred to the unknown cause of the infection Causative organism is a rickettsia microorganism (similar to chlamydia) Transmission: cattle tick to dairy herd to humans (via aerosols or unpasteurized milk) Endemic in Western US

HIV—human immunodeficiency virus.

the cell wall of procaryotic bacteria. As a result, direct toxicity to eucaryotic host cells is minimal because human cells lack cell walls. Drugs such as these are called **bactericidal** because their mechanism of action results in death of susceptible bacteria. **Bacteriostatic** drugs, such as the sulfonamides, suppress bacterial growth and allow host defenses to clear the bacteria from the body.

Differential Staining

Inoculation of microorganisms on suitable growth media and incubation of media under appropriate conditions are routinely carried out by microbiology laboratories. Microorganisms in a mixed sample may be detected by a characteristic staining reaction when treated with colored dyes. Microorganisms can be separated into several broad categories on the basis of such differential reactions.

The most widely employed **differential stain** technique is called Gram's stain. Microorganisms designated gram-positive exhibit an affinity for the primary stain used in the procedure, reject the counterstain, and remain a purplish color. Gram-negative microorganisms fail to retain the purple stain but show an affinity for a pinkish-red counterstain used in the process.

A differential stain especially useful for spu-

TABLE 16-4 COMPARISON OF PROCARYOTIC AND EUCARYOTIC CELLS AND VIRUSES

Characteristic	Procaryotic Cells	Eucaryotic Cells	Viruses
Nucleic acids*	+	+	+
Chromosomes	+	+	−
True nucleus	−	+	−
Mitosis	−	+	−
Independent metabolic processes†	+	+	−
Ribosomes‡	+	+	−
Enzymes	+	+	−
Cell wall§	+	+	−

+—found; −—not found.
*Viruses possess either DNA or RNA; procaryotic and eucaryotic cells possess both nucleic acids.
†Viruses are obligate parasites; that is, they require a host cell for survival.
‡Procaryotic and eucaryotic ribosomes differ structurally (see Box 16-2).
§Most procaryotic cells have cell walls; some eucaryotic cells (eg, plants) possess a cell wall, but it differs structurally from that of procaryotic cells.

tum samples suspected of harboring the etiologic (causative) agent of tuberculosis is the acid-fast stain (or Ziehl-Neelsen stain). In this technique, the microbes are first colored with a red dye and then treated with an acid-alcohol wash. If the organisms resist the acid decolorizing step and retain the pinkish-red stain, they are said to be acid resistant, or acid fast. Organisms designated non–acid fast are decolorized and lose their pink color. The significance of the reaction is that the *Mycobacterium* genus, which includes the etiologic agent of tuberculosis (*M. tuberculosis*), is distinctly acid fast. Although the reaction is not a positive indication of active tuberculosis, it is a means of rapidly screening a number of suspected samples. Culturing of samples, additional laboratory tests, and chest radiographs are used for a positive identification. The reader is encouraged to consult general microbiology texts listed in the chapter bibliography if additional information is sought concerning microbiologic staining procedures.

ANTIBACTERIAL AGENTS

β-Lactams

There are more similarities than differences among members of the β-lactam group of antibiotics. The classic antibiotics, such as penicillins and cephalosporins, and the newer, nonclassic β-lactams, such as monobactams and carbapenems, share a common structural configuration and exhibit similar bactericidal mechanisms of action.

Penicillins

The bactericidal activity of penicillin resides in the β-lactam ring structure of the parent molecule. Treatment with amidase enzyme causes side chains to be split off naturally occurring penicillins to produce a nucleus called 6-APA (6-aminopenicillanic acid). Semisynthetic penicillins are produced by attaching different side chains to the 6-APA molecule (Fig. 16–1). This effort has brought us a whole family of penicillins. Some have longer durations of action, others exhibit a wider spectrum of activity, and still others possess penicillinase resistance. **Penicillinase** is a β-lactamase enzyme that inactivates benzyl penicillin (see Fig. 16–1).

The mechanism of action of the penicillins is very specific because it is directed at a unique structure—the bacterial cell wall. Penicillin inhibits a transpeptidase enzyme, resulting in impairment of cell wall synthesis in young, actively growing cultures of susceptible bacteria. The en-

6-Aminopenicillanic acid (6-APA) nucleus

FIGURE 16–1 Site of amidase and β-lactamase activity.

zyme is needed to properly cross-link and strengthen a structural carbohydrate called peptidoglycan. Peptidoglycan content is higher in gram-positive than in gram-negative bacteria (50% vs 10%); therefore, the "original" natural penicillin (benzylpenicillin below) is most effective against gram-positive bacteria. With a weakened cell wall, the bacterium is highly susceptible to osmotic pressure gradients. This allows osmotic damage to ultimately lyse the cell and produce a bactericidal effect. In addition, normal host cellular defenses are able to clear the weakened bacterial cells from the body.

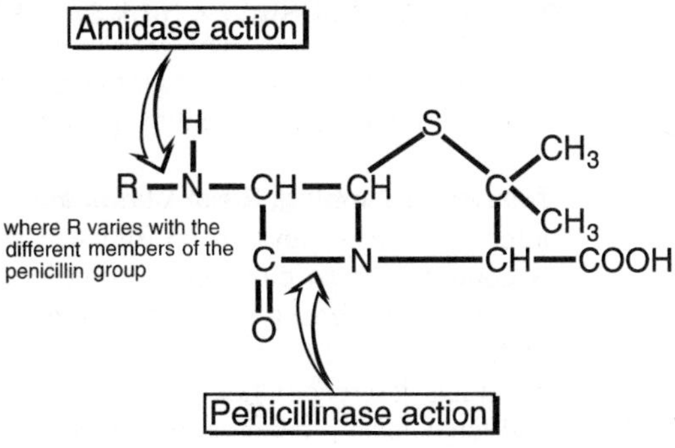

Natural Penicillins

BENZYL PENICILLIN (PENICILLIN G) (Many Manufacturers). Penicillin G or benzyl penicillin (available as a sodium or potassium salt), is the original penicillin that revolutionized medicine half a century ago (Box 16–1). It is the only naturally occurring penicillin still in use and is currently extracted from *Penicillium chrysogenum* rather than from the original *P. notatum* mold. Benzyl penicillin is still used today against a variety of infections, but it possesses several shortcomings. Disadvantages of so-called simple penicillin include a short duration of action (half-life approximately 90 minutes), lack of acid stability (unsuitable for oral administration), penicillinase susceptibility, and a relatively narrow spectrum of activity (it is effective against some of the cocci). Successive modifications of the basic drug structure over the years have minimized each of these weaknesses and resulted in the development of a versatile family of penicillin derivatives, a few of which are discussed below.

INDICATIONS. Benzyl penicillin is indicated in

BOX 16–1 USHERING IN A NEW ERA: PENICILLIN

Some of the most fascinating stories in the history of pharmacotherapeutics are associated with the development of antimicrobial drugs in the decade 1935–1945.

Alexander Fleming, Ernst Chain, and Howard Florey

Intense effort to develop an effective antibiotic with which to treat casualties of the Second World War culminated in the development of commercially available penicillin. Sir Alexander Fleming's original observations in 1928 regarding the antibacterial activity of the mold *Penicillium notatum,* and identification of the substance he named *penicillin,* eventually led researchers Ernst Chain and Howard Florey to the extraction, purification, and large-scale production of penicillin. Penicillin was the miracle drug that ushered in the modern antibiotic age beginning in 1940. Fleming, Florey, and Chain received the Nobel Prize for Medicine or Physiology in 1945 for their pioneering work.

Berquist LM: Microbiology for the Hospital Environment. Harper and Row, New York, 1981.
Jawetz E: Penicillins and Cephalosporins. In Katzung BD (ed): Basic and Clinical Pharmacology. Lange Medical Publications, Los Altos, 1982.
Jensen MM and Wright DN: Introduction to Microbiology for the Health Sciences. Prentice-Hall, Englewood Cliffs, NJ, 1989.
Tortora GJ, Funke BR, and Case CL: Microbiology: An Introduction. Benjamin/Cummings, Redwood City, CA, 1992.

the treatment of infections caused by nonpenicillinase-producing *Staphylococcus aureus,* and of infections caused by *Streptococcus pyogenes, Strep. pneumoniae, Corynebacterium diphtheriae,* and *Neisseria meningitidis.*

CONTRAINDICATIONS. Penicillin antibiotics are contraindicated in persons with known hypersensitivity to the drug.

ADVERSE REACTIONS. Because of the nature of the mechanism of action of the penicillins, direct toxicity to mammalian cells is virtually nonexistent. Intramuscular or intravenous injections of high concentrations, however, can cause direct tissue irritation. Hapten formation can occur and penicillin drug allergies exist in about 5%–10% of the population (see Fig. 9–1). Allergic responses range in severity from skin rash, pruritus, and fever to bronchoconstriction and anaphylactic shock.

Note: The indications, contraindications, precautions, and adverse reactions for the following penicillins are the same as those described for benzyl penicillin unless stated otherwise.

PROCAINE PENICILLIN G (Duracillin). The short duration of action of simple penicillin was improved with the addition of *procaine* to the penicillin nucleus. Procaine penicillin G, like benzyl penicillin, is classified as a natural penicillin. It is absorbed at a slower rate, with the blood plasma acting as a storage depot to result in a prolonged duration of action. Renal excretion is still rapid, but tissue levels remain higher for a longer period compared with benzyl penicillin.

PHENOXYMETHYL PENICILLIN (PENICILLIN V) (Pen-Vee). Addition of phenoxyacetic acid to the penicillin growth medium results in the production of an acid-stable, orally active natural penicillin known as penicillin.

INDICATIONS. The indications for use are similar to those described for *benzyl penicillin.* However, *Neisseria meningitidis* is not sensitive.

Penicillinase-Resistant Penicillins

METHICILLIN SODIUM (Staphcillin). The ability of some microorganisms, especially certain strains of *Staphylococcus aureus,* to produce the enzyme β-lactamase enables them to disrupt the β-lactam ring and inactivate simple penicillin. The value of benzyl penicillin in treating suppurative infections caused by the staphylococci is greatly reduced because of this bacterial enzyme. Addition of other *Penicillium* species to the growth medium results in the production of methicillin sodium, a penicillinase-resistant penicillin. Similar penicillinase-resistant derivatives include cloxacillin (Cloxapen), nafcillin sodium (Nafcil), oxacillin (Bactocill), and dicloxacillin (Dynapen).

INDICATIONS. The penicillinase-resistant penicillins are effective against *Streptococcus* and *Staphylococcus* species, including penicillinase-producing strains of *Staphylococcus aureus.*

TABLE 16–5 ANTIMICROBIAL ACTIVITY OF PENICILLINS

Respiratory Infection	Benzyl Penicillin	Procaine Penicillin G	Phenoxymethyl Penicillin	Penicillinase-Resistant Penicillins*	Broad-Spectrum Penicillins†
Streptococcus pyogenes	+	+	+		
Streptococcus pneumoniae	+	+	+		
Streptococcus sp				+	+
Nonpenicillinase Staphylococcus aureus	+	+	+		
Staphylococcus sp				+	+
Corynebacterium diphtheriae	+	+	+		
Neisseria meningitidis	+	+			+
Haemophilus influenzae					+
Escherichia coli					+
Proteus sp					+
Salmonella sp					+
Pseudomonas sp					+
Some protozoa					+

+—antimicrobial activity.
*methicillin, cloxacillin, nafcillin, oxacillin, dicloxacillin
†ampicillin, amoxicillin, carbenicillin, ticarcillin, mezlocillin, piperacillin

Broad-Spectrum Penicillins

AMPICILLIN (Penbritin, Polycillin). In the mid-1960s, the spectrum of activity of simple penicillin was greatly expanded through modification of the penicillin side chains. The result was a broad-spectrum, orally active derivative known as ampicillin. Other broad-spectrum penicillins include amoxicillin (Amoxil), carbenicillin (Geopen), ticarcillin (Ticar), mezlocillin (Mezlin), and piperacillin (Pipracil).

INDICATIONS. Ampicillin and related extended-spectrum penicillins are effective against a few protozoa, the gram-positive cocci (*Streptococcus* and *Staphylococcus* sp), gram-negative pathogens, such as *Neisseria meningitidis* and *Haemophilus influenzae,* and other important gram-negative bacteria, such as *Escherichia coli, Proteus* species, and *Salmonella* species. Carbenicillin and ticarcillin are especially active against *Pseudomonas* infections.

Consult Table 16–5 for a summary of the antimicrobial activity of the penicillins.

Cephalosporins

Like the penicillins, the cephalosporins are classified as β-lactam antibiotics. They are semisynthetic derivatives of the mold *Cephalosporium acremonium.* Cephalosporins possess a nucleus (similar to 6-APA of penicillin), a β-lactam ring, and different side chains, which confer different antibiotic properties on the various derivatives.

The mechanism of action of the cephalosporins is bactericidal, with inhibition of bacterial cell wall synthesis and resulting osmotic stress to susceptible bacteria. The mechanism is especially effective in actively growing populations of sensitive bacteria because the cells are continually laying down new cell walls.

The spectrum of activity of the cephalosporins is directed against mild to severe infections caused by both gram-positive and gram-negative organisms. Originally, a marketing concept of "first-generation," "second-generation," and "third-generation" cephalosporins was promoted, but now the classifications pertain more to the spectrum of activity of the various cephalosporin derivatives (Fig. 16–2). As a general trend, in discussing the cephalosporins from first- to second- to third-generation drugs, there is increasing effectiveness against gram-negative microbes and decreasing effectiveness against gram-positive organisms.

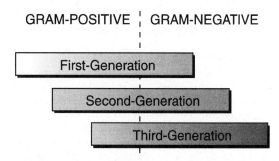

FIGURE 16–2 Spectrum of activity—cephalosporin generations.

TABLE 16–6 ANTIMICROBIAL ACTIVITY OF CEPHALOSPORINS

Respiratory Infection	First-Generation (eg, cephalothin)	Second-Generation (eg, cefaclor)	Third-Generation (eg, cefotaxime)
Streptococcus pneumoniae	+	+	(minimal)
Streptococcus pyogenes		+	(minimal)
Group A β-hemolytic streptococci	+	+	(minimal)
Staphylococcus aureus	+	+	(minimal)
Staphylococcus sp	+	+	(minimal)
Klebsiella sp	+	+	+
Haemophilus influenzae	+	+	+
Neisseria meningitidis			+
Pseudomonas aeruginosa			+

+—antimicrobial activity.

Discussion of individual pharmacologic features of the staggering number of cephalosporin derivatives is beyond the scope of this chapter. No single cephalosporin adequately serves as a prototype drug because bacterial sensitivity to individual cephalosporin drugs varies. Instead, a representative sample from each cephalosporin generation is presented.

First-Generation Cephalosporins

CEPHALOTHIN (Keflin). A first-generation cephalosporin, such as cephalothin, has a relatively narrow spectrum of activity and is effective mainly against gram-positive organisms and very few gram-negative species.

INDICATIONS. Infections of the genitourinary tract, bones, and joints are often treated with the cephalosporins. The respiratory pathogens responding to first-generation cephalosporins include *Streptococcus pneumoniae,* group A β-hemolytic streptococci, *Staphylococcus aureus,* other staphylococci, *Klebsiella* species, and *Haemophilus influenzae.*

CONTRAINDICATIONS. Known hypersensitivity to the cephalosporins is a contraindication to use.

ADVERSE REACTIONS. Hypersensitivity reactions are similar to those described for the penicillins. In addition, nausea, cramps, headache, and dizziness are occasionally observed.

Second-Generation Cephalosporins

CEFACLOR (Ceclor). Second-generation cephalosporins, such as cefaclor, are active against a variety of gram-negative organisms compared with the first-generation drugs.

INDICATIONS. The spectrum of activity includes the respiratory pathogens listed above for first-generation cephalosporins, and acitivity against *Streptococcus pyogenes,* which causes streptococcal pharyngitis and pneumonia.

CONTRAINDICATIONS AND ADVERSE REACTIONS. See Cephalothin.

Third-Generation Cephalosporins

CEFOTAXIME (Claforan). Third-generation cephalosporins, exemplified by cefotaxime, are more broad spectrum than the other cephalosporin classifications. They are effective against even more gram-negative microbes and a few anerobes, but less effective against the gram-positive cocci.

INDICATIONS. Activity against gram-positive *Streptococcus* and *Staphylococcus* species is minimal, but the drugs are effective against infections caused by *Neisseria meningitidis, Haemophilus influenzae, Klebsiella* species, and *Pseudomonas aeruginosa.*

CONTRAINDICATIONS AND ADVERSE REACTIONS. See Cephalothin.

Table 16–6 summarizes the antimicrobial activity of the cephalosporins.

Monobactams

The monobactams of medical importance are synthetic compounds, although some naturally occurring monobactams are produced by certain soil bacteria. Antibiotics such as aztreonam (Azactam) have a single β-lactam ring structure that resists the enzymatic action of β-lactamase in gram-negative organisms. The drug has an antimicrobial spectrum of activity similar to that of gentamicin and tobramycin but lacks the nephrotoxicity common with the aminoglycosides (see below). Monobactams are active against gram-negative organisms and are especially useful in *Pseudomonas* infections, but are inactive against the gram-positive microbes.

Carbapenems

Carbapenems, such as imipenem, exhibit an extremely broad spectrum of activity against most

(98%) of the gram-negative and gram-positive organisms recovered from hospital patients. Primaxin consists of the β-lactamase–resistant antibiotic imipenem and cilastatin, a drug that inhibits renal metabolism of the antibiotic.

Table 16–7 summarizes the antimicrobial activity of the newer nonclassic β-lactam drugs such as the monobactams and carbapenems.

Aminoglycosides

Streptomycin is the prototype aminoglycoside and is derived by the fermentation of *Streptomyces griseus,* one of the members of the *Actinomycetes* group of soil organisms. With the exception of the versatile penicillins and a handful of drugs produced by the *Bacillus* genus of bacteria, most of the antibiotics in use today are derivatives of the *Streptomyces* genus, an otherwise unremarkable group of free-living soil microbes.

The aminoglycosides inhibit protein synthesis in susceptible bacteria by combining with bacterial ribosomes and causing misreading of messenger RNA. The result is the production of nonfunctional proteins. Human host cells are far less susceptible because they have a slightly different type of ribosome. Mammalian ribosomes associated with mitochondria, however, are similar to the bacterial variety and can be adversely affected by certain antibiotics that interfere with bacterial ribosomes (Box 16–2). The ribosomal interference exhibited by the aminoglycosides is bactericidal, whereas other inhibitors of protein synthesis, such as erythromycin and chloramphenicol, produce a bacteriostatic action at normal concentrations (Box 16–2).

Interference with eucaryotic cell metabolism by the aminoglycosides may produce relatively serious toxicity problems, such as VIII cranial nerve (acoustic or vestibulocochlear nerve) neuritis. This ototoxicity in turn results in hearing and balance dysfunction. In addition, the development of nephrotoxicity may result in proteinuria. Finally, neuromuscular blockade caused by the aminoglycosides may potentiate the action of nondepolarizing blockers, such as pancuronium. The resulting skeletal muscle relaxation can depress ventilation by decreasing diaphragmatic function.

STREPTOMYCIN. Streptomycin is the prototype drug of the aminoglycoside family of antibiotics. It is a broad-spectrum antibiotic used in a variety of respiratory infections and in severe, complicated gram-negative infections of other body systems. As a general rule, the aminoglycosides are not used for trivial infections that are treatable with less toxic antibiotics.

INDICATIONS. Streptomycin is used in combination with other antituberculosis drugs to treat *Mycobacterium tuberculosis* infections. It is also used to combat infections caused by *Streptococcus* species, *Haemophilus influenzae,* and *Klebsiella* species.

CONTRAINDICATIONS. Known hypersensitivity to the aminoglycosides is a contraindication to their use.

Note: Indications, contraindications, precautions, and adverse reactions for the following aminoglycosides are the same as those described for streptomycin unless stated otherwise.

GENTAMICIN (Garamycin). Gentamicin is structurally similar to but produces less ototoxicity than streptomycin. The derivative is especially useful in severe gram-negative infections but is not a drug of first choice if less toxic antibiotics produce the desired control.

INDICATIONS. Gentamicin is used to treat infections caused by *Klebsiella* species, *Pseudomonas aeruginosa,* and *Staphylococcus* species. The drug exhibits synergistic action and is effective in antipseudomonal therapy when combined with the carbenicillin-ticarcillin group of penicillins.

KANAMYCIN (Kantrex). The general pharmacologic activity described for the aminoglycosides applies to kanamycin. It is occasionally aerosolized for the treatment of respiratory infections.

INDICATIONS. The spectrum of activity of kana-

TABLE 16–7 ANTIMICROBIAL ACTIVITY OF NEWER β-LACTAMS

Respiratory Infections	Monobactams (eg, aztreonam)	Carbapenems (eg, imipenem*)
Staphylococcus sp	+	+
Staphylococcus aureus	+	+
Klebsiella sp	+	+
Pseudomonas aeruginosa	+	+

+—antimicrobial activity.

*Effective against most (98%) of the gram-positive and gram-negative microorganisms recovered from patients in a hospital.

BOX 16–2 RIBOSOMES: SUBTLE DIFFERENCES

The aminoglycosides inhibit protein synthesis in susceptible bacteria by combining with bacterial ribosomes at the 30S subunit of the 70S ribosome and causing misreading of messenger RNA. This effect in turn results in production of nonfunctional proteins. Human host cells are far less susceptible to this action because they have a slightly different type of cytoplasmic ribosome, designated an 80S ribosome. Such ribosomes do not possess the 30S subunit common to procaryotic cells and are not as sensitive to antibiotic effects directed against the 30S subunit (see figure). Mammalian ribosomes

Eucaryotic Ribosome

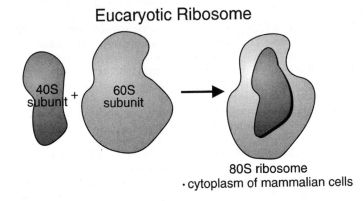

Procaryotic Ribosome

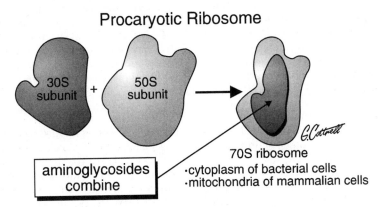

associated with mitochondria, however, are of the 70S variety and can be adversely affected by certain antibiotics that interfere with the 70S bacterial ribosomes. (Note: *S* is the symbol for *Svedberg* units, a measurement of the relative sedimentation rate in ultra–high-speed centrifugation. Sedimentation of a particle is affected by characteristics such as size, shape, and mass.)

Tortora GJ, Funke BR, and Case CL: Microbiology: An Introduction. Benjamin/Cummings, Redwood City, CA, 1992.

mycin includes treatment of infections caused by *Haemophilus influenzae, Klebsiella* species, and *Staphylococcus aureus.*

Newer Aminoglycosides

Several newer aminoglycosides have been developed and are important because antibiotic resistance is not yet widespread. In addition, they are effective against *Staphylococcus* and *Pseudomonas* species of bacteria. A semisynthetic derivative of kanamycin known as amikacin (Amikin) is resistant to metabolic inactivation. Some strains of bacteria, such as *Staphylococcus, Pseudomonas,* and *Klebsiella* species, that resist the earlier aminoglycosides may respond to amikacin. Tobramycin (Nebcin) is similar to gentamicin but exhibits less nephrotoxicity and greater activity against *Pseudomonas* species. In addition, it is active against *Klebsiella* and *Staphylococcus* species, including *S. aureus.* One of the new additions to the growing aminoglycoside family is netilmicin (Netromycin). Less bacterial resistance is seen and the drug exhibits less auditory and renal impairment than the other aminoglycosides. Antibacterial activity is directed against *Pseudomonas, Staphylococcus,* and *Neisseria* species.

For a review of the spectrum of activity of the more commonly used aminoglycosides, consult Table 16–8.

Antituberculosis Drugs

Antitubercular therapy is unique in that it is of long duration, typically 9 months or more. The lengthy therapy is necessary for the drugs to penetrate the poorly perfused tubercles. Tubercles are small nodulelike structures produced by body cells in response to the bacterium. Tubercles may grow in size to become draining abscesses that can spread the bacteria. The prolonged drug therapy necessary in tuberculosis treatment requires the use of drugs having the fewest toxic effects.

Rapid development of antibiotic resistance is another feature of tuberculosis infections. For this reason, typical drug therapy involves concurrent administration of two or more antituberculosis drugs. Multiple drug combinations minimize the development of antibiotic resistance in the mycobacteria.

The risk for tuberculosis increases with HIV (human immunodeficiency virus) infections. This increase is due to a compromised immune system, which increases host susceptibility to most opportunistic infections, including bacterial, fungal, and protozoal invaders. In addition,

multidrug-resistant tuberculosis is emerging. Some strains are resistant to all frontline antitubercular drugs and to many second- and third-line agents. Combination therapy with as many as three or four different drugs provides some control. Related mycobacteria such as *Mycobacterium avium-intracellulare,* also known as the *M. avium* complex, may invade persons in late stages of HIV infections. These opportunists also exhibit multidrug resistance and are very difficult to treat.

STREPTOMYCIN. Streptomycin, the drug that revolutionized the treatment of tuberculosis, has already been discussed in regard to the aminoglycosides. Compared with the currently used antitubercular drugs, streptomycin is of lesser benefit, but is still combined with several of these drugs to produce effective control of *Mycobacterium tuberculosis* walled off within tubercles in the lungs (Box 16–3). The mechanism of action involves bactericidal ribosomal interference to cause production of nonfunctional proteins in the target cells (Box 16–3).

INDICATIONS. The primary indication for use is in the treatment of tuberculosis infections.

CONTRAINDICATIONS. Known hypersensitivity is a contraindication to use of the drug.

PRECAUTIONS AND ADVERSE REACTIONS. Renal damage and serious neuritis involving the eighth cranial nerve can occur with streptomycin therapy (see ''Aminoglycosides'').

Note: Indications, contraindications, precautions, and adverse reactions for the following antituberculosis drugs are the same as those described for streptomycin unless stated otherwise.

ISONIAZID (Nydrazid[US], Isotamine[CAN]). The mechanism of action of isoniazid (isonicotinic acid hydrazide, or INH) involves inhibition of cell wall synthesis in the mycobacteria. The mechanism is one of competitive inhibition but is not fully understood. Isoniazid is most effective against actively growing mycobacterial pop-

TABLE 16–8 ANTIMICROBIAL ACTIVITY OF AMINOGLYCOSIDES

Respiratory Tract Infection	Streptomycin	Gentamicin	Kanamycin	Amikacin	Tobramycin	Netilmicin
Streptococcus sp	+					
Staphylococcus sp		+		+	+	+
Staphylococcus aureus			+		+	
Haemophilus influenzae	+		+			
Klebsiella sp	+	+	+	+	+	
Pseudomonas aeruginosa		+		+	+	+
Neisseria sp						+
Mycobacterium tuberculosis	+					

+—antimicrobial activity.

BOX 16-3 TAMING THE WHITE PLAGUE: STREPTOMYCIN

Albert Schatz and Selman Waksman

In 1944, streptomycin became available as a revolutionary new antibiotic belonging to the aminoglycosides, a group of compounds having a complex chemical configuration of connected amino sugars. Streptomycin quickly gained "wonder drug" status because of its ability to control *Mycobacterium tuberculosis* infections. The suffering alleviated by this single drug has been truly incalculable since its debut. In the early 1940s, Albert Schatz was working with tubercle bacilli samples and screening strains of *Streptomyces* for possible antibiotic activity against the tuberculosis organism. *Streptomyces* belongs to the *Actinomycetes*, a group of filamentous bacteria that live in the soil. One strain was found to produce an effective, natural antibiotic called streptomycin. After appropriate clinical trials, development and commercial production of the drug began. Selman Waksman received the Nobel Prize for Medicine or Physiology in 1952 for his role in the development and production of the world's first effective antitubercular drug.

Berquist LM: Microbiology for the Hospital Environment. Harper and Row, New York, 1981.
Jawetz E: Aminoglycosides and Polymyxins. In Katzung BD (ed): Basic and Clinical Pharmacology. Lange Medical Publications, Los Altos, 1982.
Jensen MM and Wright DN: Introduction to Microbiology for the Health Sciences. Prentice-Hall, Englewood Cliffs, NJ, 1989.
Ryan F: The Forgotten Plague: How the Battle Against Tuberculosis Was Won and Lost. Little, Brown, New York, 1993.
Scott F: Streptomycin: A magic bullet that tamed TB. Advance for Respiratory Care Practitioners:6–7, 1993.
Tortora GJ, Funke BR, and Case CL: Microbiology: An Introduction. Benjamin/Cummings, Redwood City, CA, 1992.

ulations. It is a synthetic chemotherapeutic agent normally administered with one or two other antitubercular drugs.

INDICATIONS. Isoniazid has very little activity against nonmycobacteria and is classified as a primary drug (along with rifampin) in antitubercular therapy. Secondary drugs are generally less effective and more toxic, but are often included in dosage regimens to reduce the development of antibiotic resistance.

PRECAUTIONS AND ADVERSE REACTIONS. Some individuals inactivate isoniazid very slowly; therefore, dosages must be tailored to the individual. Neurotoxicity may include headaches or convulsions. In addition, hepatotoxicity may occur in some patients.

RIFAMPIN (Rifadin). Rifampin belongs to the rifamycin group of antibiotics. It exerts a bactericidal effect against susceptible microorganisms by inhibiting RNA synthesis. Antibiotic resistance can develop rapidly; therefore, rifampin must be given concurrently with other antitubercular drugs. Rifampin is valuable because it can penetrate tissues and reach therapeutic levels within tubercles.

INDICATIONS. The most important use is in the treatment of *Mycobacterium tuberculosis* infections, where it is considered a primary drug (along with isoniazid). Rifampin is also effective against a variety of gram-positive and gram-negative organisms but is not used for trivial infections if another drug will work.

PRECAUTIONS AND ADVERSE EFFECTS. Gastrointestinal upsets are the most common toxicities noted although central nervous system symptoms such as headache and dizziness may occur.

ETHAMBUTOL (Myambutol). The mechanism of action of the synthetic antibacterial ethambutol is not fully understood. The mechanism is bacteriostatic and involves interruption of cell wall synthesis through a competitive inhibition mechanism.

INDICATIONS. Ethambutol is effective only against *Mycobacterium tuberculosis* and is used as a secondary drug with isoniazid, rifampin, or both.

PRECAUTIONS AND ADVERSE REACTIONS. Anaphylaxis and peripheral neuritis are occasional toxicity problems with ethambutol use.

Table 16–9 summarizes the antimicrobial activity of the antituberculosis drugs.

TABLE 16–9 ANTIMICROBIAL ACTIVITY OF ANTITUBERCULOSIS DRUGS

Respiratory Infection	Streptomycin	Isoniazid	Rifampin	Ethambutol
Mycobacterium tuberculosis	+	+	+	+

+—antimicrobial activity.

Miscellaneous Antibacterials

Inhibitors of Cell Wall Synthesis

An extremely toxic antibiotic that inhibits cell wall synthesis is vancomycin (Vancocin). It is unrelated to any other antibiotic and has a narrow bactericidal spectrum of activity directed against gram-positive organisms, such as the streptococci and staphylococci. In spite of adverse reactions such as fever, chills, ototoxicity, and nephrotoxicity, vancomycin is a very important drug for use against penicillinase-producing *Staphylococcus* species and in special situations such as streptococcus endocarditis.

The pharmacologic activity of miscellaneous antibacterials acting as inhibitors of cell wall synthesis is summarized in Table 16–10.

Inhibitors of Protein Synthesis

The tetracyclines are broad-spectrum antibiotics, effective against a variety of gram-positive, gram-negative, and spirochete bacteria in addition to mycoplasma, amebae, and some *chlamydia* and *rickettsia* species. Major respiratory uses include treatment of infections caused by *Mycoplasma pneumoniae, Chlamydia* species, and *Coxiella burnetii,* and sinobronchial infections caused by susceptible strains of *Streptococcus pneumoniae, Haemophilus influenzae,* and *M. pneumoniae.* Tetracyclines exhibit a bacteriostatic mechanism of action by preventing the addition of amino acids to form a polypeptide chain of the protein being synthesized. The tetracyclines are naturally derived from the *Streptomyces* genus of soil bacteria. The group includes short-acting

TABLE 16–10 MISCELLANEOUS ANTIBACTERIALS
Inhibitors of Cell Wall Synthesis: Antimicrobial Activity

Respiratory Tract Infection	Vancomycin
Penicillinase-producing *Staphylococcus* sp	+
Streptococcus sp	+

+—antimicrobial activity.

tetracycline (Polycycline), oxytetracycline (Terramycin), and chlortetracycline (Aureomycin) in addition to long-acting semisynthetic tetracyclines such as doxycycline (Vibramycin). The most common adverse effects include hepatotoxicity and deposition of the tetracyclines in teeth and bones. The brownish discoloration of tooth enamel is most prevalent in fetuses and in children under 7 years of age.

Chloramphenicol (Chloromycetin) is a relatively simple molecule that is cheaper to synthesize than to extract from its natural *Streptomyces* source. It inhibits protein synthesis at bacterial ribosomes and prevents binding of new amino acids. Protein synthesis in mammalian mitochondria can also be adversely affected. The bacteriostatic action of chloramphenicol is broad spectrum and the drug is particularly useful in the treatment of *H. influenzae* meningitis or laryngotracheitis. Chloramphenicol is not normally employed for trivial infections. This is due to its usefulness in meningitis therapy and the low incidence of chloramphenicol resistance. The high toxicity of the drug (bone marrow depression and potential development of anemia) also limits its use. Chloramphenicol is used if other drugs cannot be given to a particular patient.

The major macrolide antibiotic in clinical use is erythromycin, a drug derived from the *Streptomyces* genus. Erythromycin exhibits a bacteriostatic mechanism of action at bacterial ribosomes, but at high concentrations it exerts a bactericidal action. Oral administration can be irritating to tissues, with production of gastrointestinal tract symptoms such as nausea and vomiting. Most gram-negative organisms are impervious to the drug, but it is useful in a variety of gram-positive infections, such as those caused by *Streptococcus pneumoniae* and *S. pyogenes.* Erythromycin is also active against *Corynebacterium diphtheriae, Mycoplasma pneumoniae,* and some important gram-negative organisms, such as *Legionella pneumophila* and some species of *Neisseria.* Erythromycin is often used as a penicillin substitute in penicillin-allergic patients and is used against some penicillin-resistant strains of organisms. A special caution in regard to erythromycin and a similar macrolide antibiotic, troleando-

TABLE 16–11 MISCELLANEOUS ANTIBACTERIALS
Inhibitors of Protein Synthesis: Antimicrobial Activity

Respiratory Tract Infection	Tetracyclines*	Chloramphenicol†	Macrolides‡	Lincosamides§
Mycoplasma pneumoniae	+		+	
Chlamydia sp	+			
Coxiella burnetii	+			
Streptococcus pneumoniae	+		+	
Streptococcus pyogenes			+	+
Staphylococcus aureus				+
Haemophilus influenzae	+	+		
Corynebacterium diphtheriae			+	+
Neisseria sp			+	
Legionella pneumophila			+	
Bacteroides fragilis				+

+—antimicrobial activity.
*Tetracycline, oxytetracycline, chlortetracycline, doxycycline.
†Chloramphenicol exhibits a broad spectrum of activity but is generally reserved for *H. influenzae* infections.
‡Erythromycin, troleandomycin.
§Clindamycin is generally reserved for serious respiratory infections such as anaerobic pneumonitis and lung abscesses.

mycin, concerns the concurrent use of the macrolide antibiotic and a nonsedating H₁-histamine blocker, such as terfenadine (Chapter 10). Macrolide antibiotics may inhibit hepatic microsomal enzymes and prolong the time required to metabolize the recommended dose of terfenadine. As a result, cardiotoxicities such as prolonged QT intervals and ventricular arrhythmias may occur. These adverse effects are similar to those caused by overdose levels of terfenadine.

The lincosamide antibiotics include clindamycin (Cleocin). Clindamycin produces a bacteriostatic action against susceptible bacteria. Therefore, it is reserved for serious respiratory infections such as anaerobic pneumonitis and lung abscesses caused by *Staphylococcus aureus*. In addition, *Streptococcus pyogenes* and other β-hemolytic streptococci, *Corynebacterium diphtheriae,* and certain anaerobic bacteria are sensitive to the drug. Anerobes are often implicated in cases

of "aspiration pneumonia" caused by inhalation of gastrointestinal tract contents. Anaerobic bacteria such as *Bacteroides fragilis* are often recovered in such cases and are sensitive to clindamycin. Because of its value in the special situations outlined above, clindamycin is not routinely used against gram-positive cocci if more common drugs such as penicillin or erythromycin provide the desired control. Adverse reactions to clindamycin include gastrointestinal tract symptoms such as vomiting, diarrhea, and production of a very serious type of colitis.

Table 16–11 provides a summary of the pharmacologic activity of miscellaneous antibacterials acting as inhibitors of protein synthesis.

Inhibitors of Nucleic Acid Synthesis
During the 1980s, the quinolone antibiotics were introduced primarily for the treatment of urinary tract infections. One of the derivatives, called ciprofloxacin (Cipro), proved to be the most potent and is useful in a variety of respiratory infections. It inhibits an enzyme (DNA gyrase) that bacteria use to coil DNA into a double helix. The bactericidal mechanism of action interferes with synthesis of DNA in susceptible respiratory pathogens and halts bacterial reproduction. Ciprofloxacin is effective against *Streptococcus pneumoniae, S. pyogenes, Staphylococcus aureus, Klebsiella pneumoniae, Pseudomonas aeruginosa,* and *Haemophilus influenzae.* Adverse effects include nausea, diarrhea, and headache.

Consult Table 16–12 for a summary of the pharmacologic activity of the miscellaneous antibiotics used in antibacterial therapy against respiratory pathogens.

TABLE 16–12 MISCELLANEOUS ANTIBACTERIALS
Inhibitors of Nucleic Acid Synthesis: Antimicrobial Activity

Respiratory Tract Infection	Quinolones (eg, ciprofloxacin)
Streptococcus pneumoniae	+
Streptococcus pyogenes	+
Staphylococcus aureus	+
Klebsiella pneumoniae	+
Pseudomonas aeruginosa	+
Haemophilus influenzae	+

+—antimicrobial activity.

BOX 16–4 MAGIC BULLETS: PRONTOSIL AND THE SULFA DRUGS

Gerhard Domagk

In the early 1930s the death rate of women giving birth was around 20%. By the end of the decade fatalities due to puerperal fever ("childbirth fever") had dropped to about 2% through the first mass use of a chemotherapeutic agent. The synthetic drug sulfanilamide was found to have selective toxicity in humans. In other words, it had an antimicrobial action against susceptible bacterial species but produced relatively little harm to the host. In 1935, Gerhard Domagk was head of the laboratory in pathology at IG Farbenindustrie, a large German chemical cartel. He noted that a red dye called prontosil was able to cure mice infected with *Streptococcus*. The compound had been used in the dye industry and was found to have an antimicrobial action once it is metabolized to sulfanilamide in the body. The introduction of sulfanilamide led to the development of related drugs called the sulfonamides, or sulfa drugs. Domagk became known as the "father of chemotherapy" and received the Nobel Prize for Medicine or Physiology in 1939 for his discovery of the chemotherapeutic effects of prontosil.

Berquist LM: Microbiology for the Hospital Environment. Harper and Row, New York, 1981.

Jensen MM and Wright DN: Introduction to Microbiology for the Health Sciences. Prentice-Hall, Englewood Cliffs, NJ, 1989.

Modell W, Lansing A, and Editors of Time-Life Books: Drugs. Life Science Library. Time, New York, 1969.

Tortora GJ, Funke BR, and Case CL: Microbiology: An Introduction. Benjamin/Cummings, Redwood City, CA, 1992.

Sulfonamides

The sulfonamides (sulfa drugs) are synthetic antimicrobials that act as competitive antagonists, or antimetabolites, of para-aminobenzoic acid (PABA) (see Fig. 17–4). PABA is a substrate needed by some bacteria for the production of folic acid. Folic acid in turn is a vitamin needed for the synthesis of nucleic acids from nitrogenous bases. Mammalian cells use preformed dietary folic acid; therefore, the mode of action of sulfonamides is not directed against human cells. The mechanism is bacteriostatic against a few gram-positive cocci (such as the streptococci) and some gram-negative organisms. However, many microbes have developed resistance to the sulfa drugs. Allergic reactions in many patients, and development of bone marrow dysfunctions and crystalluria due to the alkaline nature of the drugs, have greatly reduced the usefulness of the sulfa drugs (Box 16–4).

The primary use of the sulfonamides today is in the treatment of certain urinary tract infections because the drugs accumulate in the urine at high concentrations (20–25 times the blood level). The only sulfa drug to be discussed in relation to the respiratory system is a combination product, co-trimoxazole, that uses sulfamethoxazole. It is introduced in the following chapter as an antiprotozoal agent useful in the treatment of *Pneumocystis carinii* pneumonia.

Table 16–13 lists the generic and trade names of the antibacterial drugs discussed in this chapter.

CHAPTER SUMMARY

In this chapter antibacterial drugs of respiratory importance are examined, as are the airborne etiologic agents responsible for common pulmonary infections. In addition, a discussion of the vulnerability of the respiratory tract and the compromised respiratory patient is integrated with an analysis of the infection risk posed by respiratory care equipment, procedures, and personnel.

Some of the drugs introduced in this chapter have been available for decades. Others are quite new and create new dilemmas for a physician treating a patient who has a serious infection. The temptation to administer the newest, most effective broad-spectrum antimicrobial drug is very strong. However, if an earlier drug provides the desired control and is equivalent in other respects, it should be the drug of choice. This strategy minimizes the development of antibiotic resistance and increases the chance that

TABLE 16–13 DRUG NAMES: ANTIBACTERIALS

Generic Name	Trade Name
β-LACTAMS	

PENICILLINS

Natural

Benzyl penicillin	*(many manufacturers)*
Procaine penicillin G	Duracillin
Phenoxymethyl penicillin (penicillin V)	Pen-Vee

Penicillinase-resistant

Methicillin	Staphcillin
Cloxacillin	Cloxapen
Nafcillin	Nafcil
Oxacillin	Bactocill
Dicloxacillin	Dynapen

Broad-spectrum

Ampicillin	Penbriten, Polycillin
Amoxicillin	Amoxil
Carbenicillin	Geopen
Ticarcillin	Ticar
Mezlocillin	Mezlin
Piperacillin	Pipracil

CEPHALOSPORINS

First-generation	
Cephalothin	Keflin
Second-generation	
Cefaclor	Ceclor
Third-generation	
Cefotaxime	Claforan

MONOBACTAMS

Aztreonam	Azactam

CARBAPENEMS

Imipenem (in combination with cilastatin)	Primaxin

AMINOGLYCOSIDES	
Streptomycin	*(many manufacturers)*
Gentamicin	Garamycin
Kanamycin	Kantrex
Amikacin	Amikin
Tobramycin	Nebcin
Netilmycin	Netromycin

ANTITUBERCULOSIS DRUGS	
Streptomycin	*(many manufacturers)*
Isoniazid	Nydrazid[US], Isotamine[CAN]
Rifampin	Rifadin
Ethambutol	Myambutol

MISCELLANEOUS ANTIBACTERIALS	

INHIBITORS OF CELL WALL SYNTHESIS

Vancomycin	Vancocin

INHIBITORS OF PROTEIN SYNTHESIS

Tetracyclines

Tetracycline	Polycycline
Oxytetracycline	Terramycin
Chlortetracycline	Aureomycin
Doxycycline	Vibramycin

TABLE 16–13 DRUG NAMES: ANTIBACTERIALS (*Continued*)

Generic Name	Trade Name
Chloramphenicol	
Chloramphenicol	Chloromycetin
Macrolides	
Erythromycin	(*many manufacturers*)
Troleandomycin	
Lincosamides	
Clindamycin	Cleocin
INHIBITORS OF NUCLEIC ACID SYNTHESIS	
Quinolones	
Ciprofloxacin	Cipro
SULFONAMIDES	
Sulfamethoxazole (combined with trimethoprim as co-trimoxazole)	Bactrim, Septra

the newer drug will be effective if and when needed.

BIBLIOGRAPHY

Aoun M and Klastersky J: Drug treatment of pneumonia in the hospital: What are the choices? Drugs 42:962–973, 1991.

Berquist LM: Microbiology for the Hospital Environment. Harper and Row, New York, 1981.

Birge EA: Modern Microbiology: Principles and Applications. William C Brown, Dubuque, IA, 1992.

Brewer NS and Hellinger WC: The monobactams. Mayo Clin Proc 66:1152–1157, 1991.

Brock TD and Madigan MT: Biology of Microorganisms. Prentice-Hall, Englewood Cliffs, NJ, 1991.

Collins T and Gerding DN: Aminoglycosides versus beta-lactams in gram-negative pneumonia. Semin Respir Infect 6:136–146, 1991.

Dudley MN: Pharmacodynamics and pharmacokinetics of antibiotics with special reference to the fluoroquinolones. Am J Med 91:45S–50S, 1991.

Duguid JP, Marmion BP, and Swain RH: Mackie and McCartney Medical Microbiology: A Guide to the Laboratory Diagnosis and Control of Infection. Churchill Livingstone, Edinburgh, 1978.

Feinberg J and Hoth DF: Current status of HIV therapy. II. Opportunistic diseases. Hosp Prac (Off Ed) 27:161–174, 1992.

Howder CL: Cardiopulmonary Pharmacology: A Handbook for Respiratory Practitioners and Other Allied Health Personnel. William and Wilkins, Baltimore, 1992.

Hughes CE and Van Scoy RE: Antibiotic therapy of pleural empyema. Semin Respir Infect 6:94–102, 1991.

Jawetz E: Aminoglycosides and polymyxins. In Katzung BD (ed): Basic and Clinical Pharmacology. Lange Medical Publications, Los Altos, 1982.

Jawetz E: Antimycobacterial drugs. In Katzung BD (ed): Basic and Clinical Pharmacology. Lange Medical Publications, Los Altos, 1982.

Jawetz E: Penicillins and cephalosporins. In Katzung BD (ed): Basic and Clinical Pharmacology. Lange Medical Publications, Los Altos, 1982.

Jensen MM and Wright DN: Introduction to Microbiology for the Health Sciences. Prentice-Hall, Englewood Cliffs, NJ, 1989.

Khan FA: Quinolones and macrolides: Roles in respiratory infections. Hosp Pract (Off Ed) 28:149–162, 1993.

Spratt JL: Antimicrobial drugs. In Conn PM and Gebhart GF (eds): Essentials of Pharmacology. FA Davis, Philadelphia, 1989.

Talaro K and Talaro A: Foundations in Microbiology. William C Brown, Dubuque, IA, 1993.

Tortora GJ, Funke BR, and Case CL: Microbiology: An Introduction. Benjamin/Cummings, Redwood City, CA, 1992.

Washington JA: Infectious disease aspects of respiratory therapy. In Burton GC, Hodgkin JE and Ward JJ (eds): Respiratory Care: A Guide to Clinical Practice, ed. 3. JB Lippincott, Philadelphia, 1984.

Weisse AB: A plague in Philadelphia: The story of Legionnaires' disease. Hosp Pract (Off Ed) 27:151–180, 1992.

CHAPTER 17

Antivirals, Antifungals, and Antiprotozoals

CHAPTER OUTLINE

Chapter Introduction
Airborne Viral Infections
   VIRAL CHARACTERISTICS
   CAUSATIVE AGENTS
Antiviral Agents

Airborne Fungal Infections
   FUNGAL CHARACTERISTICS
   TYPES OF MYCOSES
Antifungal Agents

Airborne Protozoal Infections
   PROTOZOAL CHARACTERISTICS
Antiprotozoal Agents
Chapter Summary

CHAPTER OBJECTIVES

After studying this chapter the reader should be able to:

- Outline the basic characteristics of viruses.
- Describe the pharmacologic activity of the following antivirals:
  - Amantadine, ribavirin.
- Outline the basic characteristics of the fungi.
- Describe the therapeutic problem posed by the eucaryotic structure of fungal cells.
- Describe the pharmacologic activity of the following antifungals:
  - Nystatin, amphotericin B, ketoconazole, miconazole, flucytosine.
- Outline the basic characteristics of the protozoa.
- Describe the pharmacologic activity of the following antiprotozoals:
  - Pentamidine, co-trimoxazole.

KEY TERMS

antifungal agent
antiprotozoal agent
antiviral agent
chemoprophylaxis

dimorphic fungi
superinfection (secondary
  infection)

systemic mycosis (deep-seated
  mycosis)

CHAPTER INTRODUCTION

The preceding chapter introduced the major airborne bacteria of respiratory importance and the antibacterial drugs used to combat respiratory tract infections. This chapter examines the antimicrobial drugs employed to control respiratory infections caused by other groups of microbes—the viruses, fungi, and protozoa.

Compared with bacterial infections, viral infections represent a greater percentage of respiratory ailments, whereas fungal lung infections are relatively rare but potentially very serious. Protozoal infection of the lungs was once almost unheard of but is increasing today at an alarming rate due to AIDS-related complications.

Paralleling the organization of the previous chapter, this chapter focuses on the microorganisms that present an airborne threat to the body. It also examines the major **antiviral, antifungal,** and **antiprotozoal** drugs with which the respiratory care practitioner comes into contact.

AIRBORNE VIRAL INFECTIONS

Viral Characteristics

Viruses are extremely small, obligate, intracellular parasites that invade living host cells and take over the biochemical machinery to direct production of new virus particles. Viruses exhibit several means of dissemination following their release from infected cells. Some rely on intermediate vectors such as insects, others depend on person-to-person contact, and others are spread by aerosol transmission.

There is a certain elegant simplicity in the structure of most viruses. This is evident in Figure 17–1, which shows the symmetric structure of the influenza virus. The influenza virus, an orthomyxovirus, contains several RNA mole-cules surrounded by a lipoprotein shell with characteristic surface protrusions that impart a specific antigen character to the viral particle. These surface structures can be genetically altered to produce rapid antigenic changes that allow a new viral strain to evade the immune system's attempt to clear the microorganism (Box 17–1). Viruses, unlike other microorganisms, contain a single nucleic acid and can therefore be classified as either RNA or DNA viruses (see Table 16–4).

Causative Agents

Many different viruses can enter the body through the respiratory system to cause diseases not directly affecting the respiratory tract. Examples of such diseases include rubeola, or measles (caused by a paramyxovirus), rubella or German measles (caused by a togavirus), infectious mononucleosis (caused by the Epstein-Barr virus, a herpesvirus), and smallpox (caused by a poxvirus). Most of the etiologic agents of respiratory illness are unknown, but of the known causes, viruses are the most prevalent.

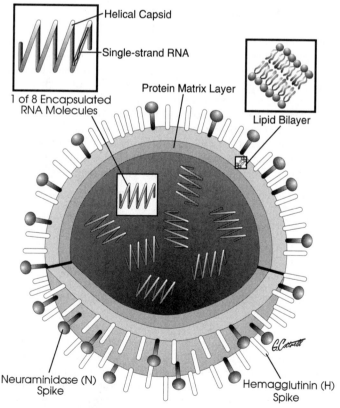

Helical Capsid

Single-strand RNA

1 of 8 Encapsulated RNA Molecules

Protein Matrix Layer

Lipid Bilayer

Neuraminidase (N) Spike

Hemagglutinin (H) Spike

FIGURE 17–1   Schematic—influenza virus.

BOX 17–1 SHIFT AND DRIFT: WHY VACCINES AND ANTIVIRALS LOSE THEIR PUNCH

Currently available antiviral agents, such as amantadine, suppress viral replication at a critical step such as viral uncoating, which exposes the viral genome (Fig. 17–2). How is it then that amantadine can lose its effectiveness in the treatment of influenza infections *in a matter of days?* Or that an effective vaccine developed for one flu season fails to provide the needed protection for high-risk populations in the following year?

The nucleic acid core of the influenza virus consists of eight RNA molecules surrounded by a protein-lipid coat. Influenza viruses are classified into groups A, B, and C on the basis of their antigenic protein coats.

Projecting from the surface of the virus are hundreds of protein molecules arranged as spikes. The makeup of these projections imparts antigenic character to the virus and allows identification of various strains. Two types of spikes exist: H (hemagglutinin) and N (neuraminidase) (Fig. 17–1). H spikes are more numerous and more antigenic than N spikes. H spikes allow viruses to recognize and attach to body cells, whereas N spikes allow the virus to separate from an infected cell after intracellular reproduction.

Different forms of the influenza virus are designated by numbers—H_1, H_2, H_3, N_1, and N_2. Each combination, such as H_2N_2 (Asian flu, 1957) or H_3N_2 (Hong Kong flu, 1968) represents a major alteration in the surface protein configuration of the virus. This substantial change is termed *antigenic shift* and allows a new strain to evade antibodies built up in the population. It also allows the new strain to resist vaccines that are developed against older strains. Recombination of the multiple RNA molecules, and recombination of RNA from influenza strains in humans with RNA from influenza strains in animals (ducks, swine) is responsible for antigenic shift and the emergence of new virulent stains.

The most infamous flu outbreak was the pandemic of 1918–1919, which claimed 20 million victims worldwide. Persons at greatest risk from influenza infection are generally the very young and the very old, but the 1918–1919 strain was especially virulent, causing the death of young adults as well as more vulnerable individuals.

Relatively minor variations in the antigenicity of the influenza virus occur between episodes of major change. Such *antigenic drift* can occur rapidly within the viral group although the nucleic acid makeup is unchanged. These fluctuations usually are caused by changes in a single amino acid within H or N spikes. Following prophylactic immunization, antibodies neutralize the viruses that have not mutated. However, this adds selection pressure and contributes to the phenomenon of decreased efficacy of flu vaccines. Intensive use of an antiviral drug in a confined population may also induce antigenic drift. Such variation reduces the efficacy of antivirals, such as amantadine.

Coles FB, Balzano GJ, and Morse DL: An outbreak of influenza A (H_3N_2) in a well-immunized nursing home population. J Am Geriatr Soc 40:589–592, 1992.

Degelau J et al: Amantadine-resistant influenza A in a nursing facility. Arch Intern Med 152:390–392, 1992.

Hayden FG and Hay AJ: Emergence and transmission of influenza A viruses resistant to amantadine and rimantadine. Curr Top Microbiol Immunol 176:119–130. 1992.

Tortora GJ, Funke BR, and Case CL: Microbiology: An Introduction. Benjamin/Cummings, Redwood City, CA, 1992.

ANTIVIRAL AGENTS

The development of **antiviral agents** is severely limited by the way in which viruses take over host cells and direct biochemical reactions. A drug that exhibits effective antiviral action must have maximal effects within *infected* cells but must not injure *uninfected* cells. This is not an easy task because viruses, in a biochemical sense, become an integral part of the host cell (see Table 16–4). Few antiviral drugs have proven beneficial in

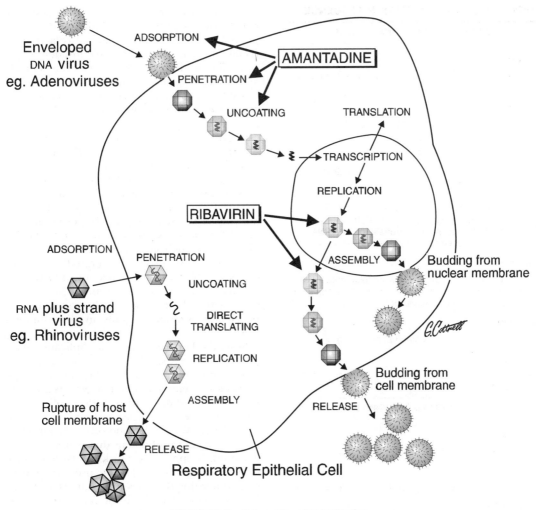

FIGURE 17–2 Schematic—viral replication.

the treatment of respiratory viral infections, or for that matter, in the treatment of any other viral illnesses. The currently available antiviral drugs are virustatic—they suppress viral activity, usually by inhibiting key steps in viral replication (Fig. 17–2). Viruses that are not actively replicating are called latent viruses. These viruses are not affected by a virustatic mode of action.

A *virion* is a fully formed virus particle, complete with a viral genome (Fig. 17–3). This nucleic acid core is surrounded by a protein coat, or *capsid*. As mentioned above, the genome may be RNA or DNA. In addition, the nucleic acid strands may be present in several configurations, such as single- or double-stranded DNA. The in-

fection sequence exhibited by a virion when it invades a host cell is unique to a particular class of viruses (Table 17–1). The numerous stages of the sequence present steps in which antiviral drugs can interfere with the process. For exam-

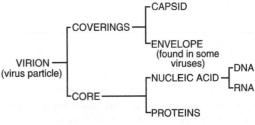

FIGURE 17–3 Viral components.

TABLE 17–1 VIRAL INFECTION SEQUENCE

DOUBLE-STRANDED DNA VIRUSES*

ADSORPTION

Adherence and fusion of viral envelope with the host cell membrane occurs.

PENETRATION

Endocytosis delivers virion to the interior of the host cell.

UNCOATIING

Capsid proteins are shed, leaving a nucleic acid core.

TRANSCRIPTION

Viral DNA is used as a template to synthesize RNA. (Some sequences involve a translation step following transcription. In translation, the RNA template is used to synthesize viral proteins.)

REPLICATION

RNA template is used to produce complementary viral DNA, resulting in the production of multiple copies of the viral genome (nucleic acid).

ASSEMBLY

New viral DNA and capsid material are joined.

RELEASE

Viruses gain a viral envelope as they are shed by the host cell through exocytosis.

PLUS STRAND RNA VIRUSES†

PENETRATION

Virion enters the host cell interior.

UNCOATING

Capsid proteins are shed, leaving the nucleic acid core.

TRANSLATION

Direct translating occurs for the production of viral RNA and proteins.

REPLICATION

RNA template is used to produce viral RNA, resulting in the production of multiple copies of the viral genome (nucleic acid).

ASSEMBLY

New viral RNA and capsid material are joined.

RELEASE

Rupture of host cell membrane sheds viruses.

*Eg, adenoviruses.
†Eg, rhinoviruses.

ple, amantadine seems to interrupt the viral adsorption, penetration, and uncoating stage, whereas ribavirin interferes with viral assembly (Fig. 17–2). In spite of the potential for disruption of the viral replication sequence, very few antiviral drugs have been developed, primarily because of the intracellular nature of the parasites. An antiviral mechanism of action directed at virions after they have invaded a host cell will most likely disrupt a key host cell mechanism such as protein synthesis.

Table 17–1 summarizes the infection sequence exhibited by double-stranded DNA viruses, such as the adenoviruses, one of several causative agents of the common cold. Viral DNA directs the multiplication of new DNA and serves directly as a template for the synthesis of RNA using host cell resources. The RNA is then used to synthesize viral proteins. The infection sequence from an RNA virus depends on the composition of the RNA strands. For example, certain RNA viruses synthesize new viral proteins directly from their single strand of RNA, whereas others must first produce intermediate strands of RNA. Table 17–1 summarizes the infection sequence exhibited by plus-strand RNA viruses, such as the rhinoviruses. Such viruses are implicated as causative agents in the common cold.

Several other pathways of multiplication exist for the various RNA viruses. The details of viral replication, however, are well beyond the scope of this text. General microbiology texts are cited in the bibliography and provide excellent discussions of the steps involved in viral replication.

AMANTADINE (Symmetrel). Amantadine has a mechanism of action that is not fully understood. It appears to block the virus particle from entering a host cell and to prevent the virus from uncoating if it does gain entry (Fig. 17–2). Uncoating of the viral nucleic acid core is a necessary step in viral replication.

INDICATIONS. Amantadine produces limited control of type A influenza virus strains. Oral amantadine is used in the **chemoprophylaxis** (prevention) and treatment of influenza and is most useful in limiting the spread of the infection in confined settings such as nursing homes (Degelau et al, 1992; Gross, 1991). Aerosolized amantadine has also proved effective against influenza A pulmonary infections (Van Voris and Newell, 1992).

PRECAUTIONS. With the expanded use of antivirals such as amantadine and rimantadine (a closely related drug), resistant viral strains are emerging with increasing frequency (Hoyden and Hay, 1992; Keating, 1992).

CONTRAINDICATIONS. Known hypersensitivity to the drug is a contraindication to its use.

ADVERSE REACTIONS. The most common adverse effects are central nervous system symptoms such as anxiety and insomnia.

RIBAVIRIN (Virazole). In 1986 the US Food and Drug Administration approved the use of aerosol ribavirin for the treatment of severe respiratory syncytial virus (RSV) infections in spontaneously breathing infants. High drug levels in bronchoalveolar fluid and alveolar macrophages (type 3 pneumocytes) are produced with administration of aerosolized ribavirin (Washkin, 1991). Ribavirin is a synthetic analogue related to guanosine. It is transported intracellularly and may persist for weeks in certain cells, such as red blood cells. Active metabolites of ribavirin inhibit viral coating during the assembly stages of viral replication (Fig. 17–2). The precise mechanism of action is not fully understood (Washkin, 1991).

AEROSOL DELIVERY AND HAZARDS. As an aerosol, ribavirin is administered by a small-particle aerosol generator (SPAG), which produces uniform, small-diameter (1.3 μm) particles (see Fig. 1–8). Small respirable particles such as these allow deep penetration of distal airways but are difficult to contain in open nebulization systems (Fallat and Kandal, 1991). As a result, medication aerosol may be released into the immediate environment. Passive ribavirin exposure may result in elevated drug levels in health care workers involved in the treatment of neonates and infants with RSV infections (Washkin, 1991). This potential exists because ribavirin, as was explained above, persists in some cells for prolonged periods. Furthermore, the manufacturer of Virazole (Viratek, Inc, Costa Mesa, CA) states that exposure to ribavirin is contraindicated in women who are or may become pregnant. Animal and *in vitro* studies suggest that teratogenic effects may exist with ribavirin (Kacmarek and Kratohvil, 1992; Washkin, 1991).

To minimize aerosol contamination of the environment by exhausted ribavirin and to reduce unnecessary risk to health care workers, equipment and treatment protocols have been developed. For example, the SPAG unit is designed to deliver ribavirin to the infant through a containment device such as an oxygen hood (Kacmarek and Kratohvil, 1992; Washkin, 1991). Exhausted aerosol is collected from around the hood by a second enclosure such as an oxygen tent, and scavenged by one or more vacuum pumps. Single-patient treatment rooms, multiple air exchanges to the outside, filters, and negative pressure in the treatment area add to the safety of caregivers (Washkin, 1991). Barrier protection such as gowns, gloves, goggles, masks, and personal respirators provide a "firstline" defense for the health care worker. Finally, minimal exposure to the treatment area and strict adherence to institution policy are required. Guidelines involving operation of the SPAG, interruption of medication administration, and removal of the infant from the double enclosure provide additional safeguards for respiratory care practitioners and others entrusted with the care of infants infected with RSV.

Aerosol delivery of antimicrobials such as ribavirin is continually being reassessed. New drug information, treatment protocols, such as for ribavirin use during mechanical ventilation, and equipment modifications, for example, the addition of mist generators in the oxygen tent, are constantly evaluated (Cefaratt and Steinberg, 1992; Kacmarek and Kratohvil, 1992; Smith et al, 1991). The Aerosol Consensus Statement for 1991 by the American Association for Respiratory Care describes such changes. Updated information will undoubtedly follow as new insight into aerosol delivery of medications is gained.

INDICATIONS. Aerosolized ribavirin possesses therapeutic efficacy against RSV and is used in severe lower respiratory infections in infants. Ribavirin is supplied as 6 g of powder per 100-mL vial for aerosol administration through the SPAG. The drug is solubilized with sterile USP water for injection or inhalation in the 100-mL vial (see Table 17–6). Sterile USP water for injection or inhalation is used to dilute further to a final volume of 300 mL for nebulization (Howder, 1992; Rau, 1989). The final concentration is 20 mg/mL, or a 2% solution. (Pharmaceutical calculations are discussed fully in Appendix A.) Ribavirin aerosol is administered 12–18 hours per day for at least 3 days and no more than 7 days (Viratek, 1986).

Aerosolized ribavirin is also effective in the treatment of severely ill patients infected with *influenza viridae A* and *B*. Oral ribavirin is slightly effective against *influenza virus A* infections and has shown promise in the treatment of *influenza virus B* infections as well (Van Voris and Newell, 1992).

CONTRAINDICATIONS. Ribavirin must not be given to pregnant women because of its potential teratogenic hazard.

PRECAUTIONS Some infants have self-limiting RSV infections and recover on their own. In these cases, ribavirin therapy may not be indicated because the normal course of treatment is 3–7 days.

Passive exposure by health care workers to ribavirin aerosol has already been discussed, including the possible teratogenic risks to a woman who is pregnant or who may become pregnant. Recommended equipment and procedures minimize the risk.

Ribavirin is not yet approved for use in infants requiring assisted ventilation. The drug may form a precipitate in the respiratory equipment and interfere with mechanical ventilation (Smith et al, 1991). Circuits and administration protocols that minimize this problem have been designed and are being evaluated (Demers, 1991; Kacmarek and Kratohvil, 1992; Smith et al, 1991).

ADVERSE REACTIONS. Cardiac instability and worsening of asthma in chronic obstructive pulmonary disease may occur with aerosol ribavirin (Washkin, 1991). Hematologic effects such as anemia may occur with oral or parenteral administration of ribavirin, but are not seen with short-term ribavirin aerosol therapy.

Airborne viruses of respiratory importance and the antiviral drugs used to treat such infections are summarized in Table 17–2.

Note: One of the few drugs available for the treatment of HIV (human immunodeficiency virus) infections in cases of AIDS (acquired immunodeficiency syndrome) is the antiviral drug zidovudine, also called azidothymidine or AZT (Retrovir). Because HIV (a retrovirus) is not an airborne viral agent, does not enter through the respiratory system, and does not directly cause respiratory illness in AIDS, the drug is not included in the preceding section although zidovudine is often in the forefront of discussions involving antiviral agents.

AIRBORNE FUNGAL INFECTIONS

Fungal Characteristics

Fungi include the molds and yeasts. On the basis of cellular organization, fungal cells differ significantly from bacteria and are classified as eucaryotic. Their structural complexity is similar to that of human cells. A serious therapeutic risk is posed by this structural similarity. As a general rule, if the mechanism of action of a chemotherapeutic drug is directed against a eucaryotic *fungal* cell structure, it will probably cause some damage to a eucaryotic *human* cell structure.

A unique type of fungal agent is able to alter its morphology depending on environmental conditions. The **dimorphic fungi** are temperature-dependent microorganisms that exist in a mycelial (mold) form at room temperature (25°C) but convert to a yeast form at body temperature (37°C). Inhalation of viable spores from the mycelial form of the fungus introduces the pathogen. Subsequent conversion to yeast cells allows dissemination of the invader within

---

TABLE 17–2 AIRBORNE VIRUSES CAUSING RESPIRATORY ILLNESS

Causative Agent	Disease	Treatment/Prevention	Comments
Orthomyxoviruses (RNA)			
Influenza viruses	Influenza A	Prophylactic immunization with multivalent vaccine for high-risk groups (65 y or more)	Classified into antigenic groups (A, B, C)
			Type B is less common, milder, and geographically limited
		Amantadine and ribavirin for chemoprophylaxis and treatment	Influenza A epidemics in large populations are often accompanied by secondary bacterial invaders (eg, *Haemophilus influenzae, Staphylococcus aureus, Streptococcus pneumoniae*)
Paramyxoviruses (RNA)			
Respiratory syncytial virus	Viral respiratory illness in infants	Ribavirin	Infections can be epidemic in hospitals; cells in culture clump together to form a syncytium
Parainfluenza viruses	Bronchitis Pneumonia Croup (in infants)	Humidity therapy; no antiviral drugs available	Croup is generally self-limiting
"Common cold" viruses			
Rhinoviruses (RNA) and Adenoviruses (DNA)	Common cold Common cold	No immunization; no antiviral drugs available	Numerous strains of viruses are involved in the infection

the body. The presence of the parasitic proteins in the body causes progressive sensitization in host tissues. The slowly developing immunologic reaction is responsible for the chronic nature of most systemic fungal infections. These infections occur primarily in persons with weakened defenses, but they may also occur as secondary infections, or **superinfections,** following antibacterial therapy. (Bacteria often provide a natural population check by producing environmental conditions unfavorable to fungal growth.)

Types of Mycoses

Fungal infections are known as mycotic infections, or mycoses. Classification of the infection is based on the depth of tissues involved. For example, athlete's foot is a type of mycotic infection known as a cutaneous mycosis, or dermatomycosis, and involves only superficial tissues. For our purposes, only the fungal agents invading deeper tissues, such as the lung, are discussed. These infections are termed **systemic mycoses,** or **deep-seated mycoses,** and are relatively serious. They are much less common than the bacterial and viral infections discussed previously and are more serious in some patients. The organisms invade subcutaneous tissues or the lungs and may metastasize (spread) to other tissues to establish disease. Many are airborne, entering through the respiratory system, but the gastrointestinal tract and skin also serve as portals of entry.

ANTIFUNGAL AGENTS

The development of effective **antifungal agents** has not been nearly as successful as the production of antibacterials. The main reason for this disparity is the difficulty involved in targeting a eucaryotic fungal structure without harming a human cell. Many antibacterials, by contrast, adversely affect procaryotic structures unique to bacteria and present little danger to eucaryotic host cells.

NYSTATIN (Mycostatin). Nystatin is classified as a polyene antibiotic and is derived from the *Streptomyces* genus of soil bacteria. The antifungal drug causes an increase in membrane permeability by combining with sterols in the fungal cell plasma membrane. The resulting osmotic stress produces the fungicidal effect. Nystatin, like amphotericin B, does not affect bacteria or viruses.

INDICATIONS. An oral form of nystatin is available to treat systemic candidiasis. (A topical form is used to treat dermal conditions involving *Candida albicans*).

CONTRAINDICATIONS. Known hypersensitivity is a contraindication to the use of this drug.

Note: The indications, contraindications, precautions, and adverse reactions of the following antifungals are the same as those described for nystatin unless stated otherwise.

AMPHOTERICIN B (Fungizone). Amphotericin B is a polyene antibiotic introduced in 1957. It is also obtained from *Streptomyces,* a genus of filamentous bacteria. It is the most versatile and effective antifungal agent available for the treatment of the deep-seated mycoses. Amphotericin B binds to sensitive fungi by combining with sterols on their membranes. The resulting membrane pores allow osmotic damage to bring about the fungicidal effect. Bacterial and viral effects are lacking because such organisms do not have sterols in their membranes. Mammalian cell membranes do possess sterols in the form of cholesterol, whereas fungal cell membranes possess ergosterol. As a result, amphotericin B produces toxicity in human cells but has a greater affinity for ergosterol; therefore, antifungal effects predominate.

INDICATIONS. The following systemic mycoses are sensitive to the antifungal action of intravenous amphotericin B: candidiasis, cryptococcosis, aspergillosis, blastomycosis, histoplasmosis, and coccidioidomycosis.

ADVERSE REACTIONS. Amphotericin B exhibits relatively serious toxicities, including anorexia, chills, fever, and anaphylaxis. Potential bone marrow depression and renal damage are especially serious. Reversible renal damage is common during amphotericin B chemotherapy, occurring in about 80% of patients. Amphotericin B is the primary drug used in systemic mycotic infections but is reserved for hospital treatment of seriously ill and debilitated patients.

KETOCONAZOLE (Nizoral). Ketoconazole is a broad-spectrum antifungal agent that interferes with the synthesis of ergosterol in fungal cell membranes, bringing about leakage of cell contents.

INDICATIONS. Ketoconazole is an orally active alternative to amphotericin B therapy and is used to treat candidiasis, blastomycosis, histoplasmosis, and coccidioidomycosis.

PRECAUTIONS. Ketoconazole suppresses hepatic microsomal enzymes and reduces the ability of the liver to metabolize compounds. Terfenadine is an H_1-histamine receptor antagonist that is extensively metabolized in the liver (see Chapter 10). Therefore, an adverse drug interaction may occur with concurrent administration of ketoconazole and terfenadine. Potential cardiotoxicity such as QT prolongation and ventricular arrhythmias is the same as that described for erythromycin-terfenadine interactions.

ADVERSE REACTIONS. Toxicities seen with ketoconazole include headache, dizziness, nausea, and vomiting, but are generally much less serious than those caused by amphotericin B.

MICONAZOLE (Monistat IV). Miconazole is a broad-spectrum antifungal agent chemically related to ketoconazole. Miconazole causes leakage of contents by altering the permeability of fungal cell membranes. It also selectively inhibits the uptake of essential nucleic acid precursors.

INDICATIONS. Miconazole is effective in cases of candidiasis, cryptococcosis, and coccidioidomycosis and is especially useful in patients who cannot be given amphotericin B because of preexisting renal insufficiency.

ADVERSE REACTIONS. The most common adverse reactions to miconazole therapy involve GI tract symptoms such as nausea, vomiting, and diarrhea.

FLUCYTOSINE (Ancobon). Flucytosine is converted *in vivo* to the compound 5-fluorouracil, which in turn inhibits DNA synthesis within fungal cells. The conversion does not occur to the same extent in human host cells.

TABLE 17–3 AIRBORNE FUNGI CAUSING RESPIRATORY ILLNESS

Causative Agent	Disease	Treatment	Comments
	UPPER RESPIRATORY INFECTIONS		
Candida albicans (kan-**DĒ**-da **AL**-bi-kans)	Candidiasis	Nystatin Amphotericin B Ketoconazole Miconazole Flucytosine	"Yeast-like fungus," normal inhabitant of mucus membranes of GI tract of many healthy persons Frequently diagnosed mycotic infection in compromised hosts Oral infections are called *thrush*
	LOWER RESPIRATORY INFECTIONS		
Candida albicans	Pulmonary moniliasis	(see above)	Most prevalent in debilitated and compromised persons
Cryptococcus neoformans (krip-tō-**KOK**-us nē-ō-**FOR**-mans)	Cryptococcosis	Amphotericin B Miconazole Flucytosine	Organism recovered from soil and droppings of caged birds (pigeons) Exact mode of transmission not understood Yeast cells metastasize throughout body Pulmonary involvement may include lobar, lobular, or nodular lesions
Aspergillus fumigatus (as-per-**GIL**-us fūm-i-**GA**-tus)	Aspergillosis (may result in necrotizing bronchopneumonia, lobar pneumonia, or lung abscesses	Amphotericin B	Second most common mycotic infection in compromised hosts Symptoms mimic pulmonary embolism
Blastomyces dermatitidis (blas-tō-**MĪ**-sēs der-ma-**TĪ**-ti-dis)	North American blastomycosis	Amphotericin B Ketoconazole	Dimorphic fungus Involvement of lungs and pleura Development of chronic, granulomatous, suppurative lesions
Histoplasma capsulatum (his-tō-**PLAZ**-ma cap-sū-**LA**-tum)	Histoplasmosis	Amphotericin B Ketoconazole	Dimorphic fungus Carried worldwide by migrating birds Calcified nodules in the lung resemble tuberculosis lesions
Coccidioides immitis (kok-sid-ē-**OID**-ēs **IM**-i-tis)	Coccidioidomycosis (also known as valley fever, desert rheumatism, San Joaquin valley fever)	Amphotericin B Ketoconazole Miconazole	Endemic in SW United States Nonproductive cough, chest pains, and dyspnea; pneumonia may occur

GI—gastrointestinal; SW—southwestern.

INDICATIONS. Flucytosine is normally given with amphotericin B to treat candidiasis and cryptococcosis infections.

ADVERSE REACTIONS. Gastrointestinal tract symptoms of nausea and vomiting are the most frequent toxicities noted.

Airborne fungi of respiratory importance and the antifungal drugs used to treat such systemic mycoses are summarized in Table 17–3.

AIRBORNE PROTOZOAL INFECTIONS

Protozoal Characteristics

Protozoa are relatively large unicellular organisms, ranging in size from 5 to 60 μm. (For comparison, a human erythrocyte measures approximately 7μm across.) Protozoa lack a cell wall but are relatively complex internally and are classified as eucaryotic cells.

Most protozoa produce disease in humans as intracellular parasites. For example, the malaria protozoan resides within red blood cells. A few protozoa, such as *Pneumocystis carinii,* invade as extracellular parasites. Modes of transmission of the protozoa group are varied, from insect- and water-borne mechanisms to airborne dispersal. Few protozoa are primary invaders of the lung, but the lung can become a site of secondary protozoal infection. *P. carinii* is an atypical protozoan, infecting the lungs as a primary invader.

ANTIPROTOZOAL AGENTS

PENTAMIDINE (Pentam 300). The mid-1940s marked the debut of pentamidine used systemically to treat protozoal infections, such as African sleeping sickness. Aerosolized pentamidine came into use in 1986 for the treatment and prevention of *Pneumocystis carinii* pneumonia (PCP). Pentamidine binds to nucleic acids and interferes with RNA and DNA synthesis (Washkin, 1991). Its mechanism, however, is not fully understood.

AEROSOL DELIVERY AND HAZARDS. Pentamidine aerosol particles of less than 5 μm diameter are needed for deep penetration of the lung (Fallat and Kandall, 1991). This is achieved by means of a small-volume nebulizer (SVN) with special internal baffling that limits delivery of large particles to the patient (see Fig. 1–7). The small particles produced by modified jet nebulizers are less irritating to the throat and trigger less bronchospasm and coughing than larger aerosol particles.

The patient's cough adds more aerosol to the environment of the respiratory care practitioner and patient (Fallat and Kandall, 1991). These aerosols in turn increase the risk of airborne infection by opportunistic pathogens. For example, *Mycobacterium tuberculosis* is common in immunocompromised HIV-positive patients. This pathogen may be released into the immediate treatment area during coughing episodes induced by aerosols. In addition, pentamidine medication aerosol may be added to the environment through patient coughing, talking, or exhalation. One-way valves in the SVN and patient-actuated inlet controls reduce unnecessary release of medication aerosol when the patient is not inhaling. Expiratory filters further limit contamination by exhausted pentamidine aerosol (Fallat and Kandall, 1991). Environmental controls such as single-patient treatment rooms, ventilation of the treatment room with multiple air exchanges, and negative air pressure in the treatment area contribute to decreased risk of contamination (Washkin, 1991). As was discussed with ribavirin administration, personal barrier protection and limited contact time further decrease the exposure of health care workers to medication aerosols. Passive exposure to pentamidine aerosol may result in toxicity in health care workers (Washkin, 1991) because the drug is deposited in tissue and persists for months (see Adverse Reactions below).

INDICATIONS. The approved indication for use of aerosolized pentamidine is the prevention and treatment of PCP. *Pneumocystis carinii* invades the alveolar spaces of the lung. Therefore, parenchymal deposition of small aerosol particles (<3 μm) is ideal for the delivery of high concentrations of pentamidine (Washkin, 1991). The drug binds to lung tissue and is slowly cleared from the body.

Recommended dosages, treatment intervals, and delivery mode for aerosolized pentamidine have undergone review and modification since the drug's introduction. Changes in pentamidine administration will undoubtedly continue to be made as better understanding of the drug is gained. At present, the typical dosage for monthly PCP prophylaxis with the small-volume jet nebulizer is 300 mg of pentamidine dissolved in 6 mL of sterile water and nebulized until the medication reservoir is dry (Vinciguerra and Smaldone, 1990; Washkin, 1991). The drug tends to become more concentrated during the latter part of the treatment as the diluent evaporates (Washkin, 1991).

PRECAUTIONS. The reader is reminded to always check the latest product information and current guidelines and protocols in the research literature for updated information on recently released drugs, such as aerosolized pentamidine. This is because new therapeutic methods are continually being evaluated and a wide degree of variation exists at different treatment facilities in regard to administration of aerosolized pentamidine.

Pentamidine binds extensively to tissues and is stored for months, thus increasing the risk of drug accumulation. The potential exists for development of systemic toxicity in patient and caregiver alike.

The risk to health care workers through passive exposure to aerosolized pentamidine and the transmission of exhaled airborne pathogens has already been discussed. Barrier protection, environmental controls, and proper equipment and technique reduce the risk.

ADVERSE REACTIONS. Recall that systemic toxicity is less common with aerosol pentamidine but that cumulative effects in a patient may occur. In addition, prolonged passive exposure to pentamidine aerosol may produce adverse reactions in an unprotected health care worker. The effects include dry mouth, metallic taste, conjunctivitis, rash, and renal insufficiency (Washkin, 1991). Hypoglycemia and diabetes are serious systemic effects that may be caused by pentamidine administration. Large aerosol particles produce irritation of the throat and promote coughing. Undesirable respiratory effects such as bronchial irritation, rhinitis, pharyngitis, and laryngitis can be minimized by pretreatment with a β_2-adrenergic agonist (Washkin, 1991).

It should be emphasized that the aerosol administration of uncommon drugs such as antivirals and antiprotozoals is currently in a state of flux. Drug dosages, acceptable levels of exposure to aerosols, safeguards for patient and caregivers, types of aerosol generators, and toxicity effects of the drugs are continually being assessed. It is the responsibility of the respiratory care practitioner to stay abreast of current standards and protocols in this dynamic area of aerosol antimicrobial therapy.

TRIMETHOPRIM - SULFAMETHOXAZOLE (TMP-SMZ) (Bactrim, Septra). Co-trimoxazole consists of trimethoprim and sulfamethoxazole in a fixed-dose combination. The mechanism of action involves drug synergism so that only *one tenth* the concentration is needed compared with each component used on its own. In addition, the development of resistant microbial strains is

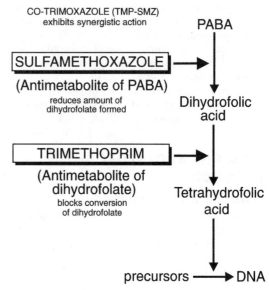

CO-TRIMOXAZOLE (TMP-SMZ)
exhibits synergistic action

FIGURE 17–4 Sequential blocking of PABA metabolic pathway by TMP-SMZ.

minimized, while the spectrum of activity is broadened.

As can be seen in Figure 17–4, the sulfonamide drug sulfamethoxazole is an antimetabolite of para-aminobenzoic acid (PABA) and competes with PABA to reduce the amount of dihydrofolic acid formed. (Dihydrofolic acid, or dihydrofolate, is an intermediate in the biosynthesis pathway.) Trimethoprim is an antimetabolite of dihydrofolate because it interferes with an enzyme needed to convert dihydrofolate to the next compound in the sequence. The end result of co-trimoxazole action is that DNA synthesis is inhibited.

INDICATIONS. Co-trimoxazole is indicated for PCP and for chronic bronchitis caused by *Streptococcus pneumoniae*.

CONTRAINDICATIONS. Known hypersensitivity to trimethoprim or to sulfamethoxazole is a contraindication to the use of co-trimoxazole.

PRECAUTIONS AND ADVERSE REACTIONS. Because co-trimoxazole is bacteriostatic, it is not indicated for the treatment of streptococcus pharyngitis ("strep throat") because of the risk for inducing bacterial mutation and thereby causing serious poststreptococcal complications (see Table 16–2).

Patients with renal or hepatic insufficiency or patients who are HIV positive show a greater incidence of undesirable side effects from co-tri-

BOX 17–2   NEWER ANTIPROTOZOALS: NEW DIRECTIONS FOR
***PNEUMOCYSTIS CARINII* PNEUMONIA THERAPY**

The current treatment of *Pneumocystis carinii* pneumonia, also known as pneumocystosis or interstitial plasma cell pneumonia, involves the administration of pentamidine and/or inhibitors of folic acid synthesis, such as trimethoprim-sulfamethoxazole (co-trimoxazole, or TMP-SMZ). This drug therapy is relatively effective but produces adverse reactions in the immunocompromised patient with AIDS. An alternative treatment being studied in animal models is a unique drug mechanism of action directed against the cyst wall of *Pneumocystis carinii*. The cyst wall is not found in human host cells, although human and protozoal cells are both classified as eucaryotic.

By inhibiting the biosynthesis of 1,3-β-glucan, an essential component of the cyst wall, experimental drugs such as aculeacin A and L-671,329 (a drug called an *echinocandin*) prevent the development of new cysts in the lung. In the rat, these novel 1,3-β-glucan synthesis inhibitors reduce cyst wall formation and inhibit cyst wall maturation. Cysts are part of the life cycle of these opportunistic protozoa and contain developing parasites that are disseminated throughout the lung. The new cyst wall–inhibitor drugs show promise in the prevention of severe pneumonia caused by *P. carinii*. Animal studies suggest that cyst clearance occurs in about 4 days, compared with 2–3 weeks with conventional pentamidine or trimethoprim-sulfamethoxazole therapy.

Matsumoto Y, Yamada M, and Amagai T: Yeast glucan of *Pneumocystis carinii* cyst wall: An excellent target for chemotherapy. J Protozool 38:6S–7S, 1991.

Schmatz DM et al: Treatment and prevention of *Pneumocystis carinii* pneumonia and further elucidation of the *P. carinii* life cycle with 1,3-beta-glucan synthesis inhibitor L-671,329. J Protozool 38:151S–153S, 1991.

moxazole therapy. The most common adverse reactions to co-trimoxazole therapy include gastrointestinal tract symptoms such as nausea and vomiting (see Box 17–2) Airborne protozoa of respiratory importance and the **antiprotozoal agents** used to treat such infections are summarized in Table 17–4.

The generic and trade names of the antiviral, antifungal, and antiprotozoal drugs discussed in this chapter are listed in Table 17–5. Drug dosages for inhalational agents are summarized in Table 17–6.

CHAPTER SUMMARY

This chapter takes a brief look at a few of the drugs employed to treat respiratory tract infections caused by microorganisms other than bacteria. From a comparison of this and the preceding chapter, the reader will note that there are far more drugs available to combat bacterial respiratory infections than there are to treat viral, fungal, or protozoal infections. Part of the reason for this disparity in numbers of chemotherapeutic agents lies with the microorganisms themselves. For example, viruses become an in-

TABLE 17–4   AIRBORNE PROTOZOA CAUSING RESPIRATORY ILLNESS

Causative Agent	Disease	Treatment	Comments
Pneumocystis carinii (nyoo-mō-**SIS**-tis ka-**RIN**-ē-ē)	Interstitial plasma cell pneumonia (also known as *Pneumocystis carinii* pneumonia [PCP] or pneumocystosis)	Trimethoprim-sulfamethoxazole (TMP-SMZ or co-trimoxazole) Pentamidine	Parasites disseminated from cysts within alveoli Presumed reservoir is nasopharynx of asymptomatic carriers Debilitated and compromised persons at greatest risk Leading cause of death in patients with AIDS

AIDS—acquired immunodeficiency syndrome.

TABLE 17–5 DRUG NAMES: ANTIVIRALS, ANTIFUNGALS, AND ANTIPROTOZOALS

Generic Name	Trade Name
ANTIVIRAL AGENTS	
Amantadine	Symmetrel
Ribavirin	Virazole
ANTIFUNGAL AGENTS	
Nystatin	Mycostatin
Amphotericin B	Fungizone
Ketoconazole	Nizoral
Miconazole	Monistat IV
Flucytosine	Ancobon
ANTIPROTOZOAL AGENTS	
Trimethoprim-sulfamethoxazole (TMP-SMZ, co-trimoxazole)	Bactrim, Septa
Pentamidine	Pentam 300

tegral part of the host cell's biochemical machinery, whereas fungal and protozoal cells have a eucaryotic structure similar to that of human cells. As a result of these constraints, researchers are faced with greater challenges to develop drugs that safely and effectively treat viral, fungal, and protozoal infections.

BIBLIOGRAPHY

Berquist LM: Microbiology for the Hospital Environment. Harper and Row, New York, 1981.

Birge EA: Modern Microbiology: Principles and Applications. Wm C Brown, Dubuque, IA, 1992.

Brock TD and Madigan MT: Biology of Microorganisms. Prentice-Hall, Englewood Cliffs, NJ, 1991.

Cefaratt BS and Steinberg MD: An alternative method for delivery of ribavirin to nonventilated pediatric patients. Respiratory Care 37:877–881, 1992.

Codish SD, Tobias JS, and Monaco AP: Systemic mycotic infections (Part 1). Hospital Medicine 14:6–19, Jun 1978.

Codish SD, Tobias JS, and Monaco AP: Systemic mycotic infections (Part 2). Hospital Medicine 14:30–48, Jul 1978.

Coles FB, Balzano GJ, and Morse DL: An outbreak of influenza A (H₃N₂) in a well immunized nursing home population. J Am Geriatr Soc 40:589–592, 1992.

Degelau J et al: Amantadine-resistant influenza A in a nursing facility. Arch Intern Med 152:390–392, 1992.

Demers, RR: Update: Ribavirin administration during mechanical ventilation. Canadian Journal of Respiratory Therapy 27(3):9–14, 1991.

Duguid JP, Marmion BP, and Swain RH: Mackie and McCartney Medical Microbiology: A Guide to the Laboratory Diagnosis and Control of Infection. Churchill Livingstone, Edinburgh, 1978.

Faculty and Writing Committee, American Association for Respiratory Care: Aerosol Consensus Statement, 1991. Respiratory Care 36:916–921, 1991.

Fallat RJ and Kandall K: Aerosol exhaust: Escape of aerosolized medication into the patient and caregiver's environment. Respiratory Care 36:1008–1016, 1991.

TABLE 17–6 DRUG DOSAGES FOR INHALATION AGENTS*

Inhalation Agent	Availability	Dosage
Ribavirin	6 g/100-mL vial for aerosol administration using the SPAG	Infants with severe RSV infections: drug is solubilized with sterile water for injection or inhalation (USP) in the 100-mL vial Sterile water for injection or inhalation (USP) is used to dilute to a final volume of 300 mL for nebulization (final concentration is 20 mg/mL or a 2% solution) Virazole is administered 12–18 h/d for 3–7 d
Pentamidine	300 mg/6 mL for aerosol administration using the SVN	Monthly PCP prophylaxis: 300 mg pentamidine is dissolved in 6 mL sterile water and nebulized at 6 L/min until the medication reservoir is dry Drug is nebulized for 20 minutes once/d; number of days of treatment is determined by the physician

Source: Data from Howder, 1992; Rau, 1989, 1991; Vinciguerra and Smaldone, 1990; Viratek, 1986; Washkin, 1991.
PCP—*Pneumocystis carinii* pneumonia; RSV—respiratory syncytial virus; SPAG—small-particle aerosol generator; SVN—small-volume nebulizer; USP—US Pharmacopeia.
*Note:The dosage information contained in this table is presented as a brief outline and summary of acceptable dosages. It is *not* meant to replace the detailed information available from manufacturers of these drugs. Package inserts provide the most current dosage information from pharmaceutical manufacturers. Guidelines describing the preparation and delivery of the drug, dosage strengths, dosage schedules, shelf life, and storage requirements are also included in the package inserts. In addition, precautions and adverse reactions are described in detail. The respiratory care practitioner is strongly urged to read this information supplied by the pharmaceutical manufacturer to provide safe and effective drug therapy.

Feinberg J and Hoth DF: Current status of HIV therapy. II. Opportunistic diseases. Hosp Pract (Off Ed) 27:161–74, 1992.

Gross PA: Current recommendations for the prevention and treatment of influenza in the older population. Drugs Aging 1:431–439, 1991.

Harrington RD et al: An outbreak of respiratory syncytial virus in a bone marrow transplant center. J Infect Dis 165:987–993, 1992.

Hayden FG and Hay AJ: Emergence and transmission of influenza A viruses resistant to amantadine and rimantadine. Curr Top Microbiol Immunol 176:119–130, 1992.

Howder CL: Cardiopulmonary Pharmacology: A Handbook for Respiratory Practitioners and Other Allied Health Personnel. Williams and Wilkins, Baltimore, 1992.

Jawetz E: Antifungal agents. In Katzung BD (ed): Basic and Clinical Pharmacology. Lange Medical Publications, Los Altos, 1982.

Jawetz E: Antiviral chemotherapy and prophylaxis. In Katzung BD (ed): Basic and Clinical Pharmacology. Lange Medical Publications, Los Altos, 1982.

Jawetz E: Sulfonamides and trimethoprim. In Katzung BD (ed): Basic and Clinical Pharmacology. Lange Medical Publications, Los Altos, 1982.

Jensen MM and Wright DN: Introduction to Microbiology for the Health Sciences. Prentice-Hall, Englewood Cliffs, NJ, 1989.

Kacmarek R: Ribavirin and pentamidine aerosols: Caregiver beware! (Editorial). Respiratory Care 35:1034–1036, 1990.

Kacmarek RM and Kratohvil J: Evaluation of a double-enclosure double-vacuum unit scavenging system for ribavirin administration. Respiratory Care 37:37–45, 1992.

Keating MR: Antiviral agents. Mayo Clin Proc 67:160–178, 1992.

Leoung GS et al: Aerosolized pentamidine for prophylaxis against *Pneumocystis carinii* pneumonia: The San Francisco community prophylaxis trial. N Engl J Med 323:769–779, 1990.

Mathewson HS: Systemic antifungal agents. Respiratory Care 35:987–989, 1990.

Medoff G and Kobayashi GS: Systemic fungal infections: An overview. Hosp Pract (Off Ed) 26:41–52, 1991.

Rau JL: Respiratory Care Pharmacology, ed 3. Yearbook Medical Publishers, Chicago, 1989.

Rau JL: Delivery of aerosolized drugs to neonatal and pediatric patients. Respiratory Care 36:514–542, 1991.

Sciacqua VC: Respiratory syncytial virus. In Wilkins RL and Dexter JR (eds): Respiratory Disease: Principles of Patient Care. FA Davis, Philadelphia, 1993.

Smith DW et al: A controlled trial of aerosolized ribavirin in infants receiving mechanical ventilation for severe respiratory syncytial virus infection. N Engl J Med 325:24–29, 1991.

Spratt JL: Antimicrobial drugs. In Conn PM and Gebhart GF (eds): Essentials of Pharmacology. FA Davis, Philadelphia, 1989.

Talaro K and Talaro A: Foundations in Microbiology. Wm C Brown, Dubuque, IA, 1993.

Tortora GJ, Funke BR, and Case CL: Microbiology: An Introduction. Benjamin/Cummings, Redwood City, Ca, 1992.

Van Voris LP and Newell PM: Antivirals for the chemoprophylaxis and treatment of influenza. Semin Respir Infect 7:61–70, 1992.

Vinciguerra C and Smaldone G: Treatment time and patient tolerance for pentamidine delivery by Respirgard II and Aerotech II. Respiratory Care 35:1037–1041, 1990.

Viratek, Inc: Virazole (ribavarin) Product Monograph. Viratek, Inc, Costa Mesa, CA, 1986.

Washkin H: Toxicology of antimicrobial aerosols: A review of aerosolized ribavirin and pentamidine. Respiratory Care 36:1026–1036, 1991.

UNIT 4

DRUGS AFFECTING THE CARDIOVASCULAR SYSTEM

UNIT INTRODUCTION

Because of the close functional association between respiratory and cardiovascular systems, pathophysiologic conditions affecting one often involve the other. The drugs used to treat dysfunctions of the *cardiopulmonary system* naturally fall into a respiratory classification (Unit 3) and a cardiovascular classification (Unit 4) but in fact have much in common. For example, symptoms of respiratory illness, such as breathlessness, can often be alleviated by drugs that improve blood flow through the lungs. The cardiovascular drugs of this unit are a diverse group: some affect the heart, others modify vessels, and others alter the blood in some way.

Interestingly, the mainstay drugs of cardiovascular therapy have been around for a comparatively long time and are still used in their original form. Digitalis (ca. 1775) is the oldest and is derived from the leaves of a flower. It is used to improve the strength of heart contractions. The nitrates (ca. 1879) are of synthetic origin and are used to relieve the pain of angina. Quinidine (ca. 1912), from the bark of a tree, stabilizes cardiac electrical activity. The catecholamines (ca. 1940) are natural neurohormones used to restore signals going to the heart. Physicians today have newer derivatives of many of the older drugs, but have few truly new agents with which to treat cardiovascular disorders.

CHAPTER 18

Cardiotonics

CHAPTER OBJECTIVES

After studying this chapter the reader should be able to:

- Define cardiotonic, chronotropic, inotropic, dromotropic, preload, afterload, congestive heart failure (CHF).
- Describe the relationship between diastolic filling and systolic ejection in terms of the length and tension of myocardial fibers.
- Explain how the following drug classes increase cardiac output and reduce cardiac preload and afterload:
    - Positive inotropic drugs, diuretics, vasodilators.
- Describe the pharmacologic activity of the following positive inotropic agents:
    - Digitalis, dopamine, dobutamine, norepinephrine, amrinone.

KEY TERMS

afterload
congestive heart failure (CHF);
  chronic congestive heart
  failure (CCHF)
chronotropic effect

diastole (Dī-a-stol or dī-AS-tō-lē);
  diastolic
dromotropic effect
Frank-Starling Law (Starling
  mechanism)

inotropic effect
preload
systole (SIS-tol or SIS-tō-lē);
  systolic

CHAPTER INTRODUCTION

The principal drugs to be discussed in this chapter are the cardiotonics. These drugs improve the tone, or tension, of heart muscle. Cardiac glycosides, catecholamines, and phosphodiesterase inhibitors are used to increase the force of myocardial contraction in congestive heart failure (CHF). The vasodilators used to decrease vascular resistance and the diuretics used to decrease plasma volume are introduced, and details of their pharmacologic activity follow in later chapters. Some of the catecholamines have been previously discussed, but this chapter concentrates on their specific cardiovascular indications.

CARDIAC OUTPUT

Continuous Circulation

The brilliant English physician Sir William Harvey radically changed our view of the function of the heart by describing its action as one of a muscular pump. He proposed that the heart undergoes a series of rhythmic squeezing and relaxing actions that develops enough pressure within blood vessels to propel blood in two endless loops, one circuit to the lungs and back and another to the other organs of the body and back again. This idea of continuous *circulation* is familiar to every student of biology, but to some of Harvey's contemporaries more than 300 years ago, the hypothesis was revolutionary. Through elegant, convincing experiments, he was able to prove that the total volume of blood ejected by the heart was too great to be replenished on a continuous basis, as was believed at the time. He clearly saw that a relatively small volume of blood was perpetually circulated to satisfy the body's metabolic needs.

Metabolically active tissues need proportionately more blood flow than their less active counterparts. The heart, being one of the most active organs in the body, has a high oxygen demand and high energy needs and produces a significant amount of carbon dioxide. If the blood supply to heart muscle is reduced, the detrimental effects of the ischemia, or lack of blood flow, are seen very quickly. Surgical procedures such as coronary bypass, assistive devices such as the intra-aortic balloon pump, or drug therapy with cardiotonics such as digitalis must be initiated to restore blood flow. Without such intervention, tissues throughout the body become deprived of oxygen; the outcome can be fatal. The drugs introduced in this chapter are used to restore the output of blood from the heart, to reduce the cardiac workload, or both. To understand how cardiotonic drugs work and why they are used to restore normal cardiac output, a basic understanding of normal hemodynamics is required.

Heart Rate and Stroke Volume

Because the left side of the heart sends blood into the coronary circuit to supply the myocardium, the volume of blood ejected per unit of time from the left ventricle is of prime concern. Cardiac output (C.O.) from the left ventricle is determined by the product of two variables: heart rate (the number of beats per minute) multiplied by the stroke volume (the amount of blood ejected with each contraction). Heart rate can be influenced by several interrelated factors, such as sympathetic and parasympathetic neuronal impulses and by hormonal influences, such as the secretion of adrenalin (Fig. 18–1). Catecholamine drugs, such as isoproterenol, mimic sympathetic autonomic impulses to increase the heart rate above a normal rate of around 70 bpm. The tachycardia produced is termed a positive **chronotropic effect.** Such an effect improves the cardiac output at a given stroke volume.

The stroke volume produced by a heart of average size is around 70 mL. Stroke volume is the difference between two different volumes in the left ventricle. The relaxation phase of the cardiac cycle is termed **diastole** and is completed just prior to contraction. The amount of blood in the chamber is called the end-diastolic volume and totals around 120 mL. **Systole** is the contraction phase of the cycle. The volume of blood present in the left ventricle immediately after contraction is known as the end-systolic vol-

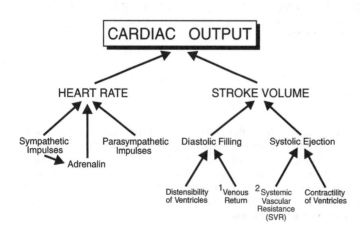

FIGURE 18–1 Cardiac output—interrelated factors. (¹The pressure of this returning blood is the filling pressure or *preload* on the ventricles. ²This resistance represents the *afterload* on the heart or the pressure against which the ventricles must work.)

ume and is approximately 50 mL. The chamber does not completely empty itself of blood, and around 70 mL is sent on its way into the systemic circulation. Figure 18–1 shows some of the variables that contribute to stroke volume. For example, the volume of blood returning to the heart contributes to diastolic filling of the heart and is affected primarily by *distensibility* of the ventricles and by *venous return* factors such as the arterial-venous pressure gradient. The pressure of this returning blood to the atria is the filling pressure, or **preload,** on the ventricles. The amount pumped out again is referred to as systolic ejection and is influenced by factors such as myocardial *contractility* and *vascular resistance.* Systemic vascular resistance is the pressure against which the ventricles must work. This resistance is the **afterload** on the heart.

Digitalis glycosides and catecholamines that increase the force of myocardial contraction have a positive **inotropic effect.** Negative inotropic effects reduce the strength of contraction and can be produced by parasympathetic (vagal) nerve impulses, cholinergic drugs, such as methacholine, and β-adrenergic blockers, such as propranolol. With positive inotropism, the stroke volume of the heart increases and cardiac output improves at a given heart rate. The strength of contraction is directly proportional to the end-diastolic tension of the myocardial fibers. In this length-tension relationship, known as the **Frank-Starling Law** or **Starling mechanism,** cardiac output is regulated by the ventricular end-diastolic volume. This volume changes the tension of the myocardial fibers in the heart wall, thus affecting the strength of contraction. The end-diastolic pressure, therefore, is generated within the heart chamber and is achieved through optimal myocardial fiber length.

CONGESTIVE HEART FAILURE

Characteristics

Chronic congestive heart failure (CCHF) is characterized by low cardiac output, widespread and severe edema, and elevated preload and afterload. Cardiac muscle becomes larger when subjected to an increased workload. In this response, the ventricular fibers increase in size, the heart dilates, the walls become rigid, and the organ enlarges. This hypertrophy is termed *cardiomegaly* and is characteristic of CHF. Elevated preload increases the filling pressures of the right and left ventricles. Increased central venous pressure raises the right atrial pressure, which increases the preload, or filling pressure, of the

right ventricle. Meanwhile, elevated left atrial pressure (represented by the pulmonary capillary wedge pressure) increases the preload, or filling pressure, of the left ventricle. The resulting high pressure in the pulmonary circuit causes plasma to leak from pulmonary capillaries into surrounding lung tissue to cause pulmonary congestion. Finally, the edematous condition of the tissue spaces begins to impair alveolar gas exchange to result in dyspnea. With elevated filling pressures, the heart dilates and the resulting wall rigidity further impairs the action of the ventricular pump. Elevated afterload in the left ventricle is produced by increased systemic vascular resistance (SVR).

Compensation

The following compensatory mechanisms in CHF result in tachycardia in the body's attempt to restore cardiac output:

1. Increased sympathetic nervous activity and circulating catecholamines stimulate the sinoatrial node to increase heart rate. The neural mechanism also causes vasoconstriction, especially of arterioles. Vasoconstriction helps maintain blood pressure but raises the systemic vascular resistance and afterload against which the left ventricle must pump.
2. Activation of the renin-angiotensin-aldosterone pathway results in sodium retention and increased plasma volume. These changes help maintain systemic blood pressure but also increase the circulatory loads on the weakened heart. (The renin-angiotensin-aldosterone pathway is detailed in Chapter 21.)

Treatment of Chronic Congestive Heart Failure

Congestive heart failure is managed clinically by lifestyle changes designed to reduce the workload on the heart. For example, weight reduction, restricted sodium intake, and control of hypertension have the effect of minimizing cardiac work. If these changes fail to achieve the desired results, diuretics, cardiac glycosides, and vasodilators are indicated.

To restore normal cardiac output in cases of CCHF, drug therapy has three goals.

Improvement in Myocardial Contractility

Drugs with a pronounced positive inotropic effect are given to increase the force of myocardial contractions and improve the stroke volume. Although operating through different mechanisms of action, cardiac glycosides such as digoxin, catecholamines such as dobutamine, and newer inotropic agents such as amrinone accomplish this therapeutic goal.

Reduction of Cardiac Preload

Reduction of plasma volume through the administration of diuretic agents effectively reduces some of the load on the right side of the heart. Similarly, the use of vasodilators with either combined arteriolodilation and venodilation properties or selective venodilation activity relieves some of the ventricular filling pressure and wall rigidity seen in some cases of CCHF.

Reduction of Cardiac Afterload

Decreasing plasma volume through diuretic action reduces cardiac afterload. This improves the low left ventricular output seen in some CCHF patients. Vasodilators with mixed action (on arterioles and veins) or specific vasodilating action on the arteriolar system reduces some of the systemic vascular resistance against which the heart must pump. Figure 18–2 depicts the anatomic sites at which various drugs used in CHF therapy are active.

THERAPEUTIC AGENTS

The following section is limited to a discussion of the positive inotropic agents used in the treatment of CCHF. The role of blood vessels and vasodilators, such as the nitrates, are covered in Chapter 19. The site and mechanism of action of diuretics such as furosemide are detailed in Chapter 20.

Cardiac Glycosides

DIGITALIS. Digitalis is the parent drug of the glycosidic group of positive inotropes. A typical cardiac glycoside, such as the prototype drug di-

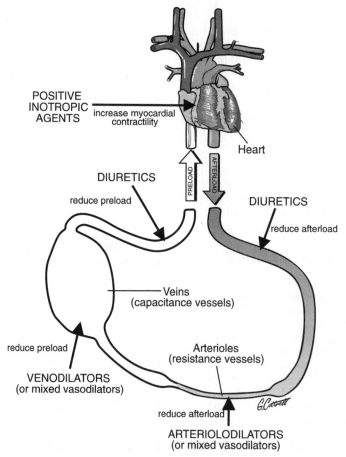

FIGURE 18–2 Sites of action of drugs used in CHF.

BOX 18–1 AN AFFAIR OF THE HEART

Around 1766, in the small English town of Stafford, a young doctor fell in love with one of his patients. Miss Helena Cookes was an artist who painted flowers, but for a time was too ill to collect them for herself. Her physician, William Withering, disliked botany as a student but enthusiastically collected native plants from the surrounding English countryside for his convalescing patient. Withering also immersed himself in the study of plants, presumably impressed Helena by his efforts, and eventually published a botany textbook that became a standard in the field. It was not unusual for physicians of the day to be part-time botanists or herbalists because nearly all available medications were of plant origin. Withering just happened to not derive particular pleasure from the study. That is, until he met Helena. They were married in 1772.

Three years later, Withering was asked for his opinion concerning a local folk remedy employed to rid the body of excess fluid and treat dropsy (the name given to a severe edematous condition). An anonymous old woman from Shropshire had a recipe for a herbal tea containing more than 20 ingredients. Because of Withering's recently acquired botanic background (thanks to Helena), he was able to study the mixture and identify the leaves of the purple foxglove flower *(Digitalis purpurea)* as the active substance in the concoction.

Over the next decade, Withering investigated *digitalis,* the drug responsible for the dropsy ''cure.'' He eventually recognized that digitalis improved the heart's action in cases of congestive heart failure and aided the kidneys in the removal of accumulated fluid. His observations were published in 1785 in *An Account of the Foxglove and Some of Its Medical Uses: With Practical Remarks on Dropsy and Other Diseases.* In this classic work, Withering states that digitalis ''. . . has power over the motion of the heart to a degree yet unobserved in any other medicine.''

Two hundred years after its discovery, digitalis remains one of the most effective cardiotonic drugs. It also provides us with one of medicine's more romantic tales.

Clark WG, Brater DC, and Johnson AR: Goth's Medical Pharmacology, ed 12. CV Mosby, St Louis, 1988.
Kreig M: Green Medicine. Rand McNally, New York, 1964.
Modell W, Lansing A, and Editors of Time-Life Books: Drugs. Life Science Library. Time, New York, 1969.

goxin (Lanoxin), has a complex chemical structure consisting of a steroid nucleus and a series of glucose molecules linked together. Digitoxin (Crystodigin) is a closely related member of the glycoside family. Cardiac glycosides possess similar pharmacologic activity, differing mainly in potency and duration of action (Box 18–1).

The positive inotropism exhibited by digitalis is due to a unique mechanism of action that increases intracellular stores of calcium to increase contractility. The drug inhibits the enzyme Na^{1+}, K^{1+}–ATPase (sodium-potassium–adenosine triphosphatase), which causes an increase in the intracellular levels of Na^{1+}. The elevated Na^{1+} then exchanges with extracellular calcium to increase the intracellular level of Ca^{2+}.

A **dromotropic effect** is an alteration in conduction velocity. Complex electrophysiologic effects in the heart can be caused by low doses of digitalis. These include a negative dromotropic effect, or slowing of atrioventricular (AV) conduction velocity, and shortening of the duration of the action potential in the ventricles. Bradycardia results from slowing of AV conduction velocity. In cases of CHF, digitalis also slows the heart rate by an indirect mechanism operating through the positive inotropic effect of the drug. For example, as cardiac output improves with the increased force of myocardial contraction, sympathetic impulses going to the sinoatrial (SA) node are slowed. As a result, the heart rate decreases.

(Note: Structures such as the SA node are part of the conducting tissue of the heart responsible for initiating and synchronizing myocardial activity. The role of these components is discussed in Chapter 22.)

INDICATIONS. The cardiac glycosides are the frontline inotropic drugs used in cases of CHF. They increase contractility and improve cardiac output, which in turn decreases elevated ventricular pressure, pulmonary congestion, and venous pressure. The pressure decreases are accomplished by means of a secondary diuresis, which reduces plasma volume. The positive inotropic effect of digitalis on the normal and weakened myocardium is described as "the whip that beats the tired horse." Like nearly all drug therapies, digitalis does nothing to correct the underlying cause of the dysfunction.

The use of digitalis in cases of myocardial infarction (MI) with heart failure is controversial (Clark et al, 1988). The drug can worsen arrhythmias and increase the oxygen demand of myocardium, but it can also relieve heart failure and therefore *reduce* oxygen demands and arrhythmias being triggered by the ischemia. Patients are closely monitored for toxicity signs when digitalis therapy is initiated (see Toxicity below).

Additional uses include the treatment of certain electrical abnormalities originating in the atria. Digitalis preparations are useful for slowing AV conduction in cases of atrial fibrillation and atrial flutter.

CONTRAINDICATIONS. Preexisting bradycardia can be made worse by digitalis therapy.

PRECAUTIONS. Because the mechanism of action of digitalis increases intracellular Ca^{2+} levels within heart muscle cells, calcium must not be administered concurrently because of the irritating effect on myocardium of the combined Ca^{2+} levels.

The antiarrhythmic agent quinidine dramatically increases the plasma level of digitalis when it is given concurrently. Quinidine presumably acts by displacing digitalis from tissue-binding sites, but the mechanism is not fully understood.

The caution regarding slowing of heart rate in cases of CHF has been discussed above.

TOXICITY. Digitalis poisoning is one of the most common adverse drug reactions seen in hospitals (Clark et al, 1988). The toxicity is due to several factors. For example, digitalis has a very small margin of safety, with a therapeutic index less than 2. This "therapeutic window," or difference in the dose producing therapeutic and toxic effects, is not only narrow, but variable among different patients. Another factor contributing to digitalis toxicity is the concomitant use of diuretics in cases of CHF. Such combination therapy is routine. However, many diuretics cause potassium and magnesium depletion, which worsen the digitalis toxicity.

At low doses, symptoms of digitalis toxicity include anorexia and bradycardia and progress to nausea, vomiting, and premature ventricular contractions. Higher doses lead to ventricular tachycardia and fibrillation (Clark et al, 1988).

Catecholamines

In addition to their many pharmacologic uses, such as the treatment of bronchial asthma, nasal congestion, and acute allergic emergencies, some catecholamines are employed as cardiotonic drugs.

DOPAMINE (Intropin). Dopamine is a quarternary amine that does not readily cross the blood-brain barrier. Therefore, cardiovascular effects are maximized and central nervous system (CNS) effects are minimal. Dopamine exhibits a dose-dependent action at peripheral receptors. At low dosages it stimulates peripheral dopaminergic (DA_1) receptors to improve renal blood flow. Increasing the dosage stimulates cardiac β_1-adrenergic receptors to produce a powerful inotropic effect. Even higher dosages cause α_1-adrenergic stimulation and increased vascular resistance. These features make dopamine particularly useful for increasing cardiac output while maintaining systemic vascular resistance and perfusion of tissues.

The adrenergic stimulation produced by dopamine is due to two mechanisms: direct stimulation of DA_1-, β_1-, and α_1-receptors, and indirect stimulation by causing the release of norepinephrine from adrenergic nerve fibers. (Norepinephrine then stimulates the appropriate adrenoceptors.) Dilation of renal blood vessels by stimulation of DA_1-receptors results in improved renal blood flow. This in turn facilitates diuresis, leading to reduced circulatory volume and reduced cardiac workload.

Dopamine is administered by intravenous infusion and has a short duration of action (approximately 10 minutes) due to rapid enzymatic degradation by endogenous COMT (catechol-*O*-methyltransferase).

INDICATIONS. Dopamine is useful in the treatment of CHF and cardiogenic shock caused by MI. In addition, dopamine is indicated in cases of hypotension occurring in the absence of hypovolemia.

CONTRAINDICATIONS. Preexisting cardiac abnormalities such as tachyarrhythmias can be worsened by the positive inotropic effects of dopamine. The presence of pheochromocytoma is also a contraindication to the use of the catecholamines because of increased hypertensive risk. Recall that pheochromocytoma is a tumor of catecholamine-producing tissue, such as the adrenal medulla. Widespread vasoconstriction and heightened blood pressure are seen with the pathologic condition and may be worsened by catecholamine drugs.

PRECAUTIONS. Administration of catecholamines reverses the effects of β-adrenergic blockers, such as propranolol. In addition, dopamine is used cautiously in patients with evidence of myocardial ischemia because positive inotropism may increase myocardial oxygen demand.

ADVERSE REACTIONS. Adverse reactions caused by catecholamine administration include tachycardia, anginal pain, palpitations, and headache.

DOBUTAMINE (Dobutrex). Dobutamine is a derivative of isoproterenol, producing a similar increase in myocardial contractility but causing less tachycardia and fewer peripheral arterial effects. It is a direct-acting, positive inotropic agent delivered as an intravenous infusion. Dobutamine exhibits relatively selective β$_1$-adrenergic activity, with only mild β$_2$- and α$_1$-adrenergic activity. It causes increased stroke volume and cardiac output but has minimal effects on peripheral vasculature.

INDICATIONS. In the absence of pronounced hypotension, dobutamine is indicated for the management of severe CCHF. It is also used in cases of pulmonary congestion with low cardiac output.

CONTRAINDICATIONS. Because dobutamine lacks appreciable α$_1$-adrenergic activity and does not significantly increase systemic vascular resistance, it is contraindicated in cases of cardiogenic shock accompanied by severe hypotension.

Dobutamine does not significantly increase heart rate; therefore, preexisting bradycardia can be worsened by the fall in rate that usually accompanies improved stroke volume.

PRECAUTIONS. The chronic use of any β-adrenergic stimulant can lead to the development of tachyphylaxis.

Through its positive inotropic effect and the increase in myocardial oxygen demand, dobutamine has the potential to aggravate preexisting ischemia and must be used with caution in patients having evidence of angina.

ADVERSE EFFECTS. Undesirable effects of dobutamine therapy include tachycardia, anginal pain, hypotension, and headache.

NOREPINEPHRINE (NORADRENALIN) (Levophed). The most active vasopressor for use in the therapy of shock is norepinephrine. This naturally occurring catecholamine is derived from dopamine in the biosynthesis of catechol-

amines and is 20 times more potent than dopamine in its ability to elevate mean arterial pressure. Norepinephrine produces pronounced α$_1$- and β$_1$-adrenoceptor stimulation to increase blood pressure and increase the force of myocardial contraction and cardiac output. Heart rate is not appreciably increased with norepinephrine because the increase in mean arterial pressure due to α$_1$ vasoconstriction triggers the baroreceptor (pressoreceptor) reflex. This stretch reflex monitors blood pressure. Sensory cells in the arch of the aorta and carotid body are stimulated by the norepinephrine-induced hypertension and send afferent impulses into the CNS. The medulla responds by reducing the sympathetic outflow to the heart to decrease the heart rate. Norepinephrine is delivered as an intravenous infusion and the rate of infusion is adjusted according to observed changes in the mean arterial pressure.

INDICATIONS. Norepinephrine is indicated in cases of shock, including cardiogenic shock, in which it is used to increase blood pressure.

CONTRAINDICATIONS. Norepinephrine is not administered to patients with hypotension caused by hypovolemia, nor is it given in cases of MI or ischemia. As with other catecholamines, hypertension due to pheochromocytoma can be aggravated by norepinephrine administration.

PRECAUTIONS. The catecholamines must be used with caution in patients with occlusive vascular disease. This is because there may be an increase in myocardial oxygen demand due to the positive inotropic effect of the drugs. In addition, care must be exercised during intravenous infusion to ensure that none of the drug is delivered extravascularly. An intense local vasoconstriction effect may cause tissue necrosis. As a general caution, it must be remembered that development of tachyphylaxis is always a possibility with the β-adrenergic stimulants such as norepinephrine, and that β-blockers can reduce the efficacy of β-stimulants.

ADVERSE REACTIONS. Intense vasoconstriction produced by α$_1$-stimulation may cause hypertension, which can then result in bradycardia due to activation of the baroreceptor reflex. In addition, norepinephrine may produce cardiac arrhythmias, chest pain, and headache.

Cyclic AMP Phosphodiesterase Inhibitors

Research to develop positive inotropic drugs with less cardiac irritation than digitalis and fewer effects on heart rate than the β-adrenergic agonists has led to the development of a group of inotropic agents that are unrelated to either the cardiac glycosides or the catecholamines.

AMRINONE (Inocor). The first drug in the new series of inotropic agents is called amrinone. It is available as an oral or parenteral preparation and acts directly on myocardial contractility to increase cardiac output. Its mechanism of action is not related to the release of catecholamines. Amrinone causes cAMP (cyclic adenosine-3′,5′-monophosphate) phosphodiesterase inhibition, resulting in elevated cAMP levels within myocardial cells. Its mode of action also involves an increase in the rate of Ca^{2+} influx into myocardial cells to provide additional intracellular calcium for contraction. In addition to its positive inotropic effects, amrinone causes peripheral vasodilation to reduce cardiac preload and afterload. Increased myocardial oxygen consumption due to the positive inotropic effect of amrinone is offset by the vasodilation produced by the drug.

INDICATIONS. Amrinone is used in patients with severe CHF who are refractory to other agents normally used in CHF therapy. These drugs include other inotropic agents, vasodilators, and diuretics.

CONTRAINDICATIONS. Hypersensitivity to the drug is a contraindication to its use.

ADVERSE REACTIONS. Untoward side effects include hepatotoxicity, arrhythmias, hypotension, fever, and nausea.

OTHER INOTROPIC VASODILATORS. Initial enthusiasm over alternative inotropic agents led to the development of amrinone and several related agents, such as milrinone, enoximone, and piroximone, all of which are at various stages of investigation. Like amrinone, these three agents are available in oral or intravenous form. They also exhibit local specific phosphodiesterase inhibition within heart muscle cells to elevate cAMP levels. In general, they are more potent than amrinone in regard to positive inotropic effects but suffer from the same shortcomings (see Chronic Use below).

INDICATIONS. The positive inotropic vasodilators (''inodilators'') are most useful in the acute management of heart failure symptoms in conjunction with cardiac surgery (Wood and Hess, 1989). They are used prior to cardiac surgery to stabilize heart failure while a patient is awaiting heart transplantation. In addition, these drugs are used following cardiopulmonary bypass surgery to manage problems such as pulmonary hypertension, pulmonary congestion, and right ventricular heart failure. The drugs are safe for low-output states often associated with cardiac surgery and produce acute hemodynamic improvements, discussed below.

ACUTE USE. The inotropic vasodilators are more potent than dobutamine in regard to acute improvements in stroke volume, cardiac output, and peripheral vasodilation (Bauman et al, 1991; Installe et al, 1991; Mager at el, 1991).

By promoting vasodilation, the inodilators reduce loadings on the heart. Hemodynamic measurements of vascular resistance, therefore, are decreased by the action of the inotropic vasodilators. For example, preload on the right ventricle is lowered by reduced right atrial pressure and central venous pressure, whereas that on the left ventricle is decreased by a drop in the pulmonary capillary wedge pressure. Afterload on the right ventricle is decreased by a fall in the mean pulmonary artery pressure, whereas afterload on the left ventricle is decreased by reduced systemic vascular resistance. These are reliable indicators of effective and widespread vasodilation. The problems arise in the chronic use of the drugs.

CHRONIC USE. In general, long-term studies of the inotropic vasodilators have not been promising because these drugs show rapid loss of hemodynamic effectiveness and little improvement over conventional CHF therapy (glycosides, diuretics, vasodilators) (Wood and Hess, 1989). In addition, an increase in mortality and serious reactions such as hypotension have been noted with chronic therapy (Packer et al, 1991). In spite of the potential benefit of the inotropic vasodilators in treating symptoms of *acute* heart failure, the safety and efficacy of the drugs have not been confirmed in longer controlled trials (Vernon et al, 1991).

TABLE 18–1   DRUG NAMES: CARDIOTONICS

Generic Name	Trade Name
GLYCOSIDES (DIGITALIS DERIVATIVES)	
Digoxin (di-**JOX**-in)	Lanoxin
Digitoxin (dij-i-**TOX**-in)	Crystodigin
CATECHOLAMINES	
Dopamine (**DŌP**-a-mēn)	Intropin
Dobutamine (dō-**BŪT**-a-mēn)	Dobutrex
Norepinephrine (noradrenalin)	Levophed
CYCLIC AMP PHOSPHODIESTERASE INHIBITORS	
Amrinone (**AM**-ri-nōn)	Inocor
Milrinone (**MIL**-ri-nōn)	(investigational)
Enoximone (e-**NOX**-i-mōn)	(investigational)
Piroximone (pir-**OX**-i-mōn)	(investigational)

Table 18–1 lists the generic and trade names of the cardiotonics discussed in this chapter.

CHAPTER SUMMARY

Heart failure is the inability of the heart to meet the oxygen needs of the body. In such a condition, the myocardial fibers fail to develop the force necessary to eject a sufficient amount of blood to sustain the required cardiac output. The sluggish circulatory condition may cause fluid to move out of blood vessels and into surrounding tissues to result in congestion of organs such as the lungs. For this reason, the pathophysiologic condition is referred to as congestive heart failure (CHF). The therapeutic goal in conditions of CHF is the restoration of cardiac output. Cardiotonics having positive action on the heart are useful for improving stroke volume. In addition, the judicious use of vasodilators and diuretics alters blood vessels and plasma volume to aid in the restoration of normal cardiac preload and afterload.

BIBLIOGRAPHY

Antman EM and Smith TW: Current concepts in the use of digitalis. Adv Intern Med 34:425–454, 1989.

Baumann G et al: Piroximone, dobutamine and nitroprusside: Comparative effects on haemodynamics in patients with congestive heart failure. Eur Heart J 12:533–540, 1991.

Beck RK: Pharmacology for Prehospital Emergency Care. FA Davis, Philadelphia, 1992.

Brody MJ, Feldman RD, and Hermsmeyer RK: Cardiovascular drugs. In Conn PM and Gebhart GF (eds): Essentials of Pharmacology. FA Davis, Philadelphia, 1989.

Butterworth JF et al: Calcium inhibits the cardiac stimulating properties of dobutamine but not of amrinone. Chest 101: 174–180, Jan 1992.

Clark WG, Brater DC, and Johnson AR: Goth's Medical Pharmacology, ed 12. CV Mosby, St Louis, 1988.

Des Jardins TR: Cardiopulmonary Anatomy and Physiology. Delmar, Albany, 1988.

Hines RL: Management of acute right ventricular failure. J Card Surg 5(Suppl 3):285–287, 1990.

Installe E et al: Comparison between the positive inotropic effects of enoximone, a cardiac phosphodiesterase III inhibitor, and dobutamine in patients with moderate to severe congestive heart failure. Eur Heart J 12:985–993, 1991.

Katzung BG and Parmley WW: Cardiac glycosides and other drugs used in the treatment of congestive heart failure. In Katzung BD (ed): Basic and Clinical Pharmacology. Lange Medical Publications, Los Altos, 1982.

Mager G et al: Phosphodiesterase III inhibition or adrenoreceptor stimulation: Milrinone as an alternative to dobutamine in the treatment of severe heart failure. Am Heart J 121:1974–1983, 1991.

McCance KL and Richardson SJ: Structure and function of the cardiovascular and lymphatic systems. In McCance KL and Huether SE (eds): Pathophysiology: The Biologic Basis for Disease in Adults and Children. CV Mosby, St Louis, 1990.

Packer M et al: Effect of oral milrinone on mortality in severe chronic heart failure. N Engl J Med 325:1468–1475, Nov, 1991.

Smith TW and Kelly RA: Therapeutic strategies for CHF in the 1990s. Physiology in Medicine Series. Hosp Pract (Off Ed) 26:127–150, 1991.

Tortora GJ and Grabowski SR: Principles of Anatomy and Physiology, ed 7. HarperCollins, New York, 1993.

Vernon MW, Heel RC, and Brogden RN: Enoximone: A review of its pharmacological properties and therapeutic potential. Drugs 42:997–1017, 1991.

Wood MA and Hess ML: Long-term oral therapy of congestive heart failure with phosphodiesterase inhibitors. Am J Med Sci 297:105–113, 1989.

CHAPTER 19

Antianginals

CHAPTER OUTLINE

CHAPTER OBJECTIVES

After studying this chapter the reader should be able to:

- Describe heart muscle in relation to the balance between oxygen requirements and oxygen supply.
- Describe angina pectoris and differentiate among the following types of angina:
  - classic angina, variant angina, unstable angina.
- Describe the pharmacologic activity of the following nitrates used an antianginals:
  - Nitroglycerin, isosorbide dinitrate, pentaerythritol tetranitrate.
- Briefly outline the mechanism of action of the calcium channel–blocking drugs at cardiac and smooth muscle.
- Describe the pharmacologic activity of the following calcium channel blockers used as antianginals:
  - Verapamil, nifedipine, diltiazem, nicardipine.
- Define cardioselective and explain how β-adrenergic blocking agents produce their antianginal activity.
- Describe the pharmacologic activity of the following beta-blockers used as antianginals:
  - Propranolol, nadolol, metoprolol, atenolol.

KEY TERMS

angina pectoris (an-**JĪ**-na pek-**TOR**-is)

classic angina (effort angina, angina of effort)
unstable angina

variant angina (Prinzmetal's angina, angiospastic angina, vasospastic angina)

CHAPTER INTRODUCTION

Portions of the myocardium can become ischemic when there is an imbalance between oxygen supply and oxygen consumption. The coronary circulation may fail to deliver a sufficient volume of blood or the myocardial oxygen demand may exceed the supply. Either way, the referred pain of myocardial ischemia is acutely felt as an excruciating, crushing sensation in the thorax. *Angina* is derived from the Latin word *an-gere,* which means "to choke." **Angina pectoris,** therefore, is "a choking or strangling of the chest." Depending on the severity of the condition, the relief of anginal symptoms is accomplished through reduction in physical activity, cardiac revascularization surgery (to repair or bypass restricted coronary vessels), or drug therapy.

Drug therapy to relieve angina is directed at increasing the oxygen supply to myocardium, reducing the oxygen demand of the tissue, or both. These goals are accomplished through the use of nitrates or calcium channel blockers, which promote vasodilation, or through the use of beta blockers, which decrease myocardial oxygen demand. This chapter briefly outlines the pathophysiology and classification of angina and examines the different mechanisms of action by which antianginal drugs exert their beneficial effects in ischemic heart muscle.

MYOCARDIAL TISSUE

Characteristics

Compared with other subtypes of muscle tissue, cardiac muscle is unique in several functional respects. First, myocardial cells do not have the luxury of accumulating oxygen debt during strenuous activity. They cannot repay an oxygen debt later, as is the case with skeletal muscle cells. Myocardial cells must be able to handle the metabolic stress of exertion *as it happens*. Accumulated metabolic waste products simply cannot be tolerated in myocardial tissue.

Second, oxygen needs are not only significant, but relatively constant. Heart muscle cells get to "rest" only between beats. Unlike blood flow and oxygen delivery to skeletal muscle, which vary according to blood vessel diameter and metabolic needs, heart muscle cells extract about three quarters of the available oxygen in coronary blood flow even during rest conditions.

Finally, nearly all coronary blood flow occurs during diastole. The time period to complete systole is relatively uniform whether the heart is at rest, beating 60 times per minute, or under stress, contracting at three times that rate. The period of relaxation, however, becomes progressively shorter with increasing heart rate. This allows more contractions to be completed per unit time (Fig. 19–1). Therefore, coronary blood flow and oxygen delivery, by being linked to diastole, are progressively diminished as the heart rate increases.

Intolerance to metabolic wastes, continual and high oxygen demand, and vulnerability to reduced blood flow at faster heart rates add up to a tissue that is particularly susceptible to ischemia. Conditions such as obstructed coronary vessels or exercise-related increases in oxygen demand can further stress mycoardial tissue.

Oxygen Supply and Demand

In terms of myocardial oxygen supply and demand, the key word is *balance*. Supply is handled

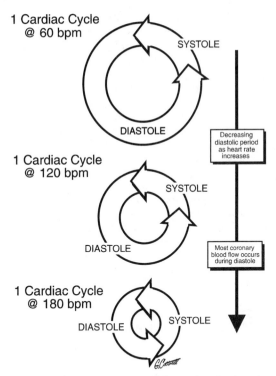

FIGURE 19–1 Schematic—cardiac cycle, showing decreasing diastolic period as heart rate increases.

primarily by coronary blood flow, whereas demand is determined mainly by cardiac activity. Mismatches result from an imbalance between the oxygen available and that consumed during cardiac work. If the imbalance is significant, the suffocating pain of angina immediately appears as the clinical symptom of cardiac ischemia.

Under normal atmospheric conditions, the partial pressure of oxygen delivered to the myocardium by coronary arteries is constant. In addition, extraction of oxygen by the myocardium occurs at near-maximal levels even when the heart is at rest. The only means, therefore, by which an increase in oxygen demand in the myocardium can be met is through an increase in coronary blood flow. Coronary blood flow in turn is inversely proportional to the vascular resistance of coronary blood vessels. Clearly the key to increasing oxygen supply in the myocardium lies in increasing the dilation of coronary blood vessels. Vasodilators termed calcium channel blockers improve coronary blood flow and diminish ischemia. Nitrates also accomplish that goal and are sometimes called "coronary vasodilators." The reference is a misnomer because the vasodilating abilities of the nitrates are not limited to coronary blood vessels. The vasodilating action of nitrates not only increases coronary blood flow to improve oxygen supply, but reduces cardiac preload, thereby lowering ventricular wall stress and reducing myocardial oxygen demand.

The oxygen requirement of the myocardium increases in response to several cardiac changes, especially to increases in heart rate and contractility. In addition to these positive chronotropic and inotropic effects, increases in ventricular wall stress can cause significant increases in myocardial oxygen needs. Elevated arterial pressure and increased ventricular volume are hemodynamic changes capable of increasing ventricular wall stress. All such hemodynamic changes occur in response to exercise and can often trigger an anginal attack in persons with obstructed coronary blood vessels (see Types of Angina below). β-Blockers are useful in reducing oxygen needs because they decrease the activity of the heart. Such antianginal drugs have *negative* chronotropic and inotropic effects. These drugs work by antagonizing norepinephrine at cardiac β1-adrenoceptors.

ANGINA PECTORIS
Types of Angina

Classic Angina

In the majority of patients diagnosed with **classic angina** (also known as **angina of effort**), the perfusion of the myocardium at rest is nominal. The oxygen supply to the heart muscle is adequate to meet the oxygen demand of the organ in a no-stress situation. Adding a physiologic stress such as the effort of exercise, however, exceeds the ability of the supply system to deliver an adequate amount of oxygen. The most common cause of such an imbalance is obstructive artery disease, such as atherosclerosis, which is characterized by the deposition of a plaquelike material on the luminal wall of blood vessels, including the coronary arteries. This is the condition commonly referred to as "hardening of the arteries." It results in reduced flow rates and the inability of blood vessels to expand rather than in an actual "hardening" of the vessel wall. Classic angina is treated mainly by antianginal drugs, such as the nitrates, that decrease myocardial oxygen demand.

Variant Angina

The classic anginal symptom of intense chest pain is present with **variant angina (Prinzmetal's angina).** However, the attack is often prolonged,

occurs cyclically, and is unrelated to effort. The ischemia occurs in the absence of activity and may be accompanied by myocardial infarction and sudden death. In variant angina, the reduced coronary flow is caused by an abrupt spasm of coronary arteries. This **angiospastic,** or **vasospastic,** form of angina is not triggered by an increase in oxygen demand by the myocardium. Variant angina responds well to antianginal drugs, such as the calcium channel blockers, that reduce coronary vascular spasm and improve myocardial oxygen supply.

Unstable Angina

Angina of changing intensity, duration, or frequency is called **unstable angina.** In this type of ischemia, prolonged anginal symptoms occur at rest. Endothelial factors such as the tearing of plaque on the lining of coronary blood vessels, platelet aggregation, and thrombosis are part of the pathogenesis of unstable angina (Boden, 1991; Spinler and Davis, 1991). Spasm of coronary arteries and increased myocardial oxygen demand are both seen with this type of angina. Antianginals such as the nitrates and calcium channel blockers are effective in the management of unstable angina because they simultaneously reduce oxygen demand and increase oxygen supply through improved coronary blood flow. In addition, calcium channel blockers decrease platelet aggregation to help reverse the course of unstable angina. Table 19–1 summarizes the characteristics of different types of angina.

THERAPEUTIC AGENTS
Nitrates

NITROGLYCERIN (GLYCERYL TRINITRATE) (Nitrostat, Nitrolingual, Nitrodisc). Nitroglycerin is the prototype for the vasodilators known as organic nitrates. It was released in 1879 as an antianginal agent and is still a first-line drug used to treat myocardial ischemia. Nitroglycerin is produced by many manufacturers and is available in several formulations, including sublingual, oral, buccal, and transcutaneous forms. Other nitrates (discussed below) are also available in multiple forms. The nitrates are roughly divided into a short-acting and a long-acting group. These classifications reflect the relative rates of absorption of drug rather than basic differences in their pharmacologic activity. As a general guide, a short-acting nitrate, such as sublingual nitroglycerin, has an onset of action of around 1–3 minutes and a duration of action

TABLE 19–1 TYPES OF ANGINA

Type of Angina	Characteristics	Drug Treatment
Classic angina (angina of effort)	Perfusion of myocardium at rest is normal Stress such as exercise exceeds oxygen 　supply system Often associated with atherosclerosis	Nitrates
Variant angina (Prinzmetal's 　angina, angiospastic angina, 　or vasospastic angina)	Angina attack is prolonged, cyclic, and 　unrelated to effort Spasm of coronary arteries	Nitrates Calcium channel blockers
Unstable angina	Prolonged anginal symptoms at rest Changing intensity, duration, or frequency Often associated with vascular effects 　such as plaque release, platelet 　aggregation, thrombosis Coronary artery spasm and increased 　myocardial oxygen demand	Nitrates Calcium channel blockers β-Blockers (used in 　conjunction with 　nitrates)

of 10–30 minutes. Long-acting preparations, such as sustained-action oral forms of nitroglycerin, have a duration of action of around 6–8 hours.

Nitroglycerin and related nitrates are extremely specific, acting at smooth muscle cells with virtually no effect at cardiac or skeletal (striated) muscle cells. All the organic nitrates form, or donate, nitric oxide (NO) in vascular smooth muscle cells. The NO then stimulates guanylate cyclase. The resulting increase in cGMP (cyclic guanosine-3′,5′-monophosphate) activates a protein kinase that decreases the intracellular concentration of free calcium ions in smooth muscle cells. The decrease in intracellular Ca^{2+} causes the relaxation of muscle fibers and promotes vasodilation (Brady et al, 1989; Kukovetz et al, 1991). Inhaled NO shows promise as a *selective* pulmonary vasodilator (Box 21–1). The mechanism of action of nitroglycerin and the nitrates is not fully understood, but does not involve a direct action at autonomic receptors. However, autonomic reflexes such as tachycardia are usually evoked as blood vessels undergo widespread vasodilation (see Precautions below).

The nitrates cause vasodilation of arteries and veins. The vascular smooth muscle–relaxing effect of the nitrates on large-diameter veins is greater than that produced at the arterioles. The resulting venodilation increases venous storage (capacitance) and reduces ventricular preload. This in turn decreases ventricular wall stress and myocardial oxygen needs. Reduction of preload is also beneficial in the restoration of cardiac output in conditions of heart failure (see Chapter 18).

INDICATIONS. Nitrates, such as nitroglycerin, are used to relieve myocardial ischemia in various angina syndromes.

■ Classic, or effort, angina responds to the nitrates through a reduction in myocardial oxygen requirements. This effect is brought about by venodilation leading to venous pooling and reduced venous return to the heart. The reduction in cardiac volume relieves ventricular wall stress and lowers oxygen demand by the heart muscle.
■ Variant, or angiospastic, angina improves following treatment with nitrates because of the vasodilating effect of the drugs on coronary arteries. Vascular spasm is lessened and perfusion of myocardium is improved to relieve the ischemia.
■ Unstable angina responds favorably to nitrates, such as nitroglycerin. This is due to a combined effect of improved oxygen delivery and reduced oxygen demand. Dilation of coronary arteries improves the oxygen supply. Dilation of systemic veins reduces the oxygen demand by decreasing cardiac preload.

In cases of congestive heart failure, nitroglycerin and other nitrates are used in combination with cardiotonics, such as digitalis, to reduce preload and afterload (Chapter 18).

CONTRAINDICATIONS. Because the nitrates effectively reduce vascular resistance and blood pressure through their vasodilating effects, they are contraindicated in patients in shock and in conditions of hypovolemia or hypotension.

PRECAUTIONS. Tachycardia and hypotension are produced by the nitrates. Nitroglycerin and the other nitrates have no *direct* effect on myocardial cells, but an increase in heart rate is routinely noted. The reflex tachycardia occurs through activation of stretch receptors involved in the baroreceptor reflex. Vasodilation caused by the nitrates produces rapid hypotension, which in turn triggers the tachycardia response. Tachycardia may increase oxygen demand and offset some of the benefits derived from nitroglycerin's ability to lower oxygen requirements.

ADVERSE REACTIONS. Undesirable effects of the nitrates are related to their therapeutic vasodilating action. These effects include not only tachycardia as described above, but also orthostatic hypotension, a low blood pressure state exaggerated by postural changes that occur when the patient rises to a standing position from a recumbent, or horizontal, position.

Throbbing, migrainelike headaches can occur following nitroglycerin administration and are due to dilation of cerebral arteries. Vasodilation also produces a characteristic redness ("blush") superior to the clavicles.

Tolerance to headaches caused by the nitrates is seen in patients, but tolerance and cross-tolerance to antianginal effects among the nitrates is a controversial topic. It has been discussed since the introduction of nitroglycerin in the late 19th century, but agreement is still lacking on the concept of tolerance (Box 19–1).

OTHER NITRATES. The pharmacologic ac-tivity of the entire group of nitrates is very similar to that described for nitroglycerin. Differences exist in the available formulations and durations of action of the various members of the group. The differences between short- and long-acting nitrates have already been discussed.

Short-acting formulations of isosorbide dini-trate (Isordil) are used in the acute treatment of an angina attack. Such nitrates can usually alleviate myocardial ischemia within minutes. Prophylaxis of angina is possible with longer-acting forms of nitroglycerin, isosorbide dinitrate, and pentaerythritol tetranitrate, or PETN (Peritrate), a nitrate with a duration of action of 6–8 hours.

Calcium Channel Blockers

VERAPAMIL (Isoptin). The prototype drug of the calcium channel–blocking agents or calcium influx–blocking drugs is verapamil (Isoptin). It was developed from papaverine, a powerful vasodilator found in the opium poppy. The calcium channel blockers have found their place in the treatment of angina pectoris, certain cardiac arrhythmias, and hypertension. These drugs are orally active and have a half-life of approximately 4 hours.

The drugs bind to structures called calcium

BOX 19–1 DYNAMITE AND THE SPLITTING HEADACHE (OR, *IF YOU FEEL AWFUL, IT'S PROBABLY MONDAY!*)

Where volatile organic nitrates, such as nitroglycerin, contaminate the workplace in the explosives industry, workers may be exposed to high levels of the compounds. Munitions workers find that severe headaches and dizziness are common complaints early in the work week, owing to the vasodilation produced by the nitrates. After a couple of days, however, tolerance to the headaches develops and the symptoms disappear. Over the weekend, away from the nitrate exposure, tolerance gradually fades so that the headaches reappear with a vengeance each Monday.

The most serious long-term toxicity problem related to industrial nitrate contamination is the development of physical dependency and the appearance of variant angina, complete with coronary artery vasospasm. This condition typically occurs after a few days away from the nitrate source. After months or years of repeated exposure, a worker might experience the chest pain of angina on Sunday night followed by a migrainelike headache Monday morning. Such a worker, no doubt, looks forward to the middle of the week.

Dependency does not develop with therapeutic doses of the nitrates. In addition, the formulation of "nitro" for medical use is stable and nonexplosive, although nitroglycerin is used in the manufacture of dynamite.

Ben-David A: Cardiac arrest in an explosives factory worker due to withdrawal from nitroglycerin exposure. Am J Ind Med 15:719–722, 1989.

Katzung BG and Chatterjee MB: Vasodilators and the treatment of angina pectoris. In Katzung BD (ed): Basic and Clinical Pharmacology. Lange Medical Publications, Los Altos, 1982.

ion channels located on the muscle cell membrane, and act on the inner side of the membrane to prevent the entry of Ca^{2+} into the muscle cell. By blocking transmembrane Ca^{2+} influx, the drugs are able to halt muscle contraction and produce relaxation in smooth and cardiac muscle cells. (Striated muscle cells have their own intracellular stores of Ca^{2+} and are, therefore, not dependent on extracellular Ca^{2+} for contraction.)

INDICATIONS. Calcium channel blockers, such as verapamil, are useful in the management of angina symptoms, especially variant angina. They are also employed to treat some types of cardiac arrhythmias (Chapter 22). Their effectiveness as antianginals is related to their activity at smooth muscle and at cardiac muscle. For example, vascular smooth muscle is the most sensitive to the effects of calcium influx–blocking drugs, although smooth muscle found in the bronchioles and gastrointestinal tract also undergoes relaxation. Within the vascular smooth muscle group, arterioles are more sensitive than veins, with the result that systemic vascular resistance (SVR) is decreased and ventricular afterload is lessened. This hemodynamic change reduces myocardial oxygen demand and is especially useful in the treatment of classic angina. Calcium channel blockers are important drugs in the treatment of variant angina because they are able to decrease coronary artery tone and thereby improve blood flow to ischemic heart muscle.

Additionally, cardiac muscle contractility and cardiac output are decreased by the calcium channel blockers, as is impulse generation in the sinoatrial (SA) node and conduction in the atrioventricular (AV) node. These effects on cardiac muscle decrease the oxygen requirements of the myocardium and are useful in the treatment of angina.

CONTRAINDICATIONS. Sinus bradycardia can be worsened by the administration of calcium channel blockers. This occurs because cardiac output is decreased further. In a similar fashion, severe cases of congestive heart failure (CHF) can be worsened by the negative inotropic effects of verapamil.

PRECAUTIONS. The calcium influx–blocking drugs must be used with caution in patients with mild CHF. In addition, verapamil can interact with and decrease the activity of digitalis.

ADVERSE REACTIONS. See Toxicity, below.

OTHER CALCIUM CHANNEL BLOCKERS. Other orally active calcium influx–blocking drugs have been developed and are used in antianginal, antihypertensive, and antiarrhythmic therapy. Their pharmacologic activity is similar to that described for verapamil. Clinical differences between the various drugs reflect their relative activity at either cardiac muscle or vascular smooth muscle and their potencies at those calcium channel sites.

Nifedipine (Adalat) produces virtually no depression of cardiac activity at the SA and AV nodes, but is the most potent arteriolar dilator of the calcium channel–blocking agents (Brody et al, 1989). It is able to decrease SVR and ventricular afterload, but may worsen a preexisting condition of hypotension. In addition, nifedipine does not specifically antagonize sympathetic effects at the heart; therefore, reflex tachycardia due to hypotension is more pronounced with this drug than with the other calcium channel blockers.

Diltiazem (Cardizem) is similar to verapamil in that it produces significant blockade at SA and AV nodes. However, it produces less arteriolar dilation than nifedipine. In addition, diltiazem produces more sympathetic antagonism at the heart than verapamil and nifedipine; therefore, reflex tachycardia is very slight. Diltiazem is undergoing clinical trials for possible intravenous use in the management of unstable angina (Boden, 1991).

Nicardipine (Cardene) is a second-generation calcium channel blocker approved for oral use in the United States and under review for intravenous use (Lambert, 1992). It is the most vascular-selective of the calcium channel blockers and is especially well suited for combination therapy with β-blockers in patients having decreased left ventricular function (Lambert, 1992). Such patients require drugs belonging to both classes.

TOXICITY. In conditions of low blood pressure, diltiazem and verapamil may be better tolerated than nifedipine because they produce the least arteriolar dilation. In combination with β-blockers, however, diltiazem or verapamil may produce atrioventricular block due to their pronounced blocking effects at the SA and AV nodes. Nifedipine and nicardipine can be used with more safety in conjunction with β-blockers because they have fewer cardiodepressant effects.

As is outlined above, the effective arteriolar dilating activity of nifedipine or nicardipine can cause a more pronounced fall in blood pressure than the other drugs. Finally, any of the calcium influx inhibitors can worsen heart failure due to negative inotropism, but the potent arteriolar dilating properties of nifedipine or nicardipine may counter some of the effect.

Beta-Blockers

Beta-blockers are used to manage symptoms of angina pectoris, but they are also used in a variety of other pathophysiologic conditions. These uses include the treatment of high blood pressure with β-blockers, such as labetalol (Chapter 21) and the treatment of cardiac arrhythmias with acebutolol (Chapter 22). In addition, some nonselective β-receptor antagonists, such as timolol, are used to reduce the formation of aqueous humor and lower intraocular pressure in certain types of glaucoma. The following section focuses on β-blockers used as antianginal agents.

PROPRANOLOL (Inderal). The prototype for the group of β-adrenergic receptor blockers is propranolol. These drugs are pharmacologic antagonists of norepinephrine and other β-agonists at β-adrenoceptors. The resulting tissue response reflects the occupancy of the receptors by either agonist or antagonist molecules. Propranolol is nonselective in its receptor activity, occupying β_1- and β_2-receptors with equal ease.

Propranolol exhibits negative chronotropic, inotropic, and dromotropic effects on the heart to significantly reduce myocardial oxygen demands. The decrease in heart rate also increases diastolic perfusion time, which has a beneficial effect on myocardial perfusion.

Propranolol significantly lowers blood pressure through several mechanisms acting both centrally and peripherally at the heart and blood vessels, and through blockade of the release of renin from the kidney. These mechanisms for the control of hypertension are examined in Chapter 21.

INDICATIONS. Propranolol is useful in the management of unstable angina in patients who do not respond to routine antianginal therapy, such as sublingual nitroglycerin. Propranolol decreases oxygen demand in the myocardium by reducing heart rate and force. However, propranolol also exhibits detrimental effects in the heart. These effects can be minimized through the concomitant use of nitrates (see Adverse Reactions below).

Additional uses of propranolol include the treatment of hypertension, certain cardiac arrhythmias, and glaucoma.

CONTRAINDICATIONS. Variant angina and angina of effort may be aggravated by propranolol because the drug can increase ventricular wall stress and myocardial oxygen requirements (see Adverse Reactions).

Due to the lack of β-adrenergic receptor specificity, propranolol can block β_2-receptors in the airways. Therefore, it is contraindicated in patients with asthma.

Negative chronotropic and inotropic effects preclude the use of propranolol in CHF.

PRECAUTIONS. A transient rise in blood pressure occurs through blockade of β_2-mediated vasodilation. This leaves α_1-receptors unopposed and free to produce vasoconstriction.

Increased airway resistance is produced by the nonselective β-blockade exhibited by propranolol. The use of cardioselective agents, such as metoprolol, reduces the risk of bronchospasm.

Drugs such as propranolol that have pronounced negative chronotropic and inotropic effects dramatically reduce cardiac output and can trigger congestive heart failure in susceptible persons.

Prolonged use of β-blockers leads to upregulation of β-adrenergic receptors. Therefore, withdrawal of β-blockers is done gradually to avoid cardiac stimulation due to heightened β-adrenoceptor response.

ADVERSE REACTIONS. Undesirable effects of propranolol use are related to its ability to lower heart rate and thereby increase the end-diastolic volume of the heart. The left ventricular volume increase leads to increased ventricular wall stress and increased oxygen consumption. The increase in myocardial oxygen requirement partially negates the beneficial effects resulting from negative chronotropism and inotropism. The undesirable effects of increased oxygen demand can be minimized, however, through the concurrent use of nitroglycerin. Recall that the nitrates lower cardiac preload through their venodilating action, thus reducing wall stress and oxygen demand.

NADOLOL (Corgard). Nadolol is a nonselective β-blocker with pharmacologic activity similar to that of propranolol. It has a long duration of action, with a half-life of 14–24 hours compared with 3–4 hours for propranolol.

INDICATIONS. Treatment of hypertension and angina pectoris are recognized indications for use.

CONTRAINDICATIONS, PRECAUTIONS, AND ADVERSE REACTIONS. See Propranolol.

CARDIOSELECTIVE BETA BLOCKERS. Beta-adrenergic blockers such as metoprolol (Betaloc[CAN], Lopressor[US], Lopresor[CAN]) and atenolol (Tenormin) are relatively selective for cardiac β_1-adrenergic receptors. These antagonists are not pure β_1-adrenoceptor blockers because higher doses elicit β_2-blocking responses. These responses include bronchospasm due to unopposed cholinergic effects and hypertension due to unopposed α-effects in the blood vessels. At lower doses, however, these drugs exhibit a "preference," or selectivity, for cardiac β_1-receptors.

INDICATIONS. See Nadolol.

CONTRAINDICATIONS AND PRECAUTIONS. Because the cardioselective β-blockers exhibit a degree of β_1-specificity, their action at β_2-adrenergic receptors is less pronounced than that seen with the nonselective blockers, such as propranolol and nadolol. For this reason, therapeutic doses of cardioselective blockers, such as metoprolol and atenolol, are better tolerated by asthmatics when β_1-blockade is needed but β_2-blockade obviously is undesirable.

The caution concerning use of β-blockers in CHF applies to the newer cardioselective agents in addition to the prototype propranolol.

ADVERSE REACTIONS. See Propranolol.

Table 19–2 lists the generic and trade names of the antianginals discussed in this chapter.

TABLE 19–2   DRUG NAMES: ANTIANGINALS

Generic Name	Trade Name
NITRATES	
Nitroglycerin (**NI**-trō-**GLIS**-er-in) (glyceryl trinitrate)	Nitrostat, Nitrolingual, Nitrodisc
Isosorbide dinitrate (ī-sō-**SOAR**-bīd)	Isordil
Pentaerythritol tetranitrate (penta-**ERE**-thri-tol)	Peritrate
CALCIUM CHANNEL BLOCKERS	
Verapamil (vir-**RAP**-a-mil)	Isoptin
Nifedipine (nī-**FED**-i-pēn)	Adalat
Diltiazem (dil-**TI**-a-zem)	Cardizem
Nicardipine (nī-**KAR**-di-pēn)	Cardene
β-BLOCKERS	
Nonselective β-blockers (β_1, β_2)	
Propranolol (prō-**PRAN**-o-lol)	Inderal
Nadolol (**NA**-do-lol)	Corgard
Cardioselective β-blockers ($\beta_1 > \beta_2$)	
Metoprolol (me-**TO**-pro-lol)	Betaloc[CAN], Lopressor[US], Lopresor[CAN]
atenolol (a-**TEN**-o-lol)	Tenormin

CHAPTER SUMMARY

Antianginal drugs are employed clinically to reduce myocardial oxygen demand or improve the supply of oxygen. Some antianginals accomplish both tasks. The antianginals discussed in this chapter attain a common therapeutic goal, but do so through different modes of action. The vasodilators, such as nitrates and calcium channel blockers, improve the oxygen supply by dilating blood vessels, including the coronary vessels. In addition, the venodilating effect of the nitrates reduces cardiac preload and thereby reduces myocardial oxygen requirements. Oxygen needs are further reduced by the action of β-blockers which decrease the force of contraction as well as heart rate. β-Blockers also inhibit the renin-angiotensin-aldosterone system to reduce blood pressure and ventricular wall stress, thereby reducing myocardial oxygen consumption.

BIBLIOGRAPHY

Beck RK: Pharmacology for Prehospital Emergency Care. FA Davis, Philadelphia, 1992.

Boden WE: New concepts for the treatment of unstable angina: Role for intravenous diltiazem. J Cardiovasc Pharmacol 18 (Supply 9):S1–S6, 1991.

Brody MJ, Feldman RD, and Hermsmeyer RK: Cardiovascular drugs. In Conn PM and Gebhart GF (eds): Essentials of Pharmacology. FA Davis, Philadelphia, 1989.

Clark WG, Brater DC, and Johnson AR: Goth's Medical Pharmacology, ed 12. CV Mosby, St Louis, 1988.

Hoffman BB: Adrenergic receptor–blocking drugs. In Katzung BD (ed): Basic and Clinical Pharmacology. Lange Medical Publications, Los Altos, 1982.

Katzung BG and Chatterjee MB: Vasodilators and the treatment of angina pectoris. In Katzung BD (ed): Basic and Clinical Pharmacology. Lange Medical Publications, Los Altos, 1982.

Kukovetz WR, Holzmann S, and Schmidt K: Cellular mechanisms of action of therapeutic nitric oxide donors. Eur Heart J 12 (Suppl E):16–24, 1991.

Lambert CR: Combination therapy with nicardipine and beta-adrenergic blockade for angina pectoris. Clin Cardiol 15:231–234, 1992.

Spinler SA and Davis LE: Advances in the treatment of unstable angina pectoris. Clin Pharm 10:825–838, 1991.

Zharov EI et al: Comparative evaluation of intravenous isosorbide dinitrate and nitroglycerin in patients with acute myocardial infarction. Cardiology 79 (Suppl 2):63–69, 1991.

CHAPTER 20

Diuretics

CHAPTER OUTLINE

CHAPTER OBJECTIVES

After studying this chapter the reader should be able to:

- Describe the structure and function of nephrons.
- Describe the following stages of diuresis:
  - Glomerular filtration, tubular reabsorption, tubular secretion.
- Define electrolyte and describe the action of a primary and secondary active transport pump in the transfer of electrolytes in the nephrons.
- Define symporter and antiporter.
- Explain how Na^{1+}, K^{1+}, H^{1+}, Cl^{1-}, and $HCO_3{}^{1-}$ movements in the nephrons affect pH.
- Define the following terms:
  - Natriuretic, saluretic, chloruretic, antikaliuretic, low-ceiling diuretic, high-ceiling diuretic.
- Describe the pharmacologic activity of the carbonic anhydrase inhibitor diuretic acetazolamide.
- Describe the pharmacologic activity of the following thiazide and related diuretics:
  - Chlorothiazide, hydrochlorothiazide, benzthiazide, methyclothiazide.
- Describe the pharmacologic activity of the following loop diuretics:
  - Furosemide, ethacrynic acid, torasemide.
- Describe the pharmacologic activity of the following potassium-sparing diuretics.
  - Spironolactone, triamterene, amiloride.
- Describe the pharmacologic activity of the following osmotic diuretics:
  - Mannitol, urea.

KEY TERMS

antikaliuretic effect (an-tē-**KAL**-i-
  ū-re-tik)
antiporter (countertransport)

Bowman's capsule (glomerular
  capsule)
chloruretic effect (**KLŌR**-ū-re-tik)

collecting duct
distal convoluted tubule
diuresis

CHAPTER INTRODUCTION

The distressed patient experiencing cardiopulmonary symptoms such as dyspnea, pulmonary congestion, or low cardiac output is familiar to most respiratory care practitioners. Nothing reinforces the functional connection between cardiovascular and respiratory systems quite so dramatically. Pathophysiologic conditions of the lungs, circulation, or heart can be involved in a variety of combinations to produce the observed symptoms of labored breathing, cyanosis, and edema. How then does the urinary system fit into this overall scheme, and how are **diuretics,** which act on the kidneys, used to alleviate clinical symptoms involving other organs?

This chapter answers that question by providing an overview of renal physiology focusing on the role of microscopic functional units in the kidneys. The functional overview is followed by discussion of several classes of diuretics used to stimulate urine production. Diuretics are used in cardiovascular conditions such as congestive heart failure and high blood pressure. The diuretic action in the kidneys decreases plasma volume and reduces excess water in the tissues. The resulting reduction in cardiac preload and afterload helps restore normal cardiopulmonary function. Diuretics are invaluable as adjuncts in cardiotonic and antihypertensive therapy. In addition, diuretics are administered to reduce cerebral edema and are also used to prevent renal failure.

apex of a renal pyramid and enters a series of hollow collecting structures within each kidney before being conveyed to the bladder.

Through microscopic branches, each nephron has a vascular connection with the abdominal aorta. The kidneys are highly perfused organs, receiving 20%–25% of the cardiac output. This translates into a flow rate through renal circulation of approximately 1–1.5 L of blood per minute. Therefore, individual nephrons are exposed to a substantial volume of blood in a day's time. (The total blood volume pushed through the entire population of nephrons is around 1500 L/d, enough to fill ten 40-gallon drums!) The nephrons, therefore, have ample opportunity to regulate not only the volume of urine eliminated each day, but also its chemical and physical characteristics. Adjustments can be made to the plasma concentration of constituents such as sodium, potassium, chloride, bicarbonate, and hydrogen ions and to the concentrations of glucose, urea, and uric acid. Diuretics, by modifying the action of nephrons, increase the rate of formation of urine by the kidneys and thereby decrease the volume of plasma remaining in circulation. This action has the effect of lowering total body water and is especially useful in pathophysiologic states such as congestive heart failure and hypertension. These conditions are aggravated by high plasma volumes and respond favorably to the use of diuretics.

THE ROLE OF NEPHRONS

At the microscopic level, the kidney is composed of functional units known as **nephrons.** Cortical nephrons are located within the cortex, or outer layer, of the kidney while juxtamedullary nephrons are found at the interface between the cortex and medulla. Triangular-shaped regions within the medullary, or core, region of the kidney are called renal pyramids and consist of a parallel array of microscopic tubules belonging to many nephrons (Fig. 20–1). Urine leaves the

DIURESIS

Although the constituents found in urine and blood are basically the same, the concentrations of the substances are different. Therefore, in a chemical and physical sense, urine mimics the composition of the blood. This is one of the reasons laboratory urinalysis is such a valuable diagnostic tool in medicine.

We now examine the stages of **diuresis,** the formation of urine. Diuresis depends on three stages: (1) **glomerular filtration,** which initially

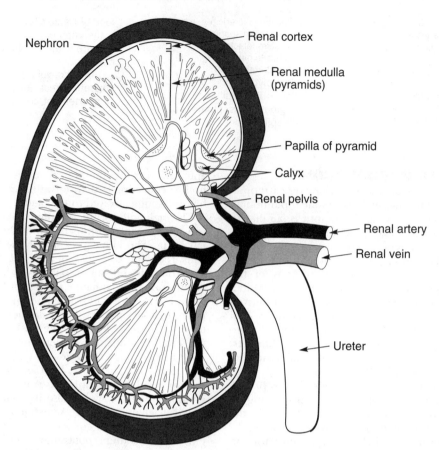

FIGURE 20–1 Structural features of the kidney (frontal section). An individual nephron is depicted in the upper part of the kidney. (From Scanlon VC and Sanders T: Essentials of Anatomy and Physiology. FA Davis Co, 1991, Philadelphia, p. 423, with permission.)

filters blood to form a protein- and erythrocyte-free fluid called *glomerular filtrate,* or *ultrafiltrate,* (2) **tubular reabsorption,** which must follow filtration and is responsible for selectively removing valuable substances such as glucose from the ultrafiltrate and returning them to the bloodstream, and (3) **tubular secretion,** which operates independently of the other two stages and actively transfers substances such as hydrogen ions (H^{1+}) from the bloodstream into the ultrafiltrate. From here they are eliminated with the urine. (See Fig. 20–7 for the locations in the nephron where glomerular filtration, tubular reabsorption, and tubular secretion occur, with the primary sites of action of diuretics.)

Glomerular Filtration

Highly perfused and under approximately twice the pressure of other capillaries in the body, the

glomerular capillaries allow small-diameter substances to leave the bloodstream through pores between endothelial cells. These substances, including a large volume of water (approximately 170 L/d), are also filtered as they pass through pores between adjacent epithelial cells of a hollow spherical structure called the **glomerular capsule (Bowman's capsule)** (Fig. 20–2). Glomerular ultrafiltrate, containing a mixture of valuable products such as water and glucose and waste products such as ammonia and urea, enters the **proximal convoluted tubule** and proceeds to the **loop of the nephron (loop of Henle).** Finally, the ultrafiltrate enters the **distal convoluted tubule** and **collecting duct** to be eliminated. Along the way, important adjustments are made to the concentrations of substances found in the ultrafiltrate. The mechanisms that remove (reabsorb) substances from and those that add (secrete) substances into the ultrafiltrate are discussed below.

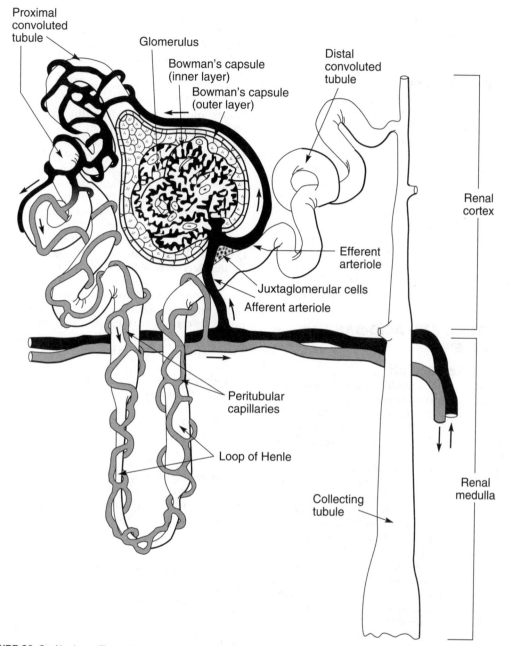

FIGURE 20–2 Nephron. The arrows indicate the direction of blood flow. (From Scanlon VC and Sanders T: Essentials of Anatomy and Physiology. FA Davis Co, Philadelphia, 1991, p. 424, with permission.)

Tubular Reabsorption

Adjustments to the glomerular ultrafiltrate occur as various substances such as water, glucose, and sodium ions (Na^{1+}) are removed from the tubules and returned to the bloodstream (see Fig. 20–7). Movement of substances from the ul-trafiltrate into adjacent blood vessels known as peritubular capillaries is called tubular reabsorption. This represents a recovery step because anything left in the ultrafiltrate "becomes" urine once it leaves the nephron. For something to be reabsorbed from the ultrafiltrate, however, it must have been already filtered. Therefore, tubular reabsorption *must* follow glomerular filtration.

Tubular Secretion

All of the substances to be eliminated by the kidneys do not necessarily enter the ultrafiltrate during glomerular filtration. Some may simply have been missed on a first pass through the glomerular capillaries. These substances, however, can be selectively removed from the peritubular capillaries and transferred into the filtrate for removal. Tubular secretion involves the movement of substances such as H^{1+}, potassium ions (K^{1+}), and ammonia from the plasma into the filtrate (see Fig. 20–7). This stage in diuresis occurs independently of filtration and reabsorption and represents the last opportunity for nephrons to get rid of wastes or make adjustments in the concentration of plasma constituents.

DIURETICS AND ACID-BASE BALANCE

Electrolytes and pH

Electrolytes are substances that separate into ions in aqueous solution and are able to conduct electricity. Because electrolytes are dissolved in and suspended in plasma, the number of electrolytes presented to the kidney is affected by the total fluid load passing from the blood through the kidney. Diuretics can affect overall electrolyte levels in the body by altering the amount of water eliminated by the kidney. Some of the electrolytes are important in homeostasis of pH, therefore, changes in electrolyte levels brought about through diuretic drug action may affect the pH of the blood. For example, the diuretic acetazolamide causes the excretion of bicarbonate ion (HCO_3^{1-}) through the urine. This drug side effect is significant because bicarbonate is one of the most important physiologic buffers of acids. Therefore, the pH of the blood may decrease and metabolic acidosis may occur if excessive numbers of HCO_3^{1-} are eliminated in the urine.

Active Transport Pumps

Different active transport mechanisms are operative in different parts of the nephron. These active transport pumps move electrolytes through cell membranes against concentration gradients. Many diuretics operate by inhibiting these transport pumps.

The primary active transport pump is the Na^{1+}-K^{1+} pump that is discussed at length in Chapter 4. It uses the energy derived from splitting ATP (adenosine triphosphate) to transport Na^{1+} into extracellular fluid and K^{1+} into intracellular fluid.

Secondary active transport pumps rely indirectly on ATP to move substances through membranes. In these mechanisms, the Na^{1+} concentration gradient established by the primary Na^{1+}-K^{1+} pump represents a form of stored energy. Cell membranes are only slightly permeable to Na^{1+}, but secondary active transport pumps provide special pathways for Na^{1+} movement. Sodium ions then follow these pathways and transport other substances through the membrane. In cotransport, or **symporter,** mechanisms, Na^{1+} and other substances move together in the same direction through the membrane. Recovery of filtered substances, such as glucose, is accomplished by symporter mechanisms. Countertransport, or **antiporter,** mechanisms move Na^{1+} and another substance in opposite directions through the membrane. For example, exchange of Na^{1+} for H^{1+} allows H^{1+} to be expelled in the urine while Na^{1+} is recovered.

A diuretic mechanism that interferes with Na^{1+} symporters or antiporters will dramatically affect Na^{1+} availability in the kidney. A change in Na^{1+} concentration can affect both primary and secondary transport pumps. Therefore, Na^{1+} levels influence the levels of electrolytes that normally interact with Na^{1+} in transport mechanisms. We now examine the fate of electrolytes in the kidney and the resulting effect on acid-base balance when these electrolyte levels are altered by diuretics.

Reabsorption of Electrolytes and Water

Sodium ions are a major constituent of glomerular filtrate. The concentration of Na^{1+} in proximal and distal convoluted tubule cells is relatively low and the interior of the cells is negative with respect to the outside. As a result of these gradient conditions, Na^{1+} in the filtrate diffuses passively into the tubule cells. Primary active transport through the action of the sodium pump (also known as the Na^{1+}-K^{1+}-ATPase pump) moves Na^{1+} from the tubule cells into the interstitial fluid around the blood vessels of nephrons. From here, Na^{1+} is reabsorbed into the blood vessels (Fig. 20–3). Potassium ions are transported by the Na^{1+}-K^{1+} pump into the tubule cells as Na^{1+} is expelled. Numerous leakage

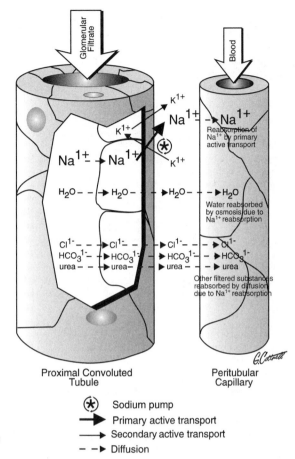

FIGURE 20–3 Primary active transport of Na^{1+} in proximal convoluted tubule.

Sodium pump

➤ Primary active transport

→ Secondary active transport

– –▶ Diffusion

channels for K^{1+}, however, simply allow K^{1+} to diffuse passively back out of the tubule cells. Therefore, reabsorption of Na^{1+} is the overall effect of primary active transport (Tortora and Grabowski, 1993).

Once primary active transport has caused Na^{1+} to be reabsorbed, passive reaborption of water by osmosis occurs. Therefore, water moves from the glomerular filtrate into peritubular capillaries. The loss of water from the filtrate, however, increases the concentration of solutes left behind. This creates a concentration gradient for ions such as chloride (Cl^{1-}) and HCO_3^{1-} and promotes their reabsorption into blood vessels through passive diffusion (Fig. 20–3).

Although not employed clinically as a diuretic drug, caffeine has a well-known diuretic effect. It increases urine output by inhibiting Na^{1+} reabsorption. Carbonic anhydrase inhibitor diuretics, such as acetazolamide, also reduce Na^{1+} reabsorption to inhibit water reabsorption

and promote diuresis. (The role of carbonic anhydrase is discussed below.)

Reabsorption of ions in the loop of the nephron (loop of Henle) occurs through a secondary active transport mechanism. The Na^{1+}-K^{1+}-$2Cl^{1-}$ symporter is a cotransport system that moves one Na^{1+}, one K^{1+}, and two Cl^{1-} from the filtrate into interstitial fluid and the peritubular capillaries (Fig. 20–4). Like other secondary active transport pumps, this symporter depends on the sodium pump to maintain a low Na^{1+} concentration within tubule cells. Leakage channels allow K^{1+} to pass into interstitial fluid and back into the filtrate; therefore, the net effect of this symporter activity is reabsorption of Na^{1+} and Cl^{1-}. Loop diuretics, such as furosemide, inhibit the Na^{1+}-K^{1+}-$2Cl^{1-}$ symporter. This interference with the reabsorption of several ions produces a powerful diuresis. Such diuretics having a high maximal efficacy are called **high-ceiling diuretics.** They promote Cl^{1-} and K^{1+} loss through their mechanism of action and may

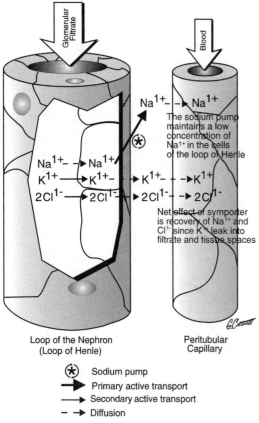

Loop of the Nephron
(Loop of Henle)

Peritubular
Capillary

✱   Sodium pump
➡   Primary active transport
→   Secondary active transport
-→   Diffusion

FIGURE 20–4 Na^{1+}-K^{1+}-$2Cl^{1-}$ symporter in loop of the nephron.

cause hypochloremia and hypokalemia. In addition, *metabolic alkalosis* may develop. This occurs because the large number of Na^{1+} left in the ultrafiltrate exchange for H^{1+}, which are then excreted. Consequently, the urine becomes more acidic and the blood pH becomes greater. (This exchange mechanism is described in the discussion on Secretion, which follows.)

Sodium-chloride (Na^{1+}- Cl^{1+}) symporters operating in distal portions of the nephron continue to bring about reabsorption of Na^{1+}, Cl^{1-}, and water. Thiazide diuretics, such as chlorothiazide, inhibit this Na^{1+}- Cl^{1-} symporter to accelerate fluid loss. These diuretics exhibit low maximal efficacy and are termed **low-ceiling diuretics.** As is outlined above for the loop diuretics, Cl^{1-} or K^{1+} depletion by the thiazide diuretics may lead to hypochloremia and hypokalemia. *Metabolic alkalosis* may occur due to excessive H^{1+} excretion. Table 20–1 shows the percentage of filtered substances reabsorbed in different parts of the nephron.

Secretion of Electrolytes and Control of Blood pH

Final adjustments to K^{1+} levels in the filtrate are made by the cells of the collecting ducts. Here an exchange with Na^{1+} occurs. The movement of K^{1+} into the lumen is due to an electrochemical gradient. As the level of Na^{1+} in the filtrate increases, more K^{1+} is secreted to be eliminated with the urine. This is why so many diuretics exhibit a side effect of K^{1+} depletion. As stated at the outset, most diuretics promote water loss by interfering with Na^{1+} reabsorption. If Na^{1+} re-

TABLE 20–1   REABSORPTION OF FILTERED SUBSTANCES

Filtered Substance	Proximal Convoluted Tubule†‡	Loop of the Nephron‡§	Distal Convoluted Tubule¶**	Collecting Ducts
Na^{1+}	65%	25%	5%	*
K^{1+}	50%	40%	5%	*
Cl^{1-}	50%	25%	20%	*
HCO_3^{1-}	80%–90%	0%	5%	*
Water	65%	15%	15%	*
Nutrients	100%	0%	0%	0%

Data from Tortora and Grabowski, 1993.

*Approximately 95% of all filtered solutes have been returned to the bloodstream. Final adjustments are made in the collecting ducts, especially "fine-tuning" of sodium and water levels by the action of aldosterone and antidiuretic hormone.
†Carbonic anhydrase inhibitor diuretics (eg, acetazolamide)
‡Osmotic diuretics (eg, mannitol)
§Loop diuretics (eg, furosemide)
¶Thiazide diuretics (eg, chlorothiazide)
**Potassium-sparing diuretics (eg, spironolactone)
Cl^{1-}—chloride ion; HCO_3^{1-}—bicarbonate ion; K^{1+}—potassium ion; Na^{1+}—sodium ion.

absorption is inhibited, Na^{1+} remain in the filtrate. Once this filtrate reaches the collecting ducts, the high Na^{1+} concentration triggers the secretion (and loss) of K^{1+}. Potassium-sparing diuretics, such as spironolactone, inhibit aldosterone, and therefore, inhibit this exchange of Na^{1+} and K^{1+}. Aldosterone normally promotes reabsorption of Na^{1+}, passive reabsorption of water, and secretion of K^{1+}. (See Chapter 14.)

Tubule cells adjust urine pH over a wide range (5.0–8.0). This in turn helps maintain normal blood pH within its narrow physiologic range (7.35–7.45). The tubule cells raise blood pH in several ways. With the exception of the osmotic diuretics, such as mannitol, virtually all diuretic drugs interfere with one or more of these renal mechanisms that control blood pH. For this reason, we briefly examine the way in which the kidney maintains blood pH.

First, the tubule cells *acidify* the urine by secreting H^{1+} directly into the filtrate by means of a countertransport mechanism. Sodium-hydrogen (Na^{1+}/H^{1+}) antiporters are secondary active transport pumps that move one H^{1+} into the filtrate in exchange for one Na^{1+} (Fig. 20–5). The H^{1+} are liberated in tubule cells through the dissociation of carbonic acid (H_2CO_3). A di-

uretic that inhibits Na^{1+} reabsorption will produce a filtrate rich in Na^{1+}. These Na^{1+}, therefore, promote secretion of H^{1+}, and the urine becomes acidic, whereas the blood pH is increased. Such a mechanism may result in *metabolic alkalosis*. Hydrogen ions that enter the filtrate through such a mechanism are normally buffered by HCO_3^{1-} to form carbonic acid. Figure 20–5 shows the pathway that results in the reabsorption of HCO_3^{1-} by the peritubular capillaries.

In the distal convoluted tubules, H^{1+} from the dissociation of carbonic acid are secreted directly into the filtrate by a primary active transport pump (Fig. 20–6). Within the filtrate fluid, nearly all the HCO_3^{1-} have already been reabsorbed. However, ammonia (NH_3) is present and is converted to ammonium ion (NH_4^{1+}) by the addition of H^{1+} ($NH_3 + H^{1+} \rightarrow NH_4^{1+}$). Monohydrogen phosphate (HPO_4^{2-}) also serves as an H^{1+} buffer in the filtrate, being converted to dihydrogen phosphate ($H_2PO_4^{1-}$) in the process ($HPO_4^{2-} + H^{1+} \rightarrow H_2PO_4^{1-}$) (Fig. 20–6). In the tubule cells, HCO_3^{1-} from the dissociation of carbonic acid is reabsorbed through the action of a HCO_3^{1-}/Cl^{1-} antiporter (Fig. 20–6).

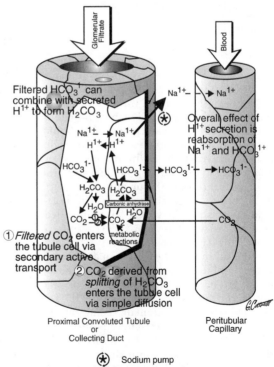

FIGURE 20–5 Na^{1+}/H^{1+} antiporter and reabsorption of HCO_3^{1-} in proximal convoluted tubule.

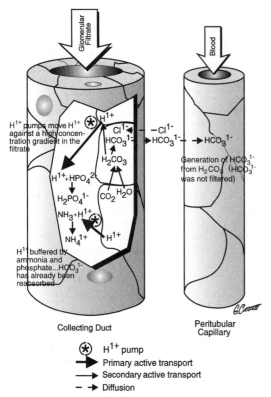

Collecting Duct

Peritubular Capillary

✱ H^{1+} pump
➡ Primary active transport
→ Secondary active transport
- -▸ Diffusion

FIGURE 20–6 Primary active transport of H^{1+}, HCO_3^{1-}/ Cl^{1-} antiporter, and reabsorption of HCO_3^{1-} in distal convoluted tubule.

In addition to secretion of hydrogen ions, tubule cells can raise blood pH through the reabsorption of filtered HCO_3^{1-}. The bicarbonate is generated through the dissociation of carbonic acid. This acid is formed when carbon dioxide from metabolic reactions in the tubule cells or carbon dioxide in the filtrate combines with water in the presence of carbonic anhydrase (Fig. 20–5). Therefore, for each carbonic acid molecule that dissociates, one HCO_3^{1-} is reabsorbed and one H^{1+} is secreted. The HCO_3^{1-} buffers the blood; the H^{1+} exchanges with Na^{1+} and acidifies the urine (Fig. 20–5). When a carbonic anhydrase inhibitor diuretic, such as acetazolamide, is given, there is a decrease in the amount of H^{1+} available for the Na^{1+}/H^{1+} antiporter. Therefore, Na^{1+} remain in the filtrate and exert an osmotic effect. There is also a decrease in HCO_3^{1-} available for reabsorption. In addition, because carbonic anhydrase *in the tubule lumen* is also inhibited by these drugs, filtered HCO_3^{1-} does not combine with H^{1+} to form carbonic acid. As a result, loss of HCO_3^{1-} is a side effect that accompanies the di-

uretic action of carbonic anhydrase inhibitors. *Metabolic acidosis* may occur as a result of this loss of buffering capacity.

In conditions of hypochloremia, there are fewer Cl^{1-} entering the glomerular filtrate from the bloodstream. Therefore, fewer Cl^{1-} are available for cotransport with Na^{1+} by the Na^{1+}-K^{1+}-$2Cl^{1-}$ symporter in the loop of the nephron and the Na^{1+}-Cl^{1-} symporter in the distal parts of the nephron. As a result, Na^{1+} tend to remain in the ultrafiltrate. In the collecting ducts, the countertransport action of the Na^{1+}/H^{1+} antiporter reabsorbs Na^{1+} and moves H^{1+} from the bloodstream into the ultrafiltrate, acidifying the urine. Thus, in a very indirect manner, hypochloremia promotes *metabolic alkalosis*. Similarly, hypokalemia results in fewer K^{1+} available for cotransport out of the ultrafiltrate with Na^{1+} by the Na^{1+}-K^{1+}-$2Cl^{1-}$ symporter. Consequently, the Na^{1+} concentration in the ultrafiltrate remains high. In addition, the Na^{1+} are not able to exchange with K^{1+} in the collecting ducts because the K^{1+} levels are depressed. The Na^{1+}/H^{1+} antiporter, as is described above, exchanges these large numbers of Na^{1+} for H^{1+}, thus producing an acidic urine and raising blood pH. Therefore, in an indirect way, hypokalemia can also bring about *metabolic alkalosis*.

THERAPEUTIC AGENTS

The accumulation of extravascular extracellular fluid is called edema and is a hallmark of low-output conditions, such as heart failure. Diuretics are used to increase the production of urine to bring about a decrease in this extravascular fluid volume. The more fluid is shifted out of the vascular compartment and into the formation of urine, the more fluid can leave the tissue spaces to enter the bloodstream. This fluid shift reduces edema and congestion in the tissues. Thus:

$$\text{tissue fluid} \rightarrow \text{plasma} \rightarrow \text{glomerular filtrate} \rightarrow \text{urine}$$

The concurrent administration of cardiotonics such as digitalis and diuretics such as furosemide reduces edema more effectively than either agent on its own. The cardiotonic improves cardiac output and delivers more blood to the kidneys, and the diuretic increases the formation of urine and unloads excess fluid from circulation (Chapter 18). Diuretics are also employed to reduce plasma volume in hypertension. Antihypertensive drugs are fully discussed in Chapter 21.

Carbonic Anhydrase Inhibitor Diuretics

ACETAZOLAMIDE (Diamox). In the early 1940s it was noted that the chemotherapeutic agent sulfanilamide inhibited carbonic anhydrase in the kidney. Inhibition of this renal cortical enzyme resulted in increased urine output by patients. By the mid-1950s, research had led to the development of acetazolamide, a potent, orally active, and well-tolerated **carbonic anhydrase inhibitor diuretic.** It was the first of the modern diuretics but has been largely replaced by more effective drugs, such as furosemide, a loop diuretic. Acetazolamide inhibits carbonic anhydrase and prevents water and carbon dioxide from combining to produce carbonic acid (Fig. 20–7). With reduced carbonic acid available, fewer H^{1+} and HCO_3^{1-} are produced. This means there is less H^{1+} available for exchange

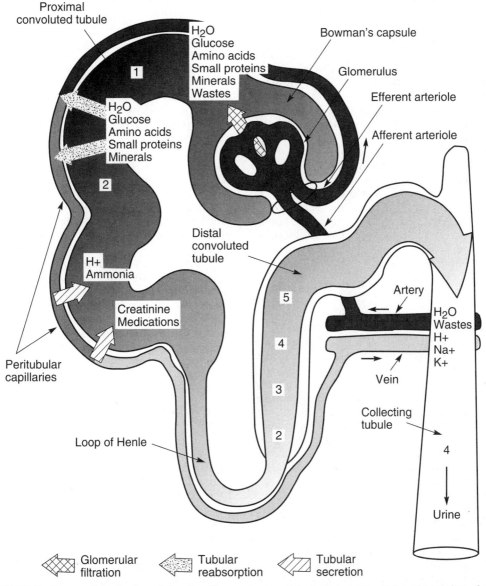

FIGURE 20–7 Primary sites of action of diuretics. The numbers on this diagram represent the primary sites of action of diuretics: 1 = carbonic anhydrase inhibitor diuretics (eg, acetazolamide); 2 = osmotic diuretics (eg, mannitol); 3 = loop diuretics (eg, furosemide); 4 = potassium-sparing diuretics (eg, triamterene); 5 = thiazide diuretics (eg, chlorothiazide). (Modified with permission from Scanlon VC, and Sanders T: Essentials of Anatomy and Physiology. FA Davis Co, Philadelphia, 1991, p. 427.)

with Na^{1+} in the filtrate (Fig. 20–5). The result of the impaired Na^{1+}/H^{1+} antiporter is that Na^{1+} remains in the glomerular filtrate, exerts an osmotic force to move additional water into the filtrate, and produces diuresis. The excretion of Na^{1+} is called a **natriuretic effect.** In addition, HCO_3^{1-} present in the filtrate remains there and is not be able to combine with H^{1+} to form carbonic acid to reenter the tubule cells (Fig. 20–5). As a consequence, urine pH increases and blood pH decreases. The net effect of carbonic anhydrase inhibition is an increase in the excretion of Na^{1+}, K^{1+}, HCO_3^{1-}, and water.

INDICATIONS. The use of acetazolamide as a primary diuretic is no longer widespread. It is, however, used in the treatment of glaucoma. Aqueous humor contains a high concentration of HCO_3^{1-}. Inhibiting carbonic anhydrase reduces the formation of HCO_3^{1-} so that less aqueous humor is formed. This in turn reduces the elevated intraocular pressure of glaucoma.

PRECAUTIONS. Continuous administration of acetazolamide causes so much HCO_3^{1-} to be excreted that a condition of metabolic acidosis may develop. Some acetazolamide is normally reabsorbed by the renal tubules. Such recovery occurs to the least extent under alkaline conditions. Therefore, the acidotic state produced by depressed HCO_3^{1-} levels increases tubular reabsorption of the drug and reduces its effectiveness.

Thiazides and Related Diuretics

CHLOROTHIAZIDE (Diuril). Certain analogues of the chemotherapeutic agent sulfanilamide cause the nephrons to excrete Cl^{1-}. This is known as a **chloruretic effect.** Chlorothiazide (Diuril) is the prototype drug for these **thiazide diuretics.** The oral and parenteral thiazide diuretics act from the luminal side of the tubule. The drugs reach their site of action in the ascending limb of the loop of the nephron through a combination of glomerular filtration and tubular secretion.

Thiazide and related low-ceiling diuretics exhibit a dual effect on the renal tubules. Through inhibition of the Na^{1+}- Cl^{1-} symporter, they reduce solute reabsorption in the distal convoluted tubules. This increases the excretion of Na^{1+}, Cl^{1-}, and water. Additionally, the thiazide diuretics cause mild inhibition of carbonic anhydrase to decrease solute reabsorption in the proximal convoluted tubule (Fig. 20–5).

A natriuretic effect is seen with all the thiazides and is unaffected by urine pH. Dozens of thiazide analogues having different dosages and durations of action have been developed. Hydrochlorothiazide (HydroDIURIL) is very similar to the prototype, and like chlorothiazide has a duration of 6–12 hours. Intermediate-acting thiazides, such as benzthiazide (Aquatag[US]), persist for 12–18 hours. The longer-acting derivatives, such as methyclothiazide (Aquatensen) have a duration of action of 24–48 hours.

INDICATIONS. Thiazide and related diuretics are valuable for treatment of the edematous patient and are often employed with other antihypertensives to lower plasma volume and reduce blood pressure.

CONTRAINDICATIONS. The thiazide diuretics are contraindicated in cases of anuria (decreased urine production) and in patients who are hypersensitive to the thiazides or other sulfonamide derivatives.

PRECAUTIONS. Potassium depletion as a result of K^{1+} excretion in the urine can lead to hypokalemia and metabolic alkalosis with prolonged diuretic therapy. In addition, patients on digitalis therapy are at greater risk for developing digitalis toxicity with concurrent administration of potassium-lowering diuretics. Recall that the mechanism of action of digitalis results in a decrease in intracellular K^{1+} available for exchange with Ca^{2+} (Chapter 18). Potassium-sparing diuretics, such as triamterene, are sometimes used concurrently with the thiazides to reduce K^{1+}-depletion.

ADVERSE REACTIONS. Volume depletion and dehydration are adverse reactions to diuretic therapy. Dizziness, orthostatic hypotension, and severe hypokalemia with muscle weakness may occur with potassium-lowering diuretics.

Loop Diuretics

Diuretics operating from the luminal side of the loop of the nephron are called **loop diuretics** (Fig. 20–7). Representative drugs of this class are furosemide, or frusemide (Lasix) and ethacrynic acid (Edecrin). These high-ceiling diuretics inhibit the Na^{1+}-K^{1+}-$2Cl^{1-}$ symporter to elevate the levels of Na^{1+}, K^{1+}, Cl^{1-}, and water in the filtrate (Fig. 20–4). They are available as oral and parenteral preparations. The loop diuretics are several times more effective than the thiazide group of diuretics.

One of the newer loop diuretics is torasemide (also called torsemide). It differs from furosemide in that it is several times more potent, has a longer duration of action, produces less K^{1+}

and Ca^{2+} depletion, and exhibits relatively mild adverse effects (Friedel and Buckley, 1991). Like the other loop diuretics, torasemide is beneficial in reducing edematous states associated with congestive heart failure (CHF). In addition, when administered at a lower dose than is used in CHF, torasemide is able to control mild-to-moderate hypertension (Achhammer and Metz, 1991).

Unlike the thiazides, the loop diuretics are 95% bound to plasma albumin; therefore, very little glomerular filtration occurs. The drugs reach their site of action in the loop of the nephron by means of secretion at the proximal segments of the renal tubules. Loop diuretics decrease the ability of the nephrons to concentrate urine. Therefore, a high volume of urine with low specific gravity is produced. Loop diuretics increase the excretion of electrolytes and depress the ability of the collecting ducts to reabsorb water.

INDICATIONS. Uses for the loop diuretics are basically the same as those discussed for the diuretics in general, namely, reduction of fluid accumulation in the edematous patient. Patients with hypertension or heart failure not controlled by the low-ceiling thiazide diuretics may respond to the more potent high-ceiling loop diuretics.

PRECAUTIONS AND ADVERSE REACTIONS. See Chlorothiazide.

Potassium-Sparing Diuretics

All of the diuretics discussed so far stimulate urine production by promoting the excretion of sodium chloride from the bloodstream. Such drugs are said to have a **saluretic effect.** They also cause a corresponding increase in K^{1+} excretion, which is why their use can often lead to hypokalemia. Drugs called **potassium-sparing diuretics** have been developed that increase Na^{1+} excretion by inhibiting its exchange with K^{1+}. This inhibition takes place in the distal convoluted tubule (Fig. 20–7). The action of preventing potassium depletion is called an **antikaliuretic effect.** Potassium-sparing diuretics are well suited for patients taking digitalis preparations concurrently. Hypokalemia is a predisposing factor in cardiac arrhythmias and is aggravated by digitalis therapy. Potassium-sparing diuretics counter the K^{1+} depletion caused by other types of diuretics. Two types of potassium-sparing diuretics exist: aldosterone antagonists and direct-acting agents that inhibit Na^{1+} reabsorption and secondary K^{1+} secretion.

Aldosterone Antagonists

SPIRONOLACTONE (Aldactone). Aldosterone is a steroid hormone produced by the adrenal cortex. Control of aldosterone secretion is detailed in the following chapter. At this point it will suffice to say that aldosterone is produced in response to hypotension or to low plasma levels of Na^{1+}. Aldosterone targets the nephrons, causing them to reabsorb Na^{1+} from the filtrate. As Na^{1+} reenter the bloodstream, they cause additional water to be reabsorbed, thus expanding the plasma volume and restoring blood pressure. Spironolactone is structurally similar to aldosterone and pharmacologically antagonizes the hormone, thus blocking Na^{1+} reabsorption. As a result, there is an increase in Na^{1+} and Cl^{1-} excretion and a decrease in K^{1+} excretion. The diuresis is slow to develop and is sustained, but is not as great as that produced by other classes of diuretics.

INDICATIONS. Hypertension caused by renin-induced aldosterone secretion responds favorably to aldosterone antagonist diuretics (Box 20–1). The renin-angiotensin-aldosterone mechanism of blood pressure control is covered in Chapter 21.

PRECAUTIONS. A normal caution with the potassium-sparing diuretics is excessive K^{1+} retention leading to hyperkalemia.

Direct-Acting Potassium-Sparing Agents

The diuretics acting directly on distal tubules to inhibit Na^{1+} reabsorption (saluretic effect) and K^{1+} secretion (antikaliuretic effect) do not depend on aldosterone. As a result, they are more reliable potassium-sparing diuretics than spironolactone. In contrast to spironolactone, the direct-acting agents produce rapid diuresis.

Direct-acting antikaliuretics such as triamterene (Dyrenium) and amiloride (Midamor) are active from the luminal side of the distal tubules and reach their site of action by being filtered at the glomeruli and secreted by the proximal tubules. In general, the direct-acting potassium-sparing diuretics are less active than the thiazides, such as chlorothiazide. Combination products such as Moduretic contain amiloride combined with hydrochlorothiazide. Such combination drugs provide an enhanced saluretic action while minimizing the change in plasma K^{1+} concentration. The thiazide in Moduretic tends to produce hypokalemia, but it is offset by the antikaliuretic produced by the potassium-sparing diuretic.

INDICATIONS. Uses such as the treatment of edematous states associated with heart failure

BOX 20-1 A DIURETIC FROM THE HEART?

Several naturally occurring hormones have an antidiuretic effect. Aldosterone, secreted by the adrenal cortex, stimulates Na^{1+} reabsorption and passive reabsorption of water. Antidiuretic hormone is produced by the hypothalamus and causes water reabsorption. Angiotensin II, derived from a plasma precursor under renin control, causes the release of both aldosterone and antidiuretic hormone. All of these hormones function to conserve body water. In the mid-1980s, however, a *diuretic hormone* was discovered—a natural substance that actually promotes fluid loss. Atriopeptin, or atrial natriuretic peptide (ANP), is released from the walls of the atria in response to stretching of the heart. The degree of stretch is proportional to the plasma volume and blood pressure. Atriopeptin promotes diuresis through several mechanisms. These include an increase in glomerular filtration rate and inhibition of secretion of the hormones that normally oppose diuresis—aldosterone, antidiuretic hormone, and renin. By causing the elimination of water and Na^{1+}, ANP lowers plasma volume, reduces stretching of the heart wall, and restores normal blood pressure. Research into the clinical use of this natural diuretic is being carried out.

Carola R, Harley JP, and Noback CR: Human Anatomy and Physiology, ed 2. McGraw-Hill, New York, 1992.

Goodman JM et al: Atrial natriuretic peptide during acute and prolonged exercise in well-trained men. Int J Sports Med 14:185–190, 1992.

Tortora GJ and Grabowski SR: Principles of Anatomy and Physiology, ed 7. HarperCollins, New York, 1993.

TABLE 20-2 DIURETICS: SUMMARY

Diuretic	Site of Action	Mechanism of Action	Effects Produced*
Carbonic anhydrase inhibitor diuretics (eg, acetazolamide)	PCT	Inhibition of carbonic anhydrase reduces amount of H^{1+} and HCO_3^{1-} produced Reduced H^{1+} impairs the Na^{1+}/H^{1+} antiporter; excretion of Na^{1+} exerts an osmotic effect to produce diuresis	Diuretic effect Natriuretic effect Alkalinization of urine
Thiazide diuretics (eg, chlorothiazide)	DCT	Inhibition of Na^{1+}-Cl^{1-} symporter reduces solute reabsorption to increase excretion of Na^{1+}, Cl^{1-}, and water Mild carbonic anhydrase inhibition	Diuretic effect Natriuretic effect Chloruretic effect
Loop diuretics (eg, furosemide)	Loop	Inhibition of Na^{1+}-K^{1+}-$2Cl^{1-}$ symporter elevates concentration of Na^{1+}, K^{1+}, Cl^{1-}, and water in the filtrate to produce diuresis	Diuretic effect Natriuretic effect Chloruretic effect Kaliuretic effect
Potassium-sparing diuretics (eg, spironolactone)	DCT CD	Pharmacologic antagonism of aldosterone inhibits Na^{1+} reabsorption; Na^{1+} and Cl^{1-} are excreted and K^{1+} is retained	Diuretic effect Natriuretic effect Chloruretic effect Antikaliuretic effect
(eg, triamterene)	DCT CD	Direct acting (aldosterone independent) Inhibition of Na^{1+} reabsorption Inhibition of K^{1+} secretion	Diuretic effect Natriuretic effect Antikaliuretic effect
Osmostic diuretics (eg, mannitol)	PCT Loop	Freely filtered Undergo limited reabsorption Exert a direct osmotic effect on the nephrons without drastically changing plasma Na^{1+} levels	Diuretic effect

*A combined natriuretic and chloruretic effect is known as a **saluretic effect.**
CD—collecting duct; Cl^{1-}—chloride ion; DCT—distal convoluted tubule; H^{1+}—hydrogen ion; HCO_3^{1-}—bicarbonate ion; K^{1+}—potassium ion; Loop—loop of the nephron (loop of Henle); Na^{1+}—sodium ion; PCT—proximal convoluted tubule.

apply to the direct-acting potassium-sparing diuretics. These indications have been described for the diuretics in general.

CONTRAINDICATIONS. See Spironolactone.

Osmotic Diuretics

MANNITOL (Osmitrol). When there is need to increase urine output but not cause an increase in the loss of Na^{1+}, **osmotic diuretics** are commonly employed. Agents such as mannitol are freely filtered at the glomerulus, undergo very limited tubular reabsorption, and are relatively resistant to metabolic change (see Fig. 20–7). As a result, osmotic diuretics may be administered in large quantities, increasing the fluid volume in the tubules and maintaining the rate of flow of relatively dilute urine. Mannitol must be administered intravenously because it is very hydrophilic and is not absorbed from the gastrointestinal tract.

INDICATIONS. Prophylaxis of acute renal failure during surgery or in response to severe trauma is one of the most important indications for use of mannitol.

Mannitol is also employed in neurosurgery because it does not penetrate the blood-brain barrier. Through its osmotic effect, mannitol causes water to leave the central nervous system. This fluid shift reduces the pressure and volume of cerebrospinal fluid and thus decreases cerebral edema.

The excretion of poisonous substances can be enhanced through the action of osmotic diuretics. Drugs such as mannitol prevent the concentration of toxic substances from reaching high levels in the glomerular filtrate. This occurs because the diuretic action promotes a steady flow of relatively dilute urine.

CONTRAINDICATIONS. Because mannitol is distributed in the extracellular fluid (ECF), high volumes are capable of shifting water from the intracellular to the extracellular fluid compartment. This shift may expand the volume of the ECF and aggravate cases of pulmonary congestion or edema. The shift may also worsen a condition of severe dehydration. Severe renal disease accompanied by anuria is also a contraindication for mannitol use.

UREA (Ureaphil). Like mannitol, urea is poorly reabsorbed in the kidney tubules and exerts an osmotic effect on tubular fluid. Adequate urine flow without a corresponding decrease in plasma levels of Na^{1+} is maintained by this mechanism. Urea is more irritating to the tissues than mannitol.

INDICATIONS. Maintenance of renal function and prevention of cerebral edema during neu-

TABLE 20–3 DRUG NAMES: DIURETICS

Generic Name	Trade Name
THIAZIDES AND RELATED DIURETICS	
Chlorothiazide (klōr-ō-**THĪ**-a-zīd)	Diuril
Hydrochlorothiazide	HydroDIURIL
Benzthiazide	Aquatag^us
Methyclothiazide	Aquatensen
LOOP DIURETICS	
Furosemide (fyoo-**RŌS**-i-mīd)	Lasix
Ethacrynic acid (eth-a-**KRIN**-ik)	Edecrin
Torasemide (tōr-**AS**-se-mīd)	
POTASSIUM-SPARING DIURETICS	
Spironolactone (spī-**RŌN**-ō-lak-tōn)	Aldactone
Triamterene (trī-**AM**-ter-ēn)	Dyrenium
Amiloride (a-**MIL**-ō-rīd)	Midamor
CARBONIC ANHYDRASE INHIBITOR DIURETICS	
Acetazolamide (a-sē-ta-**ZOL**-a-mīd)	Diamox
COMBINATION PRODUCTS	
Hydrochlorothiazide + amiloride	Moduretic
OSMOTIC DIURETICS	
Mannitol	Osmitrol
Urea	Ureaphil

rosurgery are the main indications for use of urea.

CONTRAINDICATIONS. See Mannitol.

OLDER DIURETICS. Acid-forming salts such as ammonium chloride (NH_4Cl) once served as osmotic diuretics but are now obsolete. Instead, such drugs are now used to correct metabolic alkalosis, especially in edematous patients. Following absorption, the ammonium ion (NH_4^{1+}) is converted to urea in the liver, thus freeing H^{1+} which lower the pH. Mercurial diuretics are obsolete. Xanthines are not employed as diuretics but promote urine formation through their positive inotropic and vasodilating actions (see Theophylline in Chapter 13).

Figure 20–7 shows several locations in the nephron where diuretics exert their action. Table 20–2 summarizes the type of diuretic effect produced, the site of action, and the mechanism of action for the classes of diuretics introduced in this chapter. The generic and trade names of the diuretics discussed in this chapter are listed in Table 20–3.

CHAPTER SUMMARY

This chapter examines three basic areas pertaining to the diuretics: an overview of nephron structure, the stages of diuresis and the mechanisms involved in reabsorption, secretion, and maintenance of pH, and the clinical uses of diuretics. Their uses include the treatment of cardiovascular conditions such as heart failure and hypertension. Noncardiovascular uses of diuretics include reduction of intracerebral pressure and reduction of intraocular pressure. Diuretics are also employed in cases of renal failure, but for our purposes, an understanding of cardiopulmonary applications is the most relevant.

Most diuretics, through a variety of mechanisms, accelerate the excretion of ions, especially sodium ions. This electrolyte movement exerts an osmotic effect in the kidney to increase the output of urine and lower the plasma volume. Decreased plasma volume then reduces extravascular fluid levels to alleviate the edema associated with congestive heart failure and pulmonary edema. Decreased plasma volume also reduces hypertension. By decreasing excessive fluid loads, diuretics improve cardiopulmonary performance.

BIBLIOGRAPHY

Achhammer I and Metz P: Low dose loop diuretics in essential hypertension: Experience with torasemide. Drugs 41 (Suppl 3):80–91, 1991.

Clark WG, Brater DC, and Johnson AR: Goth's Medical Pharmacology, ed 12. CV Mosby, St Louis, 1988.

Friedel HA and Buckley MM: Torasemide: A review of its pharmacological properties and therapeutic potential. Drugs 41:81–103, 1991.

Garca-Puig J et al: Hydrochlorothiazide versus spironolactone: Long-term metabolic modifications in patients with essential hypertension. J Clin Pharmacol 31:455–461, 1991.

Kruck F: Acute and long term effects of loop diuretics in heart failure. Drugs 41 (Suppl 3):60–68, 1991.

Mudge GHZ: Agents affecting volume and composition of body fluids. In Goodman AG et al (eds): Goodman and Gilman's The Pharmacologic Basis of Therapeutics, ed 7. Macmillan, New York, 1985.

Tortora GJ and Grabowski SR: Principles of Anatomy and Physiology, ed 7. HarperCollins, New York, 1993.

Warnock DG: Diuretics. In Katzung BD (ed): Basic and Clinical Pharmacology. Lange Medical Publications, Los Altos, 1982.

Weiner IM and Mudge GH: Diuretics and other agents employed in the mobilization of edema fluid. In Goodman AG et al (eds): Goodman and Gilman's The Pharmacologic Basis of Therapeutics, ed 7. Macmillan, New York, 1985.

Williamson HE: Diuretics and uricosuric drugs. In Conn PM and Gebhart GF (eds): Essentials of Pharmacology. FA Davis, Philadelphia, 1989.

CHAPTER 21

Antihypertensives

CHAPTER OUTLINE

CHAPTER OBJECTIVES

After studying this chapter the reader should be able to:

- Explain the differences between hypertension and essential hypertension.
- List two therapies described as nondrug treatment of hypertension.
- Define cardiac output (C.O.) and systemic vascular resistance (SVR) and describe the interrelated hemodynamic factors that control normal arterial blood pressure.
- List four anatomic sites at which antihypertensive drugs may act to lower elevated blood pressure.
- Describe the baroreceptor reflex and renin-angiotensin-aldosterone mechanisms for the control of blood pressure.
- Explain why combination antihypertensive therapy is more effective than treatment with a single antihypertensive agent.
- Describe how diuretics lower elevated blood pressure.
- Describe the pharmacologic activity of the following diuretics:
  - Thiazide diuretics, loop diuretics, and potassium-sparing diuretics.
- Define sympatholytic and describe how sympatholytics can lower blood pressure.
- Describe the pharmacologic activity of the following sympatholytics:
  - Methyldopa, clonidine, propranolol, nadolol, labetalol, metoprolol, atenolol, prazosin, terazosin, doxazosin.
- Describe how vasodilators can lower blood pressure.
- Describe the pharmacologic activity of the following vasodilators:
  - Hydralazine, minoxidil, nitroprusside, diazoxide, verapamil, nifedipine, diltiazem, nicardipine.
- Describe how an angiotensin-converting enzyme (ACE) inhibitor can lower blood pressure.
- Describe the pharmacologic activity of the following ACE inhibitors:
  - Captopril, enalapril, perindopril.

KEY TERMS

angiotensin-converting enzyme
  (ACE)
antihypertensives
  ACE inhibitor
  diuretic

sympatholytic
vasodilator
baroreceptor reflex
  (pressoreceptor reflex)

essential hypertension
renin-angiotensin-aldosterone
  mechanism

CHAPTER INTRODUCTION

The **antihypertensives** are a diverse group of drugs used to control elevated arterial blood pressure. Included in the therapeutic classification are diuretics, sympatholytics, vasodilators, and angiotensin-converting enzyme (ACE) inhibitors. Some of these drug classes, such as the diuretics and vasodilators, have been introduced in previous chapters, where their use in the treatment of congestive heart failure and angina pectoris is discussed.

In hypertensive individuals, the risk of damage to organ systems is directly proportional to the extent of blood pressure elevation. Therefore, the antihypertensive drugs play a vital role in lowering blood pressure. The risk of adverse effects is high with treatment because antihypertensives interfere with normal hemodynamic mechanisms. However, the risks of untreated hypertension are even greater.

HYPERTENSION

Characteristics of Hypertension

Elevated arterial pressure, or hypertension, is described as a "silent killer." It is almost always asymptomatic. Most hypertensive individuals are unaware of the insidious changes in their own bodies. Diagnosis is based on measurement of blood pressure, with readings taken repeatedly and showing consistently elevated arterial pressure. Mild hypertension in a young or middle-aged adult increases the risk of eventual damage to the heart, brain, or kidneys. Epidemiologic studies reveal positive risk factors such as excessive salt intake, smoking, hyperlipidemia, diabetes, or a family history of hypertension. In addition, the risk of eventual damage at any elevated pressure or age is greater in black patients and is somewhat less in premenopausal women than in men.

Nondrug Versus Drug Therapy

Once a positive diagnosis is made, the urgency of initiating treatment varies directly with the amount of blood pressure elevation. Some patients with mild hypertension respond dramati-

cally and favorably to nondrug therapy, including dietary salt restriction, weight reduction, and exercise. Others require a single vasodilator antihypertensive agent to reduce vascular resistance. Most require concurrent administration of several antihypertensives, such as vasodilators, β-adrenergic blockers, and diuretics, as is discussed below. Whatever treatment route is selected, patient compliance with the prescribed regimen often becomes a major problem for several reasons: (1) The disease is usually asymptomatic, (2) therapy is normally long term and provides no direct relief, and (3) the benefits of present treatment lie in preventing organ damage and death at some future date.

Causes of Hypertension

When a diagnosis of hypertension is made, there is usally no indication of the possible cause. Specific causes are known in only about 10% of hypertensive cases. For instance, renal artery constriction is a cause of hypertension that can be surgically corrected, whereas pheochromocytoma and hyperaldosteronism can be treated pharmacologically. In most patients, however, no specific abnormalities exist in autonomic nervous system function, the baroreceptor reflex, the kidneys, or the renin-angiotensin-aldosterone pathway. These patients are diagnosed as having **essential hypertension.** The term originally reflected the thinking that hypertension was *essential* in pathologic states—that an elevated arterial pressure was absolutely necessary to push blood through diseased tissues. It is now known, however, that elevated pressure is not needed for adequate perfusion of such tissues. Instead, the term conveys the fact that *essentially* little is known about the cause of most cases (90%) of hypertension (Benowitz and Bourne, 1982).

PHYSIOLOGIC CONTROL OF BLOOD PRESSURE

Compensatory Changes

Maintenance of optimal arterial blood pressure is required for the perfusion of body tissues.

Blood pressure (BP) is determined by both cardiac output (C.O.) and systemic vascular resistance (SVR), which is the resistance to blood flow through precapillary arterioles:

$$BP = C.O. \times SVR$$

As has been discussed with the cardiotonics in Chapter 18, cardiac output is varied by heart rate and stroke volume. Stroke volume in turn may be altered by blood volume or by venous capacitance tone. SVR may be varied by changes in arteriolar tone (see Fig. 18–1).

One of the conclusions to be drawn from such an interdependent mechanism is that a change in one factor may be countered by a change in several others to result in maintenance of the same blood pressure. For example, if venous capacitance tone decreases through dilation of postcapillary venules, or plasma volume decreases through hemorrhage or elimination of fluid by the kidney, there is a corresponding decrease in venous return. As a result of the Starling mechanism, the stroke volume decreases, which in turn decreases cardiac output. This hypotensive change may be minimized, however, by an immediate increase in systemic vascular resistance. The increase in SVR may occur as a result of an increase in vascular tone of precapillary arterioles or an antidiuretic effect in the kidney. There are several such compensatory negative feedback loops operating in the body to maintain homeostasis of arterial blood pressure.

Blood pressure in both normotensive and hypertensive individuals is controlled at four anatomic sites (Fig. 21–1):

- Precapillary arterioles (resistance vessels)
- Postcapillary venules (capacitance or storage vessels)
- Heart
- Kidney

Antihypertensive drugs act at one or more of these locations to restore blood pressure to its normal range.

Baroreceptor Mechanism

Continual blood pressure adjustments are carried out on a minute-to-minute basis by the **baro-**

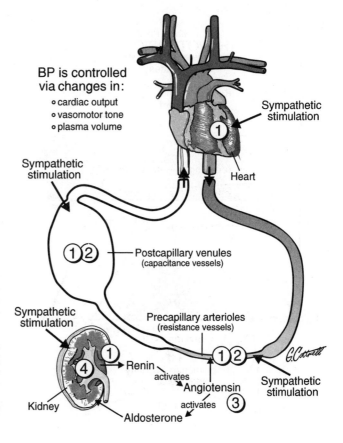

FIGURE 21–1 Control of blood pressure and antihypertensive sites of action. The numbers on the diagram represent the sites of action of antihypertensive drugs: 1 = sympatholytics—β-blockers reduce reflex tachycardia, reduce systemic vascular resistance (SVR), and reduce renin release; α_1-blockers reduce SVR; 2 = vasodilators—reduce SVR; 3 = ACE inhibitors—inhibit angiotensin, thereby reducing SVR and plasma volume expansion (see Fig. 21–2 for details of ACE inhibitor action); 4 = diuretics—reduce plasma volume expansion.

BP is controlled via changes in:
- cardiac output
- vasomotor tone
- plasma volume

Sympathetic stimulation

Sympathetic stimulation

Heart

① ② Postcapillary venules (capacitance vessels)

Sympathetic stimulation

Precapillary arterioles (resistance vessels)

① ②

Sympathetic stimulation

① Renin activates

Angiotensin

④

activates ③

Kidney

Aldosterone

receptor reflex, or **pressoreceptor reflex.** If blood pressure falls as a result of some other blood pressure–lowering mechanism, baroreceptors respond to the relative lack of stretch of major arterial walls and send sensory impulses into the central nervous system (CNS). Cardiac centers and vasomotor centers of the medulla respond by firing motor impulses to the heart and the capacitance vessels (venules). This nervous system activity stimulates the heart and increases venous return and increases cardiac output. Neural impulses are also sent to resistance vessels (arterioles) to increase SVR and thereby restore blood pressure.

Renal Mechanism

Long-term control of blood pressure is accomplished through alteration of plasma volume by the **renin-angiotensin-aldosterone mechanism** (Fig. 21–2). When the perfusion through renal arteries decreases with falling systemic blood pressure, the kidneys begin to reabsorb more salt and water to restore plasma volume and blood pressure. Additionally, *juxtaglomerular cells* in the kidneys respond to low blood pressure by secreting renin (see Fig. 20–2), which results in the production of angiotensin II. This plasma-derived substance has a direct vasoconstrictor effect on resistance vessels to increase SVR, and an indirect effect on plasma volume through stimulation of aldosterone release from the adrenal cortex. The potent mineralocorticoid action of aldosterone causes increased sodium (Na^{1+}) and water reabsorption, which decreases urine production and expands plasma volume. Restored plasma volume increases venous return and stroke volume, thereby increasing cardiac output and blood pressure. This mechanism is further explained with the antihypertensives

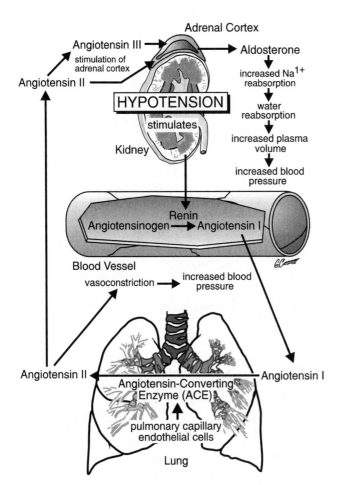

FIGURE 21–2 Schematic—renin-angiotensin-aldosterone mechanism.

known as angiotensin-converting enzyme (ACE) inhibitors. These drugs are discussed later in the chapter.

ANTIHYPERTENSIVE THERAPY

It should be obvious from the preceding section that an antihypertensive drug that suppresses a specific blood pressure–controlling mechanism may simply activate a compensatory mechanism. For example, if a diuretic is used on its own as an antihypertensive agent, it initially reduces plasma volume through increased urine output. The reduced blood pressure, however, activates the renin-angiotensin-aldosterone mechanism, which responds by causing the kidney to conserve fluid. Similarly, vasodilators used alone as antihypertensives cause a decrease in arteriolar tone and blood pressure. This decrease in turn activates the baroreceptor reflex to increase heart rate and cardiac output and raise blood pressure. The result of such monotherapy with antihypertensive drugs often is the continuation of elevated blood pressure *in spite of treatment.*

To maximize antihypertensive effects in moderate to severe hypertension, combination therapy is used. With multidrug therapy, each drug can influence a different element of the hemodynamic control system outlined above. For example, a direct vasodilator, such as hydralazine, is given to lower systemic vascular resistance, and a β-adrenergic blocker, such as propranolol, is administered to prevent reflex tachycardia. In addition, a diuretic, such as chlorothiazide, is given to prevent plasma volume expansion. Antihypertensive combination therapy is a rational approach to the control of hypertension because a compensatory mechanism can be blocked to assist the pharmacologic activity of a different antihypertensive drug.

THERAPEUTIC AGENTS

Diuretics

Following nondrug therapy, the introduction of **diuretics** may provide the desired blood pressure control (Fig. 21–1). In cases of essential hypertension, the maximal antihypertensive effect generated by diuretic monotherapy is relatively mild. However, it is actually greater than it appears because several of the compensatory mechanisms outlined above are activated by the fall in plasma volume caused by the natriuretic action of most diuretics. These pressor systems include neural mechanisms that increase SVR through an increase in sympathetic vascular

tone, and humoral mechanisms that trigger angiotensin production. In addition, antidiuretic hormone produced by the hypothalamus acts directly on the kidneys, causing them to reabsorb water and thus restore plasma volume.

For mild-to-moderate hypertension, diuretics alone are capable of decreasing blood pressure to provide satisfactory control. In severe hypertension, multidrug therapy with sympatholytic and vasodilator drugs is employed to maximize the volume-depleting action of diuretics. Drugs such as vasodilators decrease vascular responsiveness, or the ability of blood vessels to alter their diameter in response to neural impulses or other stimuli. As a result, blood pressure is intimately linked to blood volume. With the vascular response blunted, a fall in plasma volume brought about by diuretic action translates directly into a fall in blood pressure.

Low-ceiling diuretics, such as the thiazides (chlorothiazide), are well suited for patients with normal renal and cardiac function and mild-to-moderate hypertension. Severe hypertension requires the use of high-ceiling diuretics, such as the loop diuretics (furosemide). These diuretics are also indicated in patients with renal insufficiency or cardiac failure where Na^{1+} retention is marked. Loop diuretics are valuable in combination therapy when sodium-retaining drugs, such as vasodilators, are used. Potassium-sparing diuretics (spironolactone) enhance the natriuretic effect and counter the potassium (K^{1+}) depletion caused by other diuretics. Sites and mechanisms of action and other pharmacologic aspects of the diuretics are discussed fully in Chapter 20.

Sympatholytics

Drugs that block sympathetic nervous system function are called **sympatholytics.** Sympatholytic agents can interfere with neurotransmission at several locations along the sympathetic reflex arc. These locations include the CNS, autonomic ganglia, sympathetic nerve endings, and adrenergic receptors. Interference at some of these sites produces unwanted side effects, such as CNS sedation or parasympathetic ganglionic blockade.

Because of the compensatory mechanisms already discussed, it should be apparent that a sympatholytic is most effective when combined with an antihypertensive that does not operate through adrenergic nerves. For example, diuretics inhibit the Na^{1+} retention and plasma volume expansion that are triggered by a compensatory response to the sympatholytics. Sympatholytics are classified as centrally and peripherally acting agents.

Centrally Acting Sympatholytics

METHYLDOPA (Aldomet). Methyldopa is an analogue of L-dopa and is administered as a prodrug, or an inactive form that is metabolized into an active substance. The metabolic activation of methyldopa results in the production of the active metabolite α-methylnorepinephrine.

Two mechanisms are involved with the antihypertensive effects of methyldopa acting through α-methylnorepinephrine. First, reduction of sympathetic outflow from vasomotor centers in the medulla allows peripheral blood vessels to dilate reflexively. Second, binding of the drug at α_2-adrenergic receptors on presynaptic membranes of peripheral vascular sympathetic neurons prevents the release of norepinephrine at such sites. Methyldopa does not decrease the sensitivity of vasomotor centers to baroreceptor control. Therefore, orthostatic (postural) hypotension is less severe than is seen with antihypertensives such as guanethidine. (Such drugs act directly at peripheral neurons.)

INDICATIONS. The reduced systemic vascular resistance caused by methyldopa is useful in the treatment of mild-to-moderate hypertension. Heart rate and cardiac output remain at near-normal levels.

PRECAUTIONS. Volume-depleted patients are susceptible to orthostatic hypotension.

ADVERSE REACTIONS. Signs of CNS depression such as sedation and impaired mental concentration are the most serious adverse effects of methyldopa therapy.

CLONIDINE (Catapres). The centrally acting antihypertensive effect of clonidine is similar to that described for methyldopa. The effect results in depression of medullary vasomotor centers with little or no interference at brain stem baroreceptors. Orthostatic hypotension, therefore, is minimal. Through its central activity, clonidine lowers heart rate and reduces cardiac output to decrease blood pressure. In addition, clonidine causes dilation of capacitance vessels.

INDICATIONS. Mild-to-moderately severe hypertension is an indication for use of clonidine. Unlike methyldopa, clonidine does not significantly change SVR (by dilating arterioles), but instead decreases capacitance tone to dilate veins.

CONTRAINDICATIONS. Clonidine can aggravate a condition of mental depression.

PRECAUTIONS. Patients must be weaned from clonidine therapy to avoid a hypertensive crisis caused by increased sympathetic activity.

ADVERSE REACTIONS. Undesirable effects of clonidine therapy include sedation and dry mouth.

Peripherally Acting Sympatholytics

Peripherally acting sympatholytics interfere with sympathetic neuronal activity at a variety of sites: autonomic ganglia, sympathetic postganglionic neurons, and adrenergic receptors. With the advent of selective adrenergic receptor–blocking agents, such as propranolol, the popularity of ganglionic blockers and adrenergic neuronal blockers is on the decline. For example, the ganglionic blocker trimethaphan (Arfonad) and the adrenergic neuronal blocker guanethidine (Ismelin) both cause orthostatic hypotension. This is due to their venodilating effects on capacitance vessels. Such a side effect limits their usefulness compared with other antihypertensives.

Adrenergic Receptor Blockers: β-Blockade

Beta-adrenergic blockers, such as propranolol (Inderal), have already been discussed as antianginal agents (Chapter 19). Propranolol is a nonselective antagonist of catecholamines at β_1- and β_2-adrenergic receptors (Fig. 21–1). Its antihypertensive effects are due to pharmacologic actions at three locations: (1) The heart, where blockade of β_1 cardiac receptors decreases heart rate, cardiac output, and blood pressure; (2) the brain, where inhibition of sympathetic tone is initiated by medullary vasomotor centers; and (3) the kidney, where inhibition of β_2-adrenoceptor, blocks the formation of renin, which is necessary for the production of angiotensin I (Fig. 21–2).

INDICATIONS. Antihypertensives such as propranolol are normally used in combination with other drugs, such as the thiazide diuretics (chlorothiazide), to remove excess fluid and prevent volume expansion.

Other indications for use of the β-blockers include control of angina symptoms (Chapter 19) and control of cardiac arrhythmias (Chapter 22).

CONTRAINDICATIONS, PRECAUTIONS, AND ADVERSE REACTIONS. See Propranolol (Chapter 19).

A variety of other β-blocking agents are available for the treatment of essential hypertension through peripheral mechanisms. Nadolol (Corgard) is a nonselective β-blocker that differs from propranolol in that is not metabolized in the body and is excreted in the urine. These characteristics give it a relatively long half-life of up to 24 hours. Another nonselective β-blocker is labetalol (Normodyne). Unlike propranolol, it exhibits β-blockade at low concentration but α-blockade at higher concentrations. α-Adrenergic receptor block is useful in the treatment of hypertension caused by pheochromocytoma. Metoprolol (Betaloc[CAN], Lopressor[US], Lopresor[CAN]) and atenolol (Tenormin) are cardioselective β-blocking agents. At therapeutic dosages, these drugs exhibit dominant effects at $β_1$-adrenoceptors. Therefore, they are ideal for hypertensive patients who also suffer from asthma or peripheral vascular disease.

Adrenergic Receptor Blockers: α-Blockade

PRAZOSIN (Minipress). Prazosin is a selective $α_1$-adrenergic blocker acting at the postsynaptic adrenergic sites on both resistance and capacitance vessels to cause vasodilation. Its selective action at $α_1$-adrenergic sites leaves the *presynaptic* $α_2$-adrenergic sites unopposed; therefore, norepinephrine can autoregulate its own release through negative feedback (see Chapter 5). For comparison, nonselective α-blockers ($α_1$ and $α_2$), such as phentolamine (Regitine), produce more reflex tachycardia than prazosin. This is because an $α_2$-adrenergic blockade allows more norepinephrine to interact at $β_1$-receptors to produce cardioacceleration.

INDICATIONS. Prazosin is used to treat hypertension and is most effective given in conjunction with other antihypertensives, such as propranolol, and a diuretic.

CONTRAINDICATIONS. Preexisting hypotension could be worsened through blockage of the pressor ($α_1$) effect at blood vessels. Such an action leaves dilator ($β_2$) effects at blood vessels unopposed.

PRECAUTIONS. Retention of Na^{1+} and water with a corresponding expansion of plasma volume is the normal compensatory response to prazosin when it used without a diuretic.

Postural hypotension is sometimes seen with initial treatment, but is decreased as therapy progresses and dosage is individualized.

Other α-Blockers

Unlike thiazide diuretics and β-blocking agents, which tend to produce lipid, carbohydrate, and electrolyte imbalances, the selective $α_1$-adrenoceptor blockers have a beneficial effect on the plasma levels of these substances (Harper and Forker, 1992; Pool, 1991). Newer agents such as doxazosin (Cardura) and terazosin (Hytrin) are useful in the treatment of mild-to-moderate essential hypertension. Multidrug therapy with these $α_1$-blockers and antihypertensives from *any*

of the other classifications results in decreased blood pressure compared with the other agents used alone (Pool, 1991).

Vasodilators

Vasodilators, such as the nitrates (nitroglycerin) and the calcium channel blockers (verapamil) have been discussed as adjuncts to the cardiotonics in the treatment of low-output states (Chapter 18). By decreasing resistance, vasodilators decrease ventricular loadings on the heart.

Vasodilators are useful in the treatment of hypertension because they reduce vascular resistance (Fig. 21–1). All vasodilators dilate arterioles and decrease systemic vascular resistance (SVR). A few, like nitroprusside, also dilate veins to decrease venous return. By decreasing arteriolar resistance and mean arterial blood pressure, the vasodilators trigger compensatory changes through the baroreceptor reflex, the sympathetic division, and the renin-angiotensin-aldosterone pathway. For these reasons, combination therapy with other antihypertensives such as the diuretics and β-blockers makes good therapeutic sense.

Oral and parenteral vasodilators are currently available for the treatment of hypertension. Inhaled vasodilators for selective vasodilation in cases of pulmonary hypertension are being developed (Box 21–1).

Oral Vasodilators

Orally active vasodilators are used for long-term treatment of hypertension. They act at the smooth muscle of blood vessels to halt the contraction process and bring about relaxation of the vessel wall.

Hydralazine (Apresoline) is active at arterioles but not at veins. As a result, capacitance vessels are unaffected and venous return is essentially unchanged, although SVR is reduced. Tachycardia triggered by the fall in SVR can be controlled by concurrent administration of β-blockers.

Like hydralazine, minoxidil (Loniten) dilates arterioles but does not alter the diameter of veins. Minoxidil is more potent than hydralazine and is useful in patients with severe hypertension or in those who do not respond to hydralazine. Minoxidil also causes reflex sympathetic stimulation and Na^{1+} and fluid retention. It is used with a β-blocker, such as propranolol, and a loop diuretic, such as furosemide.

Parenteral Vasodilators

Parenterally administered vasodilators are used in the treatment of hypertensive emergencies

BOX 21–1   SELECTIVE VASODILATION: THE EMERGING ROLE OF INHALED NITRIC OXIDE

Dilation of blood vessels, either precapillary arterioles, postcapillary veins, or both, is an effective way to reduce vascular resistance and lower blood pressure. Antihypertensives such as β_2- and α_1-adrenergic blockers, calcium channel blockers, angiotensin-converting enzyme inhibitors, and aldosterone antagonists either bring about dilation or prevent contraction of blood vessels. What if a decrease in pulmonary vascular resistance (PVR) is desirable *without* a corresponding decrease in systemic vascular resistance (SVR)? None of the drugs listed above are suitable because they all affect vascular resistance in both circulatory loops. In fact, their lack of specificity is especially troublesome in the treatment of ARDS (adult respiratory distress syndrome) and PPHN (persistent pulmonary hypertension of the newborn).

In ARDS, acute lung injury results in physiologic derangements that include loss of surfactant function (see Chapter 15), pulmonary arterial hypertension due to vasoconstriction, and intrapulmonary shunting that results in arterial hypoxemia. Acute pulmonary hypertension may lead to pulmonary edema and increased stress on the right ventricle.

In some neonates with congenital heart defects such as persistent ductus arteriosus, PPHN may develop. In this syndrome, there is a state of fetal circulation complete with right-to-left shunting, elevated pulmonary vascular resistance, and reduced pulmonary blood flow. These conditions lead to ventilation-perfusion mismatching, hypoxemia, and a vicious cycle as pulmonary vasculature constricts further and pulmonary hypertension increases.

In theory, vasodilator therapy should improve the hemodynamic dysfunctions associated with ARDS and PPHN. The usefulness of the traditional vasodilators, however, is limited by their nonselective reduction of both SVR and PVR. For example, in the treatment of pulmonary hypertension associated with ARDS, intravenous vasodilators cause widespread dilation of systemic blood vessels, systemic arterial hypotension, and decreased venous return. Because dilation of pulmonary blood vessels also occurs, blood flow is increased to areas of intrapulmonary shunting. This increased blood flow worsens the ventilation-perfusion mismatch and further reduces arterial oxygen tension (Pao_2).

The selective vasodilation exhibited by inhaled nitric oxide (NO) at pulmonary vasculature offers a distinct advantage over conventional vasodilators. Inhaled NO is currently undergoing animal tests and clinical evaluation and may prove to be an important drug therapy in the future treatment of pulmonary hypertension associated with ARDS and PPHN. The therapeutic promise of inhaled NO is reflected in the fact that the Massachusetts General Hospital has filed for a patent (pending) on the respiratory uses of the drug (Rossaint et al, 1993).

Nitric oxide is synthesized by vascular endothelial cells from the amino acid, L-arginine. Nitric oxide functions as a local vasodilator and was originally known as endothelium-derived relaxing factor, or EDRF. Recall that NO is also the presumed inhibitory neurotransmitter in the nonadrenergic noncholinergic (i-NANC) neural control of bronchomotor tone (see Box 5–1). As a vasodilator, NO activates guanylate cyclase to elevate the levels of cGMP (cyclic guanosine-3′,5′-monophosphate). Cyclic GMP in turn activates a protein kinase that decreases free calcium (Ca^{2+}) in smooth muscle cells. As intracellular Ca^{2+} concentration decreases, relaxation of vascular smooth muscle occurs to bring about vasodilation. Although they have no effect on cardiac or skeletal muscle, nitrates, such as nitroglycerin, function as NO donors to relax vascular smooth muscle and produce widespread vasodilation in anginal therapy (see Chapter 19). Such generalized vasodilation, however, does not occur following administration of NO as an *inhaled* gas. Nitric oxide rapidly diffuses out of alveoli where its vasodilating effects are limited to ventilated areas of the lung. In addition, it binds to oxyhemoglobin and is rapidly inactivated. As a result of these actions, systemic vascular effects are minimized. By reducing PVR and improving blood flow to damaged regions of the lung, NO improves the matching of ventilation and perfusion, reduces intrapulmonary shunting, and increases Pao_2 without affecting systemic blood vessels and arterial pressure.

Bone RC: A new therapy for the adult respiratory distress syndrome (editorial). N Engl J Med 328:431–432, 1993.

Hudson LD: Pharmacologic approaches to respiratory failure. Respiratory Care 38:754–764, 1993.

Kukovetz WR, Holzmann S, and Schmidt K: Cellular mechanisms of action of therapeutic nitric oxide donors. Eur Heart J 12(Suppl E):16–24, 1991.

Malinowski C: Persistent pulmonary hypertension of the newborn. In Wilkins RL and Dexter JR (eds): Respiratory Disease: Principles of Patient Care. FA Davis, Philadelphia, 1993.

Maunder RJ and Hudson LD: Pharmacologic strategies for treating the adult respiratory distress syndrome. Respiratory Care 35:241–246, 1990.

McCarty KD: Adult respiratory distress syndrome. In Wilkins RL and Dexter JR (eds): Respiratory Disease: Principles of Patient Care. FA Davis, Philadelphia, 1993.

Pison U et al: Inhaled nitric oxide reverses hypoxic pulmonary vasoconstriction without impairing gas exchange. J Appl Physiol 74:1287–1292, 1993.

Roberts JD et al: Inhaled nitric oxide in congenital heart disease. Circulation 87:447–453, 1993.

Rossaint R et al: Inhaled nitric oxide for the adult respiratory distress syndrome. N Engl J Med 328:399–405, 1993.

Zayek M, Cleveland D, and Morin FC: Treatment of persistent pulmonary hypertension in the newborn lamb by inhaled nitric oxide. J Pediatr 122 (5 Pt 1):743–750, 1993.

rather than in the long-term treatment of hypertension. Nitroprusside (Nipride) dilates arterioles to reduce SVR and ventricular afterload. It also dilates veins to reduce venous return and ventricular preload. In patients without cardiac failure, the fall in SVR lowers blood pressure and the C.O. remains normal. However, in patients with cardiac failure, C.O. increases due to the fall in afterload. Rapid and excessive hypotension is both a precaution and an undesirable effect of nitroprusside administration.

Diazoxide (Hyperstat) is a long-acting arteriolar dilator used in the treatment of hypertensive emergencies, in which it rapidly decreases SVR and mean arterial blood pressure. Production of excessive hypotension is a potential toxicity problem with diazoxide administration.

Calcium Antagonists

Calcium channel blockers (calcium influx blockers) were discussed as antianginal drugs. Verapamil (Isoptin) is the prototype of these drugs that dilate peripheral arterioles and decrease blood pressure. Their mechanism of action inhibits calcium (Ca^{2+}) entry into muscle cells to block the contraction process (see Chapter 19).

Nifedipine (Adalat) is the most potent arteriolar dilator of the class. Its Ca^{2+}-blocking action decreases SVR and ventricular afterload. It does not antagonize sympathetic effects at the heart; therefore, reflex tachycardia is seen.

In contrast to nifedipine, diltiazem (Cardizem) produces less arteriolar block but more cardiac sympathetic antagonism. As a result, it produces only slight reflex tachycardia and is a potent antianginal agent. Diltiazem is equal in efficacy to the other antihypertensives but does not produce adverse lipid or carbohydrate metabolic effects. It is ideal in patients with concurrent angina pectoris, diabetes, or hyperlipidemia (Fagan, 1991).

A newer second-generation calcium channel blocker is nicardipine (Cardene). Like all other Ca^{2+}-influx blockers, nicardipine produces arteriolar dilation to decrease SVR. The second-generation drugs, however, also increase blood flow, reduce the oxygen requirements of the myocardium, and exhibit relatively few cardiodepressant side effects (Parmley, 1992). Compared with the first-generation calcium channel blockers, such as verapamil, the newer drugs are less prone to interaction with digoxin (see Chapter 19).

Angiotensin-Converting Enzyme Inhibitors

In the renin-angiotensin-aldosterone pathway (Fig. 21–1) renin is normally released from the renal cortex in response to low renal arterial pressure, β_2-adrenergic stimulation, or increased Na^{1+} concentration in the distal tubules. Once in the bloodstream, renin enzymatically changes an inactive plasma precursor called angiotensinogen into an intermediate compound called angiotensin I. As blood perfuses the lung, angiotensin I is changed into angiotensin II. This change is brought about by **angiotensin-converting enzyme (ACE),** which is located at the surface of capillary endothelial cells in the lung. (Chapter 2 briefly discusses this biotransformation function of the lung.) Angiotensin II is a powerful vasoconstrictor on its own and is converted finally in the adrenal cortex to angiotensin III. Angiotensin II and angiotensin III stimulate the adrenal cortex to secrete aldosterone, which brings about Na^{1+} and water retention. An expanded plasma volume helps restore blood pressure, and the increased Na^{1+} reabsorption restores the homeostasis of plasma sodium levels (see Fig. 21–2).

CAPTOPRIL (Capoten). Captopril interferes with the negative feedback mechanism described above and controls hypertension caused by excess renin release. This effect occurs because it inhibits ACE and prevents the conversion of angiotensin I to angiotensin II (Fig. 21–3). Blood pressure is lowered due to a decrease in SVR, while cardiac output and heart rate are basically unchanged.

A secondary action of captopril on blood pressure is also shown in Figure 21–3. Captopril inhibits a converting enzyme called kininase II, which normally inactivates bradykinin, a powerful vasodilator. As a result, SVR decreases as the plasma level of bradykinin rises.

INDICATIONS. Captopril is most effective in hypertensive states caused by high plasma renin levels. It does not trigger reflex sympathetic activity and is ideal for patients with ischemic heart disease. ACE inhibitors are usually reserved for hypertensive patients who do not respond to the usual sequence of dietary sodium restriction followed by diuretics, sympatholytics, and vasodilators.

ADVERSE REACTIONS. Toxicities such as bone marrow suppression and proteinuria are serious but are not common.

Enalapril (Vasotec) and perindopril are administered as prodrugs that are hydrolyzed in the body into active metabolites that inhibit ACE (Todd and Fitton, 1991). Both are relatively long acting and both have a low incidence of adverse effects. Enalapril was one of the earlier ACE in-

TABLE 21–1 DRUG NAMES: ANTIHYPERTENSIVES

Generic Name	Trade Name
DIURETICS	
Low-ceiling diuretics (thiazides)	
Chlorothiazide	Diuril
Hydrochlorothiazide	HydroDIURIL
High-ceiling diuretics (loop)	
Furosemide	Lasix
Ethacrynic acid	Edecrin
Potassium-sparing diuretics	
Spironolactone	Aldactone
Triamterene	Dyrenium
SYMPATHOLYTICS	
Centrally acting	
Methyldopa	Aldomet
Clonidine	Catapres
Peripherally acting	
β-Adrenocepter blockers	
Propranolol (β_1,β_2)	Inderal
Nadolol (β_1,β_2)	Corgard
Labetolol (β_1,β_2,α_1)	Normodyne
Metoprolol ($\beta_1>\beta_2$)	Betaloc[CAN], Lopressor[US]
Atenolol ($\beta_1>\beta_2$)	Tenormin
α_1-Adrenocepter blockers	
Prazosin	Minipress
Doxazosin	Cardura
Terazosin	Hytrin
VASODILATORS	
Oral vasodilators	
Hydralazine	Apresoline
Minoxidil	Loniten
Parenteral vasodilators	
Nitroprusside	Nipride
Diazoxide	Hyperstat
Calcium channel blockers	
Verapamil	Isoptin
Nifedipine	Adalat
Diltiazem	Cardizem
Nicardipine	Cardene
ANGIOTENSIN-CONVERTING ENZYME INHIBITORS	
Captopril	Capoten
Enalapril	Vasotec
Perindopril	

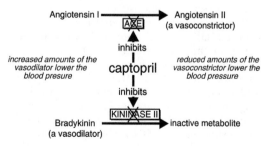

FIGURE 21–3 ACE inhibition and kininase II inhibition.

hibitors used to treat patients with mild hypertension. Although monotherapy with enalapril is often adequate, the drug can be combined with other antihypertensives to treat more serious hypertensive conditions. Perindopril is a newer agent used in monotherapy of mild-to-moderate hypertension. When combined with thiazide diuretics, it is as effective as other combinations in the treatment of severe hypertension or congestive heart failure (Todd and Fitton, 1991).

Table 21–1 lists the generic and trade names

of the antihypertensives discussed in this chapter.

CHAPTER SUMMARY

The hidden nature of hypertension makes it particularly threatening, especially for individuals with positive risk factors such as a family history of hypertension, obesity, or smoking. Symptoms are almost always lacking and the disease is unsuspected unless overt clinical signs such as kidney failure or stroke have occurred.

Once diagnosed, a determination of the cause of hypertension is usually unsuccessful. Lifestyle changes, drug therapy, or a combination all require a high degree of patient acceptance and compliance to treat symptoms that are not apparent to most people.

Antihypertensive therapy using various combinations of diuretics, sympatholytics, vasodilators, and ACE inhibitors is effective for most patients. In multidrug therapy, the antihypertensive efficacy of one drug is maximized through the inhibition of hemodynamic mechanisms by another antihypertensive drug given concurrently.

BIBLIOGRAPHY

Benowitz NL and Bourne HR: Antihypertensive agents. In Katzung BD (ed): Basic and Clinical Pharmacology. Lange Medical Publications, Los Altos, 1982.

Brody MJ, Feldman RD, and Hermsmeyer RK: Cardiovascular drugs. In Conn PM and Gebhart GF (eds): Essentials of Pharmacology. FA Davis, Philadelphia, 1989.

Clark WG, Brater DC, and Johnson AR: Goth's Medical Pharmacology, ed 12. CV Mosby, St Louis, 1988.

Clarke PF et al: Captopril and hydrochlorothiazide: A safe antihypertensive for use in general practice? J Clin Pharm Ther 16:361–363, 1991.

Fagan TC: Diltiazem: Its place in the antihypertensive armamentarium. J Cardiovasc Pharmacol 18 (Suppl 9):S26–S31, 1991.

Harper KJ and Forker AD: Antihypertensive therapy: Current issues and challenges. Postgrad Med 91:163–166, 171–174, 179–186, 1992.

Hoffman BB: Adrenergic receptor–blocking drugs. In Katzung BD (ed): Basic and Clinical Pharmacology. Lange Medical Publications, Los Altos, 1982.

Parmley WW: Efficacy and safety of calcium channel blockers in hypertensive patients with concomitant left ventricular dysfunction. Clin Cardiol. 15:235–242, 1992.

Plouin PF et al: Are angiotensin-converting enzyme inhibition and aldosterone antagonism equivalent in hypertensive patients over fifty? Am J Hypertens 4:356–362, 1991.

Pool JL: Combination antihypertensive therapy with terazosin and other antihypertensive agents: Results of clinical trials. Am Heart J 122:926–931, 1991.

Todd PA and Fitton A: Perindopril: A review of its pharmacological properties and therapeutic use in cardiovascular disorders. Drugs 42:90–114, 1991.

Warnock DG: Diuretics. In Katzung BD (ed): Basic and Clinical Pharmacology. Lange Medical Publications, Los Altos, 1982.

Wikstrand J: Reducing the risk for coronary heart disease and stroke in hypertensives: Comments on mechanisms for coronary protection and quality of life. J Clin Pharm Ther 17:9–29, 1992.

Wikstrand J, Berglund G, and Tuomilehto J: Beta-blockade in the primary prevention of coronary heart disease in hypertensive patients: Review of present evidence. Circulation. 84 (Suppl 6):VI93–VI100, 1991.

CHAPTER 22

Antiarrhythmics

CHAPTER OUTLINE

CHAPTER OBJECTIVES

After studying this chapter the reader should be able to:

- Define dysrhythmia, arrhythmia, automaticity, ectopic focus, gap junction, syncytium.
- Name the parts of the intrinsic conducting system.
- Correlate the mechanical events of the heart cycle with the electrocardiogram (ECG).
- Differentiate between a supraventricular and a ventricular arrhythmia.
- Describe the electrophysiologic events of the cardiac action potential by explaining the transmembrane movements of sodium, calcium, and potassium.
- Explain how an antiarrhythmic drug can modify the intrinsic conducting system to stabilize the rhythm of the heart.
- Describe the pharmacologic activity of the following Class I antiarrhythmics (sodium channel blockers):
  - Quinidine, procainamide, disopyramide, phenytoin, lidocaine, mexiletine, tocainide.
- Describe the pharmacologic activity of the following Class II antiarrhythmics (β-adrenergic blockers):
  - Propranolol, nadolol, metoprolol, atenolol.
- Describe the pharmacologic activity of the following Class III antiarrhythmics (drugs that prolong the action potential):
  - Bretylium, amiodarone.
- Describe the pharmacologic activity of the following Class IV antiarrhythmics (calcium channel blockers):
  - Verapamil, diltiazem.

KEY TERMS

antiarrhythmic agent
  (antidysrhythmic agent)
  class I (sodium channel blocker)
  class II (β-adrenergic blocker)
  class III (drugs that prolong the
    action potential)

class IV (calcium channel
  blocker)
arrhythmia (dysrhythmia)
  supraventricular arrhythmia
  ventricular arrhythmia
automaticity

ectopic focus
electrocardiogram (ECG, EKG)
gap junction
intrinsic conducting system
  atrioventricular bundle (bundle of
    His [**HISS**])

atrioventricular node (AV node [AVN])
bundle branches (right and left)

conduction myofiber (Purkinje [pur-**KIN**-jē] fiber)
sinoatrial node (SA node [SAN])

Purkinje system (His-Purkinje system)
syncytium (sin-**SIT**-ē-um)

CHAPTER INTRODUCTION

Abnormalities in cardiac rate or rhythm are called **arrhythmias.** The term literally means "without rhythm" and is somewhat misleading because certain abnormalities are quite rhythmic, just exceedingly fast. Some atrial tachyarrhythmias, for instance, exhibit rates well in excess of 200 bpm. A **dysrhythmia** is an abnormal rhythm. This is a more precise description, as is the term **antidysrhythmic agent,** which refers to a drug used to correct an abnormal rhythm. However, the terms **arrhythmia** and **antiarrhythmic agent** are universally used and accepted. All of these descriptive terms are used interchangeably in the following discussion. The pharmacologic characteristics of the antiarrhythmic drugs employed to reduce pacemaker activity and modify abnormal conduction in the heart are the subject of this chapter.

REGULATION OF HEARTBEAT

Automaticity

The ability of certain myocardial cells to regularly and spontaneously initiate action potentials is called **automaticity.** Such fibers are autorhythmic because no external stimuli are necessary to initiate the electrical phenomenon. This myogenic origin of heartbeat arises from within the tissue itself and accounts for the inherent rhythm. This intriguing electrophysiologic property helps explain why different locations, or foci, in myocardium have the potential to generate independent electrical rates and patterns. An **ectopic focus** is an area of electrical activity that is not in the normal location. These regions can develop abnormal self-excitability and become dominant over the heart's natural pacemaker. For example, drugs such as nicotine, caffeine, and digitalis can trigger ectopic activity. Loss of normal pacemaker control may result in an arrhythmia. Other types of arrhythmias are characterized by ectopic pacemaker activity that is superimposed on the normal sinus rhythm.

Intrinsic Conducting System

The **intrinsic conducting system** is a collection of highly specialized muscle tissue. It initiates, coordinates, and distributes electrical impulses throughout the myocardium. Extrinsic factors such as autonomic nerve impulses and hormones such as epinephrine can modify the heart's intrinsic activity but are not necessary to establish a basic rhythm.

Initiation of normal electrical activity occurs in a specialized mass of right atrial cells called the **sinoatrial (SA) node** (Fig. 22–1). This pri-

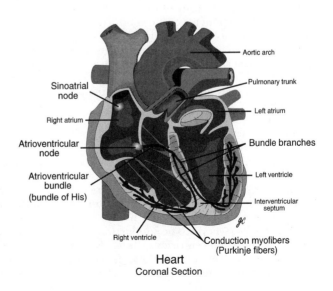

FIGURE 22–1 Intrinsic conducting system.

Heart
Coronal Section

Aortic arch
Pulmonary trunk
Left atrium
Bundle branches
Left ventricle
Interventricular septum
Conduction myofibers (Purkinje fibers)
Right ventricle
Atrioventricular bundle (bundle of His)
Atrioventricular node
Right atrium
Sinoatrial node

mary pacemaker is the site of the sinus rhythm, which drives the rest of the heart. Automaticity ranges from 60 to 100 impulses per minute. Other regions of the heart also generate action potentials, but at a slower rate. For example, specialized conduction fibers supplying the ventricles only generate approximately 35 impulses per minute. Action potentials from the SA node spread to other portions of the conducting system and stimulate them before they can generate an action potential at their own rate. In addition, impulses from the SA node spread rapidly through the interlaced atrial muscle fibers and initiate contraction of the right and left atria. The extensively branched muscle fibers contact each other physically at sarcolemma structures called *intercalated discs*. Within these thickened regions are **gap junctions**. These are electrical synapses that permit muscle action potentials to spread and allow the network of muscle fibers to contract as a group of cells, or an atrial **syncytium.** Gap junctions possess channels that provide a direct pathway for rapid ionic flow. This permits coordinated contraction. These junctions are much faster acting than chemical synapses because no neurotransmitters are required. The mass of ventricular cells also acts as a ventricular syncytium partly because of these gap junctions.

The action potential initiated by the SA node spreads to a second small mass of tissue located near the interatrial septum. This tissue is the **atrioventricular (AV) node** (see Fig. 22–1). As a secondary pacemaker, it has its own unique firing rate of approximately 50–60 impulses per minute, but does not pace the heart as long as a normal sinus rhythm is being generated by the SA node. The rate of firing of the AV node, like that of other components of the conducting system, is matched to the SA nodal rate. The AV node delays the electrical impulse before relaying it to the next component of the intrinsic conducting system. This delay allows the atria sufficient time to empty and the ventricles adequate time to fill.

Synchronization between the electrically isolated atrial syncytium and the ventricular syncytium is essential. The atrial and ventricular pumps are separated by a nonconducting band of tissue serving as the fibrous skeleton of the heart. Proper timing of atrial and ventricular events is made possible by a high-speed conduction pathway that penetrates the fibrous tissue and links the two syncytia. The conduction fibers connecting atria and ventricles collectively form the **Purkinje system,** or **His-Purkinje system.** This conducting system is made up of several

structures. The **atrioventricular bundle,** or **bundle of His,** leaves the AV node and goes a short distance into the interventricular septum. The right and left **bundle branches** travel through the interventricular septum to the apex of the heart and branch into a terminal network of **conduction myofibers (Purkinje fibers).** These fibers are distributed throughout the ventricles (see Fig. 22–1). As outlined above, gap junctions between ventricular muscle fibers allow rapid spread of ionic current and synchronized contraction of the ventricular fibers.

When an impulse arrives by way of the Purkinje fibers, ventricular contraction begins. Meanwhile, atrial contraction has already occurred, forcing blood into the two lower chambers. This primes the ventricles just before the arriving impulse in the Purkinje fibers stimulates them to contract.

ELECTROCARDIOGRAM

The Electrocardiographic Waveform

An **electrocardiogram (ECG)** is generated by a blend of action potentials produced by heart muscle fibers during a cardiac cycle. Different electrocardiographic techniques are available to produce diagnostic ECGs by means of electrodes on the skin. By altering the placement of recording electrodes, the electrical pattern of the heart can be seen from a different perspective. This is because each electrode is in a different position relative to the heart.

The typical ECG tracing shown in Figure 22–2 is a common ECG recording called a *lead II ECG*. The designation *II* refers to a particular combination of pairs of electrodes, or leads, placed on the surface of the body to measure the voltage between two points. The lead II configuration monitors the heart's electrical signals from the patient's right arm to left leg. More complex ECG techniques using multiple chest electrodes are available but are not considered here.

In Figure 22–2, the series of positive and negative waves are the electrical characteristics of different events. The P wave represents atrial depolarization, which spreads throughout both atria by means of gap junctions. The atria begin to contract shortly after the P wave begins. The QRS complex is a series of positive and negative waves that represent ventricular depolarization, or the spread of an impulse through the ventricles. Shortly after the QRS complex begins, the ventricles begin to contract. The T wave indicates repolarization of the ventricles. Immedi-

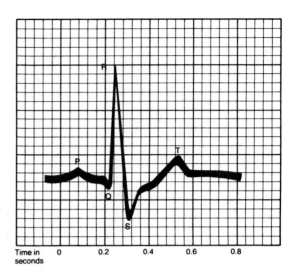

FIGURE 22–2 Lead II electrocardiogram. A heartbeat is a series of electrical events that can be detected by placing electrodes on the surface of the body. The recording is called an *electrocardiogram (ECG, EKG)*. A typical lead II ECG is a waveform that consists of three distinct waves or deflections produced by specific electrical events in the heart: *P wave*—depolarization of the atria; *QRS complex*—depolarization of the ventricles; *T wave*—repolarization of the ventricles (see text for full explanation). (From Scanlon VC and Sanders T: Essentials of Anatomy and Physiology. FA Davis Co, Philadelphia, 1991, p. 275, with permission.)

ately after the T wave begins, the ventricles start to relax. Repolarization of the atria occurs during ventricular depolarization but is hidden within the QRS complex. In addition to the basic waves of the ECG, Figure 22–2 shows the PQ (or PR) interval and the ST segment. (The R wave is not always evident; therefore, PQ is a more accurate description of this interval.) The PQ interval extends from the start of the P wave to the start of the QRS complex. Therefore, it represents the time interval from the beginning of atrial stimulation to the start of ventricular stimulation. The PQ (PR) interval is the conduction time necessary for an impulse to travel through the atria and conducting tissue to reach the ventricles. The ST segment is the period of time from the end of the S wave to the beginning of the T wave. This segment corresponds to the period of time when the ventricular fibers are fully depolarized.

Abnormalities in initiation or conduction of impulses are manifested as changes in the ECG and are of diagnostic value. For example, a rapidly firing SA node triggers multiple P waves and successive atrial contractions. Impaired conduction velocity between atria and ventricles is displayed on an ECG as a prolonged PR interval. Slow conduction through the ventricles causes a widened QRS complex. Antiarrhythmic drugs change these electrical anomalies and alter the ECG. For example, quinidine is an antiarrhythmic that suppresses the firing rate of atrial pacemaker cells. Therefore, the ECG of a patient with atrial tachyarrhythmia has fewer P waves per unit time once the dosage of quinidine has been individualized and the patient is stabilized by the drug.

Types of Arrhythmias

Classification of cardiac arrhythmias is well beyond the scope and needs of this textbook. In simplest terms, electrical abnormalities originating in the SA node, AV node, or atrial muscular are termed **supraventricular arrhythmias.** These dysfunctions, which include atrial flutter and atrial fibrillation, tend to be less serious than the **ventricular arrhythmias.** However, if left untreated, they may lead to the more serious ventricular types, such as ventricular fibrillation. Ventricular arrhythmias refer to dysfunctions originating in regions inferior to the AV node. These include electrical abnormalities in the atrioventricular bundle, bundle branches, conduction myofibers, or ventricular musculature.

CARDIAC ELECTROPHYSIOLOGY

To examine the electrophysiologic events of myocardial contraction and relaxation, we will trace an action potential from its generation in the SA node to its destination in the ventricles.

As was explained earlier, cells of the SA and AV nodes exhibit automaticity, or the ability to spontaneously generate action potentials. The generation of such impulses differs slightly from the description below for ventricular cells. To start with, the resting membrane potential (RMP) of SA node cells is around -65 mV to -70 mV. This RMP value is less negative than that of other cardiac cells (Fig. 22–3). Second, the RMP (Phase 4 in the graph) does not remain stable as it does in a ventricular cell. Instead, it slowly creeps toward threshold. In other words, every time the RMP is established in a

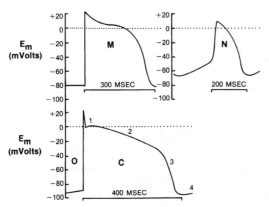

FIGURE 22–3 Cardiac action potentials. Cardiac action potentials have characteristic shapes due to differences in ion conductance across cell membranes in different parts of the heart. The phases of the cardiac action potential are labeled on the conductile cell action potential. Notice that spontaneous pacemaker depolarization is absent in muscle cells (*M*); that the cells of the conduction system (*C*), specialized for high-velocity conduction, have very rapid upstroke and long duration; and that the nodal pacemaker cells (*N*) exhibit spontaneous depolarization but have a very slow upstroke, and therefore low conduction velocity. E_m = membrane potential (mV). (Modified with permission from Brody MJ, Feldman RD, and Hermsmeyer RK: Cardiovascular drugs. In Conn PM and Gebhart GF (eds): Essentials of Pharmacology. FA Davis Co, Philadelphia, 1989, p. 238.)

nodal cell, it gradually decays until self-excitation occurs. At this point, an action potential is generated and the process repeats. Depolarization occurs because of the opening of voltage-gated slow ion channels. These permit sodium ions (Na^{1+}) and calcium ions (Ca^{2+}) to flow into the SA nodal cells through their respective channels and bring about relatively slow depolarization (Phase 0). The slow upstroke of the SA node depolarization curve is characteristic of this tissue. The interlaced atrial fibers rapidly spread the impulse to initiate atrial contraction. In addition, the action potential is relayed by the AV node into the balance of the conduction tissue. The inward current of Na^{1+} and Ca^{2+} ceases as the slow ion channels close. This is followed by repolarization (Phase 3) as voltage-gated potassium (K^{1+}) channels open to allow the outflow of K^{1+}. The increase in membrane conductance to K^{1+} prevents depolarization for a while. However, the K^{1+} conductance gradually decreases, allowing Na^{1+} and Ca^{2+} inflow to gradually erode the RMP and excite the cell again. Because these events can be completed faster by the SA node than by other regions of the heart, the SA node *paces* the heart.

The RMP of a ventricular contractile fiber is around −80 mV to −90 mV. This compares to approximately −90 mV for skeletal muscle and around −70 mV for a typical nerve cell (Table 22–1). The negative potential is maintained in part by the sodium-potassium–adenosine triphosphatase (Na^{1+}-K^{1+}-ATPase) pump that selectively moves Na^{1+} out of the cell and K^{1+} into the cell. An impulse that is fired by the SA node travels through the conducting fibers and then spreads through the ventricular contractile fibers. Figure 22–3 shows the action potentials characteristic of nodal cells such as the SA and AV nodes, conductile cells such as the Purkinje fibers, and contractile cells such as ventricular fibers.

The arrival of an impulse in the ventricles initiates the following sequence. First, a muscle fiber is brought to threshold by excitation in adjacent fibers. Rapid Na^{1+} inflow occurs because voltage-gated fast Na^{1+} channels open. This increase in membrane permeability to Na^{1+} brings about rapid depolarization (Phase 0) of the fiber. Figure 22–3 shows the vertical upstroke of ventricular depolarization through fast Na^{1+} channels, compared with the slow depolarization of nodal cells via slow Na^{1+} channels.

Next, Na^{1+} influx tapers off and the membrane starts to repolarize (Phase 1). This increase in electronegativity is short-lived, however, due to an increase in membrane permeability to Ca^{2+}. Calcium ions begin to flow inward due to the opening of voltage-gated slow Ca^{2+} channels. These cation channels allow Ca^{2+} to flow inward down a concentration gradient. Calcium ions also enter the sarcoplasm from storage sites in the sarcoplasmic reticulum. The combined effect of intracellular Na^{1+} and Ca^{2+} maintains the cardiac muscle cell in an extended depolarized state called the plateau phase (Fig. 22–3). This *transient repolarization* phase (Phase 2) contributes to the lengthy action potential of approximately 0.3 seconds (300 msec) in a ventricular fiber. By comparison, the action potential in neurons and in skeletal muscle cells lasts for only about 1 millisecond (Table 22–1).

Although the organization of cardiac muscle filaments differs slightly from that of skeletal muscle filaments, the physiologic events of contraction are similar (see Chapter 7). Briefly, free Ca^{2+} in the cardiac muscle cell sarcoplasm bind to specific muscle proteins. These proteins activate others and initiate the sliding filament action. This sliding action reduces the length of muscle fibers and develops muscle tension. Cardiac muscle contraction can be affected by alter-

TABLE 22–1 ELECTROPHYSIOLOGIC PROPERTIES OF DIFFERENT CELLS

Cell	Resting Membrane Potential (mV)	Duration of Action Potential (msec)
Nerve cell	Typical: −70	0.5–2.0
	Range: −40 to −90	
Skeletal muscle cell	−90	1.0–5.0
Smooth muscle cell*	−50 to −70	500–5000+
Heart muscle cell		
Nodal cell (eg, SA node)	−65 to −70	200
Conductile cell (eg, conduction myofiber)	−90 to −95	400
Contractile cell (eg, ventricular fiber)	−80 to −90	300
		300

Source: Data from Tortora and Grabowski, 1993; Brody et al, 1989.
*Highly variable; depends on the type of cell.

ing the amount of Ca^{2+} available. For example, norepinephrine enhances Ca^{2+} inflow through the voltage-gated slow Ca^{2+} channels and thus increases myocardial contraction. Verapamil is a calcium channel blocker that decreases myocardial contraction by decreasing Ca^{2+} inflow.

The plateau phase is followed by rapid repolarization (Phase 3) (Fig. 22–3). This phase is similar to the repolarization of nerve cells discussed in Chapter 4 and the repolarization of skeletal muscle cells discussed in Chapter 7. Voltage-gated K^{1+} channels open and K^{1+} diffuse out of the myocardial cell down a concentration gradient. During this time the Na^{1+} and Ca^{2+} channels are closing, thus restricting the inflow of these cations. As more K^{1+} exit and fewer Na^{1+} and Ca^{2+} enter, the resting membrane potential of −80 to −90 mV is restored (Phase 4) and the muscle fiber relaxes.

Modification of transmembrane ion move-ment is an effective mechanism of action for antiarrhythmic drugs. For example, quinidine blocks the fast inward Na^{1+} current, whereas verapamil (mentioned previously) blocks the slow inward Ca^{2+} current. Antiarrhythmic agents such as these are classified in one of four categories according to their primary electrophysiologic effects at myocardial cell membranes.

THERAPEUTIC AGENTS

Sodium Channel Blockers: Class I Drugs

QUINIDINE. The largest class of antiarrhythmic agents are the **sodium channel blockers,** or **Class I** drugs, which depress the fast inward Na^{1+} channels. Quinidine, sold under many trade names, is the prototype of the class (Box 22–1). It acts by depressing the Na^{1+} current of

BOX 22–1 REBELLIOUS PALPITATION

In 1749, Jean-Baptiste de Sénac, a French physician, was using powdered bark from the *cinchona* tree to treat what he described as "rebellious palpitation" of the heart. His success with the bark extract was reported but largely ignored. Many years later the active ingredient, quinine, was isolated from cinchona bark and became the mainstay of antimalarial therapy until the Second World War.

A closely related derivative named quinidine was eventually separated from quinine. Quinidine was found to have less toxicity and more efficacy than quinine in stabilizing abnormal heart rhythms. It has remained a first-line antiarrhythmic drug since its rediscovery in the early 1900s. Quinidine adverse reactions such as tinnitus and dizziness are called *cinchonism*—an obvious reference to the original botanical source of the parent compound.

Clark WG, Brater DC, and Johnson AR: Goth's Medical Pharmacology, ed 12. CV Mosby, St Louis, 1988.
Liska K: Drugs and the Human Body: With Implications for Society. Macmillan, New York, 1981.
Modell W, Lansing A, and Editors of Time-Life Books: Drugs. Life Science Library. Time, New York, 1969.

myocardial cell membranes to stabilize the heart.

INDICATIONS. Quinidine controls both supraventricular and ventricular tachyarrhythmias. It slows AV conduction and prolongs the PR interval. Quinidine also slows intraventricular conduction and widens the QRS complex. Lengthening of the QT interval is also seen with quinidine therapy.

CONTRAINDICATIONS. In patients with conduction defects, sodium channel blockers can slow conduction further and suppress automaticity to the point where the heart stops.

PRECAUTIONS. Low plasma concentrations tend to produce an anticholinergic effect that causes cardioacceleration.

ADVERSE REACTIONS. The most common adverse reactions are gastrointestinal tract effects such as diarrhea.

PROCAINAMIDE (Pronestyl). A local anesthetic called procaine (Novocain) was found to have electrical effects on the myocardium. A derivative of procaine having greater stability in the body was developed and named procainamide. Procainamide has pharmacologic properties similar to those of quinidine.

INDICATIONS, CONTRAINDICATIONS, AND PRECAUTIONS. See Quinidine.

ADVERSE REACTIONS. Relaxation of vascular smooth muscle and decreased myocardial contraction can cause hypotension.

DISOPYRAMIDE (Norpace). Disopyramide is very similar to quinidine in its pharmacologic activity but has more potent anticholinergic side effects.

INDICATIONS. See Quinidine.

CONTRAINDICATIONS. Anticholinergic effects of disopyramide can worsen paralytic ileus, urinary retention, glaucoma, and myasthenia gravis.

PRECAUTIONS AND ADVERSE REACTIONS. Disopyramide may produce hypotension and exacerbate, or worsen, congestive heart failure.

PHENYTOIN (Dilantin). The antiepileptic drug phenytoin, also known as diphenylhydantoin, was found to have limited arrhythmia-suppressing actions in addition to its main anticonvulsant effects. It suppresses automaticity in supraventricular and ventricular tissue and improves AV conduction. Phenytoin is administered only as an intravenous agent and has very limited usefulness as an antiarrhythmic.

INDICATIONS. Phenytoin is used in the treatment of digitalis-induced arrhythmias.

LIDOCAINE (Xylocaine). The main antiar-rhythmic effect of lidocaine is its depression of automaticity. Lidocaine does not slow AV conduction and does not prolong the action potential or refractory period of cardiac muscle as do the other Class I agents.

INDICATIONS. Lidocaine is only given intravenously. Its primary use is in the treatment and prevention of ventricular arrhythmias associated with myocardial infarction (MI).

CONTRAINDICATIONS. Preexisting bradycardia may be worsened by the suppressive effects of lidocaine on automaticity.

ADVERSE REACTIONS. Lidocaine can cause a variety of CNS effects such as drowsiness, convulsions, and coma.

DERIVATIVES OF LIDOCAINE. Several antiarrhythmic agents have been developed that are similar to lidocaine in regard to electrophysiologic and antiarrhythmic effects. Mexiletine (Mexitil) and tocainide (Tonocard) are available as oral agents for treatment of ventricular ectopic activity. Mexiletine is especially well suited for electrical disturbances that accompany MI, whereas tocainide is indicated in the treatment of ventricular tachyarrhythmias. Adverse reactions to the drugs include gastrointestinal tract effects such as nausea and vomiting and CNS effects such as tremors and mental confusion.

NEWER CLASS I ANTIARRHYTHMICS. In patients with ventricular tachyarrhythmia who do not respond to the usual Class I agents like quinidine, a newer group of antiarrhythmic agents may provide the desired control. They do not depress the duration of the action potential, but paradoxically, flecainide (Tambocor) and encainide (Enkaid) may *cause* tachyarrhythmia in some patients. This tendency limits their clinical usefulness. Other adverse reactions include CNS effects such as dizziness and headache.

β-Adrenergic Blockers: Class II Drugs

The **Class II** antiarrhythmic agents are the **β-adrenergic receptor antagonists.** In terms of therapeutic uses, this group is multifaceted. We have examined their use as antianginals (Chapter 19) to reduce myocardial oxygen demands and as antihypertensives (Chapter 21) to block sympathetic effects at the heart, blood vessels, and kidneys.

When used as antiarrhythmics, the nonspecific β-adrenergic blockers, such as propranolol (Inderal) and nadolol (Corgard), and the more cardioselective members, such as metoprolol (Betaloc^{CAN}, Lopressor^{US}) and atenolol (Tenormin), depress automaticity and prolong AV conduction. They also exert negative chronotropic and inotropic effects to reduce heart rate and contractility.

Beta-blockers are most effective in the treatment of tachyarrhythmia caused by increased sympathetic activity. As is discussed in Chapter 21, they are also useful for blocking reflex tachycardia that occurs as a compensatory mechanism when vasodilator antihypertensive drugs are used.

Precautions include myocardial depression, bradycardia, and use in asthmatic patients. The most common adverse reaction, especially with the nonselective β-blockers, is bronchospasm. β-Blockade caused by nonselective β-antagonists such as propranolol can also cause reflex arteriolar vasoconstriction due to unopposed α_1-adrenergic effects in the blood vessels.

Drugs that Prolong the Action Potential: Class III Drugs

Several therapeutic agents belonging to other antiarrhythmic (**Class III drugs**) classes exhibit mechanisms that **prolong the action potential** of myocardial tissue. For example, bretylium stabilizes myocardial cell membranes and prolongs the action potential. Quinidine is a Class I antiarrhythmic because of its specific sodium channel–blocking effects, but it also exhibits Class III activity because it prolongs action potentials. Specific Class III agents are relatively uncommon.

BRETYLIUM (Bretylol). Bretylium is classified pharmacologically as an adrenergic neuronal blocking drug. It interferes with the release of norepinephrine from adrenergic nerve endings and, therefore, stabilizes myocardial cell membranes. Its effects on cardiac action potentials place it in the Class III group of antiarrhythmics.

INDICATIONS. Bretylium is used in patients with severe ventricular tachyarrhythmias unresponsive to other drugs.

CONTRAINDICATIONS. A preexisting condition of bradycardia can be worsened by any of the antiarrhythmics that operate by suppressing the refractory period of myocardial cells.

ADVERSE REACTIONS. Hypotension, bradycardia, and angina pectoris are potential adverse cardiovascular reactions to bretylium. Gastrointestinal tract effects include nausea and diarrhea.

AMIODARONE (Cordarone). Amiodarone is a very toxic but effective Class III antiarrhythmic agent.

INDICATIONS. Supraventricular and ventricular tachyarrhythmias respond to amiodarone, but it is reserved for patients not responding to other, less toxic, antiarrhythmic drugs.

ADVERSE REACTIONS. Adverse reactions to amiodarone include photosensitivity, hyper- and hypothyroidism, and hepatotoxicity.

Calcium Channel Blockers: Class IV Drugs

The **calcium channel blockers (Class IV drugs)** inhibit the slow influx of Ca^{2+} through transmembrane channels. Recall that the Ca^{2+} influx blockers are also used as vasodilators in antianginal and antihypertensive therapy (Chapters 19 and 21).

VERAPAMIL (Isoptin). Verapamil is the prototype of the Class IV agents. It suppresses SA node firing, prolongs the AV refractory period, and slows AV conduction velocity to result in negative chronotropic, inotropic, and dromotropic effects.

INDICATIONS. Verapamil is useful in the treatment of some types of atrial tachyarrhythmias. Patients with atrial fibrillation can be successfully treated with calcium channel blockers because the drugs slow AV conduction and, therefore, ventricular activity.

CONTRAINDICATIONS. Preexisting bradycardia can be made worse by drugs that slow AV conduction.

DILTIAZEM (Cardizem). Diltiazem produces a negative inotropic effect on the heart like that of verapamil, but has a less pronounced effect on the slowing of conduction.

INDICATIONS AND CONTRAINDICATIONS. See Verapamil.

Table 22–2 lists the generic and trade names of the antiarrythmics discussed in this chapter.

CHAPTER SUMMARY

The remarkable ability of heart muscle cells to generate spontaneous action potentials is both a blessing and a curse. This regular, autorhythmic action allows the heart to function even without external stimuli, but it is also the reason the rhythmic action sometimes fails. The very fact that hundreds of thousands of myocardial cells have the potential to become self-excited is an

TABLE 22–2   DRUG NAMES: ANTIARRHYTHMICS

Generic Name	Trade Name
SODIUM CHANNEL BLOCKERS (CLASS I DRUGS)	
Quinidine (**QUIN**-i-dēn)	(many trade names)
Procainamide (prō-**KAN**-a-mīd)	Pronestyl
Disopyramide (dī-sō-**PEER**-a-mīd)	Norpace
Phenytoin (fe-**NIT**-ō-in)	Dilantin
Lidocaine (**LĪ**-dō-kān)	Xylocaine
Mexiletine (mex-**ILL**-e-tēn)	Mexitil
Tocainide (tō-**KAN**-īde)	Tonocard
Flecainide (flek-**KAN**-īde)	Tambocor
Encainide (in-**KAN**-īde)	Enkaid
β-ADRENERGIC BLOCKERS (CLASS II DRUGS)	
Propranolol	Inderal
Nadolol	Corgard
Metoprolol	Betaloc[CAN], Lopressor[US]
Atenolol	Tenormin
DRUGS THAT PROLONG ACTION POTENTIAL (CLASS III DRUGS)	
Bretylium (bre-**TIL**-ē-um)	Bretylol
Amiodarone (a-mē-**O**-da-rōn)	Cordarone
CALCIUM CHANNEL BLOCKERS (CLASS IV DRUGS)	
Verapamil	Isoptin
Diltiazem	Cardizem

ever-present risk should the pacemaker cells of the heart lose their dominance. Similarly, failures in conduction and failures in synchronization may have disastrous results. We have seen that drug therapy is sometimes necessary to stabilize cardiac rhythm and rate. This is done through suppression of electrical foci (natural or ectopic), suppression of conduction, or a combination of both.

BIBLIOGRAPHY

Bolognesi R: The pharmacologic treatment of atrial fibrillation. Cardiovasc Drugs Ther 5:617–628, 1991.

Brody MJ, Feldman RD, and Hermsmeyer RK: Cardiovascular drugs. In Conn PM and Gebhart GF (eds): Essentials of Pharmacology. FA Davis, Philadelphia, 1989.

Carola R, Harley JP, and Noback CR: Human Anatomy and Physiology, ed 2. McGraw-Hill, New York, 1992.

Clark WG, Brater DC, and Johnson AR: Goth's Medical Pharmacology, ed 12. CV Mosby, St Louis, 1988.

Davis WR and Schaal SF: Pharmacologic suppression of atrial flutter induced by atrial stimulation. Am Heart J 123:681–686, 1992.

Hondeghem LM and Mason JW: Agents used in cardiac arrhythmias. In Katzung BD (ed): Basic and Clinical Pharmacology. Lange Medical Publications, Los Altos, 1982.

Kulbertus HE: Antiarrhythmic treatment of atrial arrhythmias. J Cardiovasc Pharmacol 17 (Suppl 6):S32–S35, 1991.

Lewis RV, McMurray J, and McDevitt DG: Effects of atenolol, verapamil, and xamoterol on heart rate and exercise tolerance in digitalised patients with chronic atrial fibrillation. J Cardiovasc Pharmacol 13:1–6, 1989.

McCance KL and Richardson SJ: Structure and function of the cardiovascular and lymphatic systems. In McCance KL and Huether SE: Pathophysiology: The Biologic Basis for Disease in Adults and Children. CV Mosby, St Louis, 1990.

Tortora GJ and Grabowski SR: Principles of Anatomy and Physiology, ed 7. HarperCollins, New York, 1993.

Van De Graaff KM and Fox SI: Concepts of Human Anatomy and Physiology. Wm C Brown, Dubuque, IA, 1989.

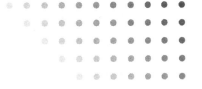

CHAPTER 23

Antithrombotics and Thrombolytics

CHAPTER OUTLINE

CHAPTER OBJECTIVES

After studying this chapter the reader should be able to:

- Define thrombus, embolus, thrombosis.
- Explain the action of blood coagulation factors by describing the cascade effect of hemostasis.
- Briefly outline the intrinsic and extrinsic pathways of hemostasis.
- Describe the pharmacologic activity of the following antithrombotics:
  - Heparin, warfarin, dicumarol, aspirin, ticlopidine, prostacyclin.
- Describe the pharmacologic activity of the following thrombolytics:
  - Streptokinase, urokinase, alteplase, anistreplase.

KEY TERMS

anticoagulant
antiplatelet
antithrombotic
cascade effect
coagulation factors

common pathway
embolus
extrinsic pathway
hemostasis

intrinsic pathway
thrombolytic
thrombosis
thrombus

CHAPTER INTRODUCTION

Thrombosis is the formation or existence of a blood clot (**thrombus**) in the circulatory system. Development of a blood clot is a beneficial process during hemorrhage because it prevents blood loss from the vascular compartment. Thrombosis occurring in the vascular system under any other circumstances is detrimental and has potentially lethal consequences. An intravascular clot that breaks away from a vessel wall is called an **embolus.** Such an object can travel away from the original site and occlude a small-caliber blood vessel. The resulting ischemia may be life threatening if vital tissues are involved. Drugs exist for the control of undesirable clot formation and for the treatment of various thromboembolic disorders. **Antithrombotics,** such as heparin, prevent thrombus formation, and **thrombolytics,** such as streptokinase, dissolve thrombi that have already formed.

Anticoagulants are substances that prevent blood clotting by interfering in some way with the hemostatic mechanism. Some, such as ethylenediamine tetraacetic acid (EDTA), are used solely for collected blood samples and have no therapeutic use in the prevention of thrombus formation. Others, such as heparin, are generally classified as anticoagulants but have specific antithrombotic effects that make them valuable therapeutic agents. In general, *anticoagulant* and *antithrombotic* are used interchangeably.

HEMOSTASIS
Role of Clotting Factors

The mechanism of **hemostasis,** or blood clotting, is vital to prevent loss of blood and to repair damaged blood vessels. The mechanism is inherently complex, involving the interaction of membrane phospholipids, calcium (Ca^{2+}), and the sequential activation of several different proteins called **coagulation factors.** Calcium is not a protein factor, but is designated as factor IV (Table 23–1). Most of the protein coagulation factors are synthesized in the liver. Interference with the hepatic synthesis of certain factors, such as prothrombin, is the mechanism of action of antithrombotics, such as warfarin. Coagulation can also be blocked in other ways. For example, interference with substances such as formed thrombin is the mechanism of action of the antithrombotic heparin, whereas blockage of platelet aggregation is the mechanism of action of the antiplatelet aspirin. We will see many more examples in which this complex hemostatic mechanism can be modified by drug action.

Cascade Effect

A detailed description of the events of hemostasis exceeds the scope of this text; however, Figure 23–1 outlines a simplified coagulation pathway. In this sequence, several basic features are apparent. For instance, the product of one reaction activates the next step in the pathway, producing a waterfall or **cascade effect.** This metaphor is a useful description of complex sequential events in which multiple reactants exist in a preformed but inactive state and are mobilized in a controlled fashion as the sequence progresses.

Second, the biochemical chain reaction can be initiated through either of two pathways: an extrinsic or an intrinsic mechanism. The **extrinsic pathway** is activated by a factor that is located extrinsic to, or outside, the plasma. For example, when the endothelial lining of blood vessels is

TABLE 23–1 NOMENCLATURE OF COAGULATION FACTORS

Factor I	Fibrinogen
Factor II	Prothrombin
Factor III	Tissue thromboplastin (tissue factor)
Factor IV	Calcium
Factor V	Labile factor (proaccelerin)
Factor VI	Not assigned
Factor VII	Stable factor (serum prothrombin conversion accelerator)
Factor VIII	Antihemophilic factor
Factor IX	Christmas factor (plasma thromboplastin component)
Factor X	Stuart-Prower factor (thrombokinase)
Factor XI	Plasma thromboplastin antecedent
Factor XII	Hageman factor (contact factor)
Factor XIII	Fibrin-stabilizing factor

Source: From Harmening, 1992; with permission.

damaged or roughened, as occurs with the deposition of plaque on the vessel wall, an endothelial cell–derived factor called tissue thromboplastin (factor III) is released. This factor, in the presence of Ca^{2+}, activates factor VII (Fig. 23–1). This activation sequence initiates a shortened pathway leading to generation of factor X and fibrin formation within a few seconds. The pathway is short because several factors are bypassed and are not activated. The mechanism is ideal for rapidly generating small amounts of thrombin, leading to rapid fibrin formation.

In the **intrinsic pathway,** however, all factors necessary for coagulation of blood have already been synthesized and are within the plasma itself. Damage to platelets, or contact of blood with a negatively charged surface such as collagen or glass, causes platelet phospholipids (PPL) (platelet factor 3 [PF3]) on the platelet membrane to function as receptor sites for the formation of an activator complex to generate factor X. In effect, the phospholipid of the platelet membrane acts as a catalytic surface to allow an interaction to occur among several different factors (Fig. 23–1). The macromolecular complex that forms on the platelet surface occurs in an environment that is "protected" from the action of natural anticoagulants, which normally circulate in the plasma. This intrinsic cascade sequence generates large quantities of thrombin on the surface of platelets, thus leading to clot formation. More coagulation factors must be activated in the intrinsic pathway. Therefore, it requires a few minutes for completion compared with the shorter-acting extrinsic pathway. Because contact of platelets with a foreign surface can activate the intrinsic pathway, this mecha-

INTRINSIC SYSTEM   EXTRINSIC SYSTEM

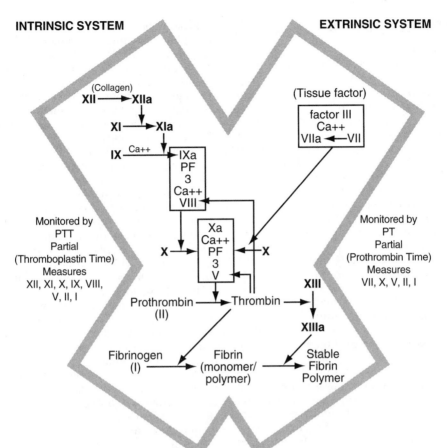

FIGURE 23–1 Hemostasis pathway. In this cascade mechanism of coagulation, intrinsic and extrinsic pathways converge into a final common pathway with the formation of activated factor X (factor Xa). (From Harmening DM: Introduction to hemostasis: An overview of hemostatic mechanism, platelet function, and extrinsic and intrinsic systems. In Harmening DM (ed): Clinical Hematology and Fundamentals of Hemostasis, ed. 2. FA Davis Co, Philadelphia, 1992, p. 427 with permission.)

nism is responsible for causing a blood sample to coagulate in a glass test tube or in plastic tubing. The coagulation mechanism occurs without the addition of any extrinsic, tissue-derived factors.

Another feature of the hemostasis mechanism is the final **common pathway,** where intrinsic and extrinsic mechanisms converge with the activation of the Stuart-Prower factor (factor X). Activated factor X (designated factor Xa) causes an inactive plasma protein called prothrombin (factor II) to be converted to thrombin. Thrombin is a protease that converts another inactive plasma protein called fibrinogen (factor I) into active fibrin. Fibrin monomers then form a complex protein meshwork (Fig. 23–1). The protein

mesh entraps erythrocytes and platelets to form a mechanical plug. The resulting blood clot is eventually dissolved and removed after tissue repair is completed.

We now examine some of the drugs that alter the latter stages of hemostasis. The cascade sequence shown in Figure 23–1 and the names of coagulation factors listed in Table 23–1 are included solely for the interest of the reader. For our purposes, most of the names of the coagulation factors will not be needed for a basic pharmacologic understanding of the drugs used to prevent and dissolve blood clots. For additional detail regarding the hemostatic mechanism, consult a hematology or anatomy and physiology textbook listed in the chapter bibliography.

THERAPEUTIC AGENTS

Antithrombotics

HEPARIN. Heparin, sold under many trade names, is located in storage granules within mast cells and basophils in our bodies and is derived from bovine liver and lung for medical use. (The name heparin is derived from *hepatic,* the liver being the natural source of the substance.) It is classified as a direct-acting anticoagulant that is effective both *in vivo* and *in vitro.* Heparin activates a plasma cofactor called antithrombin III. This protein combines naturally with thrombin in the bloodstream to prevent unnecessary clotting, but when it is induced by heparin, it combines with thrombin many times more readily. The rapid binding removes, or "neutralizes," formed thrombin so quickly that intravascular clotting is minimized. As is shown in Figure 23–2, thrombin controls the conversion of inactive fibrinogen to a fibrin intermediate. Heparin, therefore, inhibits this mechanism and prevents the formation of the fibrin clot. All the clotting factors necessary for coagulation are present in a drop of blood, whether that blood is in a blood vessel or in plastic tubing (as in a hemodialysis machine). The reason heparin is active in both locations is that it acts on preformed factors that are already in the blood. The antithrombotic effects of heparin are produced by parenteral administration (intravenous or subcutaneous) and are evident within 3–4 hours. Repeated administration is required to maintain adequate plasma levels of the drug.

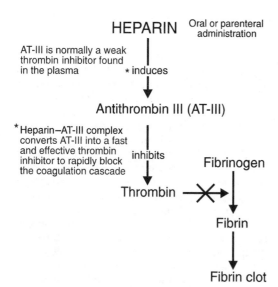

HEPARIN Oral or parenteral administration

AT-III is normally a weak thrombin inhibitor found in the plasma

* induces

Antithrombin III (AT-III)

* Heparin–AT-III complex converts AT-III into a fast and effective thrombin inhibitor to rapidly block the coagulation cascade

inhibits

Fibrinogen

Thrombin

Fibrin

Fibrin clot

FIGURE 23–2 Heparin—mechanism of action.

INDICATIONS. Blood outside the body, as in a heart-lung machine or a hemodialysis machine, is called *extracorporeal.* In a procedure known as extracorporeal membrane oxygenation (ECMO), an infant's blood is withdrawn through a venous catheter and circulated through a membrane oxygenator. After being oxygenated, the blood is returned to the infant. The technique helps reduce pulmonary vascular resistance (PVR). Tubing, filters, pumps, and other equipment that come into contact with blood during procedures such as these must be heparinized, or treated with heparin (O'Rourke, 1991). This prevents coagulation through the intrinsic pathway normally activated when blood contacts a foreign surface. Similarly, collected blood samples are placed in or on heparinized glass tubes or slides. Although not considered therapeutic drugs, other anticoagulants, such as EDTA or solutions of citrate or oxalate, are used in laboratories and blood banks to prevent clotting of collected samples. These substances bind with and inactivate Ca^{2+}. Calcium (factor IV) is used in the formation of thrombin and in all stages of coagulation.

Prevention and treatment of venous thromboembolism is the primary clinical use for heparin. Thromboembolism tends to originate in the slower-moving blood of the venous system or within the chambers of the heart. These regions are prone to clot inactivation, which may in turn release emboli into circulation. Prevention of this occurrence requires antithrombotic therapy. Pulmonary embolism and peripheral arterial thromboembolism are also indications for heparin therapy. To provide an initial antithrombotic effect, heparin is often given in combination with a slower-onset coumarin derivative. Full antithrombotic effects of coumarin derivatives, such as warfarin, take several days to develop.

CONTRAINDICATIONS. Preexisting bleeding disorders, such as hemophilia, are contraindications for use of the antithrombotics. They are also contraindicated in patients who have had recent surgery and those with active bleeding sites such as gastric ulcers.

PRECAUTIONS. Bleeding is the obvious precaution with therapy that inhibits coagulation. Reversal of heparin effects can be brought about through the administration of protamines, proteins that combine with free heparin molecules to inhibit the anticoagulant effect.

ADVERSE REACTIONS. In addition to being a precaution, bleeding is also the major adverse effect with antithrombotic therapy.

WARFARIN (Coumadin, Athrombin-K[CAN]).

Warfarin was developed from coumarin derivatives originally extracted from spoiled sweet clover hay. (Ingestion of the hay causes a hemorrhagic disease in cattle.) Warfarin is used extensively for pest control as a rodenticide in addition to being the most useful coumarin derivative antithrombotic in human medicine. Dicumarol (*bis*hydroxycoumarin) is a rarely used coumarin derivative similar to warfarin but more slowly absorbed. Warfarin is an orally active prothrombin depressant that is rapidly absorbed from the gastrointestinal tract to reach peak plasma levels quickly. Full development of its antithrombotic effect, however, takes several days until certain clotting factors are cleared from the body.

As was explained above, heparin is usually given concurrently with drugs such as warfarin. The mechanism of action of warfarin is indirect, acting on the biosynthesis of key clotting factors (Fig. 23–3). Warfarin and the other coumarin derivatives are structurally similar to vitamin K (Fig. 23–4). When one of these drugs reaches the liver, it acts as a false substrate to depress the synthesis of factors requiring vitamin K. Factors VII, IX, X, and II (prothrombin) are modified by this mechanism and synthesized in a form that is inactive (Suttie, 1990). The hemostatic pathway, therefore, is blocked at multiple sites, most notably in the prothrombin-mediated step. For this reason, coumarin derivatives are referred to as prothrombin depressant antithrombotics.

INDICATIONS. Treatment and prevention of venous thrombosis is the prime indication for use. The coumarin derivatives are inactive in extracorporeal applications because the essential clotting factors are already present in the blood. Blockade of their synthesis, therefore, is not possible.

Warfarin at very low doses and in combination with aspirin is being studied for possible use in the prevention of heart attacks (Hirsh, 1991).

CONTRAINDICATIONS. See Heparin.

PRECAUTIONS. Bleeding is a precaution with any antithrombotic therapy. In addition, caution must be used when other antithrombotics, such as aspirin, are given concurrently. Reversal of coumarin effects is brought about by introduction of large doses of vitamin K. Recovery depends largely on the biosynthetic capacity of the liver to produce active replacement clotting factors.

ADVERSE REACTIONS. Bleeding is the most common adverse reaction to coumarin therapy. Unlike heparin, the coumarin derivatives can cross the placenta to cause hemorrhagic disorders in the fetus.

ACETYLSALICYLIC ACID (ASA). Platelet aggregation plays a vital role in the hemostatic process because the clumping together, or aggregation, is partly responsible for mechanical plugging of a ruptured vessel. Acetylsalicylic acid, or aspirin, is a nonsteroidal anti-inflammatory drug (NSAID) with potent actions on the arachidonic acid pathway. Thromboxane A_2

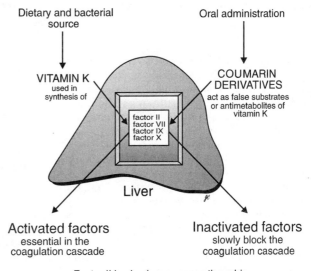

FIGURE 23–3 Warfarin—mechanism of action.

Factor II is also known as prothrombin, therefore, coumarin derivatives are called prothrombin depressant antithrombotics

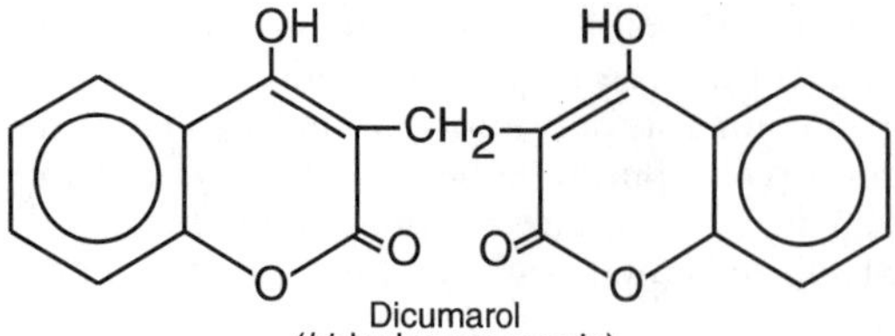

Dicumarol
(*bis*hydroxycoumarin)

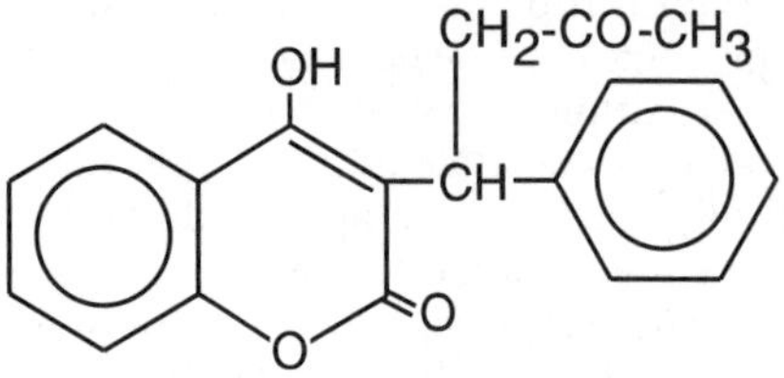

CH₂-CO-CH₃

Warfarin

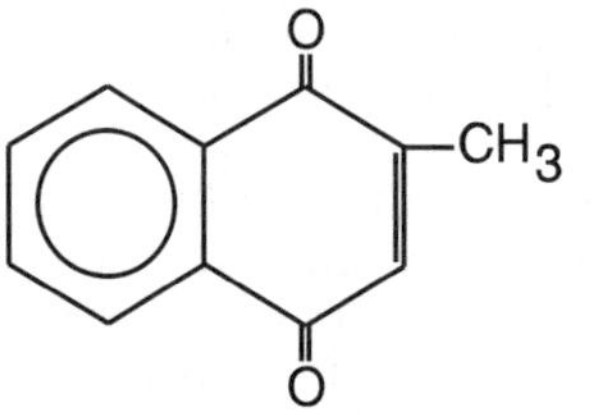

Synthetic vitamin K
(menadione)

FIGURE 23–4 Coumarin derivatives and vitamin K. The word *vitamine* was coined around 1912. It was recognized that these substances were necessary for life (*vita* = life) and it was thought that all such compounds were *amines*. When it was found that not all vitamins are amines, the *e* in the original word was dropped. *K* stands for *Koagulation*, the German word for cotting. Originally, vitamin K was known as the *Koagulation-Vitamin*, or the antihemorrhagic vitamin. (Derivation of term from Van De Graaff KM and Fox SI: Concepts of Human Anatomy and Physiology, William C. Brown Publishers, Dubuque, IA, 1989.)

minal wall respond well to antiplatelet therapy because these lesions tend to expose subendothelial collagen and activate platelets through the intrinsic pathway (Fig. 23–1).

CONTRAINDICATIONS, PRECAUTIONS, AND ADVERSE REACTIONS. See Heparin.

TICLOPIDINE (Ticlid). Ticlopidine inhibits platelet aggregation by altering the function of the platelet membrane. In animal studies, ticlopidine has been shown to decrease the number of platelet aggregates, decrease the size of the aggregates that form, and inhibit the degranulation of platelets (Morishita et al, 1991). Recall that platelets synthesize TXA₂, which in turn induces more platelet aggregation. Therefore, inhibition of platelet degranulation provides a powerful antiplatelet effect.

INDICATIONS. The major indication for use of ticlopidine is in the prevention of stroke, also called cerebrovascular accident (CVA). The drug is especially useful in patients who require an antiplatelet drug but cannot tolerate aspirin.

CONTRAINDICATIONS, PRECAUTIONS, AND ADVERSE REACTIONS. See Heparin.

PROSTACYCLIN. Antithrombotic effects through inhibition of platelets are also exhibited by prostacyclin, also known as prostaglandin I₂. Prostacyclin is normally generated within blood vessels to prevent intravascular platelet aggregation. The former process occurs when endothelial cell membrane phospholipids release arachidonic acid that is acted on through the cyclooxygenase pathway. The resulting prostaglandin synthesis produces prostacyclin, which inhibits platelet aggregation.

INDICATIONS. Prostacyclin is effective as a

(TXA$_s$) is required for normal platelet aggregation and is one of the eicosanoid mediators produced through cyclooxygenase metabolism of arachidonic acid. (This pathway is examined fully in Chapter 9.) Aspirin inhibits cyclooxygenase to block TXA₂ synthesis and, therefore, block platelet aggregation (Fig. 23–5). Aspirin is classified as an antithrombotic drug that functions through an **antiplatelet** mechanism.

INDICATIONS. Thromboprophylaxis is the main indication for use of aspirin. When used alone or in combination with antithrombotics, antiplatelet drugs are best suited for regions of high shear rates. In these areas, emboli are likely to be "sheared off" the vessel wall and released into circulation (Stein and Furster, 1989). Areas of vessel stenosis (narrowing) and areas where atherosclerotic plaque is disrupted on the lu-

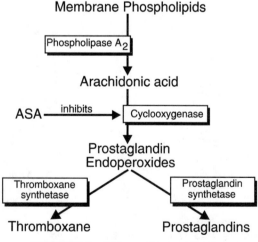

FIGURE 23–5 ASA—mechanism of action.

short-acting antithrombotic for use with extra-corporeal circulation.

PRECAUTIONS AND ADVERSE REACTIONS. Prostacyclin is limited in its usefulness because it has potent vascular smooth muscle–relaxing properties and, therefore, may cause vasodilation and hypotension.

Thrombolytics

Recall that drugs administered to break up, or lyse, thrombi after coagulation has occurred are called thrombolytics, or fibrinolytics. The following fibrinolytics all activate the thrombolytic pathway and convert plasminogen to plasmin (also called fibrinolysin). Within the boundaries of a thrombus, plasmin degrades fibrin to dissolve the clot. However, when plasmin is free in the plasma, it degrades fibrinogen and other clotting factors (Haire, 1992).

The thrombolytics currently in use are equally effective in clot dissolution and in reduction of infarct size. In addition, the fibrinolytics reduce the incidence and severity of congestive heart failure. Thrombolytic therapy has been very successful in lowering mortality due to acute myocardial infarction (White, 1991).

STREPTOKINASE (Streptase, Kabikinase). One of the first drugs of this class developed as a thrombolytic agent was streptokinase, an enzyme produced by certain virulent strains of *Streptococcus*. Bacteria producing the enzyme are able to lyse blood clots in host tissues. (Clotting is a host defense that impedes the spread of microorganisms.)

Figure 23–6 shows the thrombolysis pathway. Activated factor XII converts an inactive plasma molecule called prekallikrein to active kallikrein, which in turn changes plasminogen to plasmin. Streptokinase forms an activator complex with inactive plasminogen to result in the formation of plasmin, which lyses fibrin clots. Compared with the recombinant urokinase products discussed below, streptokinase is less effective in maintaining adequate coronary blood flow in acute myocardial infarction (MI).

INDICATIONS. Indications for use include the treatment of coronary thrombosis associated with acute MI, and the treatment of deep venous thrombosis, pulmonary embolism, and arterial embolism. Blood clot–lysing drugs are also useful for maintaining patency of cannulae and catheters.

CONTRAINDICATIONS. Preexisting bleeding tendencies, active internal bleeding, recent surgery, and severe hypertension are contraindications to the use of thrombolytics.

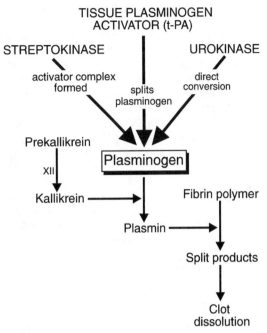

FIGURE 23–6 Fibrinolytic pathway.

PRECAUTIONS. Patients receiving concurrent antithrombotic therapy are at increased risk with thrombolytic therapy. Recent minor surgery and trauma are also precautions with use of the thrombolytics. Frequent hematologic tests must be performed to monitor the coagulation function of patients receiving fibrinolytic drugs. The drugs must also be used cautiously in patients with recent streptococcal infections because residual streptokinase may be present and produce additive effects. In addition, streptokinase exhibits significant antigenicity compared with the other thrombolytics and may be responsible for allergic reactions in some patients.

ADVERSE REACTIONS. Bleeding during therapy is the main adverse effect of the thrombolytics. Cerebral hemorrhage is one of the more common manifestations of bleeding.

UROKINASE (Abbokinase). Urokinase is an enzyme found naturally in human urine but produced commercially for medical use from kidney cell culture (Box 23–1). Its fibrinolytic activity involves direct conversion of plasminogen to active plasmin to dissolve the fibrin of blood clots (Fig. 23–6). Recombinant, or genetically engineered, urokinase products, such as pro-urokinase and urokinase plasminogen activator, have been developed and show great promise in maintaining patency of coronary blood vessels in cases of acute MI.

BOX 23–1   KEEPING COSTS DOWN . . . A HUNDRED MILES UP

The commercial feasibility and technical aspects of microgravity urokinase production aboard orbiting spacecraft has been studied by major pharmaceutical firms. Why is microgravity conducive to the production of certain pharmaceuticals?

Urokinase is difficult and expensive to make on earth. Human kidney cells produce urokinase, which must then be separated by electrophoresis. The technique is limited because heat produced by the process causes buoyancy and remixing of cells and solution. During electrophoresis in space, however, buoyancy is prevented by the microgravity environment. As a result of the more efficient separation process, drug quality and drug quantity improve.

In the mid-1980s, the cost of a standard course of therapy with urokinase was approximately US $2500 (Wall, 1982). It was believed that a space-based manufacturing enterprise could be developed that would be enormously profitable and yet provide ultra–high-quality urokinase at a cost of about US $100 per dose. Plans for urokinase production in an orbiting facility dimmed when earth-based laboratories developed commercial cell-culturing techniques for mass production of the thrombolytic. Space processing of exotic drugs, biologicals, and other materials, such as crystals and alloys, still holds promise wherever quality and performance of a product are more important than its price.

Deudney D: Space industrialization: The mirage of abundance. The Futurist:47–53, Dec 1982.
von Puttkamer J: The industrialization of space: Transcending the limits to growth. The Futurist:192–201, Jun 1979.
Wall RT: Drugs used in disorders of coagulation. In Katzung BD (ed) Basic and Clinical Pharmacology. Lange Medical Publications, Los Altos, 1982.

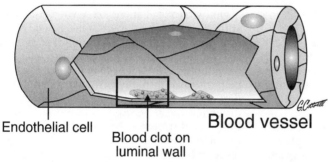

Endothelial cell

Blood clot on luminal wall

Blood vessel

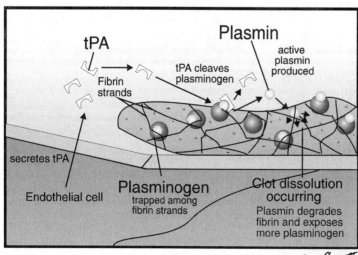

tPA

Fibrin strands

tPA cleaves plasminogen

Plasmin

active plasmin produced

secretes tPA

Endothelial cell

Plasminogen
trapped among fibrin strands

Clot dissolution occurring
Plasmin degrades fibrin and exposes more plasminogen

Detail of inset

FIGURE   23–7   tPA—mechanism of action.

BOX 23–2 LEECHES, TICKS, VAMPIRE BATS, AND GARLIC

In this day of laboratory synthesis it would seem that *all* new pharmaceuticals would be produced by such efforts. However, natural sources continue to yield promising new drugs. Just as organic sources supplied most currently used antithrombotics and thrombolytics, future drugs of these classes may soon be derived from quite novel biological sources. For example, blood-feeding organisms must keep blood flowing for several minutes to ingest a full meal from a host. This feeding method requires the production of factors that have anticoagulant, antiplatelet, or vasodilating activity.

Hirudin is a thrombin inactivator produced as a salivary enzyme by the buccal glands of the medicinal leech *(Hirudo medicinalis)*. This segmented worm now enjoys endangered species status but was used for centuries in the medical practice of bloodletting and was raised commercially in Europe in the mid-1800s. (France exported around 50 million leeches annually at that time.) Hirudin shows great promise as a future antithrombotic (see text) and in 1986 became available in sufficient quantitites as a recombinant drug to undergo further testing.

The soft tick *(Ornithodros moubata)* produces an anticoagulant in its saliva that has been identified as tick anticoagulant peptide (TAP). TAP inhibits the activity of factor X, a key clotting factor in both the intrinsic and extrinsic pathways. Tick anticoagulant peptide is presently available in recombinant form as r-TAP.

The saliva of the vampire bat *(Desmodus rotundus)* contains a thrombolytic agent called bat plasminogen activator (bat-PA). This compound has been produced through recombinant genetic techniques and has potential fibrinolytic action superior to that of tissue plasminogen activator (tPA, or alteplase). *In vitro* studies have shown that bat-PA stimulates production of plasmin and has a long duration of effect, and that the plasmin does not go on to inactivate fibrinogen. The lack of a fibrinogen-depleting effect is an advantage over current tPA therapy (see text).

Leaving the domain of saliva and blood-sucking animals, we find that the plant world offers us garlic as a platelet inhibitor. Garlic *(Allium sativum)* demonstrates antiplatelet activity and is available in several commercial preparations. The ancient cure-all contains adenosine and allicin, substances that prevent the aggregation of platelets, thereby blocking clot formation. (It is not yet known if wearing garlic around the neck has a repellant effect on vampire bats, thus providing an additional antithrombotic effect. Further experimental and clinical studies are needed . . .)

Block E: Antithrombotic agent of garlic: A lesson from 5000 years of folk medicine. In Steiner RP (ed): Folk Medicine: The Art and the Science. American Chemical Society, Washington, DC, 1986.

Fareed J et al: An objective perspective on recombinant hirudin: A new anticoagulant and antithrombotic agent. Blood Coagul Fibrinolysis 2:135–147, 1991.

Lawson LD, Ransom KD, and Hughes BG: Inhibition of whole blood platelet–aggregation by compounds in garlic clove extracts and commercial garlic products. Thromb Res 65:141–156, 1992.

Mellott MJ et al: Vampire bat salivary plasminogen activator promotes rapid and sustained reperfusion without concomitant systemic plasminogen activation in a canine model of arterial thrombosis. Arterioscler Thromb 12:212–221, 1992.

Scharfstein J and Lascalzo J: Molecular approaches to antithrombotic therapy. Physiology in Medicine Series. Hosp Pract (Off Ed) 27:77–86, 1992.

Storer TI and Usinger RL: General Zoology, ed 4. McGraw-Hill, New York, 1965.

Waxman L et al: Tick anticoagulant peptide (TAP) is a novel inhibitor of blood coagulation factor Xa. Science 248:593–597, May 1990.

INDICATIONS. Indications for use of urokinase include the treatment of massive pulmonary embolism and coronary artery thrombosis, and maintenance of patency of cannulae and catheters.

CONTRAINDICATIONS, PRECAUTIONS, AND ADVERSE REACTIONS. See Streptokinase.

ALTEPLASE (Activase, Activase rt-PA^{CAN}). Alteplase is the recombinant version of a natural enzyme called tissue plasminogen activator (tPA). This factor is produced naturally to bring about clot dissolution and retraction (Fig. 23–6). When a clot forms, plasminogen becomes incorporated in the fibrin mesh. Endothelial cells of the vessel wall release tPA, which splits plasminogen on the clot surface, releasing active plasmin. Plasmin in turn dissolves the fibrin mesh, which exposes more plasminogen to be acted on by tPA (Fig. 23–7). tPA remains active in the bloodstream for only about 10 minutes; therefore, the risk of bleeding due to fibrin activation is less than is seen with streptokinase or urokinase (Zivan and Choi, 1991). However, tPA-activated plasmin also degrades fibrinogen to result in fibrinogen depletion and greater risk of hemorrhage should wounding occur because the precursor of fibrin is in short supply.

INDICATIONS. Alteplase is used in the management of acute MI and of acute, massive pulmonary embolism. Alteplase is superior to streptokinase in maintaining adequate coronary blood flow, or patency, in acute MI. The patency declines, however, if heparin is not given concurrently (Anderson, 1991).

CONTRAINDICATIONS, PRECAUTIONS, AND ADVERSE REACTIONS. See Streptokinase.

ANISTREPLASE (Eminase). Anistreplase is also known as *anisoylated plasminogen-streptokinase activator complex* (APSAC). It consists of an inactive complex of plasminogen and streptokinase. After administration, controlled activation of the complex occurs, resulting in the conversion of plasminogen to plasmin. Plasmin, in turn, brings about lysis of blood clots. Anistreplase has a longer half-life than the fibrinolytics discussed previously (Alpert, 1991).

INDICATIONS. Acute management of coronary vessel thrombi in MI is an indication for use of anistreplase.

CONTRAINDICATIONS, PRECAUTIONS, AND ADVERSE REACTIONS. See Streptokinase. (Due to the streptokinase component of anistreplase, allergic reactions are more common than those caused by urokinase or alteplase.)

Newer Drugs

Recombinant hirudin (r-hirudin) has been developed from the saliva of the medicinal leech (Box 23–2). This salivary enzyme is a thrombin inhibitor that shows promise in animal and *in vitro* studies as an alternative to heparin therapy (Wallenga et al, 1991; Donayre, 1992). r-Hirudin has a short half-life and does not require an enzyme cofactor to produce its antithrombotic effect. In addition, r-hirudin exhibits few antigenic effects; therefore, allergic reactions are minimized (Wallenga et al, 1991).

TABLE 23–2 DRUG NAMES: ANTITHROMBOTICS AND THROMBOLYTICS

Generic Name	Trade Name
ANTITHROMBOTICS	
Heparin (**HEP**-a-rin)	(many trade names)
Warfarin (**WAR**-fa-rin)	Coumadin, Athrombin-K[CAN]
Dicumarol (dī-**KYOO**-ma-rol)	
Aspirin (acetylsalicylic acid, ASA)	
Ticlopidine (tī-**KLŌ**-pi-dēn)	Ticlid
Prostacyclin	
THROMBOLYTICS	
Streptokinase (strep-tō-**KĪ**-nās)	Streptase, Kabikinase
Urokinase (yoo-rō-**KĪ**-nās)	Abbokinase
Pro-urokinase	
Urokinase plasminogen activator	
Alteplase (**ALL**-te-plās) (tissue plasminogen activator)	Activase, Activase rt-PA[CAN]
Anistreplase (an-**Ī**-stre-plās) (anisoylated plasminogen–streptokinase activator complex)	Eminase
NEWER DRUGS	
Recombinant hirudin (hī-**RŪD**-in)	
Enoxaparin (e-**NOX**-a-pair-in)	

Enoxaparin is a member of a new group of low molecular weight heparins (LMWH) that prevent thromboembolic complications of surgery. Some studies (Donayre, 1992) indicate that LMWHs are not as effective as heparin and hirudin in anticoagulant and antiplatelet activity, whereas others report more promising results (Lassen et al, 1991).

Table 23–2 lists the generic and trade names of the antithrombotics and thrombolytics discussed in this chapter.

CHAPTER SUMMARY

Prevention of blood loss from the body is the obvious outcome of coagulation. Not quite as obvious, but equally important, is the *prevention* of coagulation. It would serve no useful purpose if slow-moving blood in a deep vein began to clot. The body produces the anticoagulant heparin to reduce the likelihood of such an occurrence. We have seen that after a blood clot forms, it is systematically removed by natural clot-dissolving chemicals, such as tissue plasminogen activator (tPA).

A variety of antithrombotic and thrombolytic

agents are currently available for clot prevention and dissolution. Nearly all were discovered as natural substances and some have been improved through cell-culturing and genetic engineering. These agents are heparin from mast cells and basophils, warfarin from coumarin compounds discovered in spoiled sweet clover hay, streptokinase from bacteria, urokinase from kidney cells, and tPA from blood vessel endothelial cells.

BIBLIOGRAPHY

Alpert JS: Importance of the pharmacological profile of thrombolytic agents in clinical practice. Am J Cardiol 68:3E–7E, 1991.

Anderson JL: Overview of patency as an end point of thrombolytic therapy. Am J Cardiol 68:11E–16E, 1991.

Benedict CR et al: Thrombolytic therapy: A state of the art review. Physiology in Medicine Series. Hosp Pract (Off Ed) 27:61–72, 1992.

Brody MJ, Feldman RD, and Hermsmeyer RK: Cardiovascular drugs. In Conn PM and Gebhart GF (eds): Essentials of Pharmacology. FA Davis, Philadelphia, 1989.

Brown BA: Hematology: Principles and Procedures, ed 6. Lea and Febiger, Philadelphia, 1993.

Carola R, Harley JP, and Noback CR: Human Anatomy and Physiology, ed 2. McGraw-Hill, New York, 1992.

Clark WG, Brater DC, and Johnson AR: Goth's Medical Pharmacology, ed 12. CV Mosby, St Louis, 1988.

Coller BS: Antiplatelet agents in the prevention and therapy of thrombosis. Annu Rev Med 43:171–180, 1992.

Cregler LL: Antithrombotic therapy in left ventricular thrombosis and systemic embolism. Am Heart J 123:1110–1114, Apr 1992.

Donayre CE: Future alternatives to heparin: Low–molecular weight heparin and hirudin. J Vasc Surg 1594:675–682, 1992.

Fareed J et al: An objective perspective on recombinant hirudin: A new anticoagulant and antithrombotic agent. Blood Coagul Fibrinolysis 2:135–147, 1991.

Fareed J et al: Experimental and clinical validation of the prophylactic antithrombotic effects of a low molecular weight heparin (enoxaparin). Semin Thromb Hemost 17(Suppl 3):319–328, 1991.

Grip L and Ryden L: Late streptokinase infusion and antithrombotic treatment in myocardial infarction reduce subsequent myocardial ischemia. Am Heart J 121:737–745, 1991.

Haire WD: Pharmacology of fibrinolysis. Chest 101(Suppl 4):91S–97S, 1992.

Harmening DM: Introduction to hemostasis: An overview of hemostatic mechanism, platelet structure and function, and extrinsic and intrinsic systems. In Harmening DM (ed): Clinical Hematology and Fundamentals of Hemostasis, ed 2. FA Davis, Philadelphia, 1992.

Hirsch J: Antithrombotic therapy in deep vein thrombosis and pulmonary embolism. Am Heart J 123:1115–1122, 1992.

Hirsch J: Oral anticoagulant drugs. N Engl J Med 324:1865–1876, 1991.

Hirsh J and Levine MN: Low molecular weight heparin. Blood 79:1–17, 1992.

Hyers TM: Venous thromboembolic disease: Diagnosis and use of antithrombotic therapy. Clin Cardiol 13:V123–V128, Apr 1990.

Imura Y, Stassen JM, and Collen D: Comparative antithrombotic effects of heparin, recombinant hirudin and argatroban in a hamster femoral vein platelet–rich mural thrombosis model. J Pharmacol Exp Ther 261:895–898, 1992.

Kelley RE: Rationale for antithrombotic therapy in atrial fibrillation. Neurol Clin 10:233–249, 1992.

Lassen MR et al: Clinical trials with low molecular weight heparins in the prevention of postoperative thromboembolic complications: A meta-analysis. Semin Thromb Hemost 17(Suppl 3):284–290, 1991.

Mangel WF: Enzyme systems: Better reception for urokinase. Nature 344:488–490, 1990.

Morishita K et al: Effect of ticlopidine and other antithrombotics on venous thrombosis induced by endothelial damage of jugular vein in rats. Thromb Res 63:373–384, 1991.

O'Rourke PP: ECMO: Where have we been? Where are we going? Respiratory Care 36:683–692, 1991.

PRIMI Trial Study Group: Randomised double-blind trial of recombinant pro-urokinase against streptokinase in acute myocardial infarction. Lancet i:863–869, 1989.

Scharfstein J and Lascalzo J: Molecular approaches to antithrombotic therapy. Physiology in Medicine Series. Hosp Pract. (Off Ed) 27:77–86, 1992.

Stein B and Fuster V: Antithrombotic therapy in acute myocardial infarction: Prevention of venous, left ventricular and coronary artery thromboembolism. Am J Cardiol 64:33B–40B, 1989.

Suttie JW: Warfarin and vitamin K. Clin Cardiol 13:V116–V118, 1990.

Tortora GJ and Grabowski SR: Principles of Anatomy and Physiology, ed 7. HarperCollins, New York, 1993.

Wallenga JM et al: Comparison of recombinant hirudin and heparin as an anticoagulant in a cardiopulmonary bypass model. Blood Coagul Fibrinolysis 2:105–111, 1991.

Wall RT: Drugs used in disorders of coagulation. In Katzung BD (ed): Basic and Clinical Pharmacology. Lange Medical Publications, Los Altos, 1982.

White HD: Comparative safety of thrombolytic agents. Am J Cardiol 68:30E–37E, 1991.

Zivin JA and Choi DW: Stroke therapy. Sci Am 265:56–63, Jul 1991.

UNIT FIVE

DRUGS AFFECTING THE CENTRAL NERVOUS SYSTEM

UNIT INTRODUCTION

The humane practice of medicine has been advanced by the discovery of many of the drugs introduced in this unit. Chemical control of various mental states, and control of pain reception, transmission, and perception, have paved the way for further developments in modern medical-surgical procedures.

The drugs affecting the central nervous system (CNS) are the subject of this unit. Most do not directly influence the respiratory system, but many are used in ways that *indirectly* modify the action of breathing. The respiratory care practitioner must be familiar with psychopharmacologic and hypnotic agents, used to decrease anxiety and stabilize ventilatory patterns, and with analgesics, used to control pain. In addition, an awareness of toxicity effects on the respiratory system is needed. The pharmacologic effects of CNS drugs acting on medullary cough control and respiratory centers will be discussed through the action of certain analgesics, general anesthetics, and ventilatory stimulants. Additionally, drugs used in surgical anesthesia, such as local anesthetics, barbiturates, and neuroleptics, are examined.

CHAPTER 24

Psychopharmacologic and Hypnotic Drugs

CHAPTER OUTLINE

CHAPTER OBJECTIVES

After studying this chapter the reader should be able to:

- Define the following terms:
  - Psychopharmacologic drug, neuroleptic, psychosis.
- Describe the mechanism and site of action of antipsychotic tranquilizers.
- Describe the pharmacologic activity of the following antipsychotic tranquilizers:
  - Chlorpromazine, haloperidol.
- Define the following terms:
  - Anxiety, anxiolytic, ataractic.
- Explain the mechanism of action of benzodiazepine tranquilizers and describe the pharmacologic activity of flumazenil as a benzodiazepine receptor–blocking agent.
- Describe the pharmacologic activity of the following antianxiety tranquilizers:
  - Diazepam, chlordiazepoxide, alprazolam, lorazepam, oxazepam, meprobamate.
- Describe the pharmacologic activity of the benzodiazepine antagonist flumazenil.
- Define depression and describe the mechanism of action of the antidepressants.
- Describe the pharmacologic activity of the following antidepressants:
  - Tranylcypromine, amitriptyline, imipramine, nortriptyline, trazodone, amoxapine.
- Describe the pharmacologic activity of the antimanic agent lithium carbonate.
- Differentiate between sedation and hypnosis.
- Describe the function of the reticular formation.
- Describe the action of the reticular activating system (RAS) in determining arousal states of the central nervous system (CNS) and describe how drugs may influence the RAS.
- Describe the pharmacologic activity of the following benzodiazepine hypnotics:
  - Flurazepam, triazolam, midazolam.
- Describe the mechanism of action of barbiturates used as hypnotics.
- Describe the pharmacologic activity of the following barbiturates:
  - Amobarbital, pentobarbital, secobarbital, butabarbital, phenobarbital.
- Describe the effects of barbiturate overdose on the respiratory system and outline the management of such toxicities.

- Describe the pharmacologic activity of the following nonbarbiturate nonbenzodiazepine hypnotics:
  - ▪ Chloral hydrate, paraldehyde, ethchlorvynol, glutethimide.

KEY TERMS

antianxiety tranquilizer
  (anxiolytic, ataractic)
antidepressant
antimanic
antipsychotic tranquilizer
  (neuroleptic)

anxiety
depression
hypnotic drug
limbic system
psychopharmacologic drug
psychosis (sī-KO-sis)

rebound anxiety
rebound insomnia
reticular activating system
  (RAS) (arousal system)
reticular formation

CHAPTER INTRODUCTION

Therapeutic agents known as **psychopharmacologic drugs** are used in the treatment of major and minor mental illnesses. **Hypnotic drugs** are used to induce sleep. Increased understanding of the chemical basis of brain function has revealed chemical imbalances responsible for certain types of mental disturbances. Specific drugs such as antipsychotic tranquilizers, antianxiety tranquilizers, antidepressants, and hypnotics have been developed for management of symptoms of schizophrenia, anxiety, depression, and insomnia. The pharmacologic activity of this diverse group of drugs and the centrally mediated effects on the respiratory system are the focus of this chapter.

ANTIPSYCHOTIC TRANQUILIZERS

Background

In the 1950s, a class of drugs was introduced that revolutionized patient care within psychiatric institutions. The **antipsychotic tranquilizers,** or **neuroleptics,** did not provide a cure. They calmed agitated patients, greatly decreased the amount of physical restraint required, and reduced the reliance on electroshock therapy. In so doing, they allowed more humane treatment of persons with debilitating mental illnesses, such as schizophrenia.

Site of Action

The antipsychotic tranquilizers act at multiple sites in the brain to quiet an agitated person. Collectively the various sites compose the **limbic system** of the brain. This system is a functional collection, or physiologically defined group of structures. It includes parts of the cerebrum, thalamus, hypothalamus, and midbrain. Figure 24–1 shows a schematic diagram of the limbic system. (The names of the individual parts mak-

ing up the limbic system are not essential for our purposes.) The limbic system is involved with memory and with emotions such as aggression, rage, fear, and sex drive. Visceral and behavioral responses, such as feeding and fighting, are also modulated by the limbic system. Antipsychotic drugs target these areas in the limbic system to cause a quieting effect on the brain. The mechanisms of action of the drugs are discussed below with the specific antipsychotic tranquilizers. In general, the antipsychotics depress dopamine neurotransmission at D_2-dopaminergic receptors in the limbic area. Excess dopamine production, faulty dopamine inactivation, heightened dopamine receptor sensitivity, or some combination of these factors is thought to be responsible for the chemical imbalance that produces major psychoses, such as schizophrenia. A

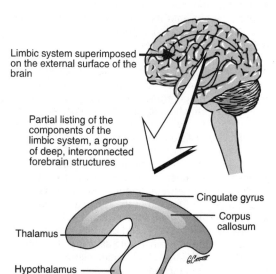

Limbic system superimposed on the external surface of the brain

Partial listing of the components of the limbic system, a group of deep, interconnected forebrain structures

Thalamus

Hypothalamus

Amygdala

Cingulate gyrus

Corpus callosum

Hippocampus

FIGURE 24–1 Limbic system.

psychosis is a serious mental disturbance characterized by delusions and hallucination. (Because of the therapeutic use in treating "major" disturbances, the antipsychotic tranquilizers have been referred to as "major tranquilizers." The term, however, is imprecise and confusing and has been generally abandoned.)

THERAPEUTIC ANTIPSYCHOTIC AGENTS

Several different families, or classes, of antipsychotic drugs have been found to have depressive activity on the dopaminergic system in the brain. A few are presented below as representative of the antipsychotic group of tranquilizers. Unfortunately, dopamine neurotransmission is also required for coordinated control of normal muscle movements. Therefore, suppression of dopmaine neurotransmission by antipsychotic drugs may produce varying degrees of unwanted parkinsonian side effects. (Parkinson's disorder is characterized by involuntary muscle movements leading to shaking and uncoordinated muscle contractions.)

Phenothiazine Derivatives

CHLORPROMAZINE (Thorazine). The phenothiazine group of antipsychotic agents includes several subgroups of drugs and is represented by chlorpromazine. Chlorpromazine was initially developed as an antihistamine and was one of the original antipsychotic tranquilizers introduced into psychiatric medicine in the early 1950s. Like all of the antipsychotics, chlorpromazine is a dopamine receptor antagonist acting in specific areas in the brain. Its pharmacologic effects can be antagonized through the administration of the dopamine precursor levodopa (L-dopa). Pharmacologic effects of the phenothiazines are related to their blocking action at cholinergic, adrenergic, and H_1-histamine receptors. For example, a related phenothiazine derivative, promethazine, is an antihistamine (Chapter 10). Many phenothiazines also exhibit a powerful antiemetic action at the chemoreceptor trigger zone.

INDICATIONS. The primary indication for use of the antipsychotic tranquilizers is in the treatment of schizophrenia. Some types of affective disorders, or mood shifts, that have a schizophrenic component may respond to the antipsychotics.

CONTRAINDICATIONS. Withdrawal from alcohol or other drugs can be aggravated through administration of the antipsychotic tranquilizers.

PRECAUTIONS. Additive effects with other central nervous system (CNS) depressants, such as alcohol, may occur and result in depression of ventilation.

ADVERSE REACTIONS. The antipsychotic tranquilizers differ in severity of adverse reactions, but all produce a variety of undesirable effects. These include muscarinic receptor blockade leading to mydriatic-cycloplegic effects, dry mouth, constipation, and α-adrenergic receptor blockade leading to orthostatic hypotension. In addition, D_2-dopaminergic receptor blockade may lead to extrapyramidal motor dysfunction, causing parkinsonian symptoms. (The extrapyramidal tract is one of the main motor pathways leading from the brain into the spinal cord.) Undesirable side effects resulting from chlorpromazine therapy are generally more pronounced than those of the newer antipsychotics that have entered therapeutic use.

Butyrophenone Derivatives

HALOPERIDOL (Haldol). Haloperidol is a newer antipsychotic possessing less severe side effects than chlorpromazine. The mechanism of action of haloperidol is one of dopamine D_2-receptor blockade, but the effects on the motor systems controlling movement are not as pronounced as those seen with the phenothiazines. A closely related butyrophenone compound is droperidol, which is used in some types of anesthesia when combined with the narcotic fentanyl. (This use is covered in Chapter 27.)

INDICATIONS, CONTRAINDICATIONS, PRECAUTIONS AND ADVERSE REACTIONS. See Chlorpromazine.

ANTIANXIETY TRANQUILIZERS
Anxiety

Anxiety, a feeling of apprehension or uneasiness, can be beneficial. It produces a state of heightened perception, or awareness, that focuses our energies in a productive way. On the other hand, when anxiety increases to the point where it diminishes or debilitates our activities, psychiatric or drug therapy may be indicated. In certain kinds of anxiety, such as panic disorder, antidepressant drugs are generally prescribed. (These drugs are described later in the chapter.) In disease states such as angina pectoris, the clinical symptom of anxiety usually disappears once the underlying cardiac condition has been controlled. In generalized anxiety disorder, however, where no organic dysfunction or psychosis is causing the anxious state, **antianxiety tranquilizers** are a prudent choice for a physician to make. These drugs are also known as **anxiolytics,** or **ataractics.** (Drugs that produce a state of mental calm and tranquility.) The term "minor tranquilizer" has been used, but like "major tranquilizer" it is inaccurate, confusing, and archaic. It is supposed to indicate that these drugs are used for "minor" mental disturbances, such as anxiety, as opposed to "major" upsets, such as schizophrenia.

Mechanism of Action

High-affinity binding sites called benzodiazepine receptors have been found on brain cells (Piercy et al, 1991) next to the binding sites for the inhibitory amino acid transmitter γ-aminobutyric acid (GABA) (Bhatnagar et al, 1989; Clark et al, 1988). These sites are associated with a chloride ion channel that allows extracellular Cl^{1-} to pass into the neuron, thus hyperpolarizing the cell membrane (Fig. 24–2). In the absence of GABA, benzodiazepines, such as diazepam, fail to open the Cl^{1-} channel, but when GABA is present, benzodiazepines bind at the receptor and promote Cl^{1-} influx (Bhatnagar et

al, 1989). Following identification of the benzodiazepine receptor, a selective benzodiazepine receptor antagonist was developed. Flumazenil (Anexate) functions as a competitive antagonist at the benzodiazepine receptor, effectively blocking the action of this class of anxiolytic (Sanders et al, 1991). Flumazenil has proven especially valuable in anesthesia, where it is used to reverse the sedation produced by benzodiazepines.

THERAPEUTIC ANTIANXIETY AGENTS

Benzodiazepines

Benzodiazepines were introduced into clinical medicine in the early 1960s. The effects of the benzodiazepines are similar, although certain members of the group are used for specific indications (Clark et al, 1988). For example, midazolam was developed specifically for use in anesthesia (Chapter 27).

DIAZEPAM (Valium, many others). Diazepam is the prototype of the benzodiazepine group of antianxiety tranquilizers. It is a long-acting psychopharmacologic agent with a duration of action in excess of 24 hours.

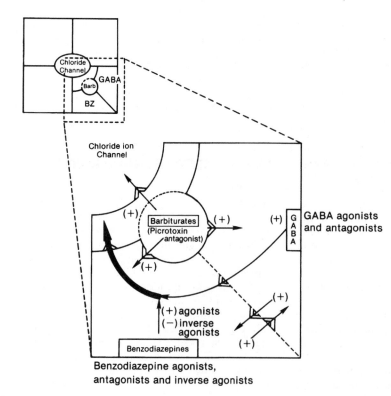

Benzodiazepine agonists, antagonists and inverse agonists

FIGURE 24–2 Chloride channel with benzodiazepine and picrotoxin receptors. (From Bhatnagar RK, Dutton GR, and Gebhart GF: Drugs acting on the central nervous system. In Conn PM and Gebhart GF (eds): Essentials of Pharmacology. FA Davis Co, Philadelphia, 1989, p. 116, with permission.)

INDICATIONS. The primary indication for use is the treatment of minor anxiety. This drug is especially useful prior to surgery and is a routine component of balanced anesthesia (Clark et al, 1988). Diazepam also has a marked skeletal muscle–relaxing effect, acting in the spinal cord to block the exit of motor impulses. The normal dosage form for producing the anxiolytic effects of benzodiazepines is the oral route. However, intravenous diazepam is available to treat seizures caused by drugs, toxins, or epilepsy.

CONTRAINDICATIONS. Known hypersensitivity to the benzodiazepines is a contraindication to the use of diazepam.

PRECAUTIONS. Chronic administration may contribute to physical and psychologic dependency. Drowsiness and additive effects, including ventilatory depression, may occur when other CNS depressants are administered concurrently with the benzodiazepines. One of the most common interactions resulting in marked ventilatory depression involves alcohol and anxiolytics such as diazepam. None of the current antianxiety tranquilizers are *pure* ataractics because all produce some measure of CNS depression in addition to their "tranquilizing" effects.

Rebound anxiety may occur with sudden benzodiazepine withdrawal (Bhatnagar et al, 1989). In this phenomenon, a significant increase in anxiety returns once the drug is removed. It is presumed that a presently unidentified endogenous benzodiazepinelike compound may be inhibited during therapy with exogenous drugs such as diazepam. Sudden withdrawal leaves the benzodiazepine receptor temporarily unoccupied and triggers the anxiety symptoms. Benzodiazepines with a short elimination half-life ($t_{1/2}$) produce the most severe effect, whereas those with a longer half-life produce the least severe rebound anxiety. Diazepam has a half-life that can persist for several days ($t_{1/2}$ = 20–200 h). Therefore, it produces less frequent and less severe effects than fast-acting triazolam ($t_{1/2}$ = 2–5 h), used primarily to induce sleep.

ADVERSE REACTIONS. Adverse reactions include drowsiness, minor skin irritations, and occasionally impotence. Ataxia (staggering gait) can also occur but is much less severe than that seen with other antianxiety tranquilizers, such as the meprobamates (discussed below).

Other antianxiety drugs of the benzodiazepine class differ from diazepam mainly in potency and duration of action. Indications, contraindications, precautions, and adverse reactions are essentially the same as those discussed with diazepam. Short-acting compounds have a duration of action of less than 24 hours and include alprazolam (Xanax), lorazepam (Ativan), and oxazepam (Serax). Long-acting benzodiazepines like diazepam have durations of action in excess of 24 hours and include chlordiazepoxide (Librium).

Carbamates

The carbamate group of antianxiety tranquilizers have more in common with the barbiturates than they do with the benzodiazepines. For example, the carbamates have a significant sedative component and an addiction potential not seen to the same extent as with the benzodiazepines. In addition, sudden discontinuation of carbamate anxiolytics may trigger serious withdrawal symptoms, including seizure activity. In general, the carbamates are not used nearly as frequently as the benzodiazepines in the treatment of minor anxiety (see Nonbarbiturate Nonbenzodiazepine Hypnotics below).

MEPROBAMATE (Equanil, Miltown). Meprobamate blocks spinal interneurons to suppress motor impulses to the skeletal muscles.

INDICATION. Meprobamate is used as an anxiolytic and sedative agent and as a centrally acting skeletal muscle relaxant.

CONTRAINDICATIONS. Known hypersensitivity to the carbamates is a contraindication to the use of meprobamate.

PRECAUTIONS AND ADVERSE REACTIONS. Drowsiness, ataxia, and residual CNS depression ("morning hangover") are precautions and undesirable effects of meprobamate therapy.

ANTIDEPRESSANTS

Depression

Slight alterations in mental outlook occur constantly and usually in a cyclical manner. Typically the swings in mood are minor, prompted by trivial changes. However, mood shifts can be significant situations of major change, such as in the death of a close family member. **Depression** in its various forms is described as a loss of interest in those things that are normally pleasurable—family, friends, hobbies, food, or sex. It is characterized as a *sadness* of long duration and of unknown cause. Reactive, or secondary, depression is the most common type of depression and is often associated with a loss in the family or a major illness such as cancer. Major, or unipolar, depression is also called endogenous depression because it has a biologic cause. Unipolar depression is typified by a continuous state of depression. Bipolar depression, or manic-depression, is characterized by alternating episodes of elation, or mania, and severe depression.

The symptoms of mania are managed with the **antimanic** drug lithium carbonate (Carbolith). This drug is not classified as an antidepressant but is briefly described in this section. Lithium is used to stabilize mood swings and decrease the severity of the manic phase of bipolar depression (manic-depression) (Hollister, 1982). It enhances the neuronal uptake and metabolism of catecholamines, such as norepinephrine and dopamine. This decreases the store of catecholamines present in nerve terminals. Lithium also interferes with sodium reabsorption and may contribute to Na^{1+} depletion. Toxicity effects include nausea, vomiting, and diarrhea and the development of polyuria and polydipsia. The combination effect of losses from the gastrointestinal and urinary systems may upset fluid and electrolyte homeostasis. CNS and cardiovascular involvement occur with more serious lithium intoxication. These effects include ataxia, mental confusion, generalized seizures, coma, cardiac arrhythmias, circulatory collapse, and death.

Effects of Antidepressants

Antidepressant drugs are used to help stabilize mood shifts. They reduce the severity of the symptoms of depression. These may include apathy, hopelessness, insomnia, fatigue, and headache. Antidepressants are not general CNS stimulants. In fact, most of the antidepressants produce very little mood elevation. Rather, they are drugs that potentiate chemical transmission in certain parts of the brain to counter the symptoms of depression.

Two major classes of antidepressants are available: the classic antidepressants, consisting of monoamine oxidase (MAO) inhibitors and tricyclic antidepressants (TCAs), and the newer second-generation antidepressants. Long-term effects of the MAO inhibitor and TCA classes of drugs result in a decrease in postsynaptic β-adrenoceptor density, a decrease in the sensitivity of presynaptic α_2-adrenoceptors to norepinephrine, and an increase in response of postsynaptic α_1-adrenoceptors to α_1-agonists and the biogenic amine serotonin. (Serotonin is also known as 5-hydroxytryptophan, or 5-HT.) Currently the neurochemical mechanism of depression is viewed as one of decreased activity of adrenergic and serotonergic systems in the CNS (Bhatnagar et al, 1989). Treatment with drugs that potentiate levels of amine transmitters in the brain is the rationale behind antidepressant pharmacotherapy.

THERAPEUTIC ANTIDEPRESSANT AGENTS

Classic Antidepressants
Monoamine oxidase inhibitors

TRANYLCYPROMINE (Parnate). Tranylcypromine is an amphetaminelike drug belonging to the MAO inhibitor group of antidepressants. These drugs are relatively toxic and have been largely replaced by the safer tricyclic antidepressants and second-generation antidepressants (discussed below). Drugs such as tranylcypromine irreversibly inhibit MAO, the effects lasting until new enzyme is synthesized.

INDICATION. Treatment of depression is the main indication for use of the MAO inhibitors.

CONTRAINDICATIONS. Concurrent therapy with vasoconstrictor drugs, such as α-adrenergic stimulants, is contraindicated because a hypertensive crisis such as stroke can be precipitated. Administration of MAO inhibitor antidepressants in conjunction with drugs that depress the CNS may cause a dangerous fall in blood pressure.

Concurrent administration of MAO inhibitors and TCAs results in severe CNS toxicity, including ventilatory depression. This is because the MAO inhibitor class of drugs slows the metabolism of the TCA class of drugs (see Adverse Reactions).

PRECAUTIONS. Foods such as wine, beer, and cheese that have been produced through fermentation contain high levels of vasoconstrictor amines such as tyramine. MAO functions in the gut and liver to metabolize such vasoactive amines. Therefore, a hypertensive crisis may occur when these foods are consumed by a patient taking MAO inhibitor antidepressants.

Barbiturates are capable of inducing hepatic microsomal enzymes. Chronic administration of barbiturates, therefore, may stimulate metabolism of drugs such as MAO inhibitor antidepressants.

ADVERSE REACTIONS. Orthostatic hypotension and drug interactions with amines are potential adverse reactions with the MAO inhibitors. These antidepressants not only inhibit MAO in the liver, but also inhibit the hepatic microsomal enzymes. These mixed-function oxidases are the most important drug-metabolizing enzymes in the liver (see Chapter 2). Therefore, the effects of most CNS depressants, including the TCA group of antidepressants, are prolonged when the hepatic microsomal enzymes are impaired. This in turn can increase the risk for producing severe ventilatory depression.

Tricyclic Antidepressants

AMITRIPTYLINE (Elavil, others). The tricyclic antidepressants such as amitriptyline are more frequently used than the MAO inhibitor class of antidepressants. Following initial therapy, the TCAs inhibit amine uptake into neurons (the "amine pump") to elevate amine levels. Recall that uptake-1 is the main mechanism for the inactivation of amines released by adrenergic neurons. Therefore, more neurotransmitter is available to act at presynaptic α_2-adrenoceptors and inhibit release of additional neurotransmitter (see Chapter 5). With prolonged therapy, adrenoceptor sensitivity returns to normal but blockage of uptake continues. The TCAs also block cholinergic muscarinic, α_1-adrenergic, and H_1-histamine receptors to produce undesirable effects such as bradycardia, urinary retention, and constipation.

INDICATIONS. The primary indication for use of the TCA group of antidepressants is in the treatment of depression. Maximal antidepressant effect takes several weeks to develop.

CONTRAINDICATIONS. Due to the anticholinergic effect produced by the TCAs, preexisting bradycardia may be worsened. In addition, the TCAs produce a quinidinelike antiarrhythmic effect. Therefore, cardiac abnormalities characterized by a prolonged QT interval or widened QRS complex may be aggravated.

PRECAUTIONS AND ADVERSE REACTIONS. Anticholinergic effects such as blurred vision, bradycardia, constipation, dry mouth, and general suppression of glandular secretion are cautions with TCA therapy. This is especially true when anticholinergic drugs are given concurrently. In addition, orthostatic hypotension may be caused by an antiadrenergic (α_1) effect. The quinidinelike effect of the drugs also warrants caution in those patients with impaired conduction. Extrapyramidal motor disturbances resembling parkinsonism and ventilatory depression may occur at higher dosages. Ventilatory depression, especially cumulative effects with other depressants, is an ever-present risk with any CNS depressant. High levels of TCAs may depress medullary centers and impair central ventilatory drive. In addition, the concurrent use of MAO inhibitor antidepressants may inhibit hepatic microsomal enzymes, thus prolonging and intensifying the effects of TCA antidepressants. Interactions may also occur with barbiturates, which can induce microsomal enzymes. This stimulates the metabolism of drugs such as the TCAs.

Tricyclic antidepressant derivatives such as imipramine (Tofranil) and nortriptyline (Aventyl) exhibit differences in cardiovascular, sedative, and anticholinergic activity (Table 24–1). Protriptyline is a low-sedative TCA useful for treatment of certain sleep apneas (see Chapter 28).

Second-Generation Antidepressants

A newer group of therapeutic agents are collectively called the second-generation antidepressants. The group includes trazodone (Desyrel), amoxapine (Asendin), and the benzodiazepine anxiolytic alprazolam (Xanax) mentioned previously. This benzodiazepine has marked antidepressant activity in addition to antianxiety activity. These newer compounds may exhibit more rapid onset of action and fewer adverse effects than other antidepressants. Extensive clinical experience has not yet been generated,

TABLE 24–1 COMPARISON OF PHARMACOLOGIC EFFECTS OF SEVERAL ANTIDEPRESSANT DRUGS

	Sedative Effects	Anticholinergic Effects	Cardiotoxic Effects*
TRICYCLIC ANTIDEPRESSANTS			
Amitriptyline	+++	+++	++
Imipramine	++	++	++
Nortriptyline	++	++	++
Protriptyline	None	++	++
SECOND-GENERATION ANTIDEPRESSANTS			
Trazodone	+++	None	Minimal
Amoxapine	++	+	Minimal

Source: Data from Bhatnagar et al, 1989.
*Cardiac effects such as orthostatic hypotension and ECG abnormalities are usually seen with high doses and may vary in severity.
+—slight; ++—moderate; +++—high.

but the drugs are now available to the physician and represent alternatives to the classic MAO inhibitor and tricyclic groups of antidepressants (Bhatnagar et al, 1989).

HYPNOTICS

Hypnotic drugs are used primarily in the treatment of insomnia. However, those having additional sedative (drowsiness) properties are valuable perioperatively. Clinical uses of hypnotics in anesthesia are covered in Chapter 27. Benzodiazepine hypnotics and barbiturates are available. Some barbiturates have pronounced sedative action. In fact, they were originally known as *sedative-hypnotics* but are currently referred to by the singular term *hypnotic.*

Reticular Activating System

A diffuse, netlike arrangement of neurons and their processes makes up the **reticular formation,** which is scattered throughout the brainstem. Vital functional groupings of cells composing the cardiac, vasomotor, and ventilatory centers are located in the reticular formation and found within specific areas of the brain such as the pons and medulla (Fig. 24–3). In addition, nonvital but important groupings such as swallowing, coughing, and emetic (vomiting) centers are found in addition to the chemoreceptor trigger zone.

Sensory impulses traveling to the cerebral cortex pass through the reticular formation and influence activities such as the rate and depth of ventilation. Continuous and regular sensory stimulation, such as the monotonous drone of a fan or the incessant hum of a fluorescent light

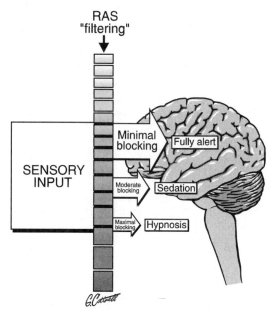

FIGURE 24–4 Function of the reticular activating system (RAS).

fixture, is not noticed after about 10–15 seconds. This sensory adaptation is called habituation and is affected by the following system.

The ascending (sensory) pathways going to the cerebrum make up the **reticular activating system (RAS),** or **arousal system.** The RAS is concerned with behavioral activities, such as the sleep-wake cycle, awareness, alertness, and the level of sensory perception at a given time. Screening of incoming sensations by the RAS prevents sensory overload of the cerebral cortex. *Arousal* of the CNS occurs if the RAS filters relatively little sensory information. However, if the RAS blocks enough sensations from reaching consciousness, *sedation* occurs. When the RAS is working maximally to filter unnecessary sensory impulses, *hypnosis,* or sleep, occurs (Fig. 24–4). The barbiturates and many opioid analgesics suppress sensations by inhibiting the pathways of the RAS.

THERAPEUTIC HYPNOTIC AGENTS

Benzodiazepine Hypnotics

The undesirable phenomenon of rebound anxiety was mentioned earlier with the main group of benzodiazepines. A similar unpleasant effect is **rebound insomnia,** in which wakefulness increases above the baseline, or normal, level for a particular patient (Bhatnagar et al, 1989). The severity of the phenomenon is inversely related

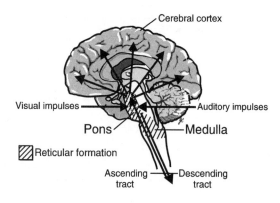

FIGURE 24–3 Reticular formation.

to the duration of effect of the benzodiazepine. Rapidly eliminated benzodiazepines, such as triazolam, produce the most rebound insomnia, whereas slowly eliminated drugs, such as diazepam, produce less severe effects.

Flurazepam (Dalmane) was introduced in 1970 as the first of the benzodiazepine hypnotics and became the most widely used hypnotic until the advent of shorter half-life benzodiazepines in the 1980s (Greenblatt, 1992). Flurazepam is more slowly absorbed but more rapidly eliminated than diazepam. Consequently, residual sedation is generally less, but rebound anxiety and insomnia are generally more. During use of flurazepam to treat insomnia, loss of hypnotic effect is very slight compared with other benzodiazepines.

Triazolam (Halcion) became available in the early 1980s as a short-acting benzodiazepine hypnotic and provided an alternative to flurazepam therapy for physicians treating sleep disorders. Triazolam is more slowly absorbed than flurazepam but has a very short elimination half-life of only a few hours compared with a few days ($t_{1/2}$ = 100 h) for flurazepam. The short time in the body results in the least amount of daytime sedation. The short elimination time, however, also results in the worst rebound insomnia side effects compared with the other benzodiazepines. In addition, triazolam exhibits rapidly developing tolerance. Other pharmacologic characteristics of flurazepam and triazolam are the same as those described for diazepam.

Midazolam (Versed) is a very water soluble, injectable benzodiazepine hypnotic specifically developed for use in clinical anesthesia. It is extremely versatile and is used as a preoperative medication, a hypnotic, and an adjunct to intravenous sedation. These and other uses relating to anesthesia are explored in Chapter 27.

INDICATIONS. Short-term management of insomnia (less than 1 month) is the main indication for use of the benzodiazepine hypnotics.

CONTRAINDICATIONS. Hypersensitivity to the benzodiazepines is a contraindication to their use. In addition, preexisting CNS depression is a contraindication to the use of benzodiazepine hypnotics.

PRECAUTIONS. Additive effects may occur between benzodiazepines and other CNS depressants, such as alcohol. As usual, there is always risk of ventilatory depression under such conditions. As a general rule, residual effects of daytime sedation ("hangover") and reduced performance are greatest with the more slowly eliminated benzodiazepines and least with those

that are rapidly eliminated (Bhatnagar et al, 1989).

ADVERSE EFFECTS. Rebound insomnia and anxiety, sedation, performance impairment, and amnesia are troublesome adverse effects with the benzodiazepine hypnotics (Greenblatt, 1992).

Barbiturates

The mechanism of action of barbiturates is very similar to that of the benzodiazepines. Both require the presence of GABA, and both increase Cl^{1-} movement into the cell to stabilize the membrane (Bhatnagar et al, 1989; Trevor and Way, 1982). Barbiturates act at a picrotoxin receptor associated with the Cl^{1-} channel on cell membranes (Fig. 24–2) and prolong the length of time the channel is open. (Picrotoxin is a CNS stimulant used in laboratories to study neurochemical transmission.) More generalized CNS depression occurs with the barbiturates than with the benzodiazepines as a result of prolonged Cl^{1-} entry and increased membrane hyperpolarization. As we will see later, this barbiturate effect on cell membranes is not restricted to cells of the CNS. Barbiturates have a particular affinity for the RAS, where they inhibit sensory arousal to produce sedation and hypnosis.

Barbiturates are synthesized from the parent compound barbituric acid, which has no hypnotic activity of its own. Chemical modification of the molecule has produced several barbiturates that differ from each other in duration of action and clinical application.

Some barbiturates have extremely high lipid-solubility and very short durations of action. The ultrashort-acting barbiturates such as thiopental are used exclusively in intravenous anesthesia and will be examined in Chapter 27. Secobarbital (Seconal) is classified as intermediate acting, whereas butabarbital (Butisol) is long acting. The classification depends on the elimination half-life of the drug. The classification of the barbiturates on the basis of their duration of effect is very imprecise. Virtually any reference source will offer a slightly different classification scheme. In general, "long-acting" implies a barbiturate with a plasma half-life in excess of 24 hours, whereas the effects of "intermediate-acting" barbiturates range from 12 to 24 hours. "Short-acting" barbiturates produce their effects for less than 12 hours, and "ultrashort-acting" are drugs acting for less than 4 hours. Remember, these times are simply measurements of *plasma* levels. Rapid-onset barbiturates used in intravenous anesthesia, for example, typically produce their desired *clinical* effect in a matter of minutes.

INDICATIONS. Therapeutic uses of the barbiturates are varied. In the context of this chapter, the intermediate-acting barbiturates such as pentobarbital (Nembutal) and amobarbital (Amytal) are valuable as hypnotics but not as useful as the benzodiazepines due to a pronounced sedative effect. As was mentioned previously, ultrashort-acting agents are employed as anesthetics and will be discussed later. All of the barbiturates are capable of suppressing convulsant activity, but the long-acting barbiturate phenobarbital (Luminal) is especially useful because it exhibits a pronounced antiepileptic effect.

CONTRAINDICATIONS. Preexisting CNS depression may be made worse by administration of barbiturates.

PRECAUTIONS. Barbiturates produce additive effects with other CNS depressants, such as tranquilizers, alcohol, and some antihistamines. As with any of the CNS depressants, barbiturates may progressively depress ventilatory controls to result in ventilatory depression. Barbiturate overdoses are discussed below. Additive effects with other CNS depressants result in typical generalized CNS depression that includes sedation, slowed speech, mental confusion, and ataxia. In addition to these cautions, the barbiturates have a significant potential for abuse.

Barbiturates induce the hepatic microsomal enzyme system and thereby modify the activity of other drugs. This important group of drug-metabolizing enzymes is discussed with pharmacokinetics in Chapter 2. The increased activity of these mixed-function oxidases stimulates metabolism of certain drugs. These include the MAO inhibitor and tricyclic classes of antidepressants, the coumarin group of anticoagulants, and phenytoin, one of the antiarrhythmic agents. Phenobarbital decreases the effect of the xanthine bronchodilator, theophylline, through the same mechanism involving induction of hepatic microsomal enzymes. Such an action enhances the clearance of theophylline and decreases its plasma half-life. This in turn reduces its bronchodilator efficacy and necessitates a dosage adjustment (see Chapter 13).

As with most drugs, hepatic metabolism and renal excretion contribute to overall reduction of plasma levels. With the barbiturates, however, these pharmacokinetic factors are especially important. Any preexisting hepatic or renal dysfunction dramatically prolongs the plasma half-life and the clinical effect of the barbiturates. Barbiturates are almost exclusively biotransformed by the hepatic microsomal enzyme system into more water-soluble metabolites. There-

fore, any drug interaction of disease such as cirrhosis that damages hepatic function prolongs barbiturate levels in the blood. In addition, adaptation of the microsomal enzymes contributes to tolerance and increased toxicity risk, and to the precipitation of withdrawal symptoms if the drug is abruptly discontinued.

The barbiturates are weak acids and are slowly excreted by the kidney in an unchanged state. The elimination of barbiturates is improved with an alkaline urine. The nonpulmonary use of sodium bicarbonate to alkalinize the urine in these instances is briefly mentioned in Chapter 15.

ADVERSE REACTIONS. Barbiturates produce generalized CNS depression and have a particular affinity for the RAS to inhibit arousal. Their effects, however, are even more widespread. Normal therapeutic doses of barbiturates are capable of depressing the RAS and the medulla, including medullary vasomotor centers. As a result, hypotension can occur. At increasing doses, sympathetic ganglia may also be depressed. This directly decreases cardiac activity and lowers blood pressure.

Barbiturates can also potentiate neuromuscular blockade caused by nondepolarizing drugs such as pancuronium or depolarizing drugs such as succinylcholine. Prolongation of neuromuscular block occurs because the mechanism of action of the barbiturates causes hyperpolarization of muscle cell membranes just as it does in the neurons of the RAS. If the neuromuscular blockade involves respiratory muscles, prolonged apnea may occur.

Paradoxically, the barbiturates may cause restlessness, excitement, and delirium in elderly patients and in patients experiencing pain (Bhatnagar et al, 1989). The sedative and hypnotic effect of the barbiturates is lacking in these individuals.

BARBITURATE TOXICITY. Barbiturate overdoses are relatively common. The delayed onset of some longer-acting barbiturates, added to sedation and perceptual time distortion, causes some patients to not remember clearly when they last took their medication. This may cause them to inadvertently overdose on barbiturates. Characteristic CNS overdose signs, such as disorientation, slowed speech, decreased mental alertness, and ataxia, are common. Accidental or intentional administration of toxic amounts of a barbiturate progressively depresses the different control mechanisms for ventilation. In addition, hypotension, renal shutdown, and circulatory collapse may occur. Initially, central ventilatory drive (hypercapnic drive) is impaired as medullary chemoreceptors become less sensitive to arterial carbon dioxide tension (Pa_{CO_2}). The central chemoreceptors indirectly monitor Pa_{CO_2} by responding to the pH of cerebrospinal fluid (CSF). Normally, as Pa_{CO_2} increases, carbon dioxide diffuses into the CSF, combines with water, and forms carbonic acid. The carbonic acid generates hydrogen ions, which lower the pH of the CSF and stimulate the medullary chemoreceptors to increase ventilatory activity. In the depressed state, however, these chemoreceptors fail to provide the stimulus needed to support ventilation.

Following the disruption of this primary CNS control, oxygen chemoreceptors in the peripheral aortic and carotid bodies take over to sustain ventilation through the hypoxic drive mechanism. In severe cases of barbiturate poisoning, however, even this final ventilatory control fails. If oxygen is given without supported ventilation to a patient depressed by toxic levels of barbiturates, these peripheral oxygen chemoreceptors may fail to provide the stimulus necessary to maintain ventilation. As a result, respiratory arrest may occur. Therefore, supplemental oxygen therapy must be administered with supported ventilation to patients intoxicated by barbiturates. In serious cases of barbiturate overdose, ventilatory depression may lead to respiratory acidosis and hypoxemia. Renal clearance of barbiturates is slowed by such acidotic conditions. Therefore, ventilatory depression has the indirect effect of prolonging barbiturate toxicity by slowing the removal of the drug from the body. The effect of barbiturate depression on vasomotor centers and sympathetic ganglia is hypotension. This in turn can lead to renal shutdown.

MANAGEMENT. The respiratory care practitioner plays a vital role in the management of barbiturate overdose. The therapeutic goal is to minimize cardiopulmonary and renal complications. This process includes endotracheal intubation to maintain airway patency and prevent aspiration of gastric contents, ventilatory support as required, and intervention to prevent collapse of the cardiovascular and urinary systems. Administration of supplemental oxygen with assisted ventilation has already been addressed.

Maintenance of an alkaline urine by means of buffers such as sodium bicarbonate minimizes tubular reabsorption to promote renal clearance of the barbiturate. This type of forced diuresis is pH dependent. An alkaline filtrate maintains the weak acid drug in an ionized form. Such ionized forms are unavailable for transfer across lipid-rich cell membranes. Therefore, the barbiturate

is excreted rather than being reabsorbed (see Chapter 2).

Hemodialysis and hemoperfusion may also aid in the removal of excess drug from the body. In hemodialysis, blood is passed through tubes composed of a semipermeable membrane. A dialyzing fluid surrounds the tubes, thus allowing the waste products in blood to diffuse into the continuously replenished dialyzing fluid. Hemoperfusion is a technique whereby the patient's blood is passed over an adsorptive surface such as activated charcoal or ion-exchange resin. No semipermeable membrane is used, and direct contact with the adsorbent material removes toxic substances from the blood.

To maintain adequate plasma volume and minimize development of a shock condition, fluid replacement in the intoxicated patient may be necessary.

Finally, because most barbiturate overdoses last many hours, the administration of a short-acting respiratory stimulant, such as doxapram, is not indicated. The limited use of such analeptics is covered in Chapter 28. Table 24–2 summarizes the effects of barbiturate toxicity and management of the intoxication.

Nonbarbiturate Nonbenzodiazepine Hypnotics

In the strictest sense, this minor group of hypnotics also includes the carbamates, such as meprobamate (Equanil). The carbamates, however, have been grouped for convenience with the antianxiety tranquilizers and were covered earlier in the chapter with the benzodiazepines. For simplicity, we will refer to the nonbarbiturate nonbenzodiazepine hypnotics as "nonbarbiturate hypnotics."

With the exception of chloral hydrate and paraldehyde, the nonbarbiturate hypnotics offer no

TABLE 24–2 BARBITURATE OVERDOSE

Effects	Supportive Therapy
Disorientation, ataxia, slowed speech	Gastric lavage (effective only within a few hours of overdose)
Ventilatory depression	Assisted ventilation
Respiratory acidosis	Supplemental oxygen
Hypoxemia	Forced diuresis (pH dependent—alkaline urine promotes elimination)
Hypotension	
Renal shutdown	Hemodialysis
	Adsorptive hemoperfusion
	Fluid and electrolyte replacement

TABLE 24–3 DRUG NAMES: PSYCHOPHARMACOLOGIC AND HYPNOTIC DRUGS*

Generic Name	Trade Name
ANTIPSYCHOTIC TRANQUILIZERS	
Phenothiazine derivatives	
Chlorpromazine (kloor-**PRŌ**-ma-zēn)	Thorazine
Butyrophenone derivatives	
Haloperidol (hal-ō-**PAIR**-i-dol)	Haldol
ANTIANXIETY TRANQUILIZERS	
Benzodiazepines	
Diazepam (dī-**AZ**-e-pam)	Valium, *others*
Alprazolam (al-**PRAZ**-ō-lam)	Xanax
Lorazepam (Lowr-**AZ**-i-pam)	Ativan
Oxazepam (Oks-**AZ**-e-pam)	Serax
Chlordiazepoxide (kloor-dī-āz-i-**POX**-īd)	Librium, *others*
Carbamates	
Meprobamate (me-**PRŌ**-ba-māt)	Equanil, Miltown
ANTIDEPRESSANTS	
Monoamine oxidase inhibitors	
Tranylcypromine (tran-il-**SĪ**-prō-mén)	Parnate
Tricyclic antidepressants	
Amitriptyline (ām-ē-**TRIP**-ti-lēn)	Elavil, *others*
Imipramine (im-**IP**-ra-mēn)	Tofranil
Nortriptyline (nōr-**TRIP**-ti-len)	Aventyl
Second-generation antidepressants	
Trazodone (**TRAZ**-ō-dōn)	Desyrel
Amoxapine (a-**MOX**-pēn)	Asendin
Alprazolam (see above)	Xanax
HYPNOTICS	
Benzodiazepine hypnotics	
Flurazepam (flyoo-**RAZ**-i-pam)	Dalmane
Triazolam (trī-**AZ**-ō-lam)	Halcion
Midazolam (mi-**DAZ**-ō-lam)	Versed
Intermediate-acting barbiturates (12–24 h)†	
Amobarbital (āmō-**BAR**-bi-tal)	Amytal
Pentobarbital (pen-tō-**BAR**-bi-tal)	Nembutal
Secobarbital (sē-kō-**BAR**-bi-tal)	Seconal
Long-acting barbiturates (>24 h)	
butabarbital (byoo-ta-**BAR**-bi-tal)	Butisol
phenobarbital (fēnō-**BAR**-bi-tal)	Luminal
Nonbarbiturate nonbenzodiazepine hypnotics	
Chloral hydrate	Noctec
Paraldehyde (pair-**AL**-de-hīd)	Paral
Ethchlorvynol (eth-kloor-**VĪ**-nol)	Placidyl
Glutethimide (glū-**TETH**-i-mīd)	Doriden
MISCELLANEOUS DRUGS	
Antimanic	
Lithium (**LITH**-ē-um) carbonate	Carbolith
Benzodiazepine antagonist	
Flumazenil (flū-**MAZ**-i-nil)	Anexate

*Ultrashort-acting barbiturates are listed in Chapter 27, "General Anesthetics."
†Also includes short-acting barbiturates.

clear therapeutic advantage over the traditional barbiturate or benzodiazepine hypnotics. One member of the group, methaqualone (Quaalude), has been withdrawn from the market because of adverse reactions and serious abuse liability (Clark et al, 1988). It produces an alcohollike intoxication and was often used in combination with other CNS depressants. As a group, the nonbarbiturate hypnotics no longer enjoy the popularity they once had. They have gradually decreased in importance with the advent of the benzodiazepine hypnotics, such as flurazepam. In general, they have greater toxicity, lower safety margins, and higher abuse potential than the benzodiazepines. (Chloral hydrate and paraldehyde are exceptions to this statement.)

Chloral hydrate (Noctec) predates the barbiturates and has been used as a sleep-inducing agent for more than 100 years. Along with paraldehyde, it is the safest of this nonbarbiturate group of hypnotics. The hypnotic activity of chloral hydrate is caused by its metabolic product, trichloroethanol. Chloral hydrate is short acting and is occasionally used in pediatric and geriatric patients because it does not produce paradoxical excitement or hyperalgesia as may occur with the barbiturates.

Good hypnotic properties are exhibited by paraldehyde (Paral). However, it has a strong disagreeable taste and produces an unpleasant breath odor. It is used primarily in the treatment of convulsion episodes triggered by alcohol withdrawal or tetanus. Ventilatory depression may be produced.

Other nonbarbiturate nonbenzodiazepine hypnotics exhibit tolerance and addiction potential as do the barbiturates. Therefore, drugs such as ethchlorvynol (Placidyl) and glutethimide (Doriden) have pharmacologic features that make them less attractive than the benzodiazepine hypnotics. Like the other CNS depressants discussed so far, the nonbarbiturate hypnotics may produce depression of ventilation.

Table 24–3 lists the generic and trade names of the psychopharmacologic and hypnotic drugs discussed in this chapter.

CHAPTER SUMARY

The psychopharmacologic and hypnotic agents discussed in this chapter have limited but important therapeutic uses. These include treatment of major and minor mental disturbances from mild anxiety and insomnia to debilitating mental states. Several of these CNS depressants produce adverse effects that include depression of ventilation. The special case of CNS depression involving barbiturate intoxication is discussed, as is the role of the respiratory care practitioner in management of such toxicities.

BIBLIOGRAPHY

Bhatnagar RK, Dutton GR, and Gebhart GF: Drugs acting on the central nervous system (CNS). In Conn PM and Gebhart GF (eds): Essentials of Pharmacology. FA Davis, Philadelphia, 1989.

Bliwise DL: Treating insomnia: Pharmacological and nonpharmacological approaches. J Psychoactive Drugs 23:335–341, 1991.

Carola R, Harley JP, and Noback CR: Human Anatomy and Physiology, ed 2. McGraw-Hill, New York, 1992.

Clark WG, Brater DC, and Johnson AR: Goth's Medical Pharmacology, ed 12. CV Mosby, St Louis, 1988.

Des Jardins TR: Cardiopulmonary Anatomy and Physiology. Delmar, Albany, 1988.

Doble A and Martin IL: Multiple benzodiazepine receptors: No reason for anxiety. Trends Pharmacol Sci 13:76–81, 1992.

Greenblatt DJ: Pharmacology of benzodiazepine hypnotics. J Clin Psychiatry 53(Suppl):7–13, 1992.

Hollister L: Antidepressants. In Katzung BD (ed): Basic and Clincial Pharmacology. Lange Medical Publications, Los Altos, 1982.

Hollister L: Antipsychotics and lithium. In Katzung BE (ed): Basic and Clinical Pharmacology. Lange Medical Publications, Los Altos, 1982.

Lenox RH et al: Adjunctive treatment of manic agitation with lorazepam versus haloperidol: A double-blind study. J Clin Psychiatry 53:47–52, 1992.

McClellan JM and Werry JS: Schizophrenia. Psychiatr Clin North Am 15:131–148, 1992.

Nicoll R: Introduction to the pharmacology of CNS drugs. In Katzung BE (ed): Basic and Clinical Pharmacology. Lange Medical Publications, Los Altos, 1982.

Piercey MF, Hoffmann WE, and Cooper M: The hypnotics triazolam and zolpidem have identical metabolic effects throughout the brain: Implications for benzodiazepine receptor subtypes. Brain Res 554:224–252, 1991.

Rau JL: Respiratory Care Pharmacology, ed 3. Yearbook Medical Publishers, Chicago, 1989.

Sanders LD et al: Reversal of benzodiazepine sedation with the antagonist flumazenil. Br J Anaesth 66:445–453, 1991.

Short TG and Galletly DC: Acute tolerance from benzodizepine night sedation. Anaesthesia 46:929–931, 1991.

Smith MC and Riskin BJ: The clinical use of barbiturates in neurological disorders. Drugs 42:365–378, 1991.

Tortora GJ and Grabowski SR: Principles of Anatomy and Physiology, ed 7. HarperCollins, New York, 1993.

Trevor AJ and Way WL: Sedative-hypnotics. In Katzung BD (ed): Basic and Clinical Pharmacology. Lange Medical Publications, Los Altos, 1982.

West JB: Respiratory Physiology: The Essentials, ed 4. Williams and Wilkins, Baltimore, 1990.

CHAPTER 25

Analgesics

CHAPTER OUTLINE

CHAPTER OBJECTIVES

After studying this chapter the reader should be able to:

- Define the following terms:
  - Narcosis, algesic, analgesic, antinociceptive, opiate, opioid, agonist-antagonist.
- Discuss pain reception, transmission, and perception by explaining the roles of nociceptors, ascending sensory tracts, thalamus, and cerebral cortex.
- Describe the function of opioid receptors.
- Describe the function of endogenous opioid peptides.
- Describe the pharmacologic activity of the following narcotic analgesics:
  - Morphine, heroin, codeine, oxycodone, hydromorphone, meperidine, propoxyphene, fentanyl, methadone, pentazocine.
- Describe the pharmacologic activity of the narcotic antagonist naloxone.
- List the toxic effects of narcotic overdose and describe the treatment of such a toxicity.
- Define the following terms:
  - Nonsteroidal anti-inflammatory drug (NSAID), antipyretic.
- Describe the pharmacologic activity of the following nonnarcotic analgesics:
  - Aspirin, ibuprofen, naproxen, indomethacin, phenylbutazone, meclofenamate, acetaminophen, phenacetin.
- Describe the symptoms of an analgesic-induced asthma syndrome (Samter's syndrome).
- List the toxicologic effects of salicylate overdose and of *p*-aminophenol overdose and describe the treatment of such toxicities.

KEY TERMS

algesic
analgesic (antinociceptive)
endogenous opioid peptides
antipyretic analgesic
narcosis
narcotic analgesic

narcotic antagonist
nociceptor
nonnarcotic analgesic
nonsteroidal anti-inflammatory
  drug (NSAID)
opiate

opioid
opioid agonist-antagonist
opioid receptors (μ—mu, δ—
  delta, κ—kappa, ϵ—epsilon,
  σ—sigma)

CHAPTER INTRODUCTION

Alleviation of pain through the use of medications occupies a sizable and significant chapter in the history of medicine. To put it mildly, pain is unpleasant. There are various degrees of pain and pain thresholds—different people perceive and react to pain differently. But most would prefer it did not exist. From a physiologic standpoint it can be argued that pain under certain circumstances plays a beneficial role. For example, we do not tend to walk on and further injure a painful sprained ankle. However, from a medical standpoint, the suppression of pain through use of **analgesics (antinociceptives)** makes certain clinical procedures possible, reduces patient discomfort during healing, and provides a humane method for managing terminal conditions. Medical terminology concerning the analgesics can be troublesome and is dealt with specifically in the following section. In general, however, the pain relievers are divided into two groups: the powerful **narcotic analgesics** reserved for the control of severe pain and the less potent **nonnarcotic analgesics** employed in the suppression of mild-to-moderate pain.

This chapter examines the pharmacologic aspects of the analgesics and briefly discusses the narcotic antagonists used to reverse the effects of narcotic agonists. In addition, the aspects of drug overdose due to narcotic and nonnarcotic analgesics are discussed, including the role of the respiratory care practitioner in the management of such toxicities.

TERMINOLOGY

Narcosis is a reversible state characterized by stupor or insensibility—a pleasant, dreamlike state with loss of sensations. Compounds that produce pain relief and sedation have traditionally been called narcotic analgesics and are similar to morphine, the prototype for the group. The nonnarcotic analgesics include aspirin and acetaminophen and are distinct from the narcotic classification. The greatest confusion in terminology centers around the word "narcotic," an imprecise term implying that a "narcotic" drug produces narcosis (or stupor). Opium, its derivatives, and synthetic compounds that resemble opium, although all capable of producing a stuporous state, can easily produce an analgesic effect without a narcotic effect. The term "narcotic," however, is commonly applied to the entire group of opium derivatives and opiumlike analgesics.

"Narcotic analgesic" is understood to include natural and synthetic derivatives of opium having pharmacologic actions similar to those of morphine. More precise terminology exists and is outlined below:

Opiates
  1. Alkaloids such as codeine, derived from opium
  2. Semisynthetic derivatives of opium, such as oxycodone

Opioids
  1. Nonopium-derived synthetic compounds, such as Demerol, that pharmacologically resemble the natural alkaloids
  2. Endogenous morphinelike compounds such as endorphins.

PAIN

Sensation refers to the arrival of an afferent (sensory) impulse in the brain. Pain sensations, like most other sensations, must be (1) detected by a specialized receptor, (2) conducted by afferent pathways from the periphery into the central nervous system (CNS), and (3) interpreted within specific parts of the brain. It might be argued that sensory inputs involved with spinal reflexes do not follow this plan because they are completed before a connection is made in the brain. Spinal reflexes aside, three sequential steps exist with pain sensations that reach the brain: *reception, transmission,* and *perception,* each providing a potential site for treatment of pain. For example, nonsteroidal anti-inflammatory drugs (NSAID) such as aspirin modify the effect of irritating chemicals that trigger the pain response. Anti-inflammatory glucocorticoids suppress the production of pain-causing chemicals. Local anesthetics alter membrane electrophysiologic characteristics to block pain reception. Surgical techniques that sever sensory nerves irreversibly block transmission of pain impulses. Finally, drugs such as morphine act in the brain to alter the perception of pain (Fig. 25–1).

Reception

Pain receptors, or **nociceptors,** are primarily cutaneous receptors classified as free nerve endings. They are located relatively close to the surface of the body in the lower layers of the epidermis. Cutaneous regions, internal tissues, and most organs are equipped with such free nerve endings, but receptor densities vary in different parts of the body. The brain, for example, is devoid of pain receptors.

Most receptors, when subjected to a continuous stimulus of constant intensity, adapt to the

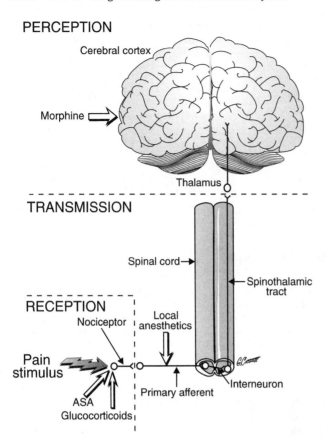

FIGURE 25–1 Control of pain—sites of action.

repetitive stimulation. When the stimulus is first applied, they respond with a burst of activity but then decrease their firing rate as the stimulus continues. A common example of such sensory accommodation is the lack of sensation of clothes against our skin after the clothes have been worn for a short time. This occurs in spite of continuous tactile stimulation of cutaneous touch and pressure receptors. Pain receptors, on the other hand, exhibit little if any adaptation to continuous stimulation. The interpretation of the sensation may be altered in the brain, but the reception of pain stimuli is fairly uniform.

Cutaneous receptors such as pressure, touch, and thermoreceptors are specialized in the detection of sensations other than pain. If they are intensely stimulated, however, they transmit afferent impulses that are perceived centrally as pain. Free nerve endings are especially sensitive to noxious chemicals produced in the tissues. (In this regard they are a type of "chemoreceptor.") Pain receptors are stimulated, for instance, by metabolic waste products such as lactic acid that can accumulate in the muscles. As is explained in Chapter 9, tissue trauma as a result

of injury may cause lysosome disruption, kallikrein release, and production of bradykinin from plasma precursors. Bradykinin causes intense stimulation of pain receptors (Box 25–1).

Transmission

Unmyelinated sensory nerve fibers conduct pain impulses from pain receptors into the spinal cord. Within the spinal cord, interneurons cross over to the opposite, or contralateral, side of the cord and travel to the brain in an ascending (sensory) pathway called the lateral spinothalamic tract (see Fig. 25–1). *Awareness* of the pain sensation occurs in the thalamus, located superiorly to the hypothalamus, but *perception* of pain occurs in specific regions of the cerebral cortex once the sensory impulses have been relayed by the thalamus to the cerebrum.

Perception

Perception of pain involves the interpretation or determination of the type and intensity of pain. It alerts the body to acute injury, disease, and

BOX 25–1 PAIN CONTROL AT THE SOURCE

Modification of peripheral pain reception rather than central pain perception may be the future trend in analgesia. Following tissue trauma, kallikrein from ruptured cells catalyses the production of bradykinin from precursor molecules. Bradykinin immediately combines at receptors on afferent nerves and initiates a powerful pain impulse. Bradykinin also combines at receptors on mast cells, causing the release of histamine, and at receptors on capillaries, causing an increase in vessel permeability. Histamine promotes vasodilation and further leakage of contents to deliver more kallikrein, bradykinin precursors, and leukocytes to the area of tissue damage. Symptoms of pain, redness, swelling, and heat are produced by these tissue events. Bradykinin binding at receptors on blood vessels also triggers the production and release of prostaglandins from endothelial cells. The prostaglandins bind to nerve cells and augment the effect of bradykinin. Thus additional pain impulses are fired and the pain signal is amplified. Meanwhile, the brain sends an impulse back down the afferent nerve fiber (an antidromic impulse), triggering the release of a neuropeptide called substance P. (Substance P was originally discovered in brain tissue and was stored in a powdered form; hence the name "substance P.") This autacoid mediator combines at mast cell receptors and induces more histamine release, prolongs the tissue response, and mediates the transmission of pain impulses in the spinal cord. The complex cascade of events just described provides many locations at which potential new drugs may modify the sequence.

The blockade of bradykinin receptors by bradykinin antagonists offers an effective way to interrupt the nociceptive, or pain-producing, system at several locations—on free nerve endings, mast cells, and endothelial cells. Such a peripheral mechanism avoids the undesirable CNS effects inherent in narcotic therapy. The search for bradykinin blockers has been going on for several decades. Dozens of such compounds have been produced and used investigationally to identify subtypes of bradykinin receptors. A promising drug in experimental animal studies is HOE 140, a very potent and long-acting B_2-bradykinin receptor antagonist.

Substance P shares several features with bradykinin because they both cause vasodilation and hypotension. However, substance P is classified as a tachykinin, a substance that induces rapid smooth muscle contraction, whereas bradykinin exhibits a slow onset of action before smooth muscle contraction begins. Substance P can be blocked by tachykinin antagonists. Experimental compounds such as CP-96345 are undergoing animal tests and show promise as competitive antagonists of substance P at specific NK_1-neurokinin receptors. Such compounds block nociception mediated by substance P, and plasma exudation, or leakage, caused by substance P.

With increased understanding of the role of mediators involved in generation and transmission of the pain impulse, researchers are able to offer us a glimpse of promising new pain relievers.

Bao G et al: HOE 140, a new highly potent and long-acting bradykinin antagonist in conscious rats. Eur J Pharmacol 200:179–182, 1991.

DeKoninck Y and Henry JL: Substance P–mediated slow excitatory postsynaptic potential elicited in dorsal horn neurons *in vivo* by noxious stimulation. Proc Natl Acad Sci USA 88:11344–11348, 1991.

Garret C et al: Pharmacological properties of a potent and selective nonpeptide substance P antagonist. Proc Natl Acad Sci USA 88:10208–10212, 1991.

Jukic D et al: Neurokinin receptors and antagonists: Old and new. Life Sci 49:1463–1469, 1991.

Lei YH, Barnes PJ, and Rogers DF: Inhibition of neurogenic exudation in guinea pig airways by CP-96,345, a new non-peptide NK_1 receptor antagonist. Br J Pharmacol 105:261–266, 1992.

McKean K: Pain. Discover 7(10):82–92, Oct 1986.

Rhaleb NE et al: Characterization of bradykinin receptors in peripheral organs. Can J Physiol Pharmacol 69:938–943, Jul 1991.

Xu XJ et al: Spantide II, a novel tachykinin antagonist, and galanin inhibit plasma extravasation induced by antidromic C-fiber stimulation in the rat hindpaw. Neuroscience 42:731–737, 1991.

occasionally organ dysfunction. Perception occurs in the somesthetic (sensory) area of the cerebral cortex. It is here that the narcotic agonist drugs produce their powerful analgesic effect and the equally powerful adverse effect of tolerance (see Fig. 25–1). Tolerance in turn contributes to a debilitating physical dependency seen with the narcotics. Other centrally mediated undesirable reactions with the narcotic analgesics include ventilatory depression and gastrointestinal tract disturbances.

Endogenous Opioid Peptides

In the early 1970s, special membrane receptors were discovered on nerve cells. It was found that these receptors mediated the effects of opiates and opioids. Around the same time, **endogenous opioid peptides** were being studied. These morphinelike compounds are synthesized within nerve cells and play a neurotransmitter or neuromodulator role, acting on the spinal cord or brain to decrease the transmission or perception of pain. The action of different endogenous compounds at different receptors has provided a clearer understanding of the pharmacologic activity of exogenously administered narcotics. Several families of endogenous opioid peptides called endorphins, enkephalins, and dynorphins have been identified (Fig. 25–2). They are unevenly distributed in the CNS. The peptides interact at different receptors but also produce a few overlapping effects. (Bhatnagar et al, 1989).

Opioid Receptors

Various subtypes of **opioid receptors** exhibit differing affinities for the endogenous opioid peptides. They also differ in affinity for exogenous opiates and opioids administered therapeutically. The receptor subtypes, like the endogenous opioid peptides, are unevenly distributed and produce overlapping as well as distinct effects. Some of the Greek letters used to designate the receptor subtypes refer to specific agonists used investigationally. For example, mu (μ) refers to morphine and kappa (κ) to ketocyclazocine, but for our purposes, the derivation of the symbols is not essential. The **μ-opioid receptor** is the most common opioid receptor and is distributed throughout the CNS. It mediates not only narcotic-induced analgesia and euphoria, but also adverse effects such as depression of ventilation and development of physical dependency. Morphine and morphine derivatives interact primarily at μ-opioid receptors on brain cells. Other opioid receptors include **delta (δ)-**,

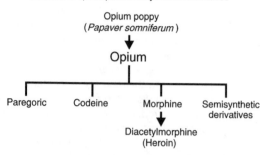

OPIATES
alkaloids in opium plus semisynthetic derivatives

Opium poppy
(*Papaver somniferum*)

Opium

Paregoric   Codeine   Morphine   Semisynthetic derivatives

Diacetylmorphine
(Heroin)

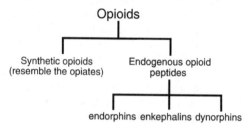

OPIOIDS
synthetics and naturally-occurring morphine-like compounds

Opioids

Synthetic opioids   Endogenous opioid
(resemble the opiates)   peptides

endorphins enkephalins dynorphins

FIGURE 25–2 Narcotic analgesics.

kappa (κ)-, epsilon (ε)-, and **sigma (σ)-opioid receptors.** The pharmacologic effects mediated by the opioid receptors, their locations, and the endogenous opioid peptides that interact with them are summarized in Table 25–1.

Mechanism of Action

Relatively little is understood of what occurs following interaction of an endogenous or exogenous compound at an opioid receptor. Several theories have been proposed, but none appear to fully explain the general inhibitory action of narcotics on the nervous system. A cyclic nucleotide mechanism mediated by cyclic adenosine-3',5'-monophosphate (cAMP) may explain the effects of chronic administration. However, electrophysiologic effects of narcotics on calcium or potassium transmembrane channels causing hyperpolarization of neurons may also provide an explanation. (The role of ion channels is discussed in Chapter 4.)

THERAPEUTIC AGENTS

Narcotic Analgesics

Opium and its derivatives, the opiates, produce narcosis in addition to a powerful analgesic ef-

TABLE 25–1 OPIOID RECEPTORS

Opioid Receptor	Distribution*	Preferentially Stimulated by Agonist[†]	Function	Comments
μ mu	CNS	Morphine	Mediate opioid-produced analgesia	"Mu" derived from morphine respiratory depression, euphoria, and physical dependency
δ delta	CNS	Enkephalins[†]	Mediate opioid effects on emotions, seizures, and respiratory depression	Respiratory depression and seizures
κ kappa	CNS	Dynorphins[†]	Mediate spinal analgesia	"Kappa" derived from ketocyclazocine, an experimental substance used in research
ε epsilon	Unknown	Endorphins[†]	Mediate opioid-produced euphoria	Minimally understood
σ sigma[§]	Unknown	Unknown	May mediate opioid-produced dysphoria and hallucinations	"Sigma" derived from SKF 10047, an experimental substance used in research. Adverse mental effects

Source: Data from Bhatnagar et al, 1989.
*Opioid receptors are distributed unevenly in the central nervous system.
[†]Neither the opioid agonists nor the receptors involved exhibit total selectivity (Bhatnager et al, 1989).
[†]Endogenous opioid peptides.
[§]The σ-opioid receptor may not be a true opioid receptor subtype because it can be stimulated by nonopioid drugs, such as phencyclidine (PCP, "angel dust").
CNS—central nervous system.

fect. The alleviation of pain, or analgesia, is the rationale for the medical use of the narcotics. The pleasurable feelings produced by the drugs contribute to their significant abuse potential.

Opium is the parent compound of the naturally occurring opiate analgesics and is the crude extract derived from the seed pod of the opium poppy *(Papaver somniferum)*. Historically, opium caused few social problems when it was smoked or ingested. However, with the advent of the hypodermic syringe (ca. 1850), intravenous administration and more pleasurable "highs" were introduced along with a very serious abuse liability. Crude dry opium contains about 10% morphine and 0.5% codeine. It is the starting point for the extraction, isolation, and production of the alkaloids morphine, heroin, and codeine, in addition to an entire family of semisynthetic derivatives (see Fig. 25–2). In addition, many opioids are produced as pure synthetic compounds. Medical use of opium itself is rare. A traditional compound, paregoric, contains tincture of opium and is occasionally used for treating acute diarrhea.

Naturally Occurring Alkaloids

MORPHINE. Morphine, sold under many trade names, is the standard analgesic by which others are judged. The principal differences among the narcotic analgesics are qualitative and reflect differences in potency more than

anything else. The analgesic effect of morphine is mediated by the μ-opioid receptor on nerve cells. For severe pain, morphine is available parenterally in intramuscular and subcutaneous preparation (Box 25–2).

INDICATIONS. The medical uses of morphine are highly restricted due to a serious abuse potential. Morphine is used primarily in patients experiencing severe pain such as occurs with certain types of cancer, severe burns, or battlefield wounds.

CONTRAINDICATIONS. Morphine and related compounds can potentially worsen preexisting head injuries because these drugs may produce marked depression of the respiratory center and retention of carbon dioxide. As a result, an elevated arterial carbon dioxide tension (Pa_{CO_2}) causes cerebral vasodilation and increases intracranial pressure. In addition, bronchial asthma can be worsened because morphine may cause contraction of bronchial smooth muscle and possible bronchoconstriction. Morphine use in undiagnosed abdominal conditions is also contraindicated because of its ability to decrease the tone of gastrointestinal tract smooth muscle and produce stasis leading to constipation. (These effects are outlined below.)

PHARMACOLOGIC EFFECTS ON ORGAN SYSTEMS: RESPIRATORY SYSTEM. The medullary respiratory center is markedly depressed by morphine. Hypoventilation occurs due to a reduction in the

BOX 25–2   SWEET DREAMS

In 1803, a German chemist named Friedrich Wilhelm Adam Sertürner became the first to successfully isolate a pure active principle from a natural source. Crude opium contains about 20 different alkaloids, but Sertürner was able to separate morphine from the rest, becoming a pioneer in alkaloid chemistry. He ingested the extract himself, shared some with friends, and everyone promptly fell asleep. He named the crystalline powder "morphine" after *Morpheus,* the Greek god of sleep and of dreams.

Clark WG, Brater DC, and Johnson AR: Goth's Medical Pharmacology, ed 12. CV Mosby, St Louis, 1988.

Liska K: Drugs and the Human Body: With Implications for Society. Macmillan, New York, 1981.

Modell W, Lansing A, and Editors of Time-Life Books: Drugs. Life Science Library. Time, New York, 1969.

sensitivity of medullary chemoreceptors to carbon dioxide. Larger doses of morphine slow the rate of respiration and produce irregular breathing so that patients are often apneic. Retention of carbon dioxide in these instances becomes severe. At even higher doses, depression of the respiratory centers may cause death (see Toxicity). As was pointed out above, morphine may cause bronchoconstriction through contraction of airway smooth muscle.

PHARMACOLOGIC EFFECTS ON ORGAN SYSTEMS: CARDIOVASCULAR SYSTEM. Morphine may induce histamine release, which can bring about peripheral vasodilation. This results in decreased venous tone and arterial resistance to reduce both ventricular preload and afterload. Therefore, these hemodynamic effects aid in reducing the ventricular workload. They are also beneficial in reducing pulmonary congestion and edema. Exaggerated vascular effects such as these may also contribute to postural hypotension.

PHARMACOLOGIC EFFECTS ON ORGAN SYSTEMS: DIGESTIVE SYSTEM. The net effect of narcotics on the digestive system is one of constipation. Morphine increases the tone of gastrointestinal tract smooth muscle and sphincters and decreases propulsive activity. Reduced fluid and electrolyte secretion into the intestinal lumen also contributes to the state of constipation. The effect of morphine on emesis is mixed. The drug can stimulate the chemoreceptor trigger zone (CTZ) of the medulla to induce emesis, but it can also depress the vomiting center. Initial doses commonly cause nausea and vomiting, whereas subsequent doses usually do not (Bhatnagar et al, 1989). (A derivative of morphine called apomorphine is used as an emetic in poisoning because of its potent CTZ-stimulating action.)

PHARMACOLOGIC EFFECTS ON ORGAN SYSTEMS: PUPILS. Of diagnostic importance in recognition of narcotic intoxication is intense miosis, or highly constricted ("pinpoint") pupils.

PRECAUTIONS AND ADVERSE REACTIONS. Precautions and undesirable reactions with narcotic administration are related to pharmacologic effects such as hypoventilation, dyspnea, nausea, and constipation, as outlined above. Additive effects with other CNS depressants, such as the barbiturates, can result in greatly exaggerated adverse effects, especially ventilatory depression.

TOXICITY. As was discussed with the barbiturates, accidental or intentional overdose with narcotics may produce death due to respiratory depression, collapse of the cardiovascular system, or both. With decreased responsiveness to $PaCO_2$, breathing patterns change to irregular periods of apnea alternating with periods of hyperpnea (Cheyne-Stokes breathing) (Des Jardins, 1993). Eventual respiratory failure occurs unless there is intervention in the form of assisted ventilation, airway management, and other supportive measures to maintain cardiovascular and renal systems. Severe narcotic toxicity is characterized by deep sleep, pinpoint pupils, and marked ventilatory depression. Retention of carbon dioxide contributes to respiratory acidosis. As with any CNS drug overdose producing a decreased level of consciousness, there is always risk for aspiration of gastric contents. This is due to an impaired swallowing mechanism and cough reflex. Aspiration may lead to acute pulmonary edema and an adult respiratory distress syndrome (ARDS) response (McCarty, 1993). Narcotic drug toxicity can also produce a generalized ARDS. In this syndrome, damage to the alveolar-capillary membrane causes an increase in pulmonary vascular permeability (see Box 21–1). This allows fluid trans-

TABLE 25–2 NARCOTIC OVERDOSE

Effects	Supportive Therapy
Decreased responsiveness to $Paco_2$ leading to Cheyne-Stokes breathing	Ventilatory support
Deep sleep (narcosis)	Supplemental oxygen therapy
Pinpoint pupils	Airway maintenance
Ventilatory depression	Support of cardiac function
Respiratory acidosis	Forced diuresis (pH-dependent; acidic urine promotes elimination)
Increased incidence of aspiration of gastric contents due to decreased consciousness. (This may lead to acute pulmonary edema and ARDS, including development of hypoxemia and hypercapnia.)	Narcotic antagonists (eg, naloxone)

ARDS—adult respiratory distress syndrome; $Paco_2$—arterial carbon dioxide tension.

fer, which results in alveolar and interstitial edema. As a result, gas exchange is impaired, causing hypoxemia and hypercapnia. Lung compliance decreases and the work of breathing increases.

MANAGEMENT. Treatment of narcotic overdose is similar to that described for barbiturate overdose (Chapter 24). Ventilatory support and airway maintenance with oxygen therapy are administered to counter the ventilatory depression and blood gas abnormalities. In addition, support of cardiac function is carried out. The use of narcotic antagonists, such as naloxone, helps reduce the adverse effects of CNS depression caused by narcotics. (This narcotic reversal agent is discussed below.) Acidic urine aids in the renal clearance of narcotics; therefore, the acidotic conditions produced by the toxicity help in the removal of the drug. This is in con-

trast to barbiturate overdose, which requires alkaline urine to force diuresis. Table 25–2 lists the effects and supportive therapy involved in morphine overdose.

HEROIN. Heroin, or diacetylmorphine, is a morphine derivative possessing a high degree of abuse potential. A pleasant, euphoric response is produced by the drug when it is injected intravenously. Psychologic dependency, tolerance, and physical dependency contribute to a significant abuse potential. Compared with morphine, heroin penetrates the blood-brain barrier with relative ease to produce its CNS effects. The medical and nonmedical uses of heroin were once fairly common. However, modern medical use is essentially nonexistent because there is generally lack of convincing evidence that heroin is superior in analgesic activity to morphine (Box 25–3).

BOX 25–3 OVER-THE-COUNTER HEROIN

Morphine was isolated from opium in 1803, codeine in 1832, and diacetylmorphine was synthesized from morphine in 1874. Diacetylmorphine was renamed *heroin* by the Bayer Company in Germany in 1898, one year before the same company released Aspirin (Box 25–4).

Around the turn of the 20th century, there were no US federal drug laws of any importance. All drug regulations were under state jurisdiction and most states allowed market considerations to dictate availability of drugs. For example, the label on a readily available heroin cough syrup marketed by the Martin H. Smith and Co., Chemists, of New York described

. . . Glyco-Heroin (Smith) . . . as a Respiratory Sedative Superior in All Respects to the Preparations of Opium, Morphine, Codeine and Other Narcotics.

There were virtually no controls on drug claims or on the ingredients contained in patent remedies. Legislation controlling mind-altering substances was eventually passed, but for a time, cocaine, morphine, heroin, and marijuana all enjoyed unrestricted sale.

Liska K: Drugs and the Human Body: With Implications for Society. Macmillan, New York, 1981.
Musto DF: Opium, cocaine and marijuana in American history. Sci Am 265(1):40–47, Jul 1991.

CODEINE. Codeine, sold under many trade names, is extracted from opium and is the least potent of the opiates. It is used as an oral drug to relieve moderate pain and is often used in combination with nonnarcotic analgesics, such as aspirin and acetaminophen. Aspirin can cause a hypersensitivity reaction in certain patients; therefore, the use of such combination analgesic products requires caution (see Aspirin, Precautions and Adverse Reactions, below). All orders for codeine require a prescription in the United States, but in Canada, low-dose combination products containing codeine are available as nonprescription controlled drugs. Codeine produces far less gastrointestinal tract and pupillary activity than morphine. In addition, tolerance and abuse are much less than with morphine and related opiates. Codeine has potent antitussive effects and is included in some cough suppressant medications. Hydrocodone is a semisynthetic opiate derivative that also has potent antitussive effects (see Chapter 15).

Semisynthetic Opiates

Opiate agonists that possess synthetic portions of the molecule but share part of their structure with the natural opiate alkaloids are termed semisynthetic opiates. Their pharmacologic activity is similar to that of morphine, but they have different potencies. Oxycodone (Percodan) has a structure very similar to that of morphine and possesses about twice the potency. In addition, oxycodone is available only in tablets that contain aspirin (Way and Way, 1982). Therefore, oxycodone should be used with caution in patients with known aspirin sensitivity (see Aspirin, Precautions and Adverse Reactions, below). A very water-soluble semisynthetic opiate suitable for intravenous administration is hydromorphone (Dilaudid). It is several times more potent than morphine in producing analgesia and is well suited for patients whose pain is not controlled by morphine.

Synthetic Opioids

A variety of narcotic agonists have been developed. All are similar to morphine and differ primarily in potency and duration of action. Abuse liability is present with all of them.

Meperidine (Demerol) is a parenteral analgesic frequently used in hospitals. It has about one tenth the potency of morphine but can still produce undesirable effects such as depression of ventilation.

Propoxyphene (Darvon) is used in the treatment of chronic pain. Like the other narcotic analgesics, it may produce drug dependency. The usual therapeutic dose of propoxyphene is approximately the same as that of codeine. Additive effects may occur with other CNS depressants such as tranquilizers, antidepressants, or alcohol. Consequently, propoxyphene is used with caution in patients who may abuse these substances. Propoxyphene is available in fixed-dose combination products, such as Darvon Compound-65. This analgesic mixture contains propoxyphene, aspirin, and caffeine. Patients who are sensitive to aspirin or caffeine must be cautioned with compounds such as these (see Salicylates, Precautions and Adverse Reactions below).

A very potent opioid related to meperidine is fentanyl (Sublimaze). It is used primarily in anesthesia in various combinations with nitrous oxide, oxygen, and neuroleptics such as droperidol. Additional synthetic opioids, such as the fentanyl derivatives alfentanil and sufentanil, are used primarily in anesthesia and are discussed in Chapter 27.

Methadone (Dolophine) was developed as a morphine substitute but is now used primarily in "methadone maintenance" programs for opioid addicts. Tolerance and dependency occur following methadone administration, but its withdrawal symptoms are, in theory at least, less severe than those caused by withdrawal from heroin addiction.

Drugs with a combination of narcotic agonist and antagonist actions have been produced. They were originally developed from mixed agonist-antagonist drugs, such as nalorphine (Nalline). Pentazocine (Talwin) is such an **opioid agonist-antagonist** drug (Bhatnagar et al, 1989). It has less potential for abuse and produces less ventilatory depression than pure agonists, such as morphine or meperidine. The antagonist effects, although less potent than those of the pure antagonists described below, are sufficient to induce withdrawal in a narcotic addict.

Narcotic Antagonists

NALOXONE (Narcan). Drugs that exhibit pharmacologic antagonism with narcotics (opiates or opioids) at opioid receptors are called **narcotic antagonists.** The most effective agent currently being used is a pure antagonist called naloxone. Earlier narcotic antagonist drugs, such as nalorphine, have been used to reverse narcotic effects. These drugs, however, produce mixed agonist-antagonist actions and have been largely replaced by the pure narcotic antagonists. Naloxone antagonizes the various subtypes of opioid receptors, but is especially effective at μ-opioid receptors.

INDICATIONS. Naloxone is particularly useful for reversing narcotic overdoses. It is also used as an investigational tool in the study of opioid receptor subtypes and endogenous opioid peptides.

PRECAUTIONS. Naloxone given to a narcotic addict may trigger a short but severe withdrawal syndrome, including production of nausea and vomiting.

Nonnarcotic Analgesics

The nonnarcotic analgesics include many different drugs having varying degrees of analgesic, antipyretic, and anti-inflammatory activity. The drugs are also called **nonsteroidal anti-inflammatory drugs (NSAID)** and **antipyretic analgesics** because of their ability to suppress inflammation and fever, respectively. (Acetaminophen lacks anti-inflammatory activity and is not an NSAID; therefore, the most useful classification for our purposes is "nonnarcotic analgesics.")

Salicylates

ASPIRIN. The salicylates are named after *Salix* species, the genus of trees that includes the willow. Aspirin, or acetylsalicylic acid (ASA), and other salicylates are converted to salicylic acid, which produces the desired pharmacologic effects. Salicylic acid is related to substances found naturally in the willow, the bark of which was originally used as a pain reliever. Aspirin is the prototype drug of the salicylate group. It is classified as an NSAID and exhibits several major pharmacologic effects—analgesic, antipyretic, anti-inflammatory, and antiplatelet. These effects determine the main indications for use of aspirin (Box 25–4).

INDICATIONS. The treatment of mild-to-moderate pain is one of the most common uses of aspirin. The mechanism of action occurs peripherally rather than in the CNS, and involves blockage of cyclooxygenase to prevent the formation of the prostanoid mediators, which include the prostaglandins and thromboxane (see Chapter 9). Tissue trauma causes bradykinin to be formed. Prostaglandins render free nerve endings (pain receptors) more sensitive to the pain-producing, or **algesic,** effects of bradykinin (McKean, 1986). Therefore, aspirin is able to blunt the algesic effect of bradykinin by suppressing prostaglandin synthesis.

Aspirin lowers an elevated temperature (hy-perthermia) caused by pyrogens, or fever-producing substances. It does not reduce normal body temperature, nor does it lower an elevated temperature that has been produced through strenuous exercise. With an infection, however, fever is often one of the symptoms. The elevated body temperature occurs when the thermoregulatory center of the hypothalamus is reset at a higher level by the presence of pyrogenic substances. The antipyretic effect of aspirin is directed at reducing the ability of endogenous pyrogens to reset the thermoregulatory center at this higher level. Normal temperature-lowering mechanisms, such as sweating and vascular shunts, are then able to reduce the fever.

The ability of aspirin to reduce the symptoms of inflammation is one of its most valuable pharmacologic effects. The anti-inflammatory effect is mediated through the cyclooxygenase pathway. The resulting decrease in prostaglandin synthesis works directly to reduce inflammatory symptoms such as swelling and hyperemia, and indirectly by suppressing bradykinin and histamine formation and release.

An antiplatelet effect of aspirin is detailed in Chapter 23. Recall that aspirin, again through the cyclooxygenase mechanism, suppresses thromboxane A_2, which is a potent mediator that promotes aggregation of platelets.

CONTRAINDICATIONS. Preexisting gastrointestinal ulcers or a history of bleeding or coagulation disorders are contraindications to the use of the salicylates.

PRECAUTIONS AND ADVERSE REACTIONS. Aspirin and aspirinlike drugs may produce a sensitivity reaction in certain asthmatics. The unusual collection of symptoms is called Samter's syndrome. This analgesic-induced asthma syndrome resembles a hypersensitivity reaction, although no specific aspirin antibodies are found. In patients with the syndrome, there is a correlation among aspirin sensitivity, asthma, and the presence of nasal polyps. The reaction is usually manifested as bronchospasm or severe rhinitis in an individual with preexisting asthma. Aspirin and other nonnarcotic analgesics, such as ibuprofen, indomethacin, phenylbutazone, and the fenamates, inhibit the enzyme prostaglandin synthetase. This slows the conversion of fatty acid precursors into prostaglandins. The decrease in prostaglandin production caused by aspirin and aspirin-type drugs may contribute to the syndrome described above. Aspirin-sensitive patients must avoid aspirin-containing products.

Gastrointestinal tract irritation is the most common adverse effect to aspirin therapy. Gas-

BOX 25–4 OLD WONDER DRUGS NEVER DIE

Aspirin is converted in the body to the active ingredient salicylic acid. A closely related, naturally occurring compound called salicin is found in the willow tree and has been prescribed since antiquity for the relief of pain and fever. Currently, about 90 million aspirin tablets per day are consumed in the United States. Symptomatic treatment of minor pain and fever are still the main indications for use of the salicylates. The following list provides a glimpse of the colorful history of one of the most common drugs in current use.

400 BC	Hippocrates (Greece) advises women in labor to chew willow leaves to reduce their pain.
Middle Ages	Meadowsweet flowers (*Spirea ulmaria*) containing natural salicylates are fermented into a home remedy used as a mild pain reliever. (Meadowsweet wine is still made today in Scotland.)
1763	Reverend Edward Stone (Oxfordshire, England) learns of a local folk remedy used to reduce fever. Bark from the white willow tree (*Salix alba*) is used as an extract in water, tea, and beer.
1830s	Salicylic acid is purified, but found to be very irritating to tissues.
1860	Salicylic acid is first synthesized.
1874	The first factory for the production of synthetic salicylates is built in Dresden. The resulting decrease in price of salicylates contributes to widespread clinical use of the drug.
1876	Salicylates are used successfully to treat inflammatory conditions such as gout and rheumatoid arthritis.
1898	Felix Hoffman (Germany) of the Friedrich Bayer–Eberfeld Division of IG Farbenindustrie produces acetylsalicylic acid (ASA), an analgesic that is less irritating than salicylic acid.
1899	ASA is marketed as Aspirin by the Bayer Company. The name *aspirin* is derived from *a* for acetyl and *spirin* from *Spirea,* the meadowsweet source of natural salicylates.
1918	The Aspirin trademark is awarded to the United States as part of Germany's World War I reparations.
1971	John Vane (Great Britain), Sune Bergström (Sweden), and Bengt Samuelsson (Sweden) discover that aspirin blocks the synthesis of thromboxane and the prostaglandins, thereby exhibiting a potent anti-inflammatory effect.
1980s	Preliminary studies indicate that the antiplatelet effect of aspirin may be useful in the prevention of stroke and heart attack.

Calrk WG, Brater DC, and Johnson AR: Goth's Medical Pharmacology, ed 12. CV Mosby, St Louis, 1988.

Grady D: Aspirin: Is the warning necessary? Discover 3(8):18–23, Aug 1982.

Modell W, Lansing A, and Editors of Time-Life Books: Drugs. Life Science Library. Time, New York, 1969.

Weissmann G: The action of NSAIDs. Hosp Pract (Off Ed) 26:60–76, 1991.

trointestinal tract irritation and bleeding occur in nearly all persons, but some individuals are more sensitive than others. Enteric-coated and buffered preparations minimize the damage to a certain extent. Two adjunctive therapies help reduce the gastric mucosal damage caused by NSAIDs such as aspirin. H_2-Histamine receptor blockers such as cimetidine, and synthetic prostaglandin E_1 drugs, such as misoprostol, are useful in the treatment or prevention of NSAID-associated gastric ulcers (Bijlsma, 1988; Cryer and Feldman, 1992; Dajani et al, 1991).

In combination products containing aspirin and other analgesics (usually codeine), caffeine is often included. The mild CNS-stimulating effects of caffeine counter some of the depression caused by the narcotic. Caffeine taken in combination with aspirin is additive with other methylxanthines. These include caffeine consumed in coffee, tea, and cola drinks, theobromine in chocolate, and theophylline used therapeutically as a bronchodilator. Patients sensitive to caffeine and the methylxanthines in general should be aware of the presence of these substances in many common analgesic mixtures. The additive effects may exaggerate the gastrointestinal and cardiovascular effects produced by the methylxanthines (see Chapter 13).

One of the most publicized but least understood precautions with aspirin therapy concerns the proposed link between aspirin and Reye's syndrome. The disorder is primarily an illness of childhood and is characterized by vomiting, encephalopathy, drowsiness, coma, and a significant mortality rate of around 35%. These complications may follow apparent recovery from acute viral infections such as influenza or chickenpox (Grady, 1982). Statistically, there is a correlation among these childhood illnesses, high fever, aspirin ingestion, and development of Reye's syndrome. The mechanism, however, is not yet understood. Aspirin substitutes, such as acetaminophen (below), are equally effective as antipyretics and have not been linked with Reye's syndrome. However, liver damage from overdoses of acetaminophen can occur.

TOXICITY. Accidental poisoning by the salicylates, especially in children, is fairly common. Mild toxicity is called salicylism and is characterized by symptoms of tinnitus, dizziness, and headache. Severe overdose symptoms include Kussmaul's breathing, a ventilatory pattern characterized by increased depth and rate of breathing (Des Jardins, 1993). In addition, hyperthermia, nausea, vomiting, acid-base disturbances, convulsions, and coma may be seen. Acid-base upsets are caused by a variety of alterations in breathing and metabolism. The effect on blood pH, therefore, depends on the stage of intoxication exhibited by the poisoning victim at the time of presentation. Initially, increased sensitivity to carbon dioxide by the medullary chemoreceptors causes hyperventilation and respiratory alkalosis. With progressive CNS depression, however, ventilatory depression and respiratory acidosis occur. Accumulation of organic acids in the tissues contributes to metabolic acidosis. The net effect of salicylate overdose in latter stages of the intoxication is acidosis, especially in infants and young children. Treatment of salicylate overdose includes ventilatory support, dialysis, and forced diuresis. Alkaline urine increases the excretion of weak acids, such as salicylate metabolites. These conditions are the same as those required for the forced diuresis of weak acid barbiturates in barbiturate overdose (Chapter 24). Buffers such as sodium bicarbonate are used to alkalinize the urine in these cases of overdose. The role of pH in the excretion and absorption of drug metabolites is discussed fully in Chapter 2. Table 25–3 outlines some of the effects of and supportive therapy for salicylate toxicity.

Propionic Acid Derivatives
Propionic acid derivatives such as ibuprofen (Motrin, Advil, Nuprin) and naproxen (Naprosyn) are classified as NSAIDs. These drugs are not completely devoid of adverse effects, but compared with aspirin produce relatively little gastrointestinal tract irritation or bleeding. They

TABLE 25–3 NONNARCOTIC OVERDOSE

ASPIRIN TOXICITY	
Effects	**Supportive Therapy**
EARLY STAGES OF INTOXICATION	Ventilatory support
	Forced diuresis (pH
Hyperventilation	dependent; alkaline urine
Respiratory alkalosis	promotes elimination)
	Hemodialysis
LATER STAGES OF INTOXICATION	
Metabolic acidosis	
Ventilatory depression	
Respiratory acidosis	

ACETAMINOPHEN TOXICITY	
Liver and kidney damage due to cytotoxic free radicals	N-acetylcysteine given within 10 h of overdose (converted into free radical–scavenging metabolites)
Jaundice	
Oliguria or anuria	Hemoperfusion

are used primarily as aspirin substitutes for the treatment of inflammatory conditions such as arthritis. Adverse effects include gastrointestinal upset, headache, and tinnitus. Ibuprofen was the first of the class, becoming available in the United States in 1975 as a prescription drug and as an over-the-counter analgesic about 10 years later (Adams, 1992).

Indole Derivatives

The indole derivatives are also NSAIDs and include the prototype indomethacin (Indocin). Newer agents, such as the propionic acid derivatives, produce fewer and less serious adverse effects than the indole derivatives. Adverse reactions to indomethacin therapy may include GI tract upset, blood disorders, and renal toxicity.

Pyrazolone Derivatives

Pyrazolone derivatives, such as phenylbutazone (Butazolidin), are more potent NSAIDs than the salicylates but produce serious adverse reactions such as GI tract disturbances, hypersensitivity, renal toxicity, and hepatotoxicity. Pyrazolone derivatives are used when other NSAIDs fail to provide the desired control of inflammatory symptoms.

Fenamates

Meclofenamate (Meclomen) is a fast-acting, potent cyclooxygenase inhibitor that suppresses the production of prostaglandins and inhibits the release of leukotriene B_4 from neutrophils. The potent anti-inflammatory effects of this NSAID are especially useful in the treatment of arthritis and mild-to-moderate pain (Conroy et al, 1991).

As mentioned with Samter's syndrome and aspirin sensitivity, some asthmatics may respond unfavorably to the NSAIDs, including propionic acid derivatives, indole derivatives, pyrazolone derivatives, and fenamates discussed above.

Para-Aminophenol Derivatives

ACETAMINOPHEN (Tylenol, Datril, Panadol). Para-aminophenol derivatives such as acetaminophen, or paracetamol, and phenacetin are aspirin substitutes that lack the adverse reactions of gastrointestinal irritation and bleeding. Following ingestion, acetaminophen is metabolized to phenacetin, so from a practical standpoint the two compounds are the same.

INDICATIONS. The p-aminophenols are equivalent to the salicylates in analgesic and antipyretic activity. These are the two most common uses for the nonnarcotic group as whole. The p-aminophenols, however, totally lack anti-inflammatory action and are not NSAIDs. They are suitable for the relief of mild-to-moderate pain and for reduction of fever. Para-aminophenols are ideal alternative antipyretic analgesics for persons with a history of gastrointestinal ulcer, bleeding disorders, or salicylate intolerance. They are also ideal for children at risk for developing Reye's syndrome.

CONTRAINDICATIONS. Known hypersensitivity to the p-aminophenols is a contraindication to their use.

PRECAUTIONS AND ADVERSE REACTIONS. Although the p-aminophenols do not cause gastrointestinal irritation, chronic overuse can lead to other adverse effects such as nephrotoxicity and hepatotoxicity. Cumulative effects can occur because a variety of prescription and over-the-counter products contain acetaminophen alone or in combination with other drugs. Acetaminophen products should be used with caution by persons with preexisting liver or kidney dysfunction.

TOXICITY. Acetaminophen, alone or in combination with other analgesics, such as aspirin or codeine, is commonly involved in analgesic overdose. Acetaminophen toxicity is caused by the accumulation of a highly reactive metabolite called N-acetylimidoquinone (Lewis and Palovcek, 1991). This compound is a cytotoxic free radical that may produce severe liver damage if not detoxified and removed. In therapeutic doses, glutathione within hepatic cells is present in adequate quantities to detoxify the free radicals, but in acute acetaminophen intoxication, glutathione levels are insufficient. The mucokinetic agent N-acetylcysteine (Mucomyst) can provide some protection for liver cells in cases of acetaminophen overdose. For maximal antidotal effect, N-acetylcysteine is administered orally or intravenously within 10 hours of acetaminophen overdose (Flanagan and Meredith, 1991; Smilkstein et al, 1991). Unlike glutathione, N-acetylcysteine crosses hepatic cell membranes. Once it is within the cells, it is converted into large quantities of glutathione, which then acts as a free-radical scavenger, or antioxidant, to protect hepatic cells (see Fig. 15–7). Chapter 15 outlines this mechanism in more detail. Table 25–3 lists the effects of acetaminophen overdose and summarizes the supportive therapy employed in such toxicities.

Table 25–4 lists the generic and trade names of the analgesics discussed in this chapter.

TABLE 25–4   DRUG NAMES: ANALGESICS

Generic Name	Trade Name
NARCOTIC ANALGESICS	
Naturally occurring alkaloids	
Morphine	(many trade names)
Diacetylmorphine (heroin)	
Codeine	(many trade names)
Semisynthetic opiates	
Oxycodone (**OKS**-ē-kō-dōn)	Percodan*
Hydromorphone (hī-drō-**MOR**-fōn)	Dilaudid
Synthetic opioids	
Meperidine (me-**PAIR**-i-dēn)	Demerol
Fentanyl (**FEN**-ta-nil)	Sublimaze
Methadone (**METH**-a-dōn)	Dolophine
Pentazocine (pen-**TAZ**-ō-sēn)†	Talwin
NARCOTIC ANTAGONISTS	
Naloxone (nal-**OKS**-ōn)	Narcan
NONNARCOTIC ANALGESICS	
Salicylates	
Aspirin (acetylsalicylic acid, ASA)	(many trade names)
Propionic acid derivatives	
Ibuprofen (ī-bū-**PRŌ**-fin)	Motrin, Advil, Nuprin
Naproxen (na-**PROX**-in)	Naprosyn
Indole derivatives	
Indomethacin (in-dō-**METH**-a-sin)	Indocin
Pyrazolone derivatives	
Phenylbutazone (fin-ill-**BUT**-a-zōn)	Butazolidin
Fenamates	
Meclofenamate (mek-lō-**FEN**-a-māt)	Meclomen
***p*-Aminophenol derivatives**	
Acetaminophen (a-sē-ta-**MIN**-ō-fin)	Tylenol, Datril, Panadol
Phenacetin (fin-**AS**-se-tin)	*(usually in combination products with aspirin and caffeine)*

*Also contains aspirin.
†An opioid agonist-antagonist (Pentazocine is also combined with naloxone as Talwin-NX).

CHAPTER SUMMARY

The control of pain in its many forms is the goal of analgesic drug therapy. The use of analgesics dates from antiquity. Early use of natural analgesic-containing products in their crude form eventually led to the extraction of pure substances. This in turn paved the way for synthesis of the analgesics and ushered in the modern era of pharmaceutical chemistry. This chapter examines the benefits and risks of the narcotic group of analgesics—drugs that provide merciful relief from severe pain, but that are very unforgiving if abused. We also discuss the nonnarcotic group of pain relievers, a group of pharmacologic agents that occupies an important niche in the clinical treatment of minor pain. The effects and management of narcotic and nonnarcotic overdoses are also examined in this chapter, including discussion of the respiratory abnormalities caused by such toxicities.

BIBLIOGRAPHY

Adams SS: The propionic acids: A personal perspective. J Clin Pharmcol 32:317–323, 1992.

Bhatnagar RK, Dutton GR, and Gebhart GF: Drugs acting on the central nervous system (CNS). In Conn PM and Gebhart GF (eds): Essentials of Pharmacology. F.A. Davis, Philadelphia, 1989.

Bijlsma JW: Treatment of NSAID-induced gastrointestinal lesions with cimetidine: An international multicentre collaborative study. Aliment Pharmacol Ther 2(Suppl 1):85–95, 1988.

Byers VL: Drugs that provide pain relief. In Kuhn MM (ed): Pharmacotherapeutics: A Nursing Process Approach, ed 2. FA Davis, Philadelphia, 1990.

Clark WG, Brater DC, and Johnson AR: Goth's Medical Pharmacology, ed. 12. CV Mosby, St Louis, 1988.

Conroy MC, Randinitis EJ, and Turner JL: Pharmacology and therapeutic use of meclofenamate sodium. Clin J Pain 7(Suppl 1): S44–S48, 1991.

Cryer B and Feldman M: Effects of nonsteroidal anti-inflammatory drugs on endogenous gastrointestinal prostaglandins and therapeutic strategies for prevention and treatment of nonsteroidal anti-inflammatory drug–

induced damage. Arch Intern Med 152:1145–1155, 1992.

Dajani EZ, Wilson DE, and Agrawal NM: Prostaglandins: An overview of the worldwide clinical experience. J Assoc Acad Minor Phys 2:23, 27–35, 1991.

Des Jardins TR: Cardiopulmonary Anatomy and Physiology: Essentials for Respiratory Care, ed 2. Delmar, Albany, 1993.

Fetrow KO: The management of pain in orthopaedics. Clin J Pain 5(Suppl 2):S26–S32, 1989.

Flanagan RJ and Meredith TJ: Use of N-acetylcysteine in clinical toxicology. Am J Med 91:131S–139S, 1991.

Grady D: Aspirin: Is the warning necessary? Discover 3(8):18–23, Aug 1982.

Lehnert BE and Schachter EN: The Pharmacology of Respiratory Care. CV Mosby, St Louis, 1980.

Lewis RK and Paloucek FP: Assessment and treatment of acetaminophen overdose. Clin Pharm 10:756–774, 1991.

McCarty KD: Adult respiratory distress syndrome. In Wilkins RL and Dexter JR (eds): Respiratory Disease: Principles of Patient Care. FA Davis, Philadelphia, 1993.

McKean K: Pain. Discover 7(10):82–92, 1986.

Smilkstein MJ et al: Acetaminophen overdose: A 48-hour intravenous N-acetylcysteine treatment protocol. Ann Emerg Med 20:1058–1063, 1991.

Way WL and Way EL: Narcotic analgesics and antagonists. In Katzung BG (ed): Basic and Clinical Pharmacology, Lange Medical Publications, Los Altos, 1982.

CHAPTER 26

Local Anesthetics

CHAPTER OUTLINE

CHAPTER OBJECTIVES

After studying this chapter the reader should be able to:

- Define regional, or conduction, anesthesia and list two subtypes of regional anesthesia.
- Briefly describe a presumed mechanism of action of the local anesthetics.
- Name the three types of nerve fibers affected by local anesthetic action and list the three types in decreasing order of sensitivity to local anesthetic action.
- Explain why an α_1-adrenergic agonist is often included with a local anesthetic to modify the duration of action of the anesthetic.
- Discuss the reason why ester- and amide-containing local anesthetics have different durations of action.
- Describe the pharmacologic activity of the following amide-containing local anesthetics:
  - Lidocaine, bupivacaine, dibucaine, etidocaine, mepivacaine.
- Describe the pharmacologic activity of the following ester-containing local anesthetics:
  - Procaine, cocaine, benzocaine, tetracaine, chloroprocaine.

KEY TERMS

local anesthesia (conduction
   anesthesia, regional
   anesthesia)
surgical anesthesia

CHAPTER INTRODUCTION

Surgical anesthesia is produced when a patient's perception of and reaction to pain are blocked. The state of surgical anesthesia can exist with or without consciousness. The general anesthetics produce surgical anesthesia with a patient in an unconscious state. These agents are discussed in Chapter 27. **Local anesthesia** produces a local, or regional, blockade of sensory impulses without loss of consciousness. Such an effect is useful for certain respiratory care procedures, such as

arterial blood gas sampling. This chapter examines a representative sample of local anesthetics used clinically.

Some local anesthetic techniques block peripheral structures such as nerves, and strictly speaking, do not affect the central nervous system (CNS). Nevertheless, the local anesthetics are included in this unit because they may influence the CNS through other procedures, such as spinal anesthesia.

LOCAL ANESTHESIA

Poorly absorbed local anesthetics, such as benzocaine, are administered topically to treat burns and abrasions. Local anesthetics, such as lidocaine, are infiltrated into the tissues using intradermal, subcutaneous, or deeper injections. Such injections produce surgical anesthesia without loss of consciousness. Figure 26–1 depicts graphically the various means of accomplishing surgical anesthesia. Because local anesthetics are introduced into a specific region, they bring about **regional anesthesia.** They also impair conduction along a nerve or a group of nerves and are said to produce **conduction anesthesia.** Several subtypes of conduction anesthesia are recognized and named according to the anatomic site used for infiltration of the local anesthetic: spinal anesthesia, epidural anesthesia, and nerve blocks. Discussion of the technical aspects of these procedures is beyond the scope of this text.

Mechanism and Sites of Action

Local anesthetics have similar pharmacologic effects. They differ slightly in potency, duration of action, selectivity, and metabolism. All are used to block sensory nerve fibers to provide pain relief. Occasionally, certain local anesthetics are employed to block sympathetic postganglionic fibers to study peripheral vasomotor tone. All local anesthetics block nerve impulses by causing hyperpolarization of neuronal membranes. The mechanism of action is under investigation and is not fully established. One explanation is that the local anesthetic passes to the internal side of the cell membrane and prevents the opening of voltage-gated sodium ion channels, thus hyperpolarizing the membrane (Hondeghem and Miller, 1982; Tortora and Grabowski, 1993). Therefore, the membrane stabilization effect of

local anesthetics may be due to interference with Na^{1+} conductance and membrane permeability. Another description of local anesthetic action is that the drug competes with calcium ions for Ca^{2+} binding sites on the nerve cell membrane (Clark et al, 1988). These sites may regulate Na^{1+} movement; therefore, Na^{1+} inflow is inhibited and the action potential is not achieved. (Neuronal action potentials and the role of ion channels in membranes are covered in Chapter 4.)

Following infiltration at an injection site, local anesthetics exhibit different affinities for different types of nerve fibers (Table 26–1). Nerve fibers are classified into three groups on the basis of axon diameter, myelination, and conduction velocity (Tortora and Grabowski, 1993). Group A fibers (several subtypes) possess large-diameter myelinated axons and conduct impulses very rapidly at velocities up to 100 meters per second. (This speed is in excess of 200 mph.) Such fibers are involved with skeletal muscle tone and with temperature, tactile (touch), proprioceptive, and sharp pain sensations. Group B fibers are smaller diameter, myelinated, and conduct at intermediate velocities of around 10 meters per second. Group B fibers are preganglionic autonomic fibers; therefore, anesthetic blockade of such fibers results in autonomic paralysis. Local anesthetics have the greatest affinity for group C nerve fibers (Hondeghem and Miller, 1982). These fibers are small diameter, unmyelinated, and conduct impulses at slow rates of less than 1 meter per second. Group C fibers include both sympathetic postganglionic fibers and nociceptive (pain) fibers. Group C fibers are preferentially targeted by local anesthetics to result in the blockade of vasoconstriction impulses and pain sensations. Local anesthetics also have a selective action at nerve fibers with high firing rates. The small-diameter group C pain fibers fall into this category because they characteristically exhibit high frequencies. Other fibers, in decreasing order of sensitivity to local anesthetic block, are associated with thermal, touch, proprioceptive, and muscle tone sensations (Clark et al, 1988; Long and Sokoll, 1989). Table 26–1 summarizes the characteristics of groups A, B, and C fibers.

The selective nature of local anesthetics makes them especially valuable in clinical medicine because they permit some types of surgical procedures to be performed without producing unwanted systemic effects. An example of this advantage is seen with overweight persons requiring surgery. In the first place, an obese patient is at increased risk because he or she requires a larger dose of general anesthetic than

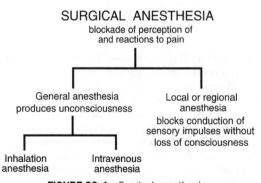

SURGICAL ANESTHESIA
blockade of perception of
and reactions to pain

General anesthesia
produces unconsciousness

Local or regional
anesthesia
blocks conduction of
sensory impulses without
loss of consciousness

Inhalation
anesthesia

Intravenous
anesthesia

FIGURE 26–1 Surgical anesthesia.

TABLE 26–1 CLASSIFICATION OF NERVE FIBERS

Group	Myelinated	Axon Diameter	Conduction Velocity (m/sec)	Location
A	Yes	Large	100	Somatic motor fibers Temperature, tactile, proprioception, and sharp pain sensory fibers
B*	Yes	Medium	10	Preganglionic autonomic fibers
C†	No	Small	1	Sympathetic postganglionic fibers Pain (nociceptive) fibers†

*Anesthetic blockade of group B fibers causes autonomic paralysis.
†Most local anesthetics preferentially target group C fibers to bring about blockade of vasoconstriction and pain impulses.
  (Cocaine *produces* vasoconstriction by blocking the amine uptake-1 mechanism.)
‡Nerve fibers exhibit differing sensitivity to local anesthetic blockade: pain > thermal > touch > proprioception > muscle
  tone.

someone of average weight. In addition, the on-set of anesthetic action is slow because some of the anesthetic is transferred into adipose tissue. Finally, recovery from anesthesia is prolonged. By contrast (and depending on the surgical procedure), the same overweight individual could be treated under spinal anesthesia and be at considerably less risk for systemic toxicity due to the selective nature of conduction anesthesia.

Absorption and Metabolism

Absorption of local anesthetic from an infiltration site adds to the potential adverse effects of regional anesthesia. To maximize the local effect at a depot site and minimize systemic effects, most local anesthetics are administered in conjunction with an α_1-adrenergic vasoconstrictor (Long and Sokoll, 1989). Drugs such as epinephrine (dilutions in the range of 1:50,000 to 1:200,000) limit the spread of the local anesthetic into general circulation (Hondeghem and Miller, 1982; Long and Sokoll, 1989). Recall that epinephrine may produce its own toxicities, including hypertension and cardiac stimulation.

Cocaine is the only local anesthetic that produces its own vasoconstrictor effect and is, therefore, self-limiting. Cocaine produces vasoconstriction through inhibition of the uptake-1 mechanism, which regulates the transport of amines such as norepinephrine into adrenergic nerve terminals. (Termination of amine action is discussed in Chapter 5.)

Cocaine was extracted from its natural source in 1860, and procaine was first synthesized in 1905. These drugs were the first local anesthetics available for clinical use. They are ester-containing local anesthetics and are characterized by an ester grouping in the intermediate chain of the molecule (Fig. 26–2). Such drugs are rapidly hy-

drolyzed by plasma pseudocholinesterase and have relatively short durations of action. (In laboratory tests, procaine is used to assess the functional activity of the cholinesterase enzyme system in patients.) With the advent of lidocaine, the amide-containing local anesthetics became available (Fig. 26–2). The amides are metabolized by the hepatic mixed-function oxidase system. The slower rate of metabolism results in longer durations of action. The local anesthetic effects of lidocaine, for example, last about three times longer than those of procaine.

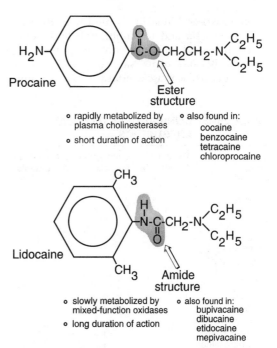

FIGURE 26–2 Procaine and lidocaine (showing typical ester and amide structures).

THERAPEUTIC AGENTS

Since the introduction of procaine as the first synthetic local anesthetic in 1905, many different local anesthetics have been produced. A few of these are reviewed below. The goal of synthesis has been to develop drugs producing less local irritation and systemic toxicity, but having a faster onset and a prolonged duration of action (Hondeghem and Miller, 1982). Physicians can choose from a variety of local anesthetic agents having different durations of action. In this way, the drug can be matched to the surgical procedure being carried out. Increased dosage, the inclusion of a vasoconstrictor agent, or a combination of the two prolongs the duration of action to provide even more versatility.

Amide-Containing Local Anesthetics

LIDOCAINE (Xylocaine, others). As was mentioned above, the introduction of the amides followed the development of the esters, such as procaine. However, because lidocaine is considered the prototype of all the local anesthestics in current use, it will be considered first. Lidocaine was synthesized in 1943, several decades after the release of procaine. It quickly became the new standard for comparison. Lidocaine is a widely used local anesthetic with more potency than procaine and far more versatility. It is used in topical, conduction, and inhalation anesthesia (Table 26–2).

INDICATIONS. Lidocaine is used both for surface anesthesia and for infiltration and nerve block. It is ideal for short-duration epidural anesthesia. Because of its Na^{1+} channel–blocking activity in cardiac muscle, lidocaine is a frontline antiarrhythmic agent used in the treatment of several cardiac electrical abnormalities (see Chapter 22). It suppresses abnormal pacemaker activity and decreases excitability and conductivity of myocardial tissue.

CONTRAINDICATIONS. Known hypersensitivity is a contraindication to the use of the local anesthetics.

PRECAUTIONS. As was explained above, epinephrine is often delivered with local anesthetics to provide localized vasoconstriction and limit spread of the anesthetic. Therefore, if the local anesthetic is inadvertently injected into a blood vessel or is absorbed in toxic amounts, epinephrine is introduced into the bloodstream along with the local anesthetic. Effects such as anxiety, widespread vasoconstriction, hypertension, and tachycardia may occur due to the action of epinephrine (Long and Sokoll, 1989).

Local anesthetics may depress neuromuscular transmission through their effect on membrane conductance of ions. This hyperpolarization effect may enhance (prolong) the action of neuromuscular blocking agents (see Chapter 7).

ADVERSE REACTIONS. If absorbed from an injection site, local anesthetics may cause undesirable systemic effects. These may involve the cardiovascular and central nervous systems. Lidocaine is the only local anesthetic with *specific* antiarrhythmic indications for use. However, the other local anesthetics may produce similar adverse reactions when absorbed systemically at excessive doses. Decreased depolarization of conduction myofibers (Purkinje fibers) and decreased conduction velocity may result in negative inotropism and blockade. Central nervous system (CNS) effects are usually produced before cardiovascular effects are seen. Because local anesthetics block C fibers, which include postganglionic sympathetic fibers, sympathetic vasomotor tone is reduced and hypotension results. Cocaine is the single exception to this statement. It blocks amine uptake into adrenergic nerve terminals, thereby raising norepinephrine levels. This induces widespread vasoconstriction and may cause hypertension.

Excessive systemic absorption of local anesthetic results in excitation, restlessness, convulsions, and ventilatory depression (Long and Sokoll, 1989). Depression of cortical inhibitory pathways leads to the excitatory symptoms. Convulsions are the most common adverse reaction and are treated with intravenous thiopental or diazepam (Hondeghem and Miller, 1982). Higher doses depress inhibitory neurons and cause ventilatory depression.

Many other amides have been developed with

TABLE 26–2 CLINICAL USES OF LOCAL ANESTHETICS

Drug	Topical Anesthesia	Conduction Anesthesia	Intravenous Anesthesia
AMIDES			
Lidocaine	+	+	+
Bupivacaine		+	
Dibucaine	+	+	
Etidocaine		+	
Mepivacaine		+	
ESTERS			
Procaine		+	
Cocaine	+		
Benzocaine	+		
Tetracaine	+	+	
Chloroprocaine		+	

+—effective.

longer durations of action than lidocaine. These include bupivacaine (Sensorcaine, Marcaine), dibucaine (Nupercaine), etidocaine (Duranest), and mepivacaine (Carbocaine). All of these agents have similar pharmacologic characteristics and are used in conduction anesthesia, as can be seen in Table 26–2.

Ester-Containing Local Anesthetics

PROCAINE (Novocain). Procaine was not the first local anesthetic to enter clinical use—cocaine was available about 20 years earlier. However, in 1905, procaine became the standard reference compound for the local anesthetics, a status it held until 1943. Procaine was synthesized in a attempt to produce a drug with the local anesthetic properties of cocaine but without the high addiction potential. Procaine is not effective topically and must be injected. It has a rapid onset of action but a relatively short duration of action (about 1 h).

INDICATIONS. Indications for use are summarized in Table 26–2.

CONTRAINDICATIONS, PRECAUTIONS, AND ADVERSE REACTIONS. See Lidocaine.

Other ester-containing local anesthetics include cocaine, which was first used in clinical medicine in 1884 as an ophthalmic anesthetic. For 25 years it was the only drug of its kind (Box 26–1). However, high abuse potential and significant toxicities, such as convulsions, eventually led to the development of more effective and safer agents. Cocaine is too toxic to be injected but is an excellent topical anesthetic, with powerful vasoconstricting effects. One of the few medical uses for cocaine today centers around

---

BOX 26–1 ENTHUSIASTIC FOLLOWERS

Since antiquity, the central nervous system–stimulant effects of cocaine have been eagerly sought. Metabolites of cocaine have recently been identified in 4000-year-old hair samples from Chilean mummies. Spanish conquistadors, in their zeal for introducing the stimulant effect of cocaine to the general population, enslaved and eventually decimated the Inca nation in South America. In the United States following the Civil War, veterans who were morphine addicts (because of war wounds) were given cocaine by physicians in the erroneous belief that cocaine would counter the narcotic addiction. Twenty years later, in 1886, the original Coca-Cola recipe contained a small amount of cocaine. (We can assume the soft drink was reasonably refreshing.) These developments were merely reflections of the prevailing attitudes of the day.

The use of cocaine as the first local anesthetic naturally evolved out of interest in its central effects. In 1860, Albert Niemann of Germany isolated cocaine from its natural source, *Erythroxylon coca*, an indigenous shrub of the Andean highlands. Sigmund Freud used cocaine for its euphoriant effects both personally and in his psychoanalysis practice. In the early 1880s, Freud invited an ophthalmologist, Carl Köller, to further investigate the drug's effects. While Freud retained his interest in the systemic effects of cocaine, Köller became intrigued with its potent local anesthetic effect on the eye. He reported his ophthalmologic findings in 1884 and is credited with introducing the concept of local anesthesia. An American surgeon, William Stewart Halsted, developed nerve blocks using cocaine and was the first to define and use regional anesthesia. Unfortunately, Halsted perfected the nerve block techniques on himself and became hopelessly addicted to cocaine in the process. The drug has had many enthusiastic followers since an anonymous person, while gazing at lush Bolivian valleys, first chewed some bright, shiny leaves from a bush that clung to an Andean hillside.

Brown RC: Perchance to Dream: The Patient's Guide to Anesthesia. Nelson-Hall, Chicago, 1981.
Carmell LW, Aufderhide A, and Weems C: Cocaine metabolites in pre-Columbian mummy hair. J Okla State Med Assoc. 84(1): 11–12, Jan 1991.
Liska K: Drugs and the Human Body: With Implications for Society. Macmillan, New York, 1981.
Meyers FH, Jawetz E, and Goldfien A: Review of Medical Pharmacology, ed 7. Lange Medical Publications, Los Altos, 1980.
Musto DF: Opium, cocaine and marijuana in American history. Sci Am 265(1):40–47, Jul 1991.
Wawersik J: History of anesthesia in Germany. J Clin Anesth 3:235–244, 1991.

its vasoconstriction activity—the treatment of epistaxis (serious blood loss from a nosebleed).

Another ester-containing local anesthetic with low solubility and excellent topical anesthetic action is benzocaine (Hurricaine, Solarcaine). Conduction anesthesia and topical use are seen with tetracaine (Pontocaine). It is more potent than procaine and has slower onset, with a longer duration of action. Tetracaine is often used in spinal anesthesia. A derivative of procaine having more potency but a shorter duration of action due to rapid hydrolysis is chloroprocaine (Nesacaine). The clinical uses of the ester-containing local anesthetics discussed above are summarized in Table 26–2.

Table 26–3 lists the generic and trade names of the local anesthetics discussed in this chapter.

**TABLE 26–3   DRUG NAMES:
LOCAL ANESTHETICS**

Generic Name	Trade Name
AMIDE-CONTAINING LOCAL ANESTHETICS	
Lidocaine (**LĪ**-dō-kān)	Xylocaine, others
Bupivacaine (byoo-**PIV**-a-kān)	Sensorcaine, Marcaine
Dibucaine (**DĪ**-byoo-kān)	Nupercaine
Etidocaine (ē-**TĪ**-dō-kān)	Duranest
Mepivacaine (me-**PIV**-a-kān)	Carbocaine
ESTER-CONTAINING LOCAL ANESTHETICS	
Procaine	Novocain
Cocaine	
Benzocaine (**BENZ**-ō-kān)	Hurricaine, Solarcaine
Tetracaine (**TET**-tra-kān)	Pontocaine
Chloroprocaine (klōr-ō-**PRŌ**-kān)	Nesacaine

CHAPTER SUMMARY

With the introduction of cocaine as the first local anesthetic used in clinical medicine, regional anesthesia could be produced. For the first time in history, painless surgery could be performed on a fully conscious patient. It was indeed a revolutionary development, but was overshadowed somewhat by the advent of the general anesthetics a few decades earlier. Local anesthesia expanded the options available to the surgeons of the day because it permitted pain control at a relatively specific anatomic site. This chapter presents an overview of the local anesthetic agents—the classic drugs and some of the newer derivatives.

BIBLIOGRAPHY

Brown BR: Pharmacology of local anesthesia: In Clark WG, Brater DC, and Johnson AR: Goth's Medical Pharmacology, ed 12. CV Mosby, St Louis, 1988.

Clark WG, Brater DC, and Johnson AR: Goth's Medical Pharmacology, ed 12. CV Mosby, St Louis, 1988.

Covino BG and Vassallo HG: Local Anesthetics: Mechanisms of Action and Clinical Use. Grune and Stratton, New York, 1976.

Hondeghem LM and Miller RD; Local anesthetics. In Katzung BD (ed): Basic and Clinical Pharmacology. Lange Medical Publications, Los Altos, 1982.

Long JP and Sokoll MD: Local anesthetic drugs. In Conn PM and Gebhart GF (eds): Essentials of Pharmacology. FA Davis, Philadelphia, 1989.

Modell W, Lansing A, and Editors of Time-Life Books: Drugs. Life Science Library. Time, New York, 1969.

Park WY and Watkins PA: Patient-controlled sedation during epidural anesthesia. Anesth Analg 72:304–307, 1991.

Tortora GJ and Grabowski SR: Principles of Anatomy and Physiology, ed 7. HarperCollins, New York, 1993.

CHAPTER 27

General Anesthetics

CHAPTER OUTLINE

CHAPTER OBJECTIVES

After studying this chapter the reader should be able to:

- Define general anesthesia and name the two types of general anesthesia.
- Define balanced anesthesia and describe its various components (control of anxiety, secretions, and muscle contractions).
- Describe the four stages of inhalation anesthesia.
- Describe the four planes of surgical anesthesia.
- Explain how alveolar and arterial tension are altered during uptake of an inhalational anesthetic by describing the role of the following:
  - Second gas effect, blood-gas partition coefficient, effect of ventilation, minimum alveolar concentration.
- Explain how distribution of an anesthetic can be changed by cardiac output.
- Describe the movement of anesthetic between compartments during elimination and recovery.
- Describe the pharmacologic activity of the following inhalational anesthetics:
  - Nitrous oxide, halothane, methoxyflurane, enflurane, isoflurane, desflurane, sevoflurane.
- Briefly discuss the drawbacks of the classic inhalational agents cyclopropane and diethyl ether.
- Describe the pharmacologic activity of the following intravenous anesthetics:
  - Barbiturates (thiopental, thiamylal, methohexital), propofol, etomidate, midazolam, fentanyl-droperidol, opioid analgesics (fentanyl, alfentanil, sufentanil), ketamine.
- Define neuroleptanalgesic, neuroleptanesthetic.

KEY TERMS

balanced anesthesia
blood-gas partition coefficient
  (λ)
general anesthesia
  inhalational anesthesia
  intravenous anesthesia
incomplete anesthetic

induction
minimum alveolar concentration
  (minimum anesthetic
  concentration [MAC])
neuroleptanalgesia (nyoo-rō-
  LEPT-a-nal-jēs-se-ah)

neuroleptanesthesia
planes of surgical anesthesia
second gas effect
stages of anesthesia
surgical anesthesia
uptake curve

CHAPTER INTRODUCTION

Drugs producing **surgical anesthesia** are capable of abolishing a patient's perception of and reaction to pain. Surgical anesthesia with loss of consciousness is called **general anesthesia.** General anesthetics are of two basic types: those entering through the respiratory system and those that must be injected. Volatile compounds, such as halothane, produce **inhalational anesthesia** following introduction through the respiratory system. **Intraveous anesthesia** results in loss of consciousness and is produced by injectable drugs, such as thiopental.

This chapter discusses a representative sample of drugs used in clinical anesthesia. These drugs include antimuscarinics, muscle relaxants, hypnotics, anxiolytics, and analgesics. The cardiopulmonary system plays an important role in the uptake, distribution, and elimination of most anesthetic agents. Therefore, the basic principles presented in this chapter should prove helpful for the respiratory care practitioner involved in the care of surgical patients.

GENERAL ANESTHESIA

For centuries the quest has continued for a drug that produces unconsciousness and alleviates pain and suffering in a patient, thus allowing a surgeon to perform longer and more complex procedures. Other desirable attributes in such a drug include production of a state of amnesia regarding the operation itself, control of secretions, and low toxicity coupled with high efficacy to provide maximum drug safety. Other requirements, such as skeletal muscle relaxation, become very important in specialized procedures in abdominal and orthopedic surgery. Most important of all, however, is the ability to reverse the state of insensibility to pain once the surgery is complete. Over the years, various drugs such as alcohol, opium, morphine, and cocaine have been tried in attempts to produce anesthesia. This experimentation fills an interesting chapter in the history of pharmacology, but none of those drugs accomplished the stated goals of anesthesia. In the mid-1800s, however, all of that changed with the introduction of ether, or more correctly, diethyl ether. Although obsolete by today's standards, diethyl ether revolutionized surgery and paved the way for the surgical techniques we now take for granted.

As is seen in Figure 26–1, **general anesthesia** may be produced by inhalational or intravenous agents. Volatile liquids or gases are used in inhalational anesthesia, in which the respiratory route permits close control of dose. In addition, rapid elimination of anesthetic is possible because the vapor is eliminated in expired air. Diethyl ether was the first of the inhalational anesthetics. It blocks the perception of and reaction to pain and produces an unconscious state. The general anesthetics that followed produce similar effects. Some of the general anesthetics provide adequate control of secretions and others provide significant skeletal muscle relaxation. Some are safer than others. None seem to meet *all* the criteria of an ideal general anesthetic. However, they do provide pain relief, with the one key feature that had been lacking in the past—reversibility of effect.

Balanced Anesthesia

In **balanced anesthesia** it is customary for physicians to administer several different drugs to produce a "balance" of deep central nervous system (CNS) depression, freedom from anxiety, control of secretions, and neuromuscular blockade. No single agent has been discovered that can accomplish all of the goals of balanced anesthesia.

Anxiety Relief

Hypnotic agents, such as pentobarbital or secobarbital are routinely used prior to surgery to ensure adequate rest and control preoperative anxiety. Benzodiazepines, such as diazepam or the newer agent midazolam are also employed to reduce anxiety prior to surgery. Naturally occurring narcotic analgesics, such as morphine, or synthetic opioids, such as meperidine, fentanyl, alfentanil, or sufentanil, are useful preoperatively because of their potent anxiolytic effects and intraoperatively for pain relief. Because all of these drugs are CNS depressants, their action is additive with the nervous system depression produced by the general anesthetic. Therefore, the amount of general anesthetic required to produce anesthesia can be reduced. This is an important consideration because general anesthetics have extremely low safety margins (T.I. ≤ 2).

Control of Secretions

The control of tracheobronchial secretions was of greater concern in the past. Diethyl ether and a few other anesthetics stimulate tracheobronchial glands. In the absence of clearance mechanisms such as the cough and swallowing reflexes (which disappear during deeper levels of anesthesia), excess glandular output can be a problem. Premedication with antimuscarinic agents such as atropine, scopolamine, or glyco-pyrrolate eliminates much of the risk associated with excess glandular activity (Clark et al, 1988). These muscarinic cholinergic blockers antagonize acetylcholine and block glandular secretion in the airways before and during surgery. The newer halogenated anesthetics, such as halothane, produce comparatively little stimulation of glands and are valuable in preventing vagal slowing of the heart, which can occur during intubation.

Neuromuscular Block

Some general anesthetics produce adequate relaxation of skeletal musculature on their own. Others require premedication with an adjunctive neuromuscular blocking agent. Certain surgical procedures require more skeletal muscle blockade than others, but in virtually all operations, a surgeon's job is made easier if skeletal muscles are somewhat flaccid. When muscle is stimulated, as occurs when a scalpel is used to make an incision, a reflex contraction occurs. In the case of abdominal muscles, the contraction may be quite violent and abdominal contents may be disturbed by its force. Flaccid muscles are not able to respond in this manner. Nondepolarizing agents, such as pancuronium, or newer agents, such as atracurium and vecuronium, are ideal skeletal muscle relaxants to accomplish these ends. Laryngospasm induced by airway secretions can be treated with depolarizing blockers, such as succinylcholine. In addition, succinylcholine is routinely used to facilitate intubation prior to surgery (see Chapter 7).

Stages and Planes of Inhalational Anesthesia

General anesthetics sequentially depress different parts of the CNS. The brain's reticular activating system is depressed first, blocking arousal mechanisms and bringing about unconsciousness. Selective areas of the cerebral cortex are affected next. These include general somesthetic and motor areas to block the perception of sensations (including pain) and the initiation of movement (Fig. 27–1). Finally, the entire cerebral cortex is depressed. At even higher doses, general anesthetics block vital centers located in the medulla oblongata.

To recognize the various levels of CNS depression produced by inhalational anesthetics, a four-stage system was developed in the early 1920s by Arthur Guedel, a pioneer in anesthesia. This classic system originally pertained only to

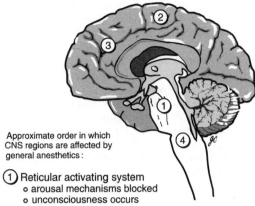

Approximate order in which CNS regions are affected by general anesthetics:

① Reticular activating system
   o arousal mechanisms blocked
   o unconsciousness occurs

② General sensory and motor areas of cerebrum
   o sensory awareness blocked
   o motor activity blocked

③ Cerebral cortex
   o general depression

④ Medulla
   o vital centers blocked

FIGURE 27–1   Regions of CNS affected by general anesthetics.

diethyl ether. However, it is still used today to describe the depth of anesthesia produced by some inhalational anesthetics. The characteristics of the four **stages** follow (Clark et al, 1988).

Stage I: Amnesia and Analgesia

Relatively light anesthesia provides relief from pain. Patients undergoing anesthesia experience anterograde amnesia. In other words, they do not remember events that occurred after the anesthetic was administered. Recall that analgesia and production of amnesia are two of the desirable features of an ideal anesthetic.

Stage II: Excitement

A period of excitement is passed through during the descent to deeper levels of anesthesia. This period of agitation and excitement occurs due to a depressant effect on cortical inhibitory pathways.

Induction is the term given to the combined events of Stage I and Stage II. The sequential nature of anesthesia stages cannot be avoided; therefore, rapid and controlled passage through the induction period is essential. Some general anesthetics slowly reach therapeutic concentrations in the brain (discussed below) and have long induction periods when used as sole agents. Therefore, specific drugs called inducing agents are often included as part of the preanesthetic regimen. Inducing agents are used as adjuncts to general anesthetics because the inducing agents have a rapid onset of action coupled with a short duration of action.

Stage III: Surgical Anesthesia

Surgical procedures are performed during this stage, which follows induction. Stage III is subdivided into four **planes,** or intermediate levels, to allow more exact determination of anesthesia depth (Fig. 27–2). Several considerations have led to the recognition and description of these planes of anesthesia. To start with, surgical procedures must be carried out during Stage III, a relatively deep level of CNS depression. Second, vital cardiopulmonary control systems fail during Stage IV of anesthesia. From this relationship it can be seen that general anesthetics are inherently unsafe. The dose required to maintain surgical anesthesia (Stage III) is only slightly less than the dose that produces medullary paralysis (Stage IV). Finally, individual differences exist among patients in regard to distribution, metabolism, and elimination of anesthetics. This

makes determination of anesthesia depth even more difficult. With these variables in mind, it became essential for anesthesiologists to be able to recognize, with as much precision as possible, just how deep within Stage III a patient has progressed. Only if the patient is deeply unconscious but vigorously alive can anesthesia-assisted surgery have any value.

From a physiologic standpoint, it is fortunate that key reflexes disappear in a more-or-less predictable manner as the CNS is progressively depressed. For example, breathing patterns shift from costal breathing (using intercostal muscles) to diaphragmatic breathing as a person descends through the various planes of surgical anesthesia. Other changes involving pupil diameter, the pupil's response to light, and tearing of the eyes are general indications of the depth of CNS depression within Stage III. Strict attention to these changes and adjustments in the concentration of anesthetic delivered, the flow rate of gas, and mechanical means of eliminating expired anesthetic allow the anesthesi-

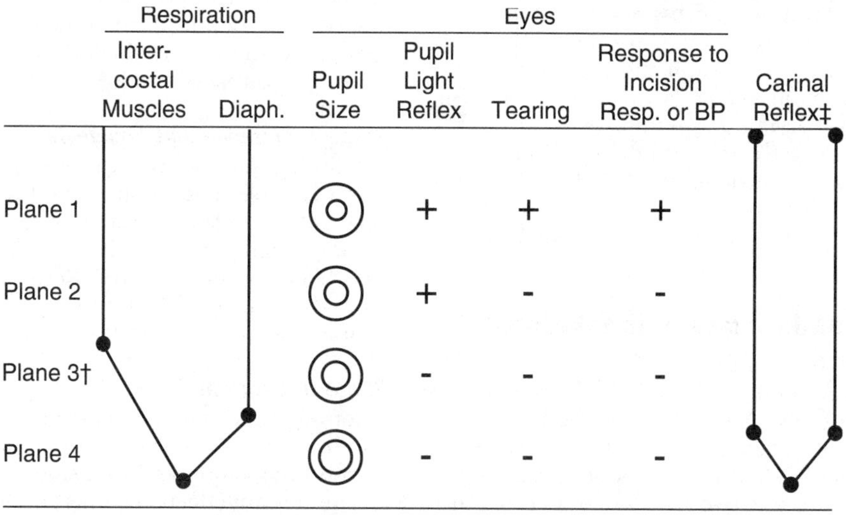

	Respiration			Eyes			
	Inter-costal Muscles	Diaph.	Pupil Size	Pupil Light Reflex	Tearing	Response to Incision Resp. or BP	Carinal Reflex‡
Plane 1			⊙	+	+	+	
Plane 2			⊙	+	-	-	
Plane 3†			⊙	-	-	-	
Plane 4			⊙	-	-	-	

*The signs of anesthesia presented here apply particularly to the halogenated agents (halothane, enflurane, and isoflurane). They have no application to intravenously administered agents.

†Although respiration is maintained to deep levels of anesthesia, the minute volume becomes inadequate in plane 3 as determined by elevated Pa_{CO_2}.

‡Note that the carinal reflex remains intact until very deep levels of anesthesia.

Diaph. = diaphragm contributions to ventilation.

FIGURE 27–2 Signs of surgical anesthesia (Stage III) seen with commonly used halogenated agents.* (From Sokoll MD and Long JP: General anesthesia and general anesthetic drugs. In Conn PM and Gebhart GF (eds): Essentials of Pharmacology. FA Davis Co, Philadelphia, 1989, p. 189, with permission.)

ologist to maintain the CNS at the desired level of depression for the length of the operation. Figure 27–2 summarizes the clinical signs of the four planes of surgical anesthesia. The signs presented are applicable to the halogenated inhalation anesthetics, such as halothane, enflurane, and isoflurane, but not to the intravenous anesthetics (Sokoll and Long, 1989).

Stage IV: Medullary Paralysis
With increasing depth of anesthesia, vital brainstem functions are finally depressed. Depression of medullary cardiovascular and respiratory centers brings about cardiopulmonary arrest and death.

Uptake, Distribution, and Elimination

Alveolar and Arterial Tension
Intravenous anesthetics establish maximal blood levels quickly and are carried rapidly in the bloodstream to highly perfused organs, such as the brain. Inhalational anesthetics reach the brain in a more indirect manner because they travel in several compartments. In addition, they are usually diluted in a background gas for delivery to the lungs and must leave the alveoli to enter circulation. Finally, they must leave circulation to enter the brain. As a result, the alveolar tension, or partial pressure, of a volatile anesthetic and the resulting arterial tension are dictated by several factors such as:

- Concentration of anesthetic in the inspired mixture
- Flow rate of anesthetic delivered into the inspired gas mixture
- Minute volume of ventilation
- Blood-gas partition coefficient
- Perfusion through the tissues

Anesthesiologists govern the delivery of anesthetic and thus alter the alveolar and arterial partial pressures of a volatile anesthetic. This is done by adjusting several variables, such as the concentration of drug in the inspired mixture, the flow rate of drug being introduced into the inspired mixture, and the minute volume of ventilation in the patient. They do not have control over physical and chemical characteristics of the anesthetic. These include solubility characteristics and diffusion between different body compartments. Anesthesiologists are also unable to control anatomic or physiologic properties such as distribution and perfusion of an agent once it enters the bloodstream.

Second Gas Effect
When a large volume of a primary gas, such as nitrous oxide, is administered in high concentration, it can affect how quickly a second gas, such as halothane, reaches equilibrium. This **second gas effect** is ideal for the concurrent administration of a more potent second gas in a low concentration (Clark et al, 1988). The second gas reaches equilibrium faster when it is "swept along" by the higher volume of primary gas.

Partition Coefficients
Inhalation anesthetics are distributed, or partitioned, in several compartments, such as inspired air, alveolar air, blood, brain, and other tissues. When a drug is at equilibrium between the blood and alveolar compartments, the **blood-gas partition coefficient (λ)** represents the ratio of the drug concentrations in the two locations. For example, at equilibrium, the anesthetic enflurane is partitioned within both the alveoli and the bloodstream. The blood-gas partition coefficient of enflurane is $\lambda = 1.80$. Therefore, at equilibrium, 1.8 times as many enflurane molecules are distributed in the blood as are found in the gas phase within the alveoli. The lower the blood-gas partition coefficient of an anesthetic, the more slowly it diffuses from the alveolus into the bloodstream. As a result of this property, the more slowly anesthetic vapor *leaves* the alveolus, the more rapidly the alveolar concentration of anesthetic increases. For all practical purposes, alveolar and arterial concentrations of anesthetic gas equilibrate within a few minutes when the inspired concentration of gas remains constant.

These kinetics determine the uptake of anesthetic from the lung. Each anesthetic agent has a characteristic **uptake curve** when the alveolar (or arterial) concentration is plotted against time (Fig. 27–3). Other factors being equal, blood-gas partition coefficients contribute to the alveolar concentration of anesthetic and its uptake curve. Increasing the amount of anesthetic delivered to the lung does not increase the partial pressure of anesthetic in the blood once equilibrium has been reached. Therefore, there exists a maximum safe concentration of drug that can be delivered to the lungs.

Other partition coefficients, such as the brain-blood partition coefficient, exist, but because the anesthetic solubility is similar in the two compartments, transfer is rapid. The greatest difference in solubility is at the air-blood interface in the lung.

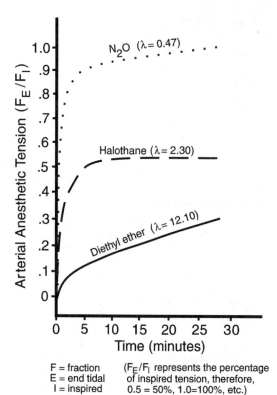

F = fraction   (F_E/F_I represents the percentage
E = end tidal   of inspired tension, therefore,
I = inspired   0.5 = 50%, 1.0=100%, etc.)

FIGURE 27–3 Anesthetic uptake curve. All else remaining constant, an anesthetic uptake curve is composed of three parts. The initial rapid rise is controlled primarily by alveolar ventilation ($\dot{V}_A$). The final, almost horizontal slope is determined by the tissue-blood solubility coefficient. The area in between, the "knee" of the curve, is determined by the uptake of anesthetic from the alveoli by the blood. This is controlled by the blood-gas partition coefficient (λ); the lower the partition coefficient, the higher the knee of the curve. (Modified with permission from Sokoll, MD and Long, JP: General anesthesia and general anesthetic drugs. In Conn, PM and Gebhart, GF (eds): Essentials of Pharmacology. F.A. Davis Co, Philadelphia, 1989, p. 191.)

The time required for an anesthetic gas to reach equilibrium between compartments depends on the relative solubility of the gas in the two compartments and the blood flow through one of the compartments. This equilibration rate, in turn, determines how rapidly the partial pressure of anesthetic vapor reaches anesthetic levels in the brain. Anesthetics with low plasma solubility (or high lipid solubility) tend to exhibit shorter induction periods because their concentration in the brain rises quickly to produce anesthesia. Recovery from anesthesia is also rapid with agents having high lipid solubility. By contrast, anesthetics with significant water solubility tend to have long induction and recovery periods.

Effect of Ventilation

Increasing the alveolar ventilation ($\dot{V}_A$) increases the rate of uptake of anesthetic because more molecules of anesthetic are "presented" to the alveoli in a given time. Anesthetics with high plasma solubility ($\lambda > 1.0$) are affected more by increases in $\dot{V}_A$ than are low-solubility ($\lambda < 1.0$) anesthetics (Clark et al, 1988).

Insoluble anesthetics reach equilibrium with relatively few molecules of drug in the blood compared with the alveoli. Increasing the alveolar ventilation results in few additional gas molecules entering the blood. This is because the blood has a low capacity for insoluble anesthetics and has already been saturated by relatively few drug molecules.

Blood has a high capacity for high-solubility anesthetics; therefore, an increase in $\dot{V}_A$ results in a more dramatic increase in anesthetic uptake. Because high-solubility anesthetics can be taken up quickly during forced artificial ventilation, they may rapidly reach dangerously high levels in the blood and tissues to cause toxic effects.

Minimum Alveolar Concentration

A measure of inhalational anesthetic potency is called the **minimum alveolar concentration** or **minimum anesthetic concentration** (MAC). It is the concentration of anesthetic measured in the alveoli at which 50% of patients will not respond to a standard noxious stimulus, such as a surgical incision (Trevor and Miller, 1982). MAC values are measured in v/v percent, or mmHg. Specifically, the MAC value is median effective dose (ED50) for a particular anesthetic agent and represents a single point on the dose-response curve. The lower the MAC, the greater the potency of the anesthetic. In a clinical setting, anesthetic doses are often stated in multiples of MAC, ranging from 0.5 to 2.5 MAC (Clark et al, 1988; Trevor and Miller, 1982). Table 27–1 presents partition coefficients and MAC values for several inhalational anesthetics.

Distribution

Once an anesthetic has reached the vascular compartment, its distribution throughout the body is governed by basic pharmacokinetic principles. For example, highly perfused tissues, such as the brain and heart, are exposed to higher amounts of anesthetic. Anesthetics with significant lipid-solubility show an affinity for ad-

TABLE 27–1 PROPERTIES OF INHALATIONAL ANESTHETICS

Anesthetic	Vapor Pressure at 20°C	Blood-Gas Partition Coefficient (λ)	Brain-Blood Partition Coefficient	Minimum Alveolar Concentration (MAC) in 100% Oxygen
Nitrous oxide	800 psi (5515 kPa)	0.47	1.1	105
Halothane	243 mmHg (32 kPa)	2.30	2.9	0.75
Methoxyflurane	22.5 mmHg (3 kPa)	13.00	2.0	0.16
Enflurane	184 mmHg (24 kPa)	1.80	1.4	1.68
Isoflurane	250 mmHg (33 kPa)	1.40	2.6	1.20

Source: Data from Sokoll and Long, 1989; Trevor and Miller, 1982.

ipose tissue and bind temporarily at such depot sites.

As cardiac output increases, there is a greater volume of blood per unit time to take up anesthetic from the alveoli and carry it into circulation. This effect is more pronounced with the high-solubility anesthetics. In depressed cardiac output states, including those produced by anesthetic action itself, sluggish blood flow through the pulmonary circuit results in more extensive uptake of high-solubility anesthetics and a rapid rise to equilibrium. The end result is that high-solubility anesthetics can alter their own uptake.

An analogy of the effect of cardiac output on anesthetic uptake is one of a moving stream with someone on the shore releasing colored dye at a constant rate into the water. If the stream is sluggish and the water is flowing very slowly, the dye concentration downstream will be high. On the other hand, a fast-moving stream will have a low concentration of dye. The dye is carried downstream so quickly the water is scarcely colored (Fig. 27–4).

Elimination

Removal of anesthetic is determined by the same factors that governed its uptake—namely, pulmonary ventilation, perfusion, partition coefficients (brain-blood and blood-gas), and the flow rate of administered anesthetic (Sokoll and Long, 1989). Partial pressures in the various partitions (compartments) decrease once the delivery of anesthetic is terminated. The anesthetic tension of inspired air decreases, followed by that of alveolar air, arterial blood, and finally other tissues. As was pointed out above, the brain is a highly perfused organ. Therefore, it is also one of the first organs cleared during recovery

as the anesthetic partial pressure begins to fall. The relatively insoluble agents, such as nitrous oxide, that have short induction times also tend to be cleared from the brain quickly to allow rapid awakening and a return to consciousness.

Patients are especially vulnerable during the recovery stage of anesthesia because several postoperative variables exist. These may include ventilatory depression, cardiovascular depression, and rapidly changing anesthetic levels as the drug vacates different compartments. Emergence time from anesthesia is also influenced by surgical trauma that may be added to the patient's preexisting pathophysiologic condition.

In summary, the blood-gas partition coefficient (λ) is the most important variable for altering the speed of induction. At a given partial pressure, the lower the partition coefficient, the faster equilibrium is reached and the faster the induction. The lower the solubility, the faster the recovery because anesthetic rapidly leaves the various compartments (brain → blood → alveoli) and is exhaled.

Induction is accelerated by concentration and the second gas effect. An increase in alveolar ventilation increases the rate of equilibrium, whereas an increase in cardiac output decreases the rate of equilibrium.

THERAPEUTIC AGENTS
Inhalational Anesthetics

NITROUS OXIDE (N_2O). Nitrous oxide, or "laughing gas," was one of the early inhalational agents used in the late 1840s. The first demonstrations of its use generally ended in failure simply because the drug is an **incomplete anesthetic.** Complete surgical anesthesia (Stage III) cannot

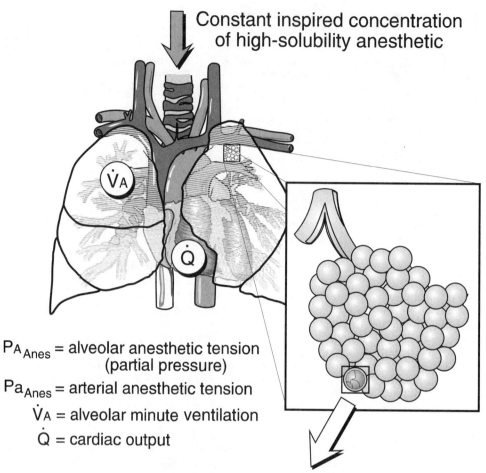

Constant inspired concentration of high-solubility anesthetic

PA_{Anes} = alveolar anesthetic tension (partial pressure)

Pa_{Anes} = arterial anesthetic tension

$\dot{V}A$ = alveolar minute ventilation

$\dot{Q}$ = cardiac output

Factors Increasing Uptake of a High-solubility Anesthetic

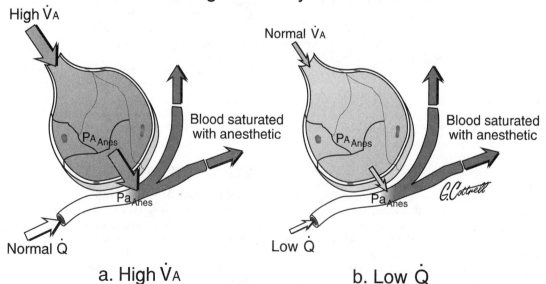

High $\dot{V}A$

Normal $\dot{V}A$

PA_{Anes}

Blood saturated with anesthetic

PA_{Anes}

Blood saturated with anesthetic

Pa_{Anes}

Pa_{Anes}

Normal $\dot{Q}$

Low $\dot{Q}$

a. High $\dot{V}A$

b. Low $\dot{Q}$

FIGURE 27–4   Schematic—effect of alveolar minute ventilation and cardiac output on anesthetic uptake.

be attained with nitrous oxide alone without causing oxygen deprivation. For example, the MAC of nitrous oxide is 100% or more, indicating that an unpremedicated patient cannot be depressed beyond Stage II (Table 27–1). Analgesia and hypnosis, however, can be produced. Nitrous oxide is commonly given with a more potent anesthetic to make use of the second gas effect. Because the analgesic action of nitrous oxide is added to that of other anesthetics, the amount of the more potent second gas can be reduced. For example, halothane delivered in oxygen has a MAC of 0.75%, but when halothane is delivered by a nitrous oxide–oxygen mixture (nitrous oxide 70%–oxygen 30%), the MAC of halothane drops to 0.3% (Sokoll and Long, 1989).

Nitrous oxide is not metabolized in the body and is eliminated within a few minutes because it has an extremely low solubility ($\lambda = 0.47$). It is compatible with all other drugs and no serious side effects are produced in the respiratory, renal, or hepatic system.

INDICATIONS. Nitrous oxide is used mainly in balanced anesthesia with analgesics, hypnotics, and muscle relaxants. It is also employed in intermittent analgesia in obstetrics and dental procedures.

PRECAUTIONS. Low-solubility anesthetics, such as nitrous oxide, are rapidly cleared from the brain, blood, and alveoli. Therefore, when nitrous oxide administration is discontinued, large volumes of anesthetic leave the brain and enter the bloodstream. From there, the anesthetic volume rapidly enters the alveoli and may displace oxygen to temporarily cause hypoxia.

HALOTHANE (Fluothane). Anesthetics that have fluorine added to their basic structure are said to be fluorinated. Such drugs exhibit reduced flammability. Halothane was the vanguard drug of the nonflammable, halogenated inhalational anesthetics introduced in 1956. Halothane has relatively low solubility ($\lambda = 2.3$) and therefore has rapid anesthetic onset. Another distinct advantage is that halothane is not irritating to the airways and does not stimulate respiratory secretions.

INDICATIONS. Halothane is used for maintenance of anesthesia. It is commonly given with nitrous oxide, but can be administered alone with oxygen.

CONTRAINDICATIONS. Halothane is contraindicated in instances in which general anesthesia is contraindicated. Use in patients with known hypersensitivity to the anesthetic is also a contraindication.

PRECAUTIONS. Alveolar ventilation is significantly decreased with halothane anesthesia. This results in a fall in tidal volume, making assisted ventilation necessary. Repeated doses of halothane sensitize the myocardium to catecholamine-induced arrhythmias. Therefore, concurrent administration of epinephrine or other sympathomimetic amines warrants special caution.

ADVERSE REACTIONS. The most common problem with halothane anesthesia is hepatotoxicity. Halothane causes liver damage in a small number of patients; however, multiple studies done over many years have failed to resolve the problem (Trevor and Miller, 1982).

METHOXYFLURANE (Penthrane). Methoxyflurane ushered in the halogenated ethers, a group of inhalational anesthetics with an ether link (–C–O–C–) common to their molecular structure. The possession of the ether link indicates that the drug does not sensitize the myocardium to catecholamines (Clark et al, 1988). It also is an indicator that the drug may have skeletal muscle–relaxing properties. Methoxyflurane does in fact exhibit far more skeletal muscle relaxation than halothane, which is not an ether. Methoxyflurane is an extremely potent anesthetic but has the drawback of high solubility ($\lambda = 13.00$). As a result, slow induction and slow recovery detract from its widespread clinical use.

INDICATIONS. Maintenance of anesthesia is the indication for use.

CONTRAINDICATIONS. See Halothane.

PRECAUTIONS. During metabolism, methoxyflurane liberates free fluoride ions (F^{1-}) that may cause renal failure. It is slightly irritating to the respiratory tract. The characteristically slow awakening during recovery may also be considered a precaution.

ADVERSE REACTIONS. Adverse cardiovascular effects are less than are seen with halothane. Depression of ventilation is produced by methoxyflurane. The potential for nephrotoxicity due to the release of free F^{1-} is discussed above.

ENFLURANE (Ethrane). Enflurane is a very potent halogenated ether. The general properties of the anesthetic are similar to those of halothane, but enflurane produces relatively little hepatic damage. It also produces better skeletal muscle relaxation than halothane, does not sensitize the myocardium to circulating catecholamines, and has a low solubility ($\lambda = 1.8$).

INDICATIONS. Enflurane is used in the maintenance of anesthesia. It is usually administered with nitrous oxide but may be given alone with oxygen.

CONTRAINDICATIONS. See Halothane.

PRECAUTIONS. Very little metabolism of enflurane occurs. Free F^{1-} are produced, but in small amounts so kidney damage is not a problem. High enflurane concentration with hypocapnia can trigger grand mal seizures. However, maintenance of normal arterial carbon dioxide tension (PaCO$_2$) reduces the risk.

ADVERSE REACTIONS. Depression of myocardial contractility is seen with enflurane administration.

ISOFLURANE (Forane). One of the most popular inhalational anesthetics in current use is isoflurane. Isoflurane is an isomer of enflurane and has a low solubility ($\lambda = 1.4$). Isoflurane entered clinical use in 1984. It produces good skeletal muscle relaxation, is nonflammable and easy to administer, and has low systemic toxicity. For example, very few free F^{1-} are released during metabolism. Anesthetics that undergo minimal biotransformation generally exhibit less systemic toxicity. This is because such anesthetics generate relatively few metabolites and the metabolites of a drug often create some of the toxicity problems seen clinically. By contrast, the intravenous anesthetics (discussed below) undergo extensive biotransformation in the body and generally have more serious toxicities than the inhalational anesthetics.

INDICATIONS. Maintenance of anesthesia is the indication for use of isoflurane.

CONTRAINDICATIONS. See Halothane.

PRECAUTIONS. Isoflurane may cause peripheral vasodilation leading to a fall in blood pressure and compensatory tachycardia. This can be a problem in patients with coronary artery disease.

ADVERSE REACTIONS. Adverse reactions are similar to those of halothane. However, the ventilatory depression is greater, whereas the cardiovascular depression is less.

NEWER HALOGENATED ETHERS. Desflurane and sevoflurane are two promising new inhalational anesthetics being investigated in animal studies and in human clinical trials (Frink et al, 1992; Rampil et al, 1991). Both are halogenated (fluorinated) ethers with low solubilities. Consistent with this physical characteristic is rapid uptake and elimination of anesthetic. Emergence and recovery from anesthesia are more rapid than observed after isoflurane administration (Smiley et al, 1991). Systemic toxicities for the drugs appear to be very low, possibly even less than seen with isoflurane.

CLASSIC INHALATIONAL ANESTHETICS. A very potent gas called cyclopropane is capable of producing complete anesthesia. Its potency is such that it can produce this anesthetic state without intravenous anesthetics used as adjuncts. It also produces extremely rapid induction. Unfortunately, cyclopropane is both flammable and explosive. It is rarely used today.

The first general anesthetic used clinically was diethyl ether. It is irritating to the respiratory tract but produces good muscle relaxation. Unfortunately, it has a high blood-gas partition coefficient and suffers from slow induction and slow elimination. In addition, the drug is a volatile liquid and is flammable. It is no longer used in clinical anesthesia. However, from a historical perspective, it is a landmark drug that opened the door to surgical anesthesia (Box 27–1).

Characteristics of inhalational anesthetics, such as effects on the respiratory and cardiovascular system, are summarized in Table 27–2.

Intravenous Anesthetics

The intravenous anesthetics lack the controllability of inhalational agents. In addition, they are often converted into active metabolites that cause postoperative complications. As was explained earlier, the various planes of surgical anesthesia (Stage III) do not apply to the clinical use of intravenous anesthetics. Also, intravenous anesthetics such as the barbiturates do not possess antinociceptive (analgesic) or skeletal muscle–relaxing properties. Therefore, they do not meet some of the criteria of surgical anesthesia.

BARBITURATES. The most useful subclass of barbiturates are the ultrashort-acting drugs such as thiopental (Pentothal), thiamylal (Surital), and methohexital (Brevital). These agents are quickly taken up into highly perfused tissues such as the brain to produce rapid induction. Recovery occurs within 15 minutes.

INDICATIONS. Barbiturates with high lipid solubility are excellent drugs for the induction of anesthesia. Modern intravenous anesthesia began with the introduction of thiopental in the 1930s.

CONTRAINDICATIONS. Preexisting shock or bronchial asthma are cautions to the use of the intravenous barbiturates.

PROPOFOL (Diprivan). Propofol is a short-acting intravenous hypnotic introduced in 1989. It is not classified as a narcotic or a barbiturate. Propofol is rapidly distributed, metabolized, and cleared from the body, allowing for quick recovery with minimal drowsiness, confusion, and amnesia (White and Negus, 1991). In addition, nausea and vomiting during recovery are minimal.

INDICATIONS. Propofol is an extremely versatile agent and may be used for both induction

BOX 27-1 HOSPITAL ANNOUNCES CUTBACKS

October 16, 1846 *(The Boston* Herald-Examiner*)*
Massachusetts General Hospital today announced the indefinite layoff of Cyrus W. Blake, long-time resident of Boston, and surgery attendant at the hospital. Officials cited substantial savings in labor costs as the reason for the layoff notice. Three other men presently working as orderlies and attendants in the operating room to immobilize patients during surgery fear similar layoffs. The hospital move comes in the wake of the successful demonstration earlier today of surgical anesthesia using diethyl ether. The burly Mr. Blake, carrying the tools of his trade—leather straps for restraint, wooden blocks for the patient to bite, and the ubiquitous bottle of alcohol—commented, ". . . it's just a fad, I'll be back."

The preceding account is fictional, but something similar probably occurred in the mid-1800s after the debut of diethyl ether anesthesia. The new drug was not a fad and in fact ushered in the era of general surgery, which permitted surgeons to perform more leisurely and complex procedures. Prior to the demonstration of anesthesia by a Boston dentist, William T.G. Morton, at Massachusettes General Hospital on October 16, 1846, surgeons had to work at breakneck speed. Strong attendants physically restrained the patient, and the only merciful relief from pain was a few ounces of liquor and swift work. Reducing the length of time of the operation was the only defense. Diethyl ether changed all that—pain perception could finally be blocked *and* the anesthetic state could be reversed. Both features, present in the same drug, had been sought for centuries.

Modell W, Lansing A, and Editors of Time-Life Books: Drugs. Life Science Library. Time, New York, 1969.
Trevor AJ and Miller RD: General Anesthetics. In Katzung BD (ed): Basic and Clinical Pharmacology. Lange Medical Publications, Los Altos, 1982.

and maintenance of anesthesia in a variety of surgical procedures (Waugaman and Foster, 1991).

CONTRAINDICATIONS. Propofol is contraindicated in instances in which general anesthesia is contraindicated. Use in patients with known hypersensitivity to propofol is a contraindication.

PRECAUTIONS AND ADVERSE REACTIONS. Hypotension, bradycardia, and apnea are cautions during propofol administration. It depresses the CNS, cardiovascular, and respiratory systems in a dose-dependent manner. Pain on injection is a common undesirable side effect of propofol administration.

ETOMIDATE (Amidate). Etomidate is an inducing agent with a very brief duration of action. It does not depress cardiovascular activity and has a wide safety margin. Etomidate has no analgesic activity.

INDICATIONS. Anesthetic induction is the indication for use of etomidate.

ADVERSE REACTIONS. Involuntary skeletal muscle contractions and pain on injection are undesirable effects of etomidate used in induction.

MIDAZOLAM (Versed). The benzodiazepines are among the most versatile drugs currently available. We discuss their use as both psychopharmacologic and hypnotic agents in Chapter 24. In the field of anesthesia, the benzodiazepine drugs such as diazepam (Valium) have been used in induction and as adjuncts since their debut in the early 1960s. Midazolam is a benzodiazepine recently developed primarily for anesthetic use. It is extremely short acting, with a half-life ($t_{1/2}$) of 2–4 hours compared with diazepam ($t_{1/2}$ = 20–200 h). Midazolam is very water soluble and is available for intravenous or intramuscular injections, in which it exhibits a potency several times greater than that of diazepam. Midazolam produces hypnotic, sedative, amnesic, and anxiolytic effects in addition to a degree of CNS-mediated skeletal muscle relaxation. Many of these effects are desirable in anesthesia.

INDICATIONS. Midazolam is remarkably versatile and is used as a preoperative medication, a hypnotic, and an adjunct to intravenous sedation.

PRECAUTIONS. Midazolam administration re-

TABLE 27–2 COMPARISON OF GENERAL ANESTHETICS: SUMMARY

Drug	Minute Ventilation	Blood Pressure*	Myocardial Contractility	Peripheral Resistance	Skeletal Muscle Relaxation	Advantages	Disadvantages
			Cardiovascular*				
Diethyl ether	Decreased	Little change	Decreased	Decreased	Marked	Cardiovascular stability	Explosive; objectionable odor
Cyclopropane	Decreased	Little change	Decreased	Increased	Moderate	Very rapid induction	Explosive; arrhythmias, especially with catecholamines
Halothane	Decreased	Decreased	Decreased	Little change	Moderate	Pleasant odor; rapid induction and recovery	Arrhythmias, especially with catecholamines; possible hepatotoxicity
Enflurane	Decreased	Decreased	Decreased	Decreased	Moderate	Pleasant odor	Marked depression of blood pressure; seizures; hepatotoxicity
Isoflurane	Decreased	Decreased	Little change	Decreased	Moderate	Stable cardiac rhythm	Somewhat objectionable odor
Nitrous oxide	Unchanged	Unchanged	Decreased	Increased	None	No odor; rapid effect	Must be combined with other agents
Thiopental	Decreased	Decreased	Little change†	Arterial resistance and venous capacity increased	None	Rapid IV induction (30 s); short duration with proper dosage	Must be combined with other agents; decreases ICP
Methohexital	Decreased	Decreased	Little change†	Arterial resistance and venous capacity increased	None	Rapid IV induction (30 s); very short duration with proper dosage	Must be combined with other agents; decreases ICP
Ketamine	Little effect	Increased	Increased	Little change	None	Can be used IV or IM for induction	May produce hallucinations
Etomidate	Decreased	Little change	Little change	Little change	None	IV induction	Purposeless movements; adrenal suppression

Source: Data from Sokoll and Long, 1989.

*Ether and cyclopropane cause little change in blood pressure in the intact animal because of elevated endogenous catecholamine.

†Blood pressure decrease with barbiturates is related primarily to venodilation and decreased venous return.

ICP—intracranial pressure; IM—intramuscular; IV—intravenous.

duces but does not remove the requirement for analgesics and inhalational agents during anesthesia (Recall that the benzodiazepines have no analgesic activity.) Postoperative ventilatory depression and CNS effects such as sedation or amnesia may occur following midazolam administration. As with all other CNS depressants, additive effects may occur and are a precaution in patients premedicated with drugs such as barbiturates or narcotics.

ADVERSE REACTIONS. Undesirable effects of midazolam administration include apnea and hypotension. Prolonged or adverse effects of midazolam postoperatively can be reversed by administration of the specific benzodiazepine antagonist flumazenil (Anexate). This antagonist competes at the benzodiazepine receptor with any of the benzodiazepines, but the action is especially useful in balanced anesthesia should reversal of benzodiazepine effect be necessary. Flumazenil and the narcotic antagonist naloxone (Narcan) provide a reassuring margin of safety in modern surgical anesthesia, a state maintained by multiple agents.

FENTANYL-DROPERIDOL (Innovar). **Neuroleptanalgesia** is a quiet state of altered awareness and analgesia. This state is produced by a fixed-dose combination product containing fentanyl (Sublimaze), a synthetic opioid analgesic, and droperidol (Inapsine), a neuroleptic agent. Neuroleptanalgesia can also be produced by concurrent administration of the two separate drugs.

INDICATIONS. The combined narcotic analgesic and antipsychotic tranquilizer is given intravenously in balanced anesthesia as a supplement to nitrous oxide–oxygen mixtures. The resulting anestheticlike state is called **neuroleptanesthesia,** in which a patient becomes totally detached and disinterested in the environment, but remains conscious (Trevor and Miller, 1982).

PRECAUTIONS. The fentanyl component of Innovar, like other narcotics, may cause depression of ventilation.

OPIOID ANALGESICS. Fentanyl (Sublimaze) has 50–100 times the potency of morphine but fails to provide complete amnesia. It has been the mainstay of narcotic administration during anesthesia but is being challenged by alfentanil and sufentanil, newer synthethic opioids having shorter durations of action and fewer side effects (Waugaman and Foster, 1991). Such drugs exhibit greater safety profiles and produce complete amnesia (Clotz and Nahata, 1991; Mehta et al, 1991).

Alfentanil (Alfenta) is less potent than fentanyl but is valuable because of its short duration

---

BOX 27–2 α_2-ADRENERGIC AGONISTS: FROM ANTIHYPERTENSIVES TO ANESTHETIC ADJUNCTS

Clonidine is a centrally acting antihypertensive agent (see Chapter 21). It acts in the CNS to stimulate presynaptic α_2-adrenoceptors and thereby reduce the stimulation of peripheral alpha receptors. Peripheral vasomotor tone is diminished and blood pressure is reduced. One of the side effects of α_2-adrenergic agonist therapy is sedation, but the mechanism is not fully understood. Clonidine is not an opioid, nor are its sedative properties blocked by naloxone. The actions of clonidine, however, can be blocked by selective α_2-adrenergic antagonists, such as yohimbine. The observation of sedative effects in α_2-adrenergic agonists led to the investigation of clonidine and similar drugs, such as dexmedetomidine, as potential preanesthetic agents in balanced anesthesia. Preliminary studies of clonidine indicate that when it is given preoperatively by the parenteral, oral, or transdermal route, it improves hemodynamic stability and reduces inhalation anesthetic requirements during anesthesia. In addition, clonidine has an antinociceptive effect that reduces the opioid requirement of anesthesia. These qualities are desirable in a preanesthetic. The mechanisms of action, however, are not completely understood. Further studies on the use of α_2-agonists as future adjuncts in anesthesia are continuing.

Bellaiche S et al: Clonidine does not delay recovery from anesthesia. Br J Anaesth 66:353–357, 1991.

Murkin JM: Central analgesic mechanisms: A review of opioid receptor physiopharmacology and related antinociceptive systems. J Cardiothorac Vasc Anesth 5:268–277, 1991.

Waugaman WR and Forster SD: New advances in anesthesia. Nurs Clin North Am 26:451–461, 1991.

of action, which is ideal for brief procedures. It has a very rapid onset of action and is ideal in the ambulatory surgical setting. Alfentanil strengthens the hypnotic and antinociceptive component of anesthetics such as thiopental (Mehta et al, 1991). A relatively small amount of hypotension is produced by alfentanil.

Sufentanil (Sufenta) is several times more potent than even fentanyl and its analgesic effects last longer (Clotz and Nahanta, 1991). The ventilatory depression effects of sufentanil are less than those produced by fentanyl. Fentanyl and other narcotics provide ideal anesthesia for cardiac surgery patients because these drugs produce adequate anesthesia (with nitrous oxide) and analgesia, in addition to greater hemodynamic stability compared with some of the inhalational agents.

KETAMINE (Ketalar). Ketamine is an incomplete anesthetic related to phencyclidine (PCP, "angel dust"). It produces a trancelike state with mild analgesia and amnesia. Such a state is called *dissociative anesthesia* (Clark et al, 1988).

INDICATIONS. Ketamine is administered intravenously or intramuscularly and is most useful in infants and children to provide analgesia during painful procedures, such as the changing of burn dressings.

PRECAUTIONS AND ADVERSE REACTIONS. Ketamine may cause vivid dreams and distortions of reality in adults. This effect is lacking in children.

A summary of the characteristics of intravenous anesthetics is given in Table 27–2, whereas newer investigational drugs in general anesthesia are briefly discussed in Box 27–2.

Table 27–3 lists the generic and trade names of the general anesthetics discussed in this chapter.

CHAPTER SUMMARY

Development of the entire field of surgery awaited the discovery of drugs that would grant freedom from pain to the patient while affording the luxury of time to the surgeon—time to perform meticulous work and time to attempt increasingly more complex procedures. Starting in the early 1840s with the debut of diethyl ether, surgical patients began to routinely survive their painless ordeal. Surgery became commonplace as newer anesthetics were introduced in an attempt to develop rapid-onset, high-potency, low-toxicity drugs that were safe not only for the patient, but for the medical staff to administer. In this chapter we examine the development, pro-

TABLE 27–3 DRUG NAMES: GENERAL ANESTHETICS

Generic Name	Trade Name
INHALATIONAL ANESTHETICS	
Nitrous oxide	
Halothane (**HAL**-ō-thān)	Fluothane
Methoxylflurane (meth-oks-ē-**FLŪ**-rān)	Penthrane
Enflurane (**IN**-flū-rān)	Ēthrane
Isoflurane (īsō-**FLŪ**-rān)	Forane
Desflurane (**DEZ**-flū-rān)	*investigational*
Sevoflurane (se-vō-**FLŪ**-rān)	*investigational*
INTRAVENOUS ANESTHETICS	
Barbiturates	
Thiopental	Pentothal
Thiamylal	Surital
Methohexital	Brevital
Propofol (**PRŌ**-pō-fol)	Diprivan
Etomidate (e-**TOM**-i-dāt)	Amidate
Benzodiazepines	
Midazolam (mi-**DAZ**-ō-lam)	Versed
Diazepam	Valium, others
Neuroleptanalgesics	
Fentanyl-Droperidol	Innovar
Opioid analgesics	
Fentanyl (**FEN**-ta-nil)	Sublimaze
Alfentanil (al-**FEN**-ta-nil)	Alfenta
Sufentanil (su-**FEN**-ta-nil)	Sufenta
Ketamine (**KET**-a-mēn)	Ketalar
α₂-Agonists (investigational)	
Clonidine (**KLON**-i-dēn)	Catapres
Dexmedetomidine (deks-me-de-**TŌ**-mi-dēn)	

gression, and clinical use of general anesthetics of the inhalational and intravenous types.

BIBLIOGRAPHY

Brown BR: Pharmacology of general anesthesia. In Clark WG, Brater DC, and Johnson AR: Goth's Medical Pharmacology, ed 12. CV Mosby, St Louis, 1988.

Cartabuke RS, Davidson PJ, and Warner LO: Is premedication with oral glycopyrrolate as effective as oral atropine in attenuating cardiovascular depression in infants receiving halothane for induction of anesthesia? Anesth Analg 73:271–274, 1991.

Clark WG, Brater DC, and Johnson AR: Goth's Medical Pharmacology, ed 12. CV Mosby, St Louis, 1988.

Clotz MA and Nahata MC: Clinical uses of fentanyl, sufentanil, and alfentanil. Clin Pharm 10:581–593, 1991.

Curtis D and Stevens WC: Recovery from general anesthesia. Int Anesthesiol Clin 29:1–11, 1991.

Dhamee, MS et al: Cardiovascular effects of pancuronium, vecuronium, and atacurium during induction of anesthesia with sufentanil and lorazepam for myocardial revascularization. J Cardiothorac Vasc Anesth 4:336–339, 1990.

Frink EJ et al: Clinical comparison of sevoflurane and isoflurane in healthy patients. Anesth Analg 74:241–245, 1992.

Korttila K et al: Randomized comparison of outcome after propofol–nitrous oxide or enflurane–nitrous oxide anaesthesia in operations of long duration. Can J Anaesth 36:651–657, 1989.

Mehta D, Bradley EL, and Kissin I: Effect of alfentanil on hypnotic and antinociceptive components of thiopental sodium anesthesia. J Clin Anesth 3:280–284, 1991.

Modell W, Lansing A, and Editors of Time-Life Books: Drugs. Life Science Library. Time, New York, 1969.

Murkin JM: Central analgesic mechanisms: A review of opioid receptor physiopharmacology and related antinociceptive systems. J Cardiothorac Vasc Anesth 5:268–277, 1991.

Ouellette RG: Midazolam: An induction agent for general anesthesia. Nurse Anesthesia 2:134–137, 1991.

Park WY and Watkins PA: Patient-controlled sedation during epidural anesthesia. Anesth Analg 72:304–307, 1991.

Rampil IJ et al: Clinical characteristics of desflurane in surgical patients: Minimum alveolar concentration. Anesthesiology 74:429–433, 1991.

Sanders LD et al: Reversal of benzodiazepine sedation with the antagonist flumazenil. Br J Anaesth 66:445–453, 1991.

Smiley RM et al: Desflurane and isoflurane in surgical patients: Comparison of emergence time. Anesthesiology 74:425–428, 1991.

Smith I, Ding Y, and White PF: Comparison of induction, maintenance, and recovery characteristics of sevoflurane-N_2O and propofol-sevoflurane-N_2O anesthesia. Anesth Analg 74:253–259, 1992.

Sokoll MD and Long JP: General anesthesia and general anesthetic drugs. In Conn PM and Gebhart GF (eds): Essentials of Pharmacology. FA Davis, Philadelphia, 1989.

Trevor AJ and Miller RD: General anesthetics. In Katzung BD (ed): Basic and Clinical Pharmacology. Lange Medical Publications. Los Altos, 1982.

Ved SA et al: Sufentanil and alfentanil pattern of consumption during patient-controlled analgesia: A comparison with morphine. Clin J Pain 5 (Suppl 1):S63–S70, 1989.

Waugaman WR and Foster SD: New advances in anesthesia. Nurs Clin North Am 26:451–461, 1991.

White PF and Negus JB: Sedative infusions during local and regional anesthesia: A comparison of midazolam and propofol. J Clin Anesth 3:32–39, 1991.

CHAPTER 28

Ventilatory Stimulants

CHAPTER OUTLINE

Chapter Introduction
Analeptics

LIMITED DRUGS
LIMITED USES

Therapeutic Agents
Chapter Summary

CHAPTER OBJECTIVES

After studying this chapter the reader should be able to:

- Define analeptic and explain why such drugs are limited in therapeutic usefulness.
- Define neonatal apnea and apnea of prematurity and explain how respiratory stimulants may be of therapeutic value.
- Differentiate between central sleep apnea, obstructive sleep apnea, and mixed apnea.
- Explain how obstructive sleep apnea may contribute to the symptoms of the pickwickian syndrome.
- Describe the pharmacologic activity of the following ventilatory stimulants:
  - Doxapram, theophylline, caffeine, progesterone, protriptyline, naloxone

KEY TERMS

analeptic
apnea of prematurity
neonatal apnea

pickwickian syndrome
sleep apnea
    central sleep apnea

mixed sleep apnea
obstructive sleep apnea

CHAPTER INTRODUCTION

A drug that causes generalized central nervous system (CNS) arousal and increases the depth and rate of ventilation is called an **analeptic.** Such drugs are active in the reticular activating system and the vital respiratory centers in the medulla. Ventilatory stimulants, often referred to as *respiratory stimulants,* are included in this category. Such drugs are relatively limited in therapeutic usefulness and are given primarily for the short-term treatment of depressed ventilatory states in infants. Several analeptics discussed in this chapter are general CNS stimulants capable of producing convulsions when present in toxic amounts. Drugs used in the management of certain sleep disorders and drugs used to reverse narcotic-induced res-

piratory depression are discussed in this chapter.

ANALEPTICS

Limited Drugs

Analeptics having nontherapeutic uses are more numerous than those with strictly clinical application. Strychnine and picrotoxin are important for their toxicologic characteristics; pentylenetetrazol is valuable in the laboratory investigation of convulsions and neurochemical transmission. Less effective analeptics, such as nikethamide and ethamivan, are seldom used clinically. All of these drugs have specific nonclinical uses, but these will not be detailed in the present chapter.

Limited Uses

Drugs of limited usefulness for the stimulation of ventilatory drive include doxapram, theophylline, caffeine, progesterone, and protriptyline. Naloxone is employed to reverse narcotic-induced ventilatory depression. Use of these analeptic drugs has always been controversial. In addition, universal access to continuous ventilatory support is available in hospitals. Therefore, justification for the use of ventilatory stimulant drugs is increasingly difficult to find.

Clinical applications such as the reversal of CNS depressant overdose are impractical. This is because of the short-lived effect of most analeptics and the characteristically long duration of most CNS depressant intoxications. Treatment of chronic ventilatory failure is ineffective for the same reason. Following general anesthesia, drug-induced CNS stimulation of breathing is possible but not practical. Supported ventilation is safer and preferable, especially in conjunction with specific reversal agents. These include neostigmine for neuromuscular blockade, naloxone for opioid narcosis, and flumazenil for benzodiazepine depression. Clinically speaking, little is left for the analeptics. Limited use of ventilatory stimulants in the treatment of certain apneic conditions is discussed below.

THERAPEUTIC AGENTS

DOXAPRAM (Dopram, Stimulexin). Doxapram is a ventilatory stimulant having a very short duration of action (3–4 minutes). Its mechanism of action is not well understood. However, it is known that doxapram stimulates carotid chemoreceptors at low doses and medullary ventilatory centers at higher doses (Stark, 1991). Doxapram has a greater safety margin than the older drugs, such as nikethamide and ethamivan, but still has serious toxicity problems (see below). Doxapram increases the depth of ventilation more than the rate.

INDICATIONS. Doxapram is indicated in the stimulation of postanesthetic ventilation, but caution is required because the drug must be administered by intravenous infusion and such administration greatly increases the risk for producing toxic effects. Doxapram has also been used to assist with weaning from mechanical ventilation (Pourriat et al, 1992). Additional indications include the cautious use of doxapram in treating **neonatal apnea** and **apnea of prematurity,** conditions that may be caused by impaired ventilatory drive (Bairam et al, 1992a).

CONTRAINDICATIONS. Hypersensitivity to doxapram is a contraindication, as is the administration of doxapram to patients with evidence of head trauma, seizures, or flail chest injuries. In addition, doxapram is contraindicated in conditions such as pulmonary embolism, pneumothorax, and acute asthma.

PRECAUTIONS. In general, ventilatory stimulants such as doxapram increase the work of breathing. This increases oxygen consumption and may further worsen hypoxia.

Continuous intravenous infusion minimizes the disadvantage of a short duration of action. Such administration, however, increases plasma levels of doxapram and increases the risk of generalized CNS stimulation and convulsions.

ADVERSE REACTIONS. Adverse reactions may occur even at dosages below the convulsant level. These undesirable effects include CNS irritability and restlessness, sweating, tachycardia, and hypertension (Stark, 1991). Convulsions are always a potential threat with generalized CNS stimulation.

THEOPHYLLINE. Theophylline is a methylxanthine exhibiting potent bronchodilating and pulmonary vasodilating effects. The bronchodilator effects of theophylline in acute and chronic airway obstruction are discussed in Chapter 13. Theophylline is also a CNS stimulant with analeptic properties. As was discussed with the xanthine bronchodilators, theophylline produces a variety of extrapulmonary effects, such as increased gastric acid secretion, a diuretic action, and positive inotropic and chronotropic effects (see Table 13–1).

INDICATIONS. In addition to the pulmonary indications, such as relief of acute and chronic bronchospasm and treatment of acute pulmonary edema, theophylline increases minute ventilation and increases central ventilatory drive by increasing carbon dioxide sensitivity. It may increase ventilatory response to hypoxia by stimulating central and peripheral chemoreceptors. In addition, theophylline increases diaphragmatic contractility, makes the diaphragm less susceptible to fatigue, and is a pharmacologic antagonist of adenosine, a neuromodulator that inhibits ventilation (Stark, 1991). (The adenosine receptor–blocking effects of the methylxanthines are discussed in Chapter 13.) Theophylline is used in the management of apnea of prematurity (Kriter and Blanchard, 1989). It decreases the frequency and duration of apneic periods, increases alveolar ventilation, and normalizes the breathing pattern of infants.

Theophylline and caffeine have been used successfully in the weaning of infants from the ventilator, presumably because the drugs decrease apnea and increase ventilatory drive (Sims et al, 1989). Improvement in respiratory muscle function and decreased pulmonary vascular resistance brought about by the methylxanthines are also useful in patients undergoing weaning. Methylxanthines are not effective in the treatment of obstructive sleep apnea in infants.

CONTRAINDICATIONS. Contraindications to theophylline therapy are well described in Chapter 13 and include conditions such as peptic ulcer and gastritis. These conditions are worsened by increased gastric acid secretion. Preexisting coronary artery disease and angina pectoris may be worsened by the cardiovascular side effects of increased cardiac output and increased myocardial oxygen consumption.

PRECAUTIONS. As is explained in Chapter 13, theophylline has a relatively narrow therapeutic margin of safety. In addition, therapeutic and toxic levels of theophylline vary among patients. Pathophysiologic states such as congestive heart failure, hepatic disease, and renal disease may alter theophylline distribution, clearance, and excretion. This may in turn produce toxic conditions even at low dosage levels. For these reasons, serum theophylline levels are determined and individual dosage adjustments made. Table 13–2 lists some of the factors that alter theophylline metabolism.

Theophylline dosage guidelines for neonatal apnea include a loading dose of 5–6 mg/kg and a maintenance dose of 1 mg/kg/dose. ''Because of changes in metabolism with postnatal age, the maintenance dose should be adjusted according to blood level monitoring'' (Blanchard and Aranda, 1992).

Theophylline causes an increase in both diuresis and basal metabolic rate. These side effects warrant caution with theophylline therapy in the treatment of apnea of prematurity. This is because the resulting homeostatic upset, such as a decrease in fluid levels and an increase in metabolic stress, is not tolerated well by a small infant with limited fluid and energy reserves (Blanchard and Aranda, 1992). In an adult, however, these theophylline side effects are not as threatening because of the significantly larger body size.

ADVERSE REACTIONS. Adverse reactions to methylxanthines are outlined in Chapter 13 (see Table 13–4). These include gastrointestinal effects such as nausea and vomiting, cardiovascular effects such as palpitations and arrhythmias, and CNS effects such as headache and agitation. At very high serum theophylline levels, seizures, convulsions, and coma may occur. Tachycardia

may occur even at therapeutic blood levels of theophylline. However, this adverse effect is relatively rare with caffeine. In addition, caffeine has a wider therapeutic range than theophylline (Blanchard and Aranda, 1992). Table 28–1 compares the pharmacologic activity of methylxanthines used as ventilatory stimulants.

CAFFEINE. Another member of the methylxanthine class of drugs is caffeine. Caffeine is available therapeutically in oral and parenteral formulations. Caffeine and theophylline both exhibit similar effects, but vary in potency. Caffeine has a long half-life ($t_{1/2}$ = 100 h). Therefore, it can be administered less frequently than theophylline (see Table 28–1).

INDICATIONS. Like theophylline, caffeine may be useful in the management of apnea in preterm infants. In large doses, caffeine stimulates medullary ventilatory centers but may trigger convulsions. In animal studies, combined caffeine and doxapram produce an interactive, dose-dependent effect on ventilatory stimulation (Bairam et al, 1992b).

Caffeine dosage guidelines for neonatal apnea include a loading dose of 10 mg/kg and a maintenance dose of 2.5 mg/kg/dose. As is explained with theophylline, postnatal adjustments to the maintenance dose must be made on the basis of therapeutic blood level monitoring (Blanchard and Aranda, 1992).

Caffeine is routinely combined with salicylates and codeine or with acetaminophen and codeine in analgesic combinations to offset depressant effects on ventilation (see Chapter 25).

CONTRAINDICATIONS, PRECAUTIONS, AND ADVERSE REACTIONS. See Theophylline.

MEDROXYPROGESTERONE (Provera). Medroxyprogesterone acetate is an oral progesterone product used to stimulate alveolar ventilation. It increases ventilatory drives by increasing

TABLE 28–1 COMPARISON OF THEOPHYLLINE AND CAFFEINE IN NEONATAL APNEA

	Theophylline	Caffeine
Efficacy	Equivalent	Equivalent
Elimination half-life	30 h	100 h
Dosing schedule	More frequent	Less frequent
Adverse effects*	More common	Less common
Therapeutic range	Narrow	Wide

Source: Data from Blanchard and Aranda, 1992.

*Adverse effects of the methylxanthines include respiratory, gastrointestinal, cardiovascular, and central nervous system effects (see Table 13–4).

the responsiveness of central ventilatory centers to hypercapnia and of peripheral chemoreceptors to hypoxia. Therefore, hypercapnic and hypoxic drives are increased. This corrects chronic carbon dioxide retention and improves hypoxemia.

INDICATIONS. **Sleep apneas** are disorders of ventilatory control in which multiple periods of apnea occur during sleep. In **central sleep apnea,** there is failure of central ventilatory drive, and therefore, muscles of ventilation are not stimulated to contract. A well-known but poorly understood syndrome that may be caused by failure of central ventilatory control is sudden infant death syndrome (SIDS, or crib death). In this untreatable disorder, death of a young infant nearly always occurs during sleep.

Medroxyprogesterone is useful in the management of **obstructive sleep apnea (OSA).** In this type of sleep disorder, central ventilatory controls are operative and inspiratory muscle effort is present. However, periodic apneic episodes occur during sleep and are caused by obstruction of the upper airway. (**Mixed apnea** has features of both central and obstructive sleep apnea.) The occlusion of the airway in obstructive sleep apnea may be caused by loss of muscle tone in structures such as the tongue, pharnyx, or larynx. During the various stages of sleep, there is a general loss of skeletal muscle tone, including the accessory muscles of breathing and those muscles associated with upper airway structures.

The apneic episode caused by the obstruction produces hypercapnia and hypoxia, which arouses the patient. On arousal, normal muscle tone returns to the upper airway structures and ventilation resumes. The patient then returns to a lighter stage of nonrapid eye movement (NREM) sleep as the arousal mechanism subsides. Progression through the different sleep stages then repeats itself. This destructive sleep cycle causes interrupted sleep, reduces the period of rapid eye movement (REM) sleep, and causes the patient to awake in an exhausted state. (NREM sleep has several subdivisions and normally alternates throughout the night with REM sleep.) This fragmented sleep pattern may lead to daytime somnolence—a state of sleepiness or unnatural drowsiness. The condition is prevalent in obese persons because excess body fat may compress the upper airway structures and contribute to obstructive sleep apnea. The complex of obesity, somnolence, hypoventilation, and polycythemia is called the **pickwickian syndrome.** (The term was inspired by an overweight character in Charles Dickens' *The Pickwick Papers.*) Sleep apnea causes low arterial oxygen saturation (SaO_2). This eventually triggers polycythemia as a compensatory mechanism. Pulmonary hypertension, right-side heart failure, cyanosis, and edema may also occur (Box 28–1).

In addition to stimulating ventilatory drives, medroxyprogesterone causes diuresis. This effect may aid saturation in patients with obstructive sleep apnea by reducing pulmonary congestion and improving oxygenation.

ADVERSE REACTIONS. Medroxyprogesterone may cause nervousness, insomnia, dizziness, nausea, and headaches. Men may experience impotency and temporary alopecia, or hair loss. (Testosterone administration can correct the impotency.)

PROTRIPTYLINE (Vivactil). Protriptyline is a tricyclic antidepressant (TCA) that has low sedative properties and moderate anticholinergic and cardiovascular side effects. By comparison, amitriptyline exhibits considerable sedative, anticholinergic, and cardiovascular effects (see Chapter 24). Protriptyline is not a respiratory stimulant in the true sense because arterial carbon dioxide tension is not affected. Protriptyline does, however, alter breathing patterns in obstructive sleep apnea. As is described in Chapter 24, the TCAs block the amine pump, or uptake-1 mechanism, to inhibit the uptake of norepinephrine and serotonin.

INDICATIONS. Protriptyline is indicated for the management of obstructive sleep apnea in patients in whom weight loss and avoidance of alcohol and sedatives do not reduce the severity of the symptoms. It suppresses REM sleep and reduces the period during which apneas are most severe. Protriptyline also increases muscle tone of the upper airway to reduce the obstruction that is common during REM sleep.

CONTRAINDICATIONS. Concurrent administration of TCAs, such as protriptyline, and monoamine oxidase inhibitors, such as tranylcypromine (Parnate) is contraindicated. The drug-drug interaction between the antidepressants may produce seizures and hypertensive crisis due to elevated amine levels (see Chapter 24).

PRECAUTIONS. Because tricyclic antidepressants can produce arrhythmias and hypotension, the use of protriptyline may be hazardous in patients with myocardial infarction. Anticholinergic drugs and barbiturates must be used cautiously with all TCAs because of potential additive effects.

ADVERSE REACTIONS. Anticholinergic effects of protriptyline include dry mouth, blurred vision, constipation, and urinary retention. Cardiovas-

BOX 28–1 IF JOE THE FAT BOY HAD BEEN A WOMAN, HE MIGHT HAVE HAD A GOOD NIGHT'S SLEEP

The object that presented itself to the eyes of the astonished clerk was a boy—a wonderfully fat boy—habited as a serving lad, standing upright on the mat, with his eyes closed as if in sleep.

"What's the matter?" inquired the clerk.

The extraordinary boy replied not a word; but he nodded once, and seemed, to the clerk's imagination, to snore feebly.

Charles Dickens, *The Pickwick Papers*, p 715

The **pickwickian syndrome** is characterized by obesity, somnolence, hypoventilation, and polycythemia. This disorder of excessive daytime sleepiness can even a cause a person to fall asleep while driving an automobile or while reading a pharmacology textbook. The pickwickian syndrome is more prevalent in men than in women—hormonal differences may provide part of the explanation.

Progesterone increases minute ventilation and may provide some protection against hypoventilation for premenopausal women. Normally, progesterone levels are increased in the last trimester of pregnancy and in the last portion of the menstrual cycle. By increasing ventilation, these elevated progesterone levels reduce arterial carbon dioxide tension. However, without such stimulation, hypoventilation may occur.

Hypoventilation can also be caused by other factors. For example, obese persons are more likely to suffer from **obstructive sleep apnea.** This condition leads to hypoventilation and may contribute to the pickwickian syndrome manifested in Joe the Fat Boy. It should be noted that Dickens' description of Joe the Fat Boy does not include other characteristics of the disorder such as apnea and cyanosis. Joe has merely coexisting obesity and somnolence—he is not a true *pickwickian* (Comroe, 1993).

"Damn that boy; he's gone to sleep again. Joe! Joe!" (Sundry taps on the head with a stick, and the fat boy, with some difficulty, roused from his lethargy.)

Charles Dickens, *The Pickwick Papers*, p 53

In a normal sleep pattern, as the reticular activating system and arousal mechanisms become less active, sleepiness is induced. The presence or absence of rapid eye movement (REM) and various electroencephalogram characteristics identify different stages of sleep. Nonrapid eye movement (NREM) sleep precedes REM sleep. Several cycles of NREM and REM sleep normally occur during the night. In each successive cycle, the time spent in NREM sleep decreases and that spent in REM sleep increases. During NREM sleep, ventilation is controlled by metabolic processes. Therefore, changes in arterial carbon dioxide and oxygen tension alter breathing. During REM sleep, however, ventilatory control is independent of metabolic needs. It is irregular due to temporary decreases in the ventilatory response to chemical stimuli. Short periods of apnea are common. Loss of voluntary muscle tone in the upper airway normally occurs during both NREM and REM stages of sleep. In obstructive sleep apnea, however, occlusion of the airway due to loss of muscle tone causes periods of apnea that decrease arterial oxygen saturation and arouse the individual. After clearing the airway, normal airflow is restored and the person begins a new cycle of NREM sleep. This pattern results in REM sleep deprivation and may lead to daytime hypersomnolence—the abnormal sleepiness of Dickens' character.

"Damn that boy," said the old gentlemen, "he's gone to sleep again."

"Very extraordinary boy, that," said Mr. Pickwick, "does he always sleep in this way?"

"Sleep!" said the old gentlemen, "he's always asleep. Goes on errands fast asleep, and snores as he waits at table."

"How very odd!" said Mr. Pickwick.

"Ah! odd indeed," returned the old gentleman; "I'm proud of that boy—wouldn't part with him on any account—damme, he's a natural curiosity! Here, Joe—Joe— take these things away and open another bottle—d'ye hear?"

Charles Dickens, *The Pickwick Papers,* p 56

Treatment of the pickwickian syndrome includes weight loss, avoidance of CNS depressants such as alcohol, and controlled oxygen therapy. Ventilatory stimulants, such as medroxyprogesterone or protriptyline, may be of therapeutic value (see text).

Comroe JH: Frankenstein, Pickwick, and Ondine (Retrospective Redux). Respiratory Care 38:940–943, 1993.

Dickens C: The Posthumous Papers of the Pickwick Club (The Pickwick Papers). MacMillan, London, 1954. First published by MacMillan, 1892.

Mallory GB and Beckerman RC: Relationship between obesity and respiratory control abnormalities. In Beckerman RC, Brouillette RT, and Hunt CE (eds): Respiratory Control Disorders in Infants and Children. Williams and Wilkins, Baltimore, 1992.

Martin RJ and Ballard RD: Respiratory stimulants. In Cherniak RM (ed): Drugs for the Respiratory System. Grune and Stratton, Orlando, FL 1986.

Schoessler M, Ludwig-Beymer P, and Huether SE: Pain, temperature regulation, sleep, and sensory function. In McCance KL and Huether SE: Pathophysiology: The Biologic Basis for Disease in Adults and Children. CV Mosby, St Louis, 1990.

Thomas CL (ed): Taber's Cyclopedic Medical Dictionary, ed 16. FA Davis, Philadelphia, 1989.

West JB: Pulmonary Pathophysiology: The Essentials, ed 4. Williams and Wilkins, Baltimore, 1992.

Wilkins RL and Dexter JR: Sleep apnea. In Wilkins RL and Dexter JR (eds): Respiratory Disease: Principles of Patient Care. FA Davis, Philadelphia, 1993.

cular effects include orthostatic hypotension, tachycardia, and arrhythmias.

NALOXONE (Narcan). Narcotic reversal agents and the narcotic analgesics are discussed in Chapter 25. Naloxone is a competitive antagonist of opiate and opioid agonists at μ-opioid receptors. Strictly speaking, naloxone is not a ventilatory stimulant. However, it can reverse respiratory depression caused by the narcotics. Naloxone is essentially a pure antagonist, whereas other narcotic reversal agents, such as nalorphine (Nalline) and levallorphan (Lorfan), are mixed agonist-antagonists. Such drugs are not as useful as naloxone because they cause some respiratory depression due to their narcotic agonist effect.

INDICATIONS. Naloxone is useful in the reversal of CNS and ventilatory depression caused by the narcotics. These analgesic drugs, such as morphine, oxycodone, and meperidine, are discussed in Chapter 25. Management of narcotic drug overdose (see Table 25–2) and reversal of postoperative narcotic depression are indications for use of naloxone.

CONTRAINDICATIONS. Hypersensitivity to naloxone is a contraindication for its use.

PRECAUTIONS. Maintenance of a patent airway and use of mechanical ventilation may be necessary with ventilatory depression caused by the narcotics. Naloxone is not an alternative to intubation and mechanical ventilation in cases of ventilatory depression. Naloxone has limited usefulness if an increase in ventilatory drive and a decrease in carbon dioxide retention are desired.

ADVERSE REACTIONS. Naloxone may bring about rapid reversal or narcotic-induced CNS depression. This effect may trigger nausea, vomiting, tachycardia, and hypertension.

Table 28–2 lists the general and trade names of the ventilatory stimulants discussed in this chapter.

CHAPTER SUMMARY

The action and use of ventilatory stimulants has always been promising from a theoretical standpoint—namely, selective stimulation of respira-

**TABLE 28–2 DRUG NAMES:
VENTILATORY STIMULANTS**

Generic Name	Trade Name
Doxapram (**DOCKS**-a-pram)	Dopram, Stimulexin
Theophylline	
Caffeine	
Medroxyprogesterone (me-**DROXY**-prō-**GES**-ter-ōn)	Provera
Protriptylline (prō-**TRIP**-ti-lin)	Vivactil
Naloxone (nal-**OKS**-ōn)	Narcan

tory centers. Practical experience with the drugs, however, has generally been disappointing. Doxapram, although effective as a ventilatory stimulant postoperatively, produces its effects for only a few minutes. Theophylline and caffeine have a useful duration of action for the treatment of apnea of prematurity but exhibit significant toxicity. The other agents discussed in this chapter are effective in only limited therapeutic applications. Medroxyprogesterone and protriptyline are useful in the management of obstructive sleep apnea. Naloxone is used exclusively to reverse narcotic-induced ventilatory depression.

BIBLIOGRAPHY

Bairam A et al: Doxapram for the initial treatment of idiopathic apnea of prematurity. Biol Neonate 61:209–13, 1992a.

Bairam A et al: Interactive ventilatory effects of two respiratory stimulants, caffeine and doxapram, in newborn lambs. Biol Neonate 61:201–208, 1992b.

Blanchard PW and Aranda JV: Pharmacotherapy of respiratory control disorders. In Beckerman RC, Brouillette RT, and Hunt CE (eds): Respiratory Control Disorders in Infants and Children. Williams and Wilkins, Baltimore, 1992.

Byers VL: Central nervous system stimulants. In Kuhn MM (ed): Pharmacotherapeutics: A Nursing Process Approach, ed 2. FA Davis, Philadelphia, 1990.

Clark WG, Brater DC, and Johnson AR: Goth's Medical Pharmacology, ed 12. CV Mosby Co, St. Louis, 1988.

Dyson M, Beckerman RC, and Brouillette RT: Obstructive sleep apnea syndrome. In Beckerman RC, Brouillette RT, and Hunt CE (eds): Respiratory Control Disorders in Infants and Children. Williams and Wilkins, Baltimore, 1992.

Finer NN et al: Obstructive, mixed, and central apnea in the neonate: Physiologic correlates. J Pediatr 121:943–950, 1992.

Henderson-Smart DJ: Apnea of prematurity. In Beckerman RC, Brouillette RT, and Hunt CE (eds): Respiratory Control Disorders in Infants and Children. Williams and Wilkins, Baltimore, 1992.

Howder CL: Cardiopulmonary Pharmacology: A Handbook for Respiratory Practitioners and Other Allied Health Personnel. Williams and Wilkins, Baltimore, 1992.

Hirnle RW: Miscellaneous respiratory agents. In Kuhn MM (ed): Pharmacotherapeutics: A Nursing Process Approach, ed 2. FA Davis, Philadelphia, 1990.

Kaake RE et al: Depressed central respiratory drive causing weaning failure. Chest 95:695–697, 1989.

Kriter KE and Blanchard J: Management of apnea in infants. Clin Pharm 8:577–587, 1989.

Martin RJ and Ballard RD: Respiratory stimulants. In Cherniak RM (ed): Drugs for the Respiratory System. Grune and Stratton, Orlando, FL, 1986.

Pourriat JL et al: Effects of doxapram on hypercapnic response during weaning from mechanical ventilation in COPD patients. Chest 101:1639–1643, 1992.

Rau JL: Respiratory Care Pharmacology, ed 3. Yearbook Medical Publishers, Chicago, 1989.

Scanlon JE et al: Caffeine or theophylline for neonatal apnoea? Arch Dis Child 67:425–428, 1992.

Sims ME et al: Comparative evaluation of caffeine and theophylline for weaning premature infants from the ventilator. Am J Perinatol 6:72–75, 1989.

Stark, AR: Disorders of respiratory control in infants. Respiratory Care 36:673–682, 1991.

Taylor AE et al: Clinical Respiratory Physiology. WB Saunders, Philadelphia, 1989.

Welborn LG et al: High-dose caffeine suppresses postoperative apnea in former preterm infants. Anesthesiology 71:347–9, 1989.

West JB: Pulmonary Pathophysiology: The Essentials, ed 4. Williams and Wilkins, Baltimore, 1992.

Wilkins RL and Dexter JR: Sleep apnea. In Wilkins RL and Dexter JR (eds): Respiratory Disease: Principles of Patient Care. FA Davis, Philadelphia, 1993.

APPENDIX A

Pharmaceutical Calculations

OUTLINE

Systems of Measurements
- METRIC SYSTEM
- APOTHECARY SYSTEM AND HOUSEHOLD SYSTEM

Equivalent Dosage Strengths
- INTERCONVERSIONS
- ZEROS

Dimensional Analysis (Unit Factor Method)

Pharmaceutial Calculations
Medication Labels
Sample Problems
Solutions

SYSTEMS OF MEASUREMENT

Several different measurement systems may be encountered in medicinal calculations. The most widespread, easy to use, and accurate system is the metric system of meters, grams, and liters. In a distant second place is the outdated **apothecary** system of grains, minims, and fluidrams, followed by the familiar but imprecise **household** measurements of drops, teaspoons, and tablespoons.

Metric System

The simplicity of the metric system lies in its reliance on the decimal system. Moving the decimal point by increments to the right to produce larger numbers, or to the left to produce smaller numbers, allows rapid and accurate calculations to be made in this system. When the ease of a decimal system is coupled with convenient units of mass, length, and volume, the metric system becomes the preferred measurement system in scientific calculations. The actual values for a gram (mass), meter (length), and liter (volume) are based on international standards but need not concern us in this discussion. Table A–1 lists some common metric units and their abbreviations. As is seen in Table A–1, additional units are used in the SI-metric system. Because some of these are cumbersome in scientific calculations, we will be using familiar metric units rather than "pure" SI units. Table A–2 gives the common prefixes used with metric units. Some of the prefixes applied to these standard measurement units are routinely used in pharmaceutical calculations and are listed in Table A–3.

Notice that only L (for liter) is capitalized. All other units are given in lowercase letters. Plural forms are not used, nor are periods used after the abbreviations. The abbreviations themselves never precede the numeric value but are always placed after the value (eg, 34.2 mg).

The Greek symbol mu (μ), although accurate in the SI–metric system, could be written incorrectly in a drug order and resemble a hastily scribbled mg. This could be misread as "milligram." A milligram delivers *one thousand times* more drug than a microgram. Therefore, for greater safety, the prefix mc is used in place of μ in pharmaceutical calculations (eg, 340 mcg).

One liter (L) contains 1000 milliliters (mL). The amount of water filling a cube that measures 1 decimeter (1 dm = 10 cm) on each side is also 1 liter. The volume of such an object is calculated as:

$$\begin{aligned} V &= \text{length} \times \text{width} \times \text{height} \\ &= (10\ \text{cm})^3 = 10^3\ \text{cm}^3 \\ \therefore V &= 1000\ \text{cm}^3 = 1\ \text{L} \end{aligned}$$

and because

$$V = 1000 \text{ mL} = 1 \text{ L},$$
$$1000 \text{ cm}^3 = 1000 \text{ mL}$$
$$\therefore 1 \text{ cm}^3 = 1 \text{ mL}$$

Common use of the term *centimeter cubed* (cm^3) is *cubic centimeter* or cc, a frequent measure used in pharmaceutical calculations. Therefore, 1 cm^3 = 1 mL = 1 cc.

(NOTE: Older non-SI abbreviations, such as K for kilogram, ℓ or l for liter (as in ml), and G or gm for gram are occasionally seen. These abbreviations are obsolete and should not be used in drug calculations.

Apothecary System and Household System

The apothecary system of measurement is the traditional system used in drug prescriptions and drug formulations. The household system contains a few commonly used measurements, such as 1 drop ≈ 1 minim (see below), 1 teaspoon = 5 mL, and 1 tablespoon = 15 mL. Both of these archaic systems have been largely replaced by the metric system. Occasionally, however, the respiratory care practitioner may encounter drug dosages given in units other than those of the metric system.

The apothecary system has no actual measure of volume. Instead, equivalent volumes based on a mass are used. The units themselves have modern metric equivalents. They also have curious origins. A grain, the basic unit of mass, was based on the mass of a grain of wheat (approximately

TABLE A–1 BASIC UNITS OF METRIC SYSTEM AND SYSTÈME INTERNATIONAL (INTERNATIONAL SYSTEM)

Base Unit	Metric System	Système International
Time	Second (s)	Second (s)
Length	Meter (m)	Meter (m)
Volume	Liter (L)*	Cubic meter (m³)
Mass	Gram (g)	Kilogram (kg)
Temperature	Degree Celsius (°C)	Kelvin (K)
Pressure	Atmosphere (atm)	Pascal (Pa)

Source: Data from Timberlake, 1992.
*Liter is a derived unit for volume. See text for explanation. Older metric abbreviations for liter include ℓ and l. Their use should be abandoned or discouraged.

equal to 60 mg). A minim is a very small measurement of volume based on the amount of water that is equal to the mass of a grain. Larger fluid measurements are the fluidram (4 mL) and the fluidounce (30 mL). Clearly, these apothecary units are somewhat obscure. In fact, the metric equivalent of a grain can range from 60 mg to 64 mg. This range of values is considered to be within acceptable accuracy limits for dosage calculations. Minims, fluidrams, and fluidounces are infrequently used. However, the respiratory care practitioner is likely to see the grain still used in medication orders. This occurs mainly with the belladonna alkaloids (eg, atropine) and the narcotics (eg, morphine). Con-

TABLE A–2 COMMON PREFIXES USED WITH METRIC UNITS*

LESS THAN BASE UNIT (SUBMULTIPLES)

Prefix	Abbreviation	Meaning	Decimal Equivalent†	Exponential (Scientific) Notation‡
Nano-	n	One billionth	0.000000001	1×10^{-9}
Micro-	μ	One millionth	0.000001	1×10^{-6}
Milli-	m	One thousandth	0.001	1×10^{-3}
Centi-	c	One hundredth	0.01	1×10^{-2}
Deci-	d	One tenth	0.1	1×10^{-1}

MORE THAN BASE UNIT (MULTIPLES)

Prefix	Abbreviation	Meaning	Decimal Equivalent†	Exponential (Scientific) Notation‡
Deka-	da	Ten	10	1×10^{1}
Hecto-	h	One hundred	100	1×10^{2}
Kilo-	k	One thousand	1000	1×10^{3}
Mega-	M	One million	1000000	1×10^{6}
Giga-	G	One billion	1000000000	1×10^{9}

*Multiples and submultiples of metric base units are obtained by multiplying the base units by powers of 10.
†Spaces instead of commas are used in the Système International to express large numbers in groupings of three digits, as in 1 000 000 rather than 1,000,000.
‡For a review of exponential notation, consult a suitable mathematics text.

TABLE A–3 PREFIXES AND METRIC UNITS COMMONLY USED IN PHARMACEUTICAL CALCULATIONS

Prefix	Abbreviation or Symbol	Example	Meaning	Decimal	Exponential or Scientific Notation*
Micro-	μ†	μg (microgram)	1/100000 g	0.000001 g	1×10^{-6} g
Milli-	m	mL (milliliter)	1/1000 L	0.001 L	1×10^{-3} L
Centi-	c	cm (centimeter)	1/100 m	0.01 m	1×10^{-2} m
Kilo-	k	kg (kilogram)	1000 g	1000 g	1×10^{3} g

*For a review of exponential notation, consult a suitable mathematics text.

†In pharmaceutical calculations, mc is commonly used in place of μ, as in "mcg" for microgram. See text for explanation.

version charts usually give *dozens* of grain—milligram interconversions such as:

$$gr\ 1/100 = 0.6\ mg$$
$$gr\ 1/60 = 1\ mg$$
$$gr\ 1/10 = 6\ mg$$
$$gr\ 1/8 = 8\ mg \ldots ad\ nauseam$$

These redundant interconversions are really quite useless because only a single equivalence is needed. "One grain equals 60 mg" is sufficient to perform all pharmaceutical calculations involving dosages given in grains. The convention used is that the abbreviation *gr* precedes the numeric value. Therefore, *one-half grain* is written as *gr 1/2*. (Do not confuse gr with g, the SI–metric abbreviation for a gram.)

Numbers in the apothecary system can be written as Arabic (eg, 1, 3, 4) or Roman (eg, I, III, IV) numerals. Lowercase Roman numerals (eg, i, iii, iv) are also seen. For accuracy, when Roman numerals are used, a horizontal line is drawn over the tops of the numbers and a dot is placed above the line over the numerals (eg, gr 3 = gr gr III = gr iii). This practice helps safeguard against a hastily written numeral, such as V, which could resemble two ones written at angles to each other (eg, \/). A final point is that the fraction one half is occassionally written as a lowercase double s with a horizontal line above (eg, gr ½ = gr s̄s̄).

Table A–4 lists some common apothecary and household measurement units and their abbreviations or symbols. Metric equivalents for the measures are also given.

EQUIVALENT DOSAGE STRENGTHS

Interconversions

Drugs encountered by the respiratory care practitioner come in a variety of dosage forms, such as oral preparations, injectables, and aerosols,

and in many different dosage strengths. The reader needing a review of basic arithmetic operations, including determination of fractions, ratios, decimals, and percentage, is directed to consult programmed self-study texts such as those listed at the back of this Appendix. The following discussion assumes the reader is familiar with such operations and is able to interconvert between different equivalent measurements. The ratio 1:200 states a relationship between two different things—one part of drug in 200 parts of solvent, for instance. This ratio is equivalent to the fraction 1/200. This fraction, expressed as a percent, is 0.5% and when the percentage is converted to a decimal, it becomes 0.005:

TABLE A–4 COMMON APOTHECARY AND HOUSEHOLD SYSTEM UNITS AND ABBREVIATIONS WITH METRIC EQUIVALENTS

APOTHECARY SYSTEM

Unit	Abbreviation	Approximate Metric Equivalent
Grain	gr	60–64 mg*
Minim	ɱ or min	†
Fluidram	fl dr or f ℨ	4 mL
Fluidounce	fl oz or f ℥	30 mL

HOUSEHOLD SYSTEM

Drop	gtt (L. *gutta*—drop)	†
Teaspoon	t or tsp	5 mL
Tablespoon	T or tbs	15 mL

*60 mg = gr 1 is acceptable for pharmaceutical calculations.

†A minim is the volume that is equal to the mass of one grain (≈ 60 mg). Also, one drop is *approximately* equal to one minim. The size of a drop varies somewhat with the viscosity of the substance being measured. A minim of water is approximately equal to one drop, whereas a minim of a low-viscosity substance, such as alcohol, is equal to more than one drop.

1:200 changed to a fraction:
1:200 means "1 part in 200 parts," or 1/200

and

1/200 converted to a percentage:

$$\frac{1}{\underset{2}{\cancel{200}}} \times \cancel{100} = \frac{1}{2}\%, \text{ or } 0.5\%$$

Finally, 0.5% expressed as a decimal:

$$0.5\% = 0.005$$

(The percent sign is omitted and the decimal point is moved two places to the left.)

As can be seen in the following list, dosage strengths of drugs are expressed in various ways. The reader must be adept at switching from one equivalent dosage to another as was described above.

Percentages   eg, 0.025% ipratropium;
               20% N-acetylcysteine
Ratios   eg, 1:200 isoproterenol; 1:1,000
               epinephrine
Mass per   eg, 5 mg/mL albuterol^{US}
volume   (salbutamol^{CAN}) nebulizer
               solution
                   50 mcg/metered dose
               beclomethasone metered-dose
               inhaler
                   10 mg/teaspoonful
               metaproterenol oral
                   25 mg/mL aminophylline
               injectable
Mass only   eg, 100 mg theophylline tablets

Zeros

The preceding list of dosage strengths illustrates the use of a variety of measurement units and the proper use of **zeros** to express drug dosages. Basic rules involving zeros in drug calculations are quite simple:

1. Do not use unnecessary zeros. Technically, their use, as in 53.0 mg, implies a measurement precision that may or may not be true. In practical terms, the use of unnecessary zeros in a medication order adds to the risk of misunderstanding. For example, the order to "administer 53 milligrams of drug" could be written as 53.0 mg. However, if the decimal point is not read properly or is carelessly written, as in 53.0 mg, the order appears to be 530 mg. The dosage delivered by this medication error will be *ten times* the dosage ordered. This magnitude of error could spell disaster. The or-

der written as *53 mg* is accurate and less subject to misinterpretation. If a zero is not needed to designate a place, as in *53.01* mg, do not use it.

2. Use a zero to represent the place of the unit (the one). For numbers less than 1, as in 0.53 mg, the zero plays an essential role and increases the accuracy of pharmaceutical calculations because it draws attention to the location of the decimal.

Summary

The zero in 0.1 g is necessary, accurate, and acceptable.

The zero in 1.0 g is unnecessary, incorrect, and risky to use.

DIMENSIONAL ANALYSIS (UNIT FACTOR METHOD)

If you grew up with the English (US) system of measurement, the following problem should be simple. *What is eighteen inches expressed in feet?* "Easy," you answer. "There are 12 inches in a foot, therefore, 18 inches equals a foot-and-a-half. One point five feet if you want a decimal answer." Correct. Now try this one. *How many feet is 21.5 inches?* The answer, of course, is not reached as quickly. Whatever "mathematical" process worked on the first problem—inspection, intuition, or familiarity— does not seem to be of much help in the second.

What do you know about this problem? You *must* ask yourself this question with every problem. One thing you know is that the answer is to be expressed in feet. Another thing you know is that the length is given as 21.5 inches. The only other thing you know is that there are 12 inches to the foot. This type of relationship, in which one thing is equivalent to another, is crucial. Without this relationship, you cannot solve the problem. The unit relationship will be given to you in the problem, be available in a conversion table, or be familiar to you because of common unit conversions within a system of measurement. For example, "One foot equals 12 inches" is a well-known equivalent in the US system.) Let us look more closely at this simple equivalence:

$$12 \text{ in} = 1 \text{ ft}$$

If both sides of the equation are divided by 12 inches, we get:

$$\frac{12 \text{ in}}{12 \text{ in}} = 1 = \frac{1 \text{ ft}}{12 \text{ in}}$$

Note that the expression *1 ft/12 in* equals 1. This is called a **unit factor.** Because 1 ft and 12 inches are exactly equal, any expression can be multiplied by this unit factor without changing its value.

Here is the second problem again. This time we will use the **unit factor method,** also known as the **dimensional analysis method,** to solve it.

A length is given as 21.5 inches. How many feet is this? Multiply the appropriate unit factor by the length in inches:

$$\frac{1 \text{ ft}}{12 \text{ in}} \times 21.5 \text{ in} = \frac{21.5}{12} \text{ ft} = 1.79 \text{ ft}$$

Note that the inch units cancel, leaving the answer expressed in feet. This is what we wanted to accomplish.

In summary, first inspect the problem to find out what you know about it. This will give you a unit factor based on information in the problem or an equivalence you should know (or can find in a reference table). Second, arrange the unit factor so that it will generate the units you want. Note that in the above problem in which 1 ft = 12 in, there are really *two* equivalent unit factors:

$$\frac{1 \text{ ft}}{12 \text{ in}} \text{ and } \frac{12 \text{ in}}{1 \text{ ft}}$$

How do you know which unit factor to use? Simply look at what is asked for in the problem and select the unit factor that has the desired *final units in the numerator.* The unwanted units will cancel. In other words, to end up with *feet,* choose the unit factor 1 ft/12 in. To convert to *inches,* select the unit factor 12 in/1 ft. We will practice using the dimensional analysis method with the following sample problems.

Example 1: *An older anatomy text states that the adult trachea is about 4.5 inches long. What is this length in centimeters? (2.54 cm = 1 in.)*

In this problem, the conversion factor between English and metric systems is given. Therefore, the unit factors available to us are 2.54 cm/1 in and 1 in/2.54 cm. Because we want to obtain an answer in centimeters, we use the 2.54 cm/1 in unit factor. (This factor has the desired final units in the numerator.) Multiplying this unit factor by the length of the trachea in inches gives us the desired final units in centimeters.

$$\frac{2.54 \text{ cm}}{1 \text{ in}} \times 4.5 \text{ in} = 11.4 \text{ cm}$$

Example 2: *During normal, quiet breathing, the diaphragm descends around 1.5 cm and generates an intrapleural pressure of approximately −3 cmH₂O. What is this pressure expressed in milli-*

meters of mercury (mmHg)? (1 mmHg = 1.36 cmH₂O).

The conversion between pressure units is given to us in the problem. We know the intrapleural pressure in centimeters of water. As usual, there are two unit conversions available to us: 1 mmHg/1.36 cmH₂O and 1.36 cmH₂O/1 mmHg. We want to be left with mmHg in the numerator. Therefore, we multiply the 1 mmHg/1.36 cmH₂O unit factor by the intrapleural pressure given in cmH₂O:

$$\frac{1 \text{ mmHg}}{1.36 \text{ cmH}_2\text{O}} \times -3 \text{ cmH}_2\text{O} = -2.21 \text{ mmHg}$$

Example 3: *Pulmonary function test (PFT) results on a particular patient reveal that the patient's total lung volume is 5.79 liters (L). What is this volume in milliliters (mL)?*

You may immediately know to multiply the given lung volume by 1000 to get the correct answer—but what are you actually doing with such an arithmetic operation? Apply the logical steps of dimensional analysis. With a little practice this method will become familiar to you. You will rely on it for all calculations involving unit conversions because it is essentially foolproof.

In this sample problem, we want to generate milliliters in our answer and we know that 1 L = 1000 mL. Therefore, to cancel liters and leave milliliters, we use the unit factor, 1000 mL/1 L:

$$\frac{1000 \text{ mL}}{1 \text{ L}} \times 5.79 \text{ L} = 5790 \text{ mL}$$

Example 4: *The mass of a drug is given as 200 micrograms (mcg). How many milligrams is this?*

Although you will become familiar with conversions between small units, it is always advisable to work from the SI-metric base units of gram (g) for mass, meter (m) for length, and liter (L) for volume. What do we know in this problem? Working from the base unit of grams, we can state that one gram (g) equals 1000 milligrams (mg). One gram is also equal to 1,000,000 micrograms (μg, or mcg in pharmaceutical calculations). We want to end up with milligrams. Therefore, the 1000 mg/1 g unit factor is used and simply multiplied by other appropriate unit factors (remember, the factors are equivalent, so multiplying any expression by them does not change their value):

$$\frac{1000 \text{ mg}}{1 \text{ g}} \times \frac{1 \text{ g}}{1000000 \text{ mcg}} \times 200 \text{ mcg} = 0.2 \text{ mg}$$

As is shown in this example, you may arrange multiple unit factors so that the unwanted units automatically cancel. This leaves the desired units as a numerator (milligrams, in this case). You can chain together as many unit factors as needed to generate the proper units for your answer. The only math required is simple multiplication of the fractions to arrive at the numeric value. The final units are generated by the dimensional analysis method. The use of scientific (exponential) notation (eg, 200 mcg = 2×10^2 mcg) streamlines the mechanics of the mathematical operation but is not absolutely necessary for solution of these problems.

PHARMACEUTICAL CALCULATIONS

Basic pharmaceutical calculations involve various combinations of known drug amount or mass, volume of drug delivered, or strength of solution. There are only a few simple guidelines to remember when performing basic pharmaceutical calculations:

1. Convert any dosage strength that is given in a percent or ratio to a mass-volume format. Ratios must first be converted to a percentage. Drug percentage strengths are given as mass/volume relationships. Therefore, a 1% solution contains 1 g of drug (solute) in 100 mL of solvent. From this relationship, further conversions to milligrams or micrograms can be easily made if required.
2. Set up the problem so that the calculation will generate the units required. The dimensional analysis approach will eliminate unnecessary reliance on rules and formulas. (Rules and formulas painstakingly memorized are surprisingly fleeting just at the moment when they are needed most.) If a dosage strength of 10 mg/mL is given in a problem but the *volume* of a drug required to deliver a certain dosage is asked for, the *volume units* (mL) must remain after all other units have been canceled through the calculations. The mg/mL relationship must be inverted so that milliliters appear in the numerator. A dosage strength of 10 mg/mL means that there are 10 milligrams of drug in 1 milliliter of solvent, but it also implies that 1 milliliter of solvent contains 10 milligrams of drugs. Therefore:

$$\frac{10 \text{ mg}}{1 \text{ mL}} \text{ is equivalent to } \frac{1 \text{ mL}}{10 \text{ mg}}$$

3. Calculate the answer.
4. Examine the answer and determine whether it seems logically correct. This step will not verify the accuracy of the arithmetic, but it will minimize the occurrence of nonsensical answers. These are most often produced if the incorrect units are used in the numerator.
5. Double-check the math. Having another person independently solve the problem and arrive at the same answer adds immensely to the accuracy of the arithmetic operations.

Example 5: *A dosage strength of 10 mg/mL is available. How many milliliters of drug are required to deliver a 4-mg dose to a patient?*

$$\frac{10 \text{ mg}}{1 \text{ mL}} = \frac{1 \text{ mL}}{10 \text{ mg}}$$

$$\therefore \frac{1 \text{ mL}}{10 \text{ mg}} \times 4 \text{ mg} = \textbf{0.4 mL}$$

In this example, the mass units (mg) have been canceled, leaving the required volume units (mL).

Example 6: *The dosage strength of a drug is given as 0.01%. What volume of this drug is required to administer a 250-mcg dose?*

$$0.01\% = \frac{0.01 \text{ g}}{100 \text{ mL}}$$

$$\therefore \frac{100 \text{ mL}}{0.01 \text{ g}} \times \frac{1 \text{ g}}{1000000 \text{ mcg}} \times 250 \text{ mcg} = \textbf{2.5 mL}$$

In Example 6 the percentage strength of of the solution generated the mass units (g), which were then converted to micrograms (mcg). Micrograms were then canceled, leaving the necessary volume units (mL).

Example 7: *A drug is available as a 1:200 solution. How much drug (in milligrams) is contained in 2 mL of this solution?*

$$1:200 = \frac{1}{200} \times 100 = 0.5\% = \frac{0.5 \text{ g}}{100 \text{ mL}}$$

$$\therefore \frac{0.5 \text{ g}}{100 \text{ mL}} \times \frac{1000 \text{ mg}}{\text{g}} \times 2 \text{ mL} = \textbf{10 mg}$$

The solution strength expressed as a ratio is converted to a percentage in this example and the percentage strength generates the mass/volume format. Grams (g) are converted to milligrams (mg), which remain after the volume units (mL) are canceled.

When these dimensional analysis problems are properly set up, the unit conversions occur more or less "automatically." Cancellation of common units generates the required units for solution of the problem. There is little to think about other than accurately carrying out the arithmetic operations.

Sample problems with solutions are presented at the end of Appendix A.

MEDICATION LABELS

Drug labels contain essential information regarding the drug name(s), dosage strength, and other instructions (Fig. A–1). **Trade names** generally are printed first and in large letters, often accompanied by the registered (®) or trademark (™) symbol used with most proprietary drugs. The **generic name** is printed in smaller type and follows the trade name. Older drugs that are well known often have only the generic name on the label, whereas combination products are described by their trade name only.

The **volume** of the container (liquids, aerosols) or the **number** of capsules or tablets is also given on the drug label. The term *multiple-use* or *single-use* is often included on parenteral medication labels (eg, "1 mL Single-Use Ampule").

The **dosage strength** is stated as a percentage, a ratio, or the mass per tablet or per volume (eg, mg/mL, mcg/mL, mg/tsp). A few drugs are offered in uncommon dosage strength formats, such as milliequivalents per volume (mEq/mL) for intravenous electrolytes, like sodium chloride and potassium chloride solutions, or in USP units per volume (eg, U/mL) for heparin and for many antibiotics and vitamins.

Additional information may include instructions or warnings such as

- May be habit forming.
- Discard if solution appears discolored.
- Keep out of light.
- Keep tightly closed.
- Store at controlled room temprature.

The **controlled substances** category is included for drugs such as the narcotics (eg, CII) and barbiturates (eg, CIV). **Product identification** (eg, Lot) and **shelf life** (expiration date) are also printed on a typical drug label along with other ingredients such as alcohol or preservatives.

Using the simulated medication label shown in Figure A–1, calculate the following:
How many milliliters of the 1:200 solution are required to deliver a dose of 500 mcg?

Solution

$$1{:}200 \text{ solution strength} = \frac{1}{\overset{200}{\underset{2}{}}} \times \overset{1}{\cancel{100}} = \frac{1}{2}\% = 0.5\%$$

$$0.5\% = \frac{0.5 \text{ g}}{100 \text{ mL}} = \frac{100 \text{ mL}}{0.5 \text{ g}}$$

$$\therefore \frac{100 \text{ mL}}{0.5 \text{ g}} \times \frac{1 \text{ g}}{1000000 \text{ mcg}} \times 500 \text{ mcg} = \textbf{0.1 mL}$$

How many milligrams of drug (in total) are contained in an unopened 20-mL bottle?

Solution

$$\frac{1000 \text{ mg}}{1 \text{ g}} \times \frac{0.5 \text{ g}}{100 \text{ mL}} \times 20 \text{ mL} = \textbf{100 mg}$$

SAMPLE PROBLEMS

(Round off answers to the nearest tenth.)

1. A drug formulation is available in the strength $gr \frac{1}{4}$ *per cc*. What volume of drug would be administered to deliver a 30-mg dose?
2. How many milliliters would be needed to prepare a 20-mg dosage of a drug that is available in an 80 mg/2 mL strength?
3. How much drug present as a 1:200 solution is needed to deliver a 5-mg dose?
4. A medication order requires a dosage of 200 mcg. The strength available is 0.3 mg in 1.5 mL. How many milliliters of drug are required?
5. A 10% solution of drug is on hand. How many milliliters of this solution are required to prepare 20 mL of a 3% solution?

20 mL ‧ Multiple Use Vial

TRADE NAME®*Nebulizer Solution*

generic name

Inhalation Solution, U.S.P. ‧ **1:200**

BRONCHODILATOR
For Oral Inhalation Only

Keep Tightly Closed ‧ Discard If Solution Appears Discolored

LOT A1124 ‧ EXP NOV 99

FIGURE A–1 Simulated medication label.

6. How many milligrams of drug are contained in 15 mL of a 2% stock solution?

7. 100 mL of a 1:100 solution strength is available. How many milliliters of solvent must be added to produce a 1:1000 solution?

8. The dosage strength on hand is 15 mg/5 mL. What volume will deliver a 500-mcg dose to a patient?

9. A drug is available as a 20 mg/3 mL solution. What is its percentage strength?

10. What is the solution strength of a 200 mg/mL drug when expressed as a ratio?

(Note: Dimensional analysis (the *unit factor method*) is used exclusively in the following solutions. There are always different ways in which to solve math problems, but the reader is urged to gain proficiency in the dimensional analysis method presented here. It is fast, accurate, and requires absolutely no memorization of formulas. Other methods for solving pharmaceutical calculations can be found in the books cited at the end of this Appendix.)

SOLUTIONS

1.

$$gr \tfrac{1}{4} \text{ per cc} = \frac{1 \text{ mL}}{gr \tfrac{1}{4}}$$

$$\therefore \frac{1 \text{ mL}}{gr \tfrac{1}{4}} \times \frac{gr \ 1}{60 \text{ mg}} \times 30 \text{ mg} = 2 \text{ mL (using gr 1 = 60 mg)}$$

2.

$$80 \text{ mg}/2 \text{ mL} = \frac{2 \text{ mL}}{80 \text{ mg}}$$

$$\therefore \frac{2 \text{ mL}}{80 \text{ mg}} \times 20 \text{ mg} = \textbf{0.5 mL.}$$

3.

$$1{:}200 = \frac{1}{200} \times 100 = 0.5\%$$

$$0.5\% = \frac{0.5 \text{ g}}{100 \text{ mL}} = \frac{100 \text{ mL}}{0.5 \text{ g}}$$

$$\therefore \frac{100 \text{ mL}}{0.5 \text{ g}} \times \frac{1 \text{ g}}{1000 \text{ mg}} \times 5 \text{ mg} = \textbf{1 mL}$$

4.

$$0.3 \text{ mg}/1.5 \text{ mL} = \frac{1.5 \text{ mL}}{0.3 \text{ mg}}$$

$$\therefore \frac{1.5 \text{ mL}}{0.3 \text{ mg}} \times \frac{1000}{1 \text{ g}} \times \frac{1}{1000000 \text{ mcg}} \times 200 \text{ mcg} = \textbf{1 mL}$$

5.

$$3\% = \frac{3 \text{ g}}{100 \text{ mL}}$$

$$\frac{3 \text{ g}}{100 \text{ mL}} \times 20 \text{ mL} = 0.6 \text{ g (the amount of drug required)}$$

$$10\% = \frac{10 \text{ g}}{100 \text{ mL}} = \frac{100 \text{ mL}}{10 \text{ g}}$$

$$\therefore \frac{100 \text{ mL}}{10 \text{ g}} \times 0.6 \text{ g} = \textbf{6 mL} \text{ (of 10\% solution)}$$

6.

$$2\% = \frac{2 \text{ g}}{100 \text{ mL}}$$

$$\therefore \frac{2 \text{ g}}{100 \text{ mL}} \times \frac{1000 \text{ mg}}{1 \text{ g}} \times 15 \text{ mL} = \textbf{300 mg}$$

7.

$$1{:}1000 = \frac{1}{1000} \times 100 = 0.1\% = \frac{0.1 \text{ g}}{100 \text{ mL}}$$

$$\frac{0.1 \text{ g}}{100 \text{ mL}} \text{ needed, or } \frac{0.1 \text{ g}}{100 \text{ mL}} \times 10 = \frac{1 \text{ g}}{1000 \text{ mL}}$$

$$1{:}100 = \frac{1}{100} \times 100 = 1\% = \frac{1 \text{ g}}{100 \text{ mL}} \text{ (on hand)}$$

$$\frac{1 \text{ g}}{100 \text{ mL}} \text{ concentration on hand}$$

$$\frac{1 \text{ g}}{1000 \text{ mL}} \text{ concentration needed}$$

$\therefore$ Add 900 mL solvent (1000 mL − 100 mL = 900 mL) to dilute the 1 g of solute and produce a 1:1000 solution.

8.

$$15 \text{ mg}/5 \text{ mL} = \frac{5 \text{ mL}}{15 \text{ mg}}$$

$$\therefore \frac{5 \text{ mL}}{15 \text{ mg}} \times \frac{1000 \text{ mg}}{1 \text{ g}} \times \frac{1 \text{ g}}{1000000 \text{ mcg}} \times 500 \text{ mcg} = \textbf{0.2 mL}$$

9.

$$\frac{20 \text{ mg}}{3 \text{ mL}} = \frac{6.67 \text{ mg}}{\text{mL}}$$

$$\therefore \frac{6.67 \text{ mg}}{1 \text{ mL}} \times 100 = \frac{667 \text{ mg}}{100 \text{ mL}} \times \frac{1 \text{ g}}{1000 \text{ mg}} = \frac{0.667 \text{ g}}{100 \text{ mL}} = \textbf{0.7\%}$$

10.

$$\frac{200}{1 \text{ mL}} \times \frac{1 \text{ g}}{1000 \text{ mg}} = \frac{0.2 \text{ g}}{1 \text{ mL}}$$

$$\frac{0.2 \text{ g}}{1 \text{ mL}} \times 100 = \frac{20 \text{ g}}{100 \text{ mL}} = 20\%$$

$$\therefore 20\% = \frac{20}{100} = \frac{1}{5} = \textbf{1:5}$$

BIBLIOGRAPHY

Curren AM and Munday LD: Math for Meds: Dosages and Solutions, ed 6. Wallcur, San Diego, 1990.

Hart LK: The Arithmetic of Dosages and Solutions: A Programmed Presentation, ed 7. CV Mosby, St. Louis, 1989.

Medici GA: Drug Dosage Calculations: A Guide for Clinical Practice, ed 2. Appleton and Lange, Norwalk, CT, 1988.

Osis M: Dosage Calculations in SI Units, ed 2. Mosby Yearbook, St Louis, 1991.

Richardson JK and Richardson LI: The Mathematics of Drugs and Solutions, ed 4. CV Mosby, St Louis, 1990.

TImberlake K: Chemistry: An Introduction to General, Organic, and Biological Chemistry, ed 5. HarperCollins, New York, 1992.

Prescriptions

OUTLINE
Parts of a Prescription
Evaluation of Drug Therapy

PARTS OF A PRESCRIPTION

In a hospital setting, doctors convey medication orders to other medical personnel by means of a chart order, or specific medication instructions entered on the patient's chart. An outpatient prescription conveys similar instructions to a pharmacist and patient outside the hospital.

In the past, there were very few effective medicines available for drug therapy. Most of the elaborate concoctions were, for the most part, harmless but ineffective. Their contents were cloaked in secrecy and hidden from the patient through extensive use of Latin abbreviations. Very few such abbreviations have survived with the advent of effective medications.

There are four parts of a typical prescription as shown in Figure B–1:

1. Superscription: written as the symbol ℞, which is derived from a Latin word meaning "recipe," or "take thou."
2. Inscription: a list of the ingredients and amounts of drug to be taken. The principal drug is listed first in a mixture of more than one drug. In modern usage, the inscription is the part of the prescription in which a drug is ordered by name (generic name, trade name, or both). In the past, the inscription gave instructions to the pharmacist as to which substances were to be included in the compound.
3. Subscription: contains directions for dispensing. Sometimes the subscription consists only of *M.* (abbreviation for the Latin *misce,* or "mix").
4. Signature: contains specific directions to the patient regarding administration of the drug. Instructions such as "external use only" or "take one tablet at bedtime" are given with the signature. Occasionally the signature is written as *Sig.* (abbreviation for *signa,* Latin for "mark" or "write").

Additional information that may be given on a prescription includes the patient's name, the current date, the prescribing physician's name and signature, and information relating to controlled substances category and number of refills permitted. Common pharmaceutical abbreviations used with prescriptions and chart order are given in Table B–1. Drug schedules used in the United States and Canada are listed in Tables B–2 and B–3.

EVALUATION OF DRUG THERAPY

Respiratory care practitioners may routinely be involved with evaluation of drug therapy. The purpose of the appraisal is to assess and report drug efficacy and patient response. The evaluation may be part of a respiratory care practitioner's normal hospital responsibilities or it may be part of the clinical testing of a drug (see Box 3–3). The methods employed are beyond the scope of this text because they are more of a practical nature, better suited to reinforcement in the clinical setting. Briefly, the techniques involve regular and methodical gathering of information related to patient response and drug effects, organization of the material, and presentation of the data to the attending physician. For example, an asthmatic patient may report that the feeling of "tightness" in the chest has not improved following bronchodilator therapy with a particular drug. In another patient, a respiratory care practitioner may note a signifi-

FAMILY PHYSICIANS, INC.

J.L Doe, M.D.
222 Generic Street
City
Telephone (911) 555-1212

Patient's Name _____ Date _____
Address _____ Age _____

① R$_x$

② *naproxen* TABS *375 mg*

③ *M. #60*

④ SIG: TAB $\frac{1}{1}$ *bid*
ō food

_____   *J. L. Doe, M.D.*
Dispense as Written   Substitution Permissible

Narcotic Reg. No. _____
Number of Refills _____

① **Superscription**
"recipe", "take thou"

② **Inscription**
name and amount of
drug to be compounded

③ **Subscription**
directions to the
pharmacist for
dispensing

④ **Signature**
directions to the
patient for taking
the medication

FIGURE B–1 Typical prescription. In this typical prescription, sixty 375-mg tablets of naproxen have been ordered. The patient is instructed to take one tablet with food twice a day.

cant change in the consistency and volume of mucus produced after administration of an aerosol mucokinetic. Pulmonary function tests performed by respiratory care practitioners provide valuable data related to changes in a patient's respiratory status following drug administration. All of this information—subjective descriptions from the patient, objective reports from the respiratory care practitioner, and the results of clinical tests—is vital in the ongoing assessment of drug therapy. The respiratory care practitioner plays a critical role in the evaluation process.

BIBLIOGRAPHY

Burt RAP: The importance of prescribing precisely. In Audet PR: Davis's Physician's Drug Guide. FA Davis, Philadelphia, 1989.

Clark WG, Brater DC, and Johnson AR: Goth's Medical Pharmacology, ed 12. CV Mosby, St Louis, 1988.

Deglin JH and Vallerand AH: Davis's Drug Guide for Nurses, ed 3. FA Davis, Philadelphia, 1993.

Howder CL: Cardiopulmonary Pharmacology: A Handbook for Respiratory Practitioners and Other Allied Health Personnel. Williams and Wilkins, Baltimore, 1992.

Lofholm PW: Prescription writing. In Katzung BD (ed): Basic and Clinical Pharmacology. Lange Medical Publications, Los Altos, 1982.

Moraca-Sawicki A: History, legislation, and standards. In Kuhn MM (ed): Pharmacotherapeutics: A Nursing Process Approach, ed 2. FA Davis, Philadelphia, 1990.

TABLE B–1 COMMON PHARMACEUTICAL ABBREVIATIONS

a.c.	Before meals (L. *ante cibum*)
b.i.d.	Twice daily (L. *bis in die*)
c̄	With (L. *cum*)
cap	Capsule
CR	Controlled release
dr or ƒ3	Dram
fl dr or ƒ3	Fluidram
fl oz or ƒ3	Fluidounce
ER	Extended release
g	Gram(s)
gr	Grain(s)
gtt	Drop(s) (L. *gutta*)
h or hr	Hour(s) (L. *hora*)
IM	Intramuscular
Inhaln	Inhalation
IV	Intravenous
L	Liter
ɱ or min	Minim
mcg or μg	Microgram
mg	Milligram
mL	Milliliter
0.9% NaCl	0.9% Sodium chloride; "normal" saline (NS)
NSAID (NSAIA)	Nonsteroidal anti-inflammatory drug (agent)
OTC	Over the counter
oz or 3	ounce(s)
p.c.	After meals (L. *post cibum*)
PO	By mouth; orally (L. *per os*)
p.r.n.	When required; as needed (L. *pro re nata*)
q.	Every (L. *quaque*)
q.d.	Every day
q.h.	Every hour
q.i.d.	Four times a day (L. *quater in die*)
q.od	Every other day
q.wk	Every week
q.2h	Every 2 hours
q.3h	Every 3 hours
s̄	Without (L. *sine*)
SC	Subcutaneous
SL	Sublingual
soln	Solution
SR	Sustained release
s̄s̄	One half (L. *semis*)
stat	Immediately
supp	Suppository
tab	Tablet
tbs or T	Tablespoon
t.i.d.	Three times a day (L. *ter in die*)
Top	Topical
tsp or t	Teaspoon
wk	Week

Source: Data from Deglin and Vallerand, 1993.

TABLE B–2 DRUG SCHEDULES: UNITED STATES*

Schedule	Remarks	Examples
I (C–I)	Potential for abuse is so high as to be unacceptable May be used for research with appropriate limitations	LSD Heroin Cocaine

II (C–II)	High potential for abuse and extreme liability for
	  physical and psychological dependence
	Outpatient prescriptions must be in writing
	No refills
		Amobarbital
		Amphetamine
		Codeine (single entity; solid dosage form or
		  injectable)
		Meperidine
		Methadone
		Methylphenidate
		Morphine
		Oxycodone
		Pentobarbital
		Secobarbital
		Sufentanil

III (C–III)	Intermediate potential for abuse and intermediate
	  liability for physical and psychological dependence
	Outpatient prescriptions can be refilled 5 times
	  within 6 months from date of issue if authorized by
	  prescriber
		Codeine (in combination with nonnarcotic
		  analgesics; solid oral dosage forms)
		Pentobarbital (rectal)
		Secobarbital (rectal)
		Thiopental

IV (C–IV)	Less abuse potential than Schedule III with minimal
	  liability for physical or psychological dependence
	Outpatient prescriptions can be refilled 5 times
	  within 6 months from date of issue if authorized by
	  prescriber
		Chloral hydrate
		Chlordiazepoxide
		Codeine (elixir or oral suspension with
		  acetaminophen)
		Diazepam
		Flurazepam
		Pentazocine
		Propoxyphene

V (C–V)	Minimal abuse potential
	Number of refills for outpatients determined by
	  prescriber
	Some products (cough suppressants with small
	  amounts of codeine, and antidiarrheals containing
	  paregoric) may be available without prescription to
	  patients > 18 years of age
		Codeine (in cough preparations; 10 mg/5 mL or
		  dosage unit)
		Paregoric

Source: Data from Deglin and Vallerand, 1993.

*Note: Classes or schedules are determined by the Drug Enforcement Agency, which is an arm of the United States Justice Department, and are based on the potential for abuse and dependence liability (physical and psychological) of the medication.

Some states may have prescription regulations that are stricter than those listed in the table. This table is a summary. For complete details, reference should be made to the official information. Drug names used in this table are for illustrative purposes only. This is not a complete listing. Legislation can change. Keep abreast of changes in prescription requirements.

Table B–3 DRUG SCHEDULES: CANADA*

Schedule	Remarks	Examples
Narcotic Drugs (N) Schedule N Drugs	All straight narcotic drugs All narcotic drugs for parenteral use All products containing hydrocodone and oxycodone Written prescription required No refills	Codeine Morphine Meperidine
Narcotic Preparations (N) (oral prescription narcotics) Schedule N Preparations	All combinations containing only 1 narcotic drug and 2 or more nonnarcotic medicinal ingredients in a recognized therapeutic dose Not intended for parenteral use Written or verbal prescriptions No refills	Codeine (15 or 30 mg) with acetaminophen and caffeine Tylenol #2, #3
Controlled Drug (C) Schedule G Drugs	All straight controlled drugs All combinations containing more than 1 controlled drug Written or verbal prescriptions No refills if original prescription is verbal; original written prescription may be refilled if prescriber has indicated in writing the number of refills and dates for, or intervals between, refills	Dextromethorphan Pentobarbital Secobarbital Pentazocine
Controlled Drug Preparations Schedule G Preparations	All combinations containing only 1 controlled drug and 1 or more medicinal ingredients in a recognized therapeutic dose See Schedule G Drugs for refill information	Darvon compound (propoxyphene with aspirin and caffeine)
Controlled drugs in Schedule to Part G of Regulation (C)	Barbituric acid (excluding secobarbital and pentobarbital) An original or verbal prescription may be refilled if the prescriber has authorized in writing or verbally the number of times and dates for, or intervals between, refills	Amobarbital Methylphenidate
Schedule E and F Drugs (Pr—prescription required)	All drugs listed in Schedule F of Food and Drug Regulations All drugs listed in Schedule E of Health Disciplines Act Prescription on regular file (in contrast to prescription on Narcotic and Controlled Drug file for drugs in other schedules) An original written or verbal prescription may be refilled if the prescriber has authorized in writing or verbally the number of times it may be refilled	Antibiotics Antidepressants Antipsychotics Steroids Oral contraceptives

Source: Data from Moraca-Sawicki, 1990.

*This is a summary. For complete details, reference should be made to the official information. Drug names used in this table are for illustrative purposes only. This is not a complete listing. Legislation can change. Keep abreast of changes in prescription requirements.

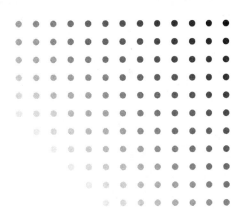

Index

A "t" following a page number indicates a table; an "f" following a page number indicates a figure.